The Lady's Stratagem.

The Lady's Stratagem.

A Repository of 1820s Directions for
the Toilet, Mantua-Making, Stay-Making,
Millinery & Etiquette.

Edited and with Additional Material by:
Frances Grimble.

Author of *After a Fashion, Reconstruction Era Fashions,*
Fashions of the Gilded Age, Vols. 1 & 2,
The Voice of Fashion, The Edwardian Modiste, &c., &c.

Translations by:
Frances Grimble.

Lavolta Press
20 Meadowbrook Drive
San Francisco, CA 94132
www.lavoltapress.com

MMIX.

The Lady's Stratagem: A Repository of 1820s Directions for the Toilet, Mantua-Making, Stay-Making, Millinery & Etiquette is a new work first published by Lavolta Press in 2009. All translations; new text and illustrations; the selection and arrangement of period text, illustrations, and patterns; and revised versions of the period materials are protected by copyright. They may not be reproduced or transmitted in any form whatsoever without prior written permission from Lavolta Press.

First edition.
ISBN: 978-0-9636517-7-8

Published by:
Lavolta Press
20 Meadowbrook Drive
San Francisco, CA 94132
www.lavoltapress.com

Book design, cover design, scanning, scan editing and colouring, page layout, and production management by Frances Grimble and Allan Terry.

Printed and bound in the United States of America.

Publisher's Cataloging-In-Publication Data.

The Lady's stratagem : a repository of 1820s directions for the toilet,
   mantua-making, stay-making, millinery & etiquette / edited and
   with additional material by Frances Grimble ; translations by Frances
   Grimble. – 1st ed.

   p. ; ill. ; cm.

   Includes translations of 19th-century instructional manuals written by
Elisabeth Celnart and Madame Burtel.
   Includes bibliographical references and index.
   ISBN: 978-0-9636517-7-8

1. Etiquette for women–History–19th century. 2. Women–Manners
and customs–History–19th century. 3. Beauty, Personal–Technique–
19th century. 4. Fashion–History–19th century. 5. Home economics–
History–19th century. I. Grimble, Frances. II. Celnart, Elisabeth, 1796-
1865. III. Burtel, Madame.

BJ1838 .L33 2008
395.1/44/09034   2008920010

Acknowledgements.

First and foremost, I would like to thank my parents, Ralph and Helen Grimble. Their constant support, encouragement, and advice for this book was invaluable. To my deep regret, neither lived to see it published.

My husband, Allan Terry, helped to design and lay out the book cover and interior, coloured the cover, created new illustrations, and helped to edit the old ones. He also did much of the work of preparing the files for the printer and of coordinating printing.

Historic knitter and technical editor Chris Laning closely reviewed the translation of Chapter XVII for technical and terminological errors.

Several people helped at different stages with a variety of questions. In more or less chronological order, they are: expert on historical units of measure Dr. Russ Rowlett, expert on historical chemical terms Dr. Carmen Giunta, French historic knitter Isabelle Pellé, British editor Joseph Harris, lawyer Benedict Mahoney, InDesign expert Kenneth Benson, and production expert Pete Masterson.

Our printer, McNaughton & Gunn, did their usual high-quality job. Our account representative, Karl Frauhammer, deserves special thanks.

To the memory of my parents,
Ralph and Helen Grimble.

Contents.

Introduction 1

Part I. The Toilet 6

Chapter I. Preservation of the Hair 7

  Modes of beautifying the Hair 8
  The Use of an Egg-yolk to de-grease the Hair 12
  The Removal of Superfluous Hair 12
    Oriental Rusma 13
    Parisian Depilatory Cream 13
    Laforest's Depilatory Preparation 14
    Additional Remarks 14
  To make the Hair grow, and prevent its falling out . . . 14
    Oil for making the Hair grow 15
  Greying Hair 16
  Diversion 1 17
    Curling-irons *vs.* Curl-papers 17
  Diversion 2 17
    The Best French Receipts 17
    Parisian Pomatum 18
    English Pomatum 18
    Italian Pomatum 18
    Palm Pomatum 19
    Rowland's Hair-oil 19
    Fragrant Hair-oil 19
    Russian Hair-oil 19
    Antique Oils 20
    Antique Oil *au Musc* 20
    Antique Oil *à l'Orange* 20
    Antique Oil *à la Rose* 20
    Antique Oil *à la Tubéreuse* 21
    Antique Oil *Verte* 21
    Macassar Oil 21
    Curling Fluid 21

Contents.

Diversion 3 22
   Arguments against washing the Hair 22
   Arguments in favour of washing the Hair 22
Diversion 4 23
   Depilatories 23
   Depilatory of Ants' Eggs 23
   Plucking and Shaving 23
Diversion 5 24
   Receipts for Dyes 24
   Composition for staining the Hair Black 25
   Tinctures for staining the Hair Black 25
   To stain Light Hair a Chestnut-colour 25
   To dye the Hair Flaxen 26

Chapter II. Preservation of the Teeth 27
The Formation of Tartar on the Teeth 27
Tooth-brushes from Marsh-mallow
   or Horse-radish Roots 29
Dentifrice Powder of M. Cadet de Gassicourt 29
Another Powder for preserving the Teeth 30
Soap Solutions to whiten and preserve the Teeth 30
Preparation to strengthen the Teeth
   or check Caries 30
Guaiac Brandy, to preserve the Teeth and Gums 30
Dental Elixer 31
Water to strengthen the Gums,
   especially when they are disposed to Scurvy 31
The Best Mode of cleansing the Teeth 31
Additional Means of preserving the Teeth 33
Diversion 1 35
   Note 35
Diversion 2 35
   Measuring-glasses 35
Diversion 3 35
   Decayed Teeth 35
   Lotion for the Tooth-ache 36
   Mucilage for the Tooth-ache 37
   Liniment for the Tooth-ache 37
Diversion 4 37
   False Teeth 37

Contents.

Chapter III. Preservation of the Complexion
and the Skin 38
  Diversion 1 42
    Bathing 42

Chapter IV. Concerning Cosmetics 45
  True Vegetable Rouge, or Rose in a Cup 47
  Cream Pomatum for the Complexion 47
  Pomatum for the Lips 47
  Angel-water to firm and refresh the Skin 47
  Rose Milk for preserving the Complexion 47
  Simple Almond-milk to make the Skin Fresh 47
  Lily-water for the Complexion 48
  Cucumber Pomatum 48
  Preparation of Dr. Withering,
      to dispel Eruptions of the Skin 48
  Cosmetic Infusion of the Same Kind for the Skin 48
  Strawberry Water to soften and whiten the Skin 49
  Veal Broth to calm Reddened Skin 49
  Oil of Bitter Almonds, to cure Sun-burn and Freckles 49
  Athenian Water to efface Wrinkles 49
  Economical Paste to whiten the Hands 49
  Almond Paste with Brandy 50
  Almond Paste with Egg-yolks 50
  Almond Paste with Honey 50
  Toilet-soap, called Lady Derby's Soap 50
  Soap with Honey, to whiten the Skin
      and dispel Sun-burn Marks 50
  Emollient Preparation for the Bath 50
  Diversion 1 51
    The Use of Paints 51
    Carmine 52
    Portuguese Rouge 53
    Spanish Wool 53
    Spanish Papers 53
    Chinese Boxes of Colours 53
    White Paints 54
    Talc White 55
  Diversion 2 55
    Receipts for Perfumed Soaps 55

Contents.

Seraglio Soap 55
Musk Soap 56
Diversion 3 56
Bath of Modesty 56

Chapter V. Remedies for the Little Faults which are injurious to Beauty 57

Remedies for Pimples 57
Round Pimples 57
Flat Pimples 58
Quick, or Living Pimples. 58
Composite Pimples 59
Black Points 59
Remedy for Mealy Skin 60
Remedies for Chaps 60
Remedy for Ruddiness 60
Modes of getting rid of Freckles 61
Remedy for Tanning 61
Remedy for Scurf Patches 61
Remedy for Wrinkles 62
Remedy for Mosquito-bites 62
Remedy for Imperfections of the Eyebrows 62
Modes of calming Redness and Inflammation of the Eyelids . . . 63
Remedy for Little Foreign Bodies which get into the Eyes 63
Weakening of the Sight 63
Falling out of the Eyelashes 64
Their Waxy Matter. 65
The Droplets of White Matter which often appear
in the Corner of the Eye 65
Remedies for Defects of the Ears 65
Remedy for Thickening of the Neck 66
Remedy for a Ropy Neck 66
The Mode of removing Pellicles and Scales from the Fingers . . 67
The Mode of curing Hang-nails 67
The Mode of ridding the Nails of the Skin
which sometimes covers them 68
Remedy for Warts 68
Corn Plaster of M. Laforest, Foot Surgeon 68
Another Mode by Potash 69

Contents.

Another Mode by Pumice-stone 69
Another Mode of curing Corns, with Ivy 69
Another Cure, by means of Starched Muslin 69
Another Corn Plaster 69
Remedy for Pain caused by Uncomfortable Shoes,
    or the Fatigue of the Dance 70
The Mode of dissipating the Coagulated Blood which
    collects under the Nails, following a Blow 70
Remedy for Broken or Very Weak Nails,
    especially those of the Feet 70
Regime to counter Leanness 70
Regime to counter Excess Embonpoint 71
Diversion 1 72
    Small-pox and Vaccination 72
Diversion 2 72
    Note 72
Diversion 3 72
    To blacken the Eyelashes and Eyebrows 72
    Wash for blackening the Eyebrows 72
    Black for the Eyebrows 73
Diversion 4 73
    To calm Needle Pricks 73
Diversion 5 73
    Remedies for Corpulence 73
    Contour of the Breasts 74
    Dr. Ure's Ointment for the Breasts 74

Chapter VI. Perfumes 75
The Mode of making Cologne Water 76
Another Mode 77
A Simple and Easy Way of perfuming Linens
    and Other Clothing 77
Fragrant Bags to perfume the Linen in Armoires
    and Ornaments in Boxes 78
Bags with Herbs *de Montpellier* 78
Bags with Powdered Scent 78
Fragrant Pastilles to burn 78
Flasks for the Mantel-piece 79
Pocket Flasks 79

Contents.

To perfume Handkerchiefs 79
To perfume Baths, General and Partial. 79
Diversion 1 79
   Note 79
Diversion 2 79
   Perfume for Gloves 79
   Another Mode 80
Diversion 3 80
   Hungary Water. 80
   Luce Water 80
   Imperial Water 80
   Lavender-water 80

Chapter VII. Hygienic Habits 81

Diversion 1 86
   Clothing in regard to Health 86
   To render Cloth Water-proof according to
      the Manner of the Chinese 87
   Pliable Varnish for Umbrellas 88
Diversion 2 88
   Stays 88
Diversion 3 90
   Padding, Bandaging, &c. to improve the Shape 90
Diversion 4 91
   Advice to Married Ladies 91

Chapter VIII. The Art of arranging the Hair, lacing the Stays, Dressing, &c. 92

Practical Directions for Hair-dressing 92
   Coiffure *à Chou* 95
   Coiffure *à Cache-peigne* 95
   Coiffure *à Chinoise* 95
   Coiffure *en Couronne*. 95
   Coiffure *en Chignon* 95
   Coiffure *à la Ninon* 96
   Coiffure *à la Nœuds d'Apollon* 96
Concerning the Stays 99
To put on your Gown 100
The Choice and Care of the Foot-wear 102

Contents.

Diversion 1 104
   The Dressing-room 104
Diversion 2 104
   Divers Operations of Hair-dressing 104
Diversion 3 106
   Fashions in Hair-dressing 106
   May 1824 106
   July 1824 106
   November 1824 106
   January 1827 107
   September 1827 107
   October 1827 107
   November 1827 107
   January 1829 107
   February 1829 108
   September 1829 108
   October 1829 109
   November 1829 109
Diversion 4 109
   To unlace your Stays 109
Diversion 5 110
   Ill-fitting Shoes 110
Diversion 6 110
   To make Gaiters 110

Chapter IX. Of the Order and Cleanliness which
must preside over the Concerns of the Toilet 113
To cleanse the Toilet Articles 113
Directions for the Garments which you are putting on
   or taking off 115
To tidy and put away Each Kind of Linen, Garment,
   and Ornament 120
To preserve Furs 126
Diversion 1 127
   The Lady's Maid 127
Diversion 2 129
   To store Pomatum 129
Diversion 3 129
   To store Clothing 129

Contents.

Diversion 4 130
    To increase the Value of Furs Tenfold,
       and beautify the Hair of Animals 130

Chapter X. The Art of Laundering and Scouring 131
The sorting of Linens 131
The rinsing out of Linens 132
To attach Pairs of Stockings, &c. 132
Directions for the Wash-liquor 133
The Art of making your own Soap by the American Mode . . . 137
A New Way to apply Wash-liquor, after the Preceding Mode . . 138
The Experiment of washing with Steam 139
The Experiment of washing with Potatoes 140
The Mode of washing with Rice 142
The Mode of washing with Soapwort 142
The Best Mode of Soaping 143
The Best Mode of Blueing 144
To compose Chemic or Liquid Blue 144
The Mode of M. Estève of Flushing for making
    Balls of Celestial Blue, called English Blue 145
The Mode of Mr. William Story for the Same Composition . . . 145
To make ironing Linens easier, with a Handsome Result 145
Preparation for restoring Scorched
    or Almost Burned Linen 146
To wash Calico or Gingham Gowns to look like new 146
To wash Nankeen when it is Soiled,
    so that it does not lose its Colour 147
To wash Unbleached Materials 147
To soap White Silks, Gauzes, Silk Tulle, Ribands, &c. 147
Suphuring 148
The Mode of cleansing Black Silk Materials 148
The Mode of cleansing Silks dyed Other than Black 149
Modes of reviving Colours 149
The Way to partially replace the Glaze
    of Materials spotted by Water 151
The Mode of raising the Nap of Velvets 151
To wash Woollen Materials or Merino Shawls 151
To wash Lace, and Linen or Cotton Tulles, to look like new . . 152
Finishing 153
The Mode of preparing Fish-glue 153

Contents.

To have Fish-glue ready to use at Any Time 154

To wash Black Lace Veils and Black Blonds 154

The Mode of cleansing Gold and Silver Lace 154

The Mode of cleansing Embroidery in general 154

The Mode of cleansing Silk Stockings 155

To cleanse Ribands 155

To whiten Unbleached Toiles 155

To size Toiles 157

To determine the Manner in which Toiles
    have been whitened 157

To scour with Sand and Bullock's Gall 158

The Mode of purifying Bullock's Gall 158

The Mode of scouring Woollens 159

To cleanse Garments of Blue, Black, or Dark Brown Drap . . . 159

The Art of removing Spots 160

Spots from Simple Grease, Tallow, Broth, &c. 160

To easily prepare Essence of Soap 161

To remove Grease-spots from All Kinds of Materials
    without wetting 162

Grease-spots 162

Spots from Grease contained in Dirty Oil,
    Sauces, Oil-paints, Ointments, &c. 163

Ink, Mud, Rust, and Dirty Oil Spots 163

The Mode of M. Rue, to remove Ink, Rust, and Other Spots . . 164

Vegetable Spots 165

Soap for removing Spots 165

Water for removing Spots 166

Spots which alter or destroy the Colour 166

To repair Spots which have altered or destroyed the Colour . . 167

Diversion 1 168

    The Washhouse 168

    The Laundry-maid 170

Diversion 2 170

    The Mode of marking Linens 170

    To obtain a Black Liquor for marking Linens
        in a Strong and Lasting Manner 170

    Preparation of the Mordant 171

    Preparation of the Ink 171

    Application of this Ink for printing
        Toile d'Orange and Other Materials 171

Contents.

Diversion 3 172
   Contagion 172
Diversion 4 172
   The Wash-water 172
Diversion 5 172
   The Choice of Soap 172
Diversion 6 172
   Note 172
Diversion 7 172
   Utensils for the Art of Dyeing 172
Diversion 8 174
   Ironing 174
Diversion 9 174
   To make Starch 174
   To make Starch from Horse Chestnuts 174
   The Best Mode of making and using Starch 175
Diversion 10 175
   To wash Fine Muslins 175
   To rinse Muslins before you starch them 176
   To starch Fine Muslins 176
   To clap Muslins before they are ironed 176
   The Proper Mode of ironing Muslins 177
   To starch Lawns 177
Diversion 11 177
   The Mode of cleansing White Satins 177
Diversion 12 178
   To wash Black Silks 178
Diversion 13 178
   To cleanse Silks of All Kinds 178
Diversion 14 178
   To keep Silks from staining in washing 178
Diversion 15 178
   To wash Lace 178
Diversion 16 179
   To cleanse Gold and Silver Lace, Stuffs, &c. 179
   To cleanse Gold and Silver Lace 179
   To cleanse Gold Lace 179
Diversion 17 179
   To wash Gold or Silver Work on Linen,
      or Any Other Stuff, to look like new 179

Contents.

Diversion 18 180
   To wash Thread and Cotton Stockings 180
Diversion 19 180
   The Best Mode of whitening Any Kind of Material 180
   To make Linen White that is turned Yellow 180
Diversion 20 180
   To prevent Scarlet Cloth from being stained Black 180
   For cleansing Scarlet Cloth 180
   Another Mode 181
   The Mode of dipping Scarlet Cloth 182
   A Cheaper Mode 182

Chapter XI. Of the Choice of Clothing 183
  Night Clothing 183
  Morning Clothing 185
  Clothing for Ordinary Days 186
  Négligé 187
  Demi-négligé 187
  The Manner of dressing for an Ordinary Walk 189
  The Manner of dressing for a Morning Repast 189
  The Manner of dressing for an Evening Repast 189
  For an Assembly Properly Speaking 190
  The Manner of dressing for a Ball 190
   The Simple Toilet 190
   The Demi-toilet 191
   The Grand Toilet 191
  Differences in the Toilet between Married Women
    and Young Ladies 193
  The Manner of wearing Mourning properly 194
  Diversion 1 195
   The Trade of the Linen-draper 195
   Calico 195
  Diversion 2 196
   Costumes for Morning Wear 196
   August 1824 196
   June 1829 197
  Diversion 3 197
   Costumes for Home Wear 197
   May 1824 198
   June 1824 198

Contents.

July 1824 198
October 1824 198
December 1824 198
March 1827 198
April 1827 199
May 1827 199
June 1827 199
August 1827 199
September 1827 199
December 1827 200
January 1829 200
August 1829 200
October 1829 200
November 1829 200
December 1829 200
Diversion 4 201
Fashions for *Négligé* 201
August 1827 201
October 1827 201
June 1829 202
August 1829 202
December 1829 203
Diversion 5 203
To open a Blocked Flask 203
Diversion 6 203
Walking and Carriage Costumes 203
February 1824 204
March 1824 204
June 1824 205
July 1824 205
August 1824 206
October 1824 207
December 1824 207
January 1827 208
March 1827 208
April 1827 208
June 1827 208
August 1827 209
September 1827 210

Contents.

November 1827 210

December 1827 211

January 1829 211

March 1829 211

May 1829 213

June 1829 213

July 1829 213

August 1829 214

September 1829 215

October 1829 215

November 1829 216

December 1829 216

Diversion 7 217

Dinner-party Dress 217

September 1827 217

November 1827 217

April 1829 217

Diversion 8 218

Costumes for Assemblies, Concerts, &c. 218

May 1824 219

January 1827 220

April 1827 220

June 1827 220

January 1829 221

February 1829 221

March 1829 221

April 1829 222

May 1829 223

June 1829 223

July 1829 223

September 1829 224

October 1829 224

November 1829 224

December 1829 224

Diversion 9 226

Costumes for the Ball 226

March 1824 226

May 1824 226

September 1824 226

Contents.

January 1827 226
March 1827 227
April 1827 228
June 1827 228
August 1827 228
November 1827 228
December 1827 229
February 1829 230
March 1829 230
August 1829 230
September 1829 231
November 1829 232
Diversion 10 232
Court Mourning 232
December 1824 233
February 1827 233
Diversion 11 235
Note 235

Chapter XII. The Conventions of Costumes 236
To choose Fashions
which are neither *Recherché* nor *Passé* 237
The Style of Gowns and the Choice of Trimmings 239
Diversion 1 242
Taste in the Colours of Dress 242
The Carnation Complexion 243
The Florid Complexion 243
The Fair Complexion 243
The Pale Complexion 244
The Sallow Complexion 244
The Brunette Complexion 244
Additional Remarks 244
The Theory of Colours 245
The Change of Colours by Light 246
Diversion 2 246
Rivalry in Dress 246
Good Housewifery 247
Propriety in Dress 247
Dress for the Lower Orders 249
The Thrifty Cottager 250

Contents.

Negro Women's Clothes,
    for Plantations in the West Indes, or in America 251
Diversion 3 251
    "Cachemiremania" 251
Diversion 4 252
    The Lady's Maid as Mantua-maker 252

**Chapter XIII. The Art of a Fine Carriage
and Proper Gestures** 254
Diversion 1 257
    To walk well 257
Diversion 2 257
    The Courtesy 257

Part II. Needle-work 260
Chapter XIV. The Art of the Stay-maker 261
The Materials for Stays 261
The Furnishings for Stays 261
Divers Kinds of Stays 262
The Parts of Stays 262
Stays with One Bosom Gore 262
    To take the Pattern 262
    To cut out the Stays 264
    To baste the Stays 265
    To try on the Stays 266
    To make up the Stays 266
    To finish the Stays 270
Stays with Two Bosom Gores 271
Kinds of Shoulder-straps which include Gores 272
Pieced Stays 274
Lined Stays 275
Half-stays, or Morning Belts 277
Stays with Straps 278
Stays *à la Paresseuse* 278
Stays for Pregnant Women 279
Elastic Stays 280
Stays made to conceal Defects of the Shape 281
Diversion 1 282
    The Art of making Stays 282

Contents.

Suitable Materials for making Stays 282
The Measures for Stays 283
To cut out a Pattern 284
Different Kinds of Stays 286
The Different Parts of Stays in general 286
Divers Furnishings, their Choice and Use 288
To lace the Stays correctly 288
To fit on the Stays 289
Seams to work on Stays 291
To make the Eyelet-holes 292
To completely prepare the Bones and secure them 294
The Modesty-piece 295
Stays with Single Gores 296
Lined Stays 296
Stays *à la Paresseuse* 297
Stays with Straps 298
Stays for Pregnant Women,
        called *Brassières de Venus*. 298
Half-stays or Morning Belts. 299
Elastic Stays 300
Night Stays or *Brassières* 301
The Mode of concealing Faults in the Shape 301
To wash Stays 302
To keep your Work clean 303
Diversion 2 303
Ladies' Stays 303

Chapter XV. The Art of the Mantua-maker
or Cutter of Gowns. 305
Common Stitches and Seams. 305
The Running Stitch 305
The Over-cast Stitch 307
The Seam *à la Reine* 308
The Lace Seam 308
The Side-stitch 309
The Mantua-maker's Hem or Seam 310
Hemming 310
The Back-stitch 311
The Herring-bone Stitch 313

Contents.

The Button-hole Stitch 313
The Chain-stitch 314
General Rules for Gowns 314
To cut out the Skirt 314
To make up the Skirt 315
To make up the Body 318
To set on the Skirt 319
Of lining a Gown 320
Divers Trimmings 323
Flounces 323
Corded Piping for the Edge of a Flounce,
or what you please 323
To sew on a Flounce 324
Rouleaux 326
Folds, or Tucks 328
Biases 329
Braid and Fringe 330
Entre-deux 330
To put *Entre-deux* on Collars 333
Draperies 333
Agrafes 334
Ruches 334
Panes 336
Diversion 1 336
The Trade of the Mantua-maker 336
Diversion 2 337
The Art of Mantua-making 337
The Work-room 338
Of the Measure 338
General Observations 339
Of cutting out the Skirt 341
Of making up the Skirt 344
Of cutting out the Body 345
Of making up the Body *en Fourreau* 347
The Best Mode of fitting a Gown 349
To make up the Gown 349
The Body *à la Raphaël* 351
Long Sleeves 351
Short Sleeves 354

Contents.

The Mode of making Separate Draperies 354

The Little Accessories
    of which Trimmings are composed 355

The Trimmings which are put
    on the Hems of Gowns 357

The Mode of cutting out a Redingote 360

The Mode of cutting out Divers Mantles for Women,
    called Pelisses *à l'Autrichienne* 361

The Mode of fringing and using Ribands
    in making Belts 362

Some Pretty Collars for *Fichus* 364

Diversion 3 366

Gentlemen's Night-shirts and Ladies' Night Jackets 366

Ladies' Shifts 369

Diversion 4 369

Marking 369

Diversion 5 369

To cut out a Gown 369

Diversion 6 371

The Trade of the Tailor 371

The Ladies' Riding Habit 372

Of the Back 374

The Front Piece 374

The Sleeve 378

Of the Pelisse and Spencer 379

Diversion 7 383

A Pattern for the Body of a Gown 383

Diversion 8 386

Tambour-work 386

Embroidery on Muslin 387

Lace-work 394

Gold-thread Embroidery 395

Divers Embroidery Patterns 396

Diversion 9 407

The Lady's Maid as Embroideress 407

Chapter XVI. The Art of mending
and renewing Garments 408

Darning 408

Patching 408

Contents.

Over-cast Patching 410
To patch with Button-hole or Blanket-stitch 410
To mend with Laced Stitches 411
To mend *à Dentelle* 413
Invisible Mending 413
To make up Gowns
    so that you may easily alter them 415
The Mode of turning Kitchen Aprons 416
The Mode of turning Merino and Silk Gowns 417
To renew Cotton Gowns without dyeing them 417
To repair and renew Woollen and Silk Gowns
    when you cannot match the Material 420
To renew Faded or Half-worn Calico Gowns 421
To discharge the Colours from Faded Calicoes
    and Printed Toiles 422
To repair and renew Furs 422
    To mend Furs 422
    To change the Style of Furs 423
The Modes of renewing Shoes 423
    To bind Shoes 424
    To re-cover Shoes 425
Diversion 1 426
    Kitchen Aprons 426
Diversion 2 426
    A Carriage Dress consisting of a Petticoat
        and a Canezou-spencer 426
Diversion 3 426
    A Walking Gown with the Body covered by
        a Canezou-spencer 426
Diversion 4 428
    Directions for changing the Colours
        of Garments, &c. already dyed 428
    For a Black Silk Gown 429
Diversion 5 430
    To make Good Children's Frocks from
        Partly-worn Gowns 430

Chapter XVII. The Art of Knitting 431
The Mode of knitting Common Stitches 431
The Mode of knitting Stockings 432

Contents.

Additional Remarks 435
The Mode of knitting Slippers 436
The Mode of knitting Gloves 438
The Mode of knitting Petticoats 439
The Mode of knitting Night Jackets 441
Of Open-work Knitting 442
Mitts 443
Knit Berets 444
A Purse knitted like a Pine-apple 445
Purses knitted with Designs 446
Purses knitted Double 447
Purses knitted in Gold and Silk, with Spaces 447
Beaded Purses 448
To line Bags and Purses 450
Purses knitted on a Mould 450
The Art of mending Stockings 452
  To pick up Loose Stitches 452
  Grafting 453
  To re-enforce Stockings 454
  To foot Stockings 456
  To re-cut Stockings 456
Diversion 1 458
  Note 458
Diversion 2 458
  Note 458
Diversion 3 458
  Knitting for the Lower Orders 458
Diversion 4 459
  The Trade of the Stocking-weaver 459
Diversion 5 459
  Note 459
Diversion 6 460
  Note 460
Diversion 7 460
  The Mode of knitting Gentlemen's Waistcoats 460
  The Waistcoat all in One Piece 461
  The Waistcoat in Three Pieces 463
Diversion 8 464
  Note 464

Contents.

Diversion 9 464
    Note 464
Diversion 10 464
    The Mode of knitting Pantaloons 464
Diversion 11 464
    Note 464
Diversion 12 465
    Note 465
Diversion 13 465
    Gold-thread Purses and Bags 465
Diversion 14 465
    To dye Thick Silks, Satins, Silk Stockings, &c.
        of a Flesh-colour 465
    For dyeing Silk Stockings Black 466

Chapter XVIII. The Art of making and mending
Elastic Bracelets and Garters 467
  Bracelets 467
  Garters 467
  Repairs 468

Chapter XIX. The Art of sewing Gloves 470
  Diversion 1 474
    To wash and tint Gloves 474
    To cleanse Gloves without wetting 474
    To dye Gloves 474
    To dye Gloves to resemble York Tan,
        Limerick Dye, &c. 475
  Diversion 2 475
    The Straight Over-cast Stitch or *Cordonnet* 475
    The Slanting Over-cast Stitch or *Cordonnet* 475

Chapter XX. The Art of the Haberdasher and Lace-woman,
or the Art of preparing Belts, *Fichus*, Caps, &c. 476
  A Round Braid for Gowns 476
  Covered Cords 477
  A Cord for Watches, &c., made with the Fingers 477
  Plaited Ribands 478
  A Round Lace, made with Bobbins 478

Contents.

The Mode of tagging Laces 478
The Mode of preparing Woollen Garters with Slip-knots 479
The Mode of pinking Ruches and Flounces
    of *Gros de Naples, Crêpe Lissé,* or *Crêpe Gaufré* 480
The Mode of Preparing Veils 480
    Veils with String-cases 481
    Veils with Tassels 481
The Mode of making Riband Bows 481
    Small and Middle-sized Bows 481
    Large Bows 482
    Half-bows 483
The Mode of making Belts 484
    Belts Fastened at the Back 484
    Belts *à Chou* 485
    Belts with Sewed Loops, without a Knot or Ends 486
    Lined Belts 486
    Belts with Metal Buckles 487
    Belts with Shoulder-straps 487
    Belts bordered with Corded Piping 489
    Elastic Belts 489
Riband *Fichus* 489
The *Fichu* or Belt *à la Duchesse* 491
The Mode of making Fancy *Fichus* 491
    Of cutting out and making up *Fichus* 492
    Standing Collars for *Fichus* 494
    Trimmings for Standing Collars 496
    Falling Collars for *Fichus* 498
Double and Single Three-cornered *Fichus* 502
Fichu-canezous 502
Somnambules and Shawls of Blond or Tulle 503
The Mode of making Cornettes and Fancy Caps 503
    Three-piece Caps 503
    Cornettes *à Casque* 504
    Caps *à la Folle* 504
    Additional Remarks 505
Trimmings *de Lingère* 505
Diversion 1 507
    Note 507
Diversion 2 508
    Belts worn with Evening Dress 508

Contents.

August 1824 508
June 1829 509
Diversion 3 509
   Ladies' Collars 509
   Gentlemen's Collars 509
Diversion 4 512
   Note 512
Diversion 5 512
   Ladies' Caps 512
   Morning Cap 512
   Dress Cap 515
   Dress or Mourning Cap 515
   Turban Cap 515
   Widow's Cap 519
   Night-cap 519

Chapter XXI. The Art of the Milliner,
   or the Mode of making Hats, Toques, &c. 522
Kinds of Head-dresses 522
The Body of the Hat 523
   To cut out and prepare the Body 524
   To cover the Brim 525
   To cover the Crown 528
   The *Coiffe*, or Crown Lining 530
   To assemble the Hat 531
Toques 532
Turbans 533
Berets 534
Caps 534
The Mode of making Hats of All Kinds of Straw,
   cutting them, trimming them, &c. 535
   Chip Hats 535
   Leghorn Straw Hats 536
   Hats of Sewed Straw and of Monaco Straw 538
Hats of Esparto 538
Hats of Gauze Woven with Straw 538
Hats of Decorated Marli 539
The Mode of making Hats of Cotton Tissue,
   Silk Tissue, and Straw Braids 539
Ornaments for Hats 541

Contents.

Bows of Riband 541
Bows of Material 541
Gathered Bows 542
Recoquillé Bows 543
Cockades 543
Fringed Bows 543
Trimmed Bows 544
Bows with Pompons 544
Bows with Thick Braids and Flattened Pompons 544
Bows Decorated with Flowers 545
Bows Decorated with Feathers 545
Bows with Metal Clasps 545
Biases 545
Ruches 546
Torsades 546
Vandykes 546
Agrafes of Material, Gauze, or Riband 546
Tulle or Satin Panes 547
Turbans 547
Blond Half-veil 547
Fichus on Hats 548
Marabouts 548
Esprits 549
Weeping Willow Plumes 549
Plumes Decorated with Gold or Steel 549
Bird-of-paradise 549
Bouquets of Feathers 549
Mixed Flowers 550
Flowers and Fruits 550
Flowers and Feathers 550
Flowers and Tinsel 550
Veiled Flowers 551
Velvet Flowers, for Winter 551
Chenille Flowers 551
Straw Flowers 551
Herbs 551
Sticks 551
Pearls 551
Steel Ornaments, such as Bees, Crescents, &c. 551
Chains and Gilded Circlets 552

Contents.

Buttons 552
Circular Garlands 552
Garlands of Foliage 552
Garlands of Bows 552
Garlands of Loops 552
Garlands *en Casque* 552
Ornaments under the Hat-brim 553
Riband Strings 553
Strings with Corded Piping 553
Gauze or Blond Strings 553
Strings Trimmed with Box-plaits 553
Double and Triple Strings 554
Diversion 1 554
To wash Straw Hats 554
Black Varnish, for Old Straw or Chip Hats 554
For dyeing Straw and Chip Bonnets 554
For dyeing Straw Bonnets Brown 555
For dyeing Straw Bonnets Black 555
Diversion 2 555
Divers Head-dresses 555
April 1827 556
Diversion 3 558
Kinds of Turbans 558
To make a Turban with a Scarf 558
Another Turban made with a Scarf 560
To make a Turban with a Shawl 560
Diversion 4 561
Dressing for Hats of *Écru* Silk
    imitating Leghorn Straw 561
Dressing for Hats formed of Braids
    of Cotton or Silk Thread 561
Diversion 5 562
To cleanse Brown, Fawn-colour, and White Feathers 562
To cleanse Black Feathers 562
For dyeing and cleansing Feathers 562
The Finest Blue on Feathers 563
Another Receipt 564
Brown Feathers 564
Chocolate and Full Rich Brown Feathers 564
For Orange, Madder, &c. Feathers 564

Contents.

Part III. Etiquette 565

Chapter XXII. Of Propriety, and its Advantages 566

  Diversion 1 568
    Differences between French and American Etiquette 568

Chapter XXIII. Propriety as regards yourself 569

  The Toilet 569
  Reputation 573
  Diversion 1 576
    Chaperons 576
  Diversion 2 577
    Conduct of a Widow 577
  Diversion 3 577
    Note 577
  Diversion 4 577
    Gossips and Scandal-mongers 577
  Diversion 5 579
    Means of avoiding Moral Contagion 579
  Diversion 6 580
    Means of avoiding Censure 580

Chapter XXIV. Propriety in Domestic Duties 582

  Propriety in Conjugal and Domestic Relations 583
  Diversion 1 586
    Evenings at Home without Company 586

Chapter XXV. Propriety in the Street and in Travelling . . 589

  Deportment in the Street 589
  Travelling 593

Chapter XXVI. Propriety in Religious Duties 596

  Respectful Deportment in Churches 596
  Religious Propriety in Social Intercourse 598
  Diversion 1 599
    Differences between Catholic
      and Protestant Churches 599

Chapter XXVII. Politeness in a Business or Profession . . . 600

  Politeness of Shop-keepers and Purchasers 600
  Politeness between Persons in Office and the Public 603

Contents.

Politeness of Lawyers and their Clients 603
Politeness of Physicians and their Patients 604
Politeness of Artists and Authors,
    and the Deference due to them 604
Politeness of Military Men 607
Propriety of Clergymen and Nuns,
    and the Deference due to them 608
Diversion 1 608
    Titles given to Members of Religious Orders 608

Chapter XXVIII. Of Visits 609

Different Kinds of Visits 609
The Manner of receiving Visitors 616
Diversion 1 619
    New Acquaintance 619
Diversion 2 619
    Morning Visits 619
Diversion 3 621
    Note 621
Diversion 4 621
    Visiting amongst Servants 621
Diversion 5 622
    Arrangement of the Drawing-room 622

Chapter XXIX. Promenades, Parties,
and Amusements 624

Promenades 624
Dinner-parties 626
Other Parties and Amusements 629
Card-parties 630
Parlour Games with Forfeits 632
Balls, Concerts, and Public Performances 632
    Balls 632
    Concerts 635
    The Theatre, Opera, Ballet, &c. 635
The Duties of Hospitality 637
Diversion 1 639
    Dinner-parties 639
Diversion 2 644
    Note 644

Contents.

Diversion 3 644
   Note 644
Diversion 4 645
   Card-parties and Conversaziones 645
Diversion 5 646
   Forfeits 646
   To kiss the Four Corners of the Room 646
   To kiss the Candlestick 646
   To kiss the Bottom of the Candlestick 646
   To kiss your Shadow 646
   To kiss the Earth 646
   To kiss the Image of God 646
   To kiss the Person you prefer, without appearing to 647
   The Deceitful Kiss 647
   To kiss the Back of the Door 647
   To kiss the Top of the House 647
   To kiss the Hare 647
Diversion 6 647
   Balls 647
Diversion 7 651
   Amusements for Servants 651
Diversion 8 652
   Evenings at Home with Company 652
Diversion 9 653
   Gifts to Servants from Visitors 653

Chapter XXX. Propriety in the Happiest
and Unhappiest Circumstances of Life 654
Weddings 654
Christenings 657
Duties to the Sick, Infirm, and Unfortunate 658
Funerals and Mourning 659
Diversion 1 661
   Love and Courtship 661
   Advice previous to Matrimony 663
   Considerations before Marriage 665

Chapter XXXI. The Art of Conversation 666
Physical Concerns 666
   Divers Faults 666
   Gestures 667

Contents.

Pronunciation 668
   Volubility 668
   Hesitancy 668
   Bad Habits 668
   Accents and Tones 669
Correct Grammar and Language 669
Customary Formalities in Conversation 671
   Inquiries concerning the Health 671
   Forms of Address 671
   Greetings, Apologies, &c. 672
Dialogues 673
   Suppositions and Comparisons 673
   Frequently Recurring Expressions 674
   Quotations and Proverbs 674
   Pleasantries 675
   Eulogiums and Complaints 676
   Tactlessness and Prejudices 678
   Questions 678
   Discussions and Disputes 678
   Narrations 679
   Literary Critiques 680
   Digressions 681
The Art of Listening 681
   Repetition 682
   Interruptions 682
   Falsehoods 683
   Additional Remarks 684
Diversion 1 684
   Swearing 684
Diversion 2 684
   Note 684
Diversion 3 685
   Of Addressing Relations in French 685
Diversion 4 685
   The Use of the Third Person
      in French 685
Diversion 5 686
   Raillery 686
Diversion 6 686
   Arguments 686

Contents.

Diversion 7 687
   Note 687
Diversion 8 687
   Listening 687
Diversion 9 687
   Exaggeration 687

Chapter XXXII. Epistolary Composition 688

General Observations 688
The Appearance of Letters 689
The Style of Letters 691
The Forms for Formal and Informal Letters 692
Billets 694
Diversion 1 695
   Time devoted to Correspondence 695
Diversion 2 696
   Expense of Correspondence 696
Diversion 3 696
   Discretion in Correspondence 696

Chapter XXXIII. Additional Rules
for the Social Relations 698

Advice 698
Discretion 698
Favours 700
Loans 701
Presents 702
Diversion 1 704
   The Manners of the French 704

Glossary 706

Bibliography 728

References 728
Further reading 732

Index 735

Introduction.

The heart of *The Lady's Stratagem* consists of six important instructional manuals originally published in France in the 1820s (and in one case, the early 1830s). Four of them, the *Manuel des dames,* the *Manuel des demoiselles,* the *Manuel complet d'économie domestique,* and the *Manuel complet de la bonne compagnie,* were written, or revised, by Mme. Celnart. This was the *nom-de-plume* of Elisabeth-Félice Bayle-Mouillard, a prolific author of instructional manuals and journal articles. The other two manuals, the *Art de la couturière en robes* and the *Art de faire les corsets, les guêtres et les gants,* were written by Mme. Burtel, about whom I have discovered little further information.

All except the *Manuel complet de la bonne compagnie* were originally written for an exclusively female audience. *Manuel des dames* translates to "manual for married ladies," whom Mme. Celnart views as the most morally appropriate users of the advice on cosmetics and hygiene which forms an important, though by no means exclusive, part of its contents. The *Manuel complet d'économie domestique,* or "complete manual of domestic economy," is a housekeeping manual for married women. The *Manuel des demoiselles* or "manual for unmarried young ladies" (probably adolescents rather than little girls), consists almost entirely of instructions for various kinds of needle-work, which was taught to females beginning at a young age. However, the same techniques were practised by them throughout life. The *Art de la couturière en robes,* or "the art of making gowns," and the *Art de faire les corsets, les guêtres et les gants,* or "the art of making stays, gaiters, and gloves," are both ostensibly aimed at the same audience as the *Manuel des demoiselles.* They stress the importance of young ladies making their own clothing—yet they also include instructions on making gowns and stays for pregnant women. The *Manuel complet de la bonne compagnie,* or "complete manual for polite society," in its sixth edition by 1832, claims to have been written for young persons of both sexes making their first appearance in adult society. Yet some advice is appropriate only for married adults, while some other advice appears to be aimed at younger adolescents. I should add, that all six manuals are written for a solidly bourgeois audience, with occasional reference to the habits of the upper and lower classes.

Early in the project, I decided to focus on the work required behind the scenes to fulfill what period works explicitly present as a duty to females of the 1820s: to be agreeable. This led to a decision not to translate the greater portion of the *Manuel complet d'économie domestique*, relating to cooking and housekeeping. I also decided to focus on the information which is most unique or most usable, as far as modern readers are concerned; which led to a decision not to translate some parts of the *Manuel des demoiselles*. The other four manuals are presented in their entirety (excepting Mme. Burtel's glove-making instructions, which add nothing to Mme. Celnart's). However, I have done some re-organization to make *The Lady's Stratagem* one core Book with some sources used as side commentary, as opposed to a disorganized and repetitive agglomeration of miscellaneous sources. This core is written as I imagine Mme. Celnart would have written it if she had combined several of her works into one. I shall explain what I did with Mme. Burtel's manuals later.

Which leads me to the Diversions. As I worked on Mme. Celnart's and Mme. Burtel's manuals, I researched every other source on related topics which I could get my hands on, whether French, English, or American. This was partly to answer a variety of questions raised by the core sources. And partly, I developed an obsession for locating every English-language source of the 1820s which contained substantial information on mantua-making or stay-making. What I discovered is that there seems to be no such English or American work. There are a few little books designed to inform school-mistresses on how to teach small children the most basic sewing stitches, and how to knit a stocking. There are some manuals which teach professional tailors how to draft patterns for men's clothing, plus how to draft a riding habit and perhaps a few other (usually outer) garments for women. Several such patterns are included in the Diversions. There is a now rare household encyclopædia titled *The Alphabetical Receipt Book and Domestic Advisor* which contains a pattern and sewing instructions for a bodice, and several patterns each for caps, collars, and embroidery, and which I have bought at great expense so I could put the patterns in *The Lady's Stratagem*. And that is all.

In short, I came across twenty-three other sources which contained information which clarifies, amplifies, comments on, supports, or contradicts the text I had originally planned to use, and which were too informative to merely ignore. Added to which (since by no means all of them are about needle-work), they present a picture of how the customs and dress of France, England, and the United States were similar to, or in some cases different from, each other. And some explain the customs and dress of the lower classes of these countries—or at least, what the middle classes thought those ought to be.

Therefore, I excerpted portions of this material, ranging from a few lines to, in the case of Mme. Burtel, entire manuals, translated them into English where necessary, and inserted them as Diversions. I would like to say that I invented the concept. However, every one who has ever used the Internet has seen it. The numbered cross-references stand in place of links, the material at the end of each Chapter is the material "linked" to, and that is all there is to it. As some Diversions are mere footnotes and others are very long, I advise glancing at them while reading the main part of the Chapter, and then if you wish, postpone reading the long ones to a convenient time. A signature line at the end of each Diversion (and for that matter at the end of the main part of each Chapter) indicates the title of its source or sources. Full bibliographic information is contained in, of course, the Bibliography.

Though much of Mme. Celnart's information on mantua-making and stay-making differs significantly from Mme. Burtel's, a few portions are so similar that either one author must have copied the other, or they both copied some other source which I have not discovered despite diligent efforts to do so. However, material on these subjects is so rare for this period, that I flattered myself that if I left any thing out, my readers would perish from curiosity. Thus the mantua-making and stay-making instructions of both authors have been presented in their entirety. Where possible, I cleared up ambiguities in the originals, assembling muslins, making trimmings, &c. as necessary.

One significant point regarding gowns, accessories, millinery, trimmings, and hair-styles, is that Mme. Celnart gives instructions for some styles which she says are long-stranding or even *passé*, and worn as long as fifteen years before she wrote about them, which extends their appropriate time-frame. In fact, many of the sources used were read longer and more widely than may at first appear, a subject covered in more depth in the Bibliography.

An American edition of the *Manuel complet de la bonne compagnie* was published in 1833 as *The Gentleman and Lady's Book of Politeness and Propriety of Deportment*. I initially hoped to use it as is; but on making what I thought would be a perfunctory check against the French edition, I discovered so many omissions and errors, and so much awkward wording, that I ended up largely re-translating it.

I cast all the translated material into 1820s English, because it seems like the most appropriate language for the subject-matter. I have, however, spared my readers the page-long sentences common to both French and English in the 19th century. I have also mostly avoided the use of the subjunctive, which was much more common in English then than now, leading to many phrases such as, "If she be a married lady," and "If she finish the day without company." In short, I have modified the entirely authentic style where modern readers would find it too obscure or bizarre. The period spelling may at first seem odd to American readers, as American spelling was closer to the British than it is now, though it is not quite modern British spelling either. I am confident that they will soon get used to it. I have used and italicized French terms where 1820s publications did so—English fashion journals were liberally peppered with French, and indeed were often translated from French, with or without attribution. French terms, and many period English ones as well, are defined in the Glossary.

I may seem at times to have spoken as if *The Lady's Stratagem* contains mostly information on needle-work. Part II, "Needle-work," does in fact focus exclusively on hand-sewing, mantua-making, stay-making, knitting, embroidery, millinery, making a variety of accessories, mending, and alterations. It is designed for the practical use of, as well as research by, historic re-enactors, living history interpreters, and film and theatre costumers. However Part I, "The Toilet," focuses on hair-dressing, beauty treatments, hygiene, choosing clothing, the process of getting dressed, cleansing and caring for clothing, and the carriage of the body. Though some of this information may be of practical use, it is largely intended for research purposes. As well as to the readers above mentioned, the intimate details about women's appearance and private life will be useful to historical and romance novelists. Part III of *The Lady's Stratagem*, "Etiquette," focuses on the public or social life of both women and men. It comprehends behaviour in daily acts such as walking, at every kind of entertainment and ceremony from balls to weddings, and the art of conversation as well. Re-enactors and living history interpreters may put this information to work in their interpretations, and novelists will find it a valuable research source.

——Frances Grimble.

Warning and Disclaimer.

Part I.
The Toilet.

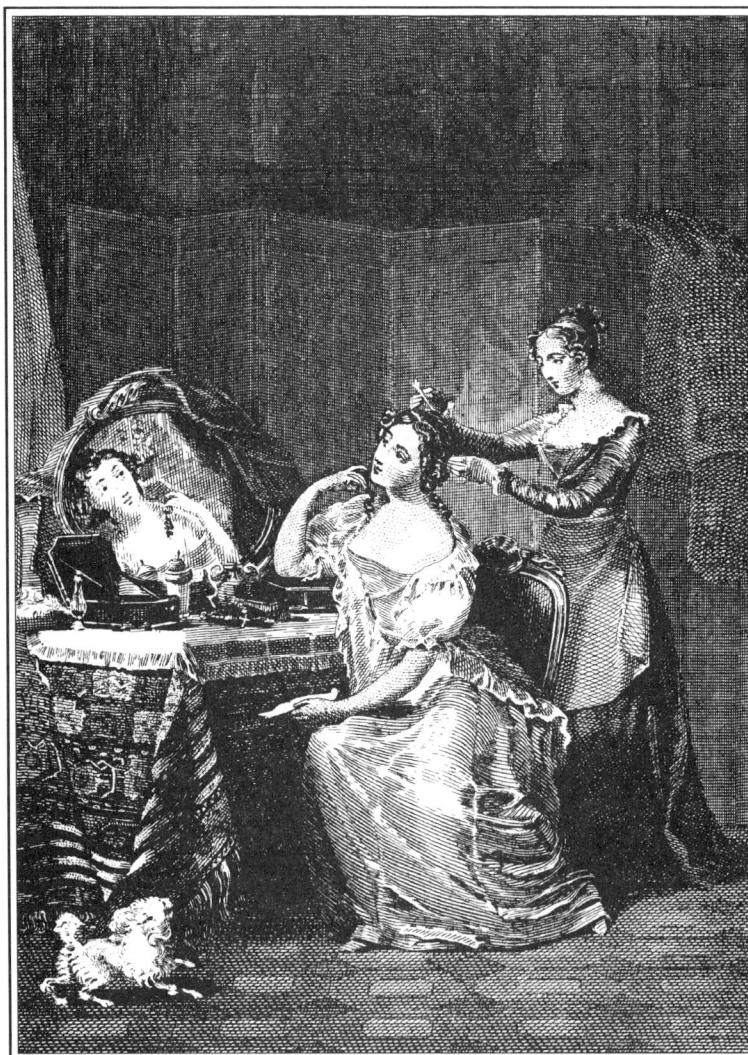

Chapter I.
Preservation of the Hair.

Ladies, let us begin our lessons in coquetry in all good conscience. The desire to please is innocent in itself, and it is even very laudable in a married woman, who should make it her principal occupation to render herself agreeable to her spouse. Doubtless the care of her person should not, without being blameable, lead her to neglect the cultivation of her mind, the governance of her home, or the education of her children. But it must accompany these important duties; it must be their crowning touch. A person who is active, careful, and not too undisciplined, may easily manage all this without being negligent.

The most estimable women would be vexed to be disesteemed by their husbands; therefore, they must strive to excite and nourish more pleasant sentiments. The neglect and infidelity so much deplored in husbands is often owing to wives' neglect of themselves. Who can gauge the consequences of the first impulses of disgust? You always present yourself clean and neat, showing your best side, to your intended, whose expectant eyes admire you incessantly. And then you appear unkempt and disordered to a husband who is disenchanted day after day by possession and habit! The care which you take now and then with your toilet to appear in society, renders your habitual negligence still more disagreeable and conspicuous, because you render to the conventions, perhaps to vanity, what you refuse to love.

Ladies, let us not imitate this discordant mixture of disorder and elegance. Let us act with a constant and thorough neatness, because neatness adorns ugliness, whereas untidiness lends ugliness to the happiest charms. Let us give rank, youth, and public appearances their due; but also, when possible, let us be less brilliant in society and prettier in our homes. Let us preserve and adorn ourselves for those whose pleasures we must care for, so as to achieve happiness. Such a respectable motive (if it may be so expressed) must sanctify our toilet and strictly proscribe all useless expense, cosmetics, and impropriety. I do not fear to advance a sophism by saying that coquetry thus practiced is a virtue, and that the moralists would readily say, "March forward, ladies, and become coquettes." So be it then, and let us first occupy ourselves with our hair.

Modes of beautifying the Hair.

To assist and care for Nature rather than aspiring to force it: that is the whole art of the toilet. This reflection, which we will have reason to recall throughout the course of this work, applies principally to the hair, a natural and precious adornment without which the richest and most elegant attire is not pleasing. You may cultivate it, preserve it from divers mishaps, and even restore it, when its colour and nature are unfavourable, and when poor health or low spirits have caused it to fall out. But in proportion as its cultivation and preservation are easy and sure, so much is restoration difficult, long, dangerous, and sometimes even impossible.

Cleanliness is the soul of the toilet as well as of health. Your principal task must be to keep your hair extremely clean. Every morning, before arranging your hair, disentangle it with a large comb, holding it upright in a straight line in order not to break the hairs. If your hair is very long or thick, divide it into two or three parts, and comb them separately. This practice is above all essential when a finer comb succeeds the large one. When your hair has been well cleansed with these two combs, rub it with a square brush with a handle, whose bristles are very soft, or better yet are replaced with fine rice roots.

It is necessary to occasionally pass a very fine ivory comb through your hair. When your hair is not greasy by nature, and when it is quite long, it is sufficient to use this comb every two or three weeks. In the contrary case, you must use the ivory comb once or twice a week. When your hair is naturally covered by a very fine scurf, it is urgent to use the ivory comb every day, and for at least twenty minutes.

Next comes the arrangement of your hair, with which we will occupy ourselves in Chapter VIII. For the present I shall confine myself to saying that to preserve your hair you should, as far as possible, avoid using a curling-iron and crimping it while wielding the comb; for one of these practices dries it out, and the other twists it, shrivels it, and removes all its gloss. (See Div. 1.) If you tie your hair with a cord, do not tie the cord too tight, or use woollen yarn, for fear of gradually wearing it away. It is also well to guard against twisting or knotting any hairs with the cord, which breaks them, causes pain, and above all prevents your coiffure from smoothing properly. Never raise your hair with a comb which has steel teeth, because the metal breaks the hairs.

When night comes, very gently undo your coiffure, first removing all the black pins which you find there, and shaking out the locks as you let them down. These steps are especially necessary when your hair has been dressed by a hair-dresser. The locks of hair unpinned, comb them well and plait them neatly, because you should never go to bed with your hair tangled and not fixed in a plait. Nothing makes hair deteriorate quicker than such negligence. This is besides extremely untidy, because your hair pushes back the cap, escapes from it, and falls tumbled and dreadfully mixed up over the pillow, which it soils. Besides these inconveniences, it occasions a lively itching of the head. I am well aware that there is no young woman who habitually neglects herself to this point. But in the season of balls and assemblies, when you return late, you may take down your hair and go to bed in haste, and all the mishaps which I have just described occur, with great damage to your hair.

When you leave a ball or any other place where your hair is necessarily covered by dust, after having taken down and combed your hair, wipe it well with a very dry towel, and the next day pass an ivory comb through it. If you have the good habit of occupying yourself with household tasks, cover your hair when you are cooking, because smoke dulls it. In the cold and damp season, press your hair now and then with a warm linen cloth. When in summer your hair is drenched with sweat, likewise wipe it with the linen, but unheated.

Finally, to give strength to your hair, and prevent it from thinning, becoming uneven, and fading at the ends, adopt the good habit of cutting it every fortnight, about half an inch above the ends. Nature will soon repair the loss. If you have neglected this practice for a long time, and if your hair has become uneven, you must cut it straight even when some locks are cut back by nearly three inches. This is called refreshing the hair. Your hairs will grow longer together, and will always be even. The ends will be the same colour as the rest of your hair, and will be rid of ugly twists which separate them. If their nature is to curl, they will form beautiful equal curls. Moreover, when raised to the summit of your head, they will cease to produce a coiffure with a rounded side and a flat side, or a plait thick at the beginning and ending in a rat's tail.

I am sure that these important tasks, which largely compose the art of preserving the hair, will appear to many of my readers as merely insignificant preliminaries, accustomed as they are to hearing the efficacy of a thousand cosmetics vaunted by the countless pretentious prospectuses of hair-dressers and perfumers. But when I have subtracted every thing superfluous or pernicious from this mass; when I have, above all, erased the pompous names and shown how, in certain cases, it is proper to use even the best pomatums with discretion, I shall have mostly proved that the use of cosmetics is only incidental to preserving your hair.

It is well to use fine pomatum, or the lightly-perfumed oils called antique (see Div. 2); but it is still necessary to consider the season, the nature of your hair, and the amount of perspiration which is given forth from your head. In winter, it is better to use antique oil than pomatum. Your hair, dried and stiffened by the cold, requires moistening by a slightly oily liquid, which makes it supple. In summer, on the contrary, hair gradually moistened by perspiration needs pomatum, but very little; for many heads of hair, it is preferable to abstain. In moist and rainy weather, oil and pomatum, used alone and in quantity, are much more hurtful than useful, in that they contribute to rendering your hair incapable of holding a curl.

This inconvenience of dampness is with reason a lively vexation for ladies, because despite all possible care, it gives the appearance of uncleanliness. To remedy this, they resort to the iron, and thus prepare their hair to fall out. Some persons are in the habit of dissolving a little gum-arabic in a few drops of water, wetting their fingers with this solution, and moistening their curls. In order to receive all the benefits of this mode, when your hair is thus glued, comb it lightly, and pass it between your dry fingers, so that the curls will not appear disagreeably stiff. When the glue has dried slightly, you may put a little pomatum on it, to prevent your hair from looking dull.

All this is a great deal of work; so I advise those of my readers who have many occupations, or whose hair always refuses to hold a curl, to wear a *tour en cheveux roulés,* which will never uncurl. It goes without saying that this must be perfectly matched to your hair, and that you do not put it on when your hair is dressed *en cheveux,* or when you must make a grand toilet. It is worn at home, under a cap or a beret, or under a hat to go out without ceremony. At this time the curls are rolled and held in place by a very short black pin, placed crossways in the middle, or a little strip of lead which remains under the *tour* much of the time, firmly holding the shape of the curls. It is well to use this mode in all seasons, on days when you are to go to a ball, because you will know quite well how to attach the *tour* so that the curls hold properly.

Some ladies leave their hair in curl-papers under the *tour.* It is enough to mention this practice to condemn it. Indeed the papers show through your hair, and put a disagreeable space between the *tour* and your forehead; and the idea of present negligence is united to that of future coquetry. Is not the point of this that we wish above all to appear to advantage in our husbands' eyes, and to show ourselves always well groomed in the home? You may well think, after this advice, that I will cry out against the curl-papers, the leaden strip alone, or the pins which hold the curls; but this negligence would be in such bad taste, that I do not suspect my amiable readers of it.

The nature of your hair demands still more imperiously that in every season you must employ each substance to the exclusion of all others. The season also regulates the quantity. Practically speaking, you need consider only this. Hair which is dry and rough, which has the property of bristling, requires much more greasy matter than hair naturally coated with it. Thus oil, and plenty of it, agrees with coarse hair, whereas other kinds merely require to be very lightly rubbed from time to time with a bit of pomatum spread over your hand. Because greasy hair is almost flattened by its own oil, you should not only abjure oil and pomatum, but often wash it with a weak solution of soap. I shall discuss this means of preserving the hair when I have exhausted the subject of pomatums.

Such greasy substances as you use, whether oils or pomatums, must always be very fine, fresh, not too thick, and lightly perfumed. Strong odours, such as musk, amber, orange-flower, tuberose, and similar things must be entirely avoided. Soft and gentle perfumes, such as heliotrope, rose, narcissus, &c. are a thousand times preferable, at least if you use only a little, because the delicate odours are lost (or at least weaken) with time: then the oils and pomatums of jasmine, carnation, and vanilla chiefly serve. They are intermediate between the weakest perfumes and the strongest, which you should abstain from completely. Frequent megrims, nervous illness (though unnoticed owing to habit), a noticeable decrease in facial colour, and the unpleasantness of appearing affected and coquettish: these are the fruits which you will gain from them.

When in winter oils congeal and pomatums harden, they should not be used in this state. Wait until a gentle heat has returned their softness and liquidity. The mode of putting them to the fire makes them rancid; rather immerse them in the lukewarm water which you used for your toilet. In summer be careful to keep them in a cool place, especially pomatums, because the heat renders them disagreeably liquid.

When by nature, or by the prolonged or exaggerated use of oils and pomatums, your hair is greasy to the point of being dull, dense, and flat, you must resort to soap solutions. (See Div. 3.) Pour a *demi-tasse* of lukewarm water into a saucer. Soak a very lightly-perfumed toilet-soap in the water for a few moments, and stir it a little. Soon the water will be foamy. Then spread the locks of your hair well apart, and with a sponge dampened with the soapy water, wash them well from all sides. If during this operation the water cools off, add enough hot water to make it lukewarm. With your hair perfectly clean, dry it well with slightly-warmed linen, then brush it several times with the rice brush. In summer you may use unwarmed linen, and even cool water, especially when you are accustomed to this. However, it is always better to warm the water a little in the sun. This practice should be more or less frequent according to your kind of hair. Blonde hair, which is rarely greasy, and whose fineness and softness prevent the use of pomatums, should above all be washed very rarely.

Guard against replacing the slight alkalinity of the soap with spirituous liquors such as Cologne water, lavender-water, &c. These spirits dry your hair, wear it away, and contribute to making it quickly break or fall out. Do not use brandy on your head except in two cases. Here is the first: when the comb which lifts your hair presses too much on the place where it rests, and hurts it, move away your hair and rub the place with a sponge or a knot of linen soaked in brandy. The pain, which is ordinarily quite acute, will abate in a little while. I shall describe the second case later.

The Use of an Egg-yolk to de-grease the Hair.

Here is a very easy means of removing grease from your hair. Take the yolk of a raw egg. Moisten your hand with it, pass it over your hair several times, then comb with a fine comb. It is well known that egg-yolk absorbs grease stains on material (see Chapter X).

The Removal of Superfluous Hair.

At times hair grows in an odd manner. Sometimes it grows down the middle of the forehead like a forelock; sometimes it descends along the ears, like a man's whiskers; sometimes also it extends over the neck, where it forms a kind of collar. All these blemishes have a disagreeable and ridiculous effect. Cutting the hair renders it thicker and stronger; plucking it out is impossible; using a depilatory is dangerous. All the depilatories which charlatans extol and sell very dearly have no effect but to dupe you, unless they attack the tissue of the skin, which they ordinarily do. Moreover, the best depilatories have only temporary success: after a certain time the hair grows back.

The famous rusma of the Orientals, which the Arabs and Persians call *nouret*, *nure*, or *nuret*, and so much used in harems, has no different effect. Here is the mode of preparing it, as given by Cadet de Gassicourt in the *Dictionnaire des sciences médicales*.

Oriental Rusma. Take two ounces of quicklime, and mix it with half an ounce of orpiment or realgar (sulphur of arsenic). Boil them with a pound of sufficiently strong alkaline washing powder. To try it, immerse a feather in it; when the barbs fall out, the rusma is properly prepared. Rub it on the parts where you wish to destroy the hair, then bathe them with warm water. This depilatory is highly caustic. It often attacks the skin at the same time as the hair: therefore you must apply it with the greatest circumspection.

To weaken the strength of this composition, content yourself with mixing the quicklime and the orpiment, and moistening them with lukewarm water at the time of using them. This is quite like the Parisian Depilatory Cream (which see below) as a very fine powder.

Instead of diluting rusma, some persons add hog's lard to it, and make a pomatum which they colour and perfume at will. In the harems of Turkey, the proportion of the mixture is varied according to the ages of the persons who will use it, the nature of their skin, and the colour of their hair. Sometimes an ounce of orpiment is put to eight ounces of quicklime, sometimes two ounces of orpiment to twelve ounces of quicklime, and sometimes three ounces of orpiment to fifteen ounces of this last substance. The third mixture is the most violent.

To temper the dangerous causticity, add an eighth part of starch or rye-flour. Make a paste with a little lukewarm water. Apply it to the desired places, and let it stay there for several minutes. Be careful to moisten it a little so that it does not dry too quickly, and try whether the hair can be removed easily and with no resistance. Ordinarily it appears burnt: then the operation is complete. Use rusma only in small quantities, because apart from alteration of your skin, you may fear absorption and therefore all the mishaps of arsenic poisoning.

Parisian Depilatory Cream. Put a few pinches of this mixture into a small vessel, such as an egg-cup, a soup-spoon (provided that it is wooden), or even a very small saucer. Pour on a few drops of lukewarm water. Dilute to it the consistency of tolerably thick gruel, and apply this on the places you wish to depilate. Leave it on for five to eight minutes. Dampen it with a little lukewarm water, then take it off while damp, lightly, with the point of a knife. Then wash with a sponge soaked in lukewarm water. Dry gently, avoiding rubbing. Always leave an interval of twenty-four hours from one application to the next. This depilatory does not produce an unfortunate effect on the skin when its application is not continual.

I use this composition for clearing my forehead. It does indeed remove hair, but this grows back after about ten days. I advise you not to repeat the application more than three times, because your skin feels a lively burning and breaks a little. However, if you absolutely must remove hair, you will do well to apply it as soon as the hairs reappear; this caustic brings them down like a razor. Blonds will find this depilatory most beneficial, because though it removes the hairs, it does not remove the slight shadow which remains after their fall, like that from the beards of dark-haired men.

Laforest's Depilatory Preparation. Take two ounces of quicksilver, an ounce of yellow orpiment, an ounce of starch, and an ounce of litharge. Pass them all through a silken sieve, and mix with soap and water until they form a paste. Put this on the place to be depilated, and proceed as I have indicated for Oriental Rusma and the Parisian Depilatory Cream.

Additional Remarks. Before applying a depilatory, it is well to cut the hairs which you wish to remove, in order to make it more effective. Some time after application, you ought to wear a strip of woollen in order to wear off the hair as it regrows. Put this bandage on at night under your bandeau, so that it does not touch your other hair, upon which it would also act. It should cover only the depilated place and be attached in the middle by two linen tapes. This bandage will not lead to any mishaps, but the results are extremely slow.

Troches of arsenic, salve of Mynsicht quicklime, and sulphur of baryte reduced in liniment, with a sufficient quantity of water, are also depilatories which may be recommended, though subject to very great precautions in using them. As for parsley juice, acacia juice, tithymal mixed with oil, cherry-tree gum dissolved in water, ants' eggs, and other such things, you should smile and leave them alone. (See Div. 4.)

To make the Hair grow, and prevent its falling out.

Whereas some ladies deplore superfluous hair and expose themselves to serious mishaps to get rid of it, others weary themselves with efforts to check the rapid loss of their hair, or to refurnish their balding heads. This natural misfortune, called alopecia, ordinarily occurs after a serious illness, or when you have let your hair go for a long time without combing it, such as during a fever, erysipelas of the face, or a confinement, when you dare not, through excess of caution, uncover your head.

Without doubt, your health is more important than mere appearance, and when you must choose between preserving your hair and recovery, do not hesitate. But in the case of less dangerous illnesses, you will do very well to comb your hair now and again, putting yourself in a comfortable position for this without quitting your bed. When you have combed it, you may rub it and blot your head with warm linen cloths. Then rearrange your hair very quickly. By this means you will avoid insupportable tangles, the torment you would suffer when disentangling your hair, and finally the total or partial loss of this precious ornament.

The hottest weather is disastrous to the hair; so from the beginning of summer you should redouble your care and cleanliness. Increase your use of soap solutions and refresh your hair often.

When in spite of all precautions, great quantities of hair continue to fall out, it is necessary to make a sacrifice: to cut it or have it shaved. Otherwise you risk your hair becoming uneven, sparse, and frayed. By this drastic measure, at the end of some years you are sure to see a magnificent head of hair, thicker and more beautiful than before. After the first month you will already see a thick growth of down, which confirms this hope. You may accelerate its growth by dipping toilet-soap in a little brandy, then rubbing your head well at night when going to bed. When your hair is a little longer, separate it so that the soap solution penetrates to the roots. I know that many people will condemn this mode, but I have tried it. You will do well to apply pomatum and soap alternately. The human and bear grease, and the beef marrow which cupidity, routine, or charlatanism promote so zealously, are no more efficacious than ordinary pomatum, or any other greasy substance. You may use the following oil for growing the hair:

Oil for making the Hair grow. Mix equal parts of oil and spirit of rosemary. Add several drops of oil of nutmeg. Every day anoint and brush your hair with a little of this liniment, increasing the amount daily.

When you may still hope to save your hair, and the falling out diminishes gradually, it is necessary, in often refreshing it, to use the preceding remedy. But when your hair falls out *en masse*, without new hairs gradually filling the bare places, the roots have perished. Nothing will revive them, and you will remain entirely bald. This complete loss of hair, called calvities, is much rarer in women than in men. Nonetheless, in both sexes acute illness, advanced age, the abuse of coffee, and irregular conduct equally produce this sorry state. When it is certain, seeking remedies is useless. A wig, well made and well matched, is the only palliative.

You may likewise be obliged to wear a wig during the first year of regrowth, unless you always wear a cap. A wig is even an excellent way to promote regrowth, because air dries the hairs and lessens their strength. The hair grows rapidly until it is about half a foot long, but after that growth is very slow. No matter, that is enough to leave off the wig and be coiffed *en cheveux*. I shall explain how in Chapter VIII. While you are waiting, I strongly recommend that you do not curl your growing hair *à la Ninon,* because the iron which you must use would be exceedingly hurtful. You must braid your hair when it is possible, and refresh it often.

Greying Hair.

Now that I have given remedies for thinning hair and baldness, I shall discuss greying hair, or canities. There are scarcely any remedies which are not false, and that is all the same to us. This condition is caused by age, debauchery, long and profound studies, and severe disorders of the mind. Well, in the first case you hide your hair, and are sensible. The second is unknown to us; the following is not very common; and the last—does it permit care for outward appearance?

But suppose you are young, gay, happy, and your hair is straw-coloured, dull black, or a perfect red! If you cut and recut overly blond hair, when it regrows it will assume a darker shade; you should cease in order to have less wavy and fine hair. For dull and dirty-looking black hair, smooth it for a long time with your hand moistened with oil, and choose head-dresses whose colour brings out the black. Finally, for red hair, wear a wig.

You see that I am not numbered amongst the partisans of hair-dye. That is because false colouring is a recurring source of annoyances, heavy expenses, and more or less great dangers. Preparations praised for dyeing the hair nearly all consist of metallic oxides, whose action on the hair and skin is exceedingly hurtful. They inhibit perspiration, and may lead to head-aches, ear-aches, and more or less serious inflammation of the eyes. These cosmetics do not even have the promised effect. They indeed dye your hair, but it soon grows, and the difference in colours betrays the deception. It is wiser and healthier to leave your hair as it is. So the physician M. Ratier expresses himself in the *Nouvelle médecine domestique.* I must add that the noxious substance in the cosmetics in question can penetrate to the interior by absorption, and case terrible illness.

Hair-dyes obtained from vegetables are nearly always ineffective. However, you may try them. Many authors recommend, as a means of dyeing the hair black, cypress-leaves crushed in vinegar. The use of a leaden comb is advised for red hair: it darkens the hair, but also soils it. Furthermore, see *l'Art de conserver et d'augmenter la beauté,* by J-M. Mossé, and *Embellissements du corps humain,* by Jean Liébault, published in

1582. After reading these, you will renounce the project of dyeing your hair. (See Div. 5.)

——*Manuel des dames.*

Diversion 1.

Curling-irons *vs.* Curl-papers. The use of curling-irons has been much decried as hurtful to the growth of hair, though I cannot see how they can produce injury, except on the portions where they are applied, and not even on these unless the irons are too hot, which you must be careful to prevent. I cannot indeed recommend their constant use, for accidents are continually happening with them from want of care.

Curl-papers, the most usual mode of curling, are apt to be more injurious than curling-irons. By being closely twisted, they not only prevent the hair from growing at the roots, but are apt to cause head-aches, tooth-aches, ear-aches, and sometimes pimples on the face. None of these consequences, however, will happen if care is taken not to overdo the thing. Every thing, indeed, which deprives the hair of its free and natural flow, and of its natural moisture, will check its growth, and make it thin and short; so that there can be no doubt that many of the fashionable modes of hair-dressing are hurtful to its beauty. The hairs naturally go out from the skin in a slanting or oblique direction. If they are twisted or pulled out of this direction, the passage of the fluid which nourishes them will be obstructed or stopped, and their fine gloss and colour will be injured. It cannot be denied, accordingly, that curling the hair by means of hard-twisted curl-papers, or twisting up the hair in a hard knot or bow on the summit of the head, or even plaiting or binding it with a riband or fillet, must all be injurious and detrimental. On the other hand, even if the hair is dressed in any of these fashions, if it is not drawn tight from the skin, but left rather loose and easy, no injury can follow.

——*The Duties of a Lady's Maid.*

Diversion 2.

The Best French Receipts. When the hair has been properly washed and thoroughly dried, it may be useful, in order to give it the requisite gloss, to have recourse to a little fine pomatum or hair-oil, which I shall now teach you how to make for yourself, according to the best French receipts which I have been able to procure.

Parisian Pomatum. Put into a proper vessel two and a half pounds of prepared hog's lard with two pounds of picked lavender-flowers, orange-flowers, jasmine, buds of sweet briar, or any other sweet-scented flower, or a mixture according to your choice, and knead the whole with your hands into a paste as uniform as possible. Put this mixture into a pewter, tin, or stone pot, and cork it tight. Place the vessel in a vapour-bath, and let it stand in it six hours, at the expiration of which time strain the mixture through a coarse linen cloth by means of a press. Now throw away the flowers which you have used as being useless, pour the melted lard back into the same pot, and add four pounds of fresh lavender-flowers. Stir the lard and flowers together while the lard is in a liquid state, in order to mix them thoroughly, and repeat the first process. Continue to repeat this until you have used about ten pounds of flowers.

After having separated the pomatum from the refuse of the flowers, set it in a cool place to congeal. Pour off the reddish-brown liquor or juice extracted from the flowers. Wash the pomatum in several waters, stirring it about with a wooden spatula to separate any remaining watery particles, until the last water remains perfectly colourless. Then melt the pomatum in a vapour-bath, and let it stand in it about an hour, in a vessel well corked, then leave it in the vessel to congeal. Repeat this last operation until the watery particles are entirely extracted, when the wax must be added, and the pomatum melted for the last time in a vapour-bath in a vessel closely corked, and suffered to congeal as before. When properly prepared it may be filled into pots. Tie the mouths of them over with wet bladder to prevent the air from penetrating. This pomatum will be very fragrant, and form an excellent preparation for improving the gloss and luxuriance of the hair.

English Pomatum. Take six ounces of common pomatum, and add to it two or three ounces of very clean white wax, scraped very fine. Melt the whole together in an earthen pan, which is immersed in a larger one containing boiling water, over a clear and steady fire. When properly incorporated take it off, and keep stirring it with a spatula until it is about half cold or congealed. Then put it into small pots, as before directed, or make it up into rolls the size of the little finger. This pomatum may be scented with whatever agreeable flavour the perfumer pleases. It will keep good, even with less wax than has been above directed, in the East Indies or any other warm climate for a long time.

Italian Pomatum. Take twenty-five pounds of hog's lard, eight pounds of mutton-suet, six ounces of oil of bergamot, four ounces of essence of lemon, half an ounce of oil of lavender, and a quarter of an ounce of oil of rosemary. These ingredients are to be combined in the same manner as those for the English pomatum, and kept in pots for use.

Palm Pomatum. Take five pounds of hog's lard, a pound of mutton-suet, three ounces of Portugal water, half an ounce of essence of bergamot, four ounces of yellow wax, and half a pound of palm-oil. Mix as directed for hard pomatum, and put it into small gallipots, which must be well covered.

Another way is to melt in a water-bath the quantity required of common pomatum, and add an equal weight of fresh orange-flowers. Let the whole remain for four hours, when it is to be passed through a linen cloth by pressure. Put this with a fresh quantity of the flowers again into the water-bath. Repeat the process in this manner five or six times, when it may be set aside to cool, and in fifteen days remelted in the water-bath, and put into pots.

Rowland's Hair-oil. Boil half a pound of green southernwood in a pint and a half of sweet oil, and half a pint of port wine. When sufficiently boiled, remove it from the fire, and strain off the liquor through a linen bag. Repeat this operation three times with fresh southernwood; and the last time add to the strained materials two ounces of bear's grease. It is excellent for promoting the growth of the hair, and preventing baldness.

Fragrant Hair-oil. Blanch a quantity of sweet almonds in hot water. When dry reduce them to powder, and sift them through a fine sieve. Strew a thin bed of almond powder, and a bed of fresh odoriferous flowers, such as lavender, jasmine, roses, &c., over the bottom of a box lined with tin. Do this alternately until the box is full, and leave them together for twelve hours. Then throw away the flowers, and add fresh ones in the same manner as before. Repeat the same operation every day for eight successive days. When the almond powder is thoroughly impregnated with the scent of the flowers, put it into a new clean linen cloth, and with an iron press extract the oil, which will be strongly scented with the fragrance of the flowers.

Russian Hair-oil. Put a gallon of salad oil into a pipkin with a bag containing four ounces of alkanet root, cut and bruised. Give the whole a good heat, but not a boiling one, until the oil is completely impregnated with the red colour. Pour the whole into a jar, and let it stand until cold. Then add four ounces of essence of bergamot, four ounces of oil of jasmine, and three ounces of mille-fleur water. When properly mixed, put the compound liquid into small bottles for use.

Antique Oils. These oils, which are sold in considerable quantity, are chiefly composed of oil of ben, or behen nuts. The oil, like that of almonds, is made first by beating, and then sifting the behen nuts through a coarse wire sieve, and expressing them by means of the press. The nuts are imported from Italy, and are of various quality, but the oil differs from that of almonds in being adapted to keep more years than the latter will months. Its principal excellence consists in its having no smell of its own, and consequently being ready to imbibe the odour of any perfume with which it may be combined.

Antique Oil *au Musc.* Pound in a glass mortar a drachm of musk with four grains of amber, while gradually adding eight ounces of oil of behen. When they are all well mixed put the mixture into a small bottle, and take up every particle of the musk and amber. Put into the mortar four ounces of fresh oil of behen, which is also to be put into the same bottle. Leave the whole for twelve or fourteen days in a warm place, shaking it every day. Leave it then to rest for one day more, pour off the oil clear, and preserve it in small bottles, well corked for use. In the same manner you may make antique oil *à l'Ambre,* by changing the proportions of the amber and the musk.

Antique Oil *à l'Orange.* With a pound of oil of behen, mix three ounces of essential oil of orange, and put it into small bottles well corked, with wax over them to preserve it from the air and prevent the perfume of the orange-oil from evaporating. In the same manner you may make antique oils *au Citron, à la Bergamote, au Cédrat, au Girofle, au Thym, à la Lavande, au Rosmarin,* &c. Take care, as a general rule, to proportion the quantity of the perfumed essence which you employ to its strength.

Antique Oil *à la Rose.* Procure a tin or white iron box, about a foot square, opening by a grating on one side, and divided in the middle by a portion of white iron drilled full of small holes close together. Fold a cotton towel in quarters, soak it in oil of behen, and place it on the grating, so as to exactly fit the box. Upon this cloth place your rose-leaves fresh gathered, leave them for about twenty-four hours, and then replace them with fresh rose-leaves. The cloth may then be removed, and the oil now charged with the perfume, carefully expressed. This may be mixed with fresh oil of behen and bottled for use. In the same manner you may make antique oils *à la Fleur d'Orange, à la Violette, à la Jonquille, au Jasmin,* &c. and by means of various mixtures—*à l'Héliotrope, aux Mille-fleurs, au Pot-pourri,* &c.

Antique Oil *à la Tubéreuse.* Mix the flowers with ground blanched bitter almonds, and then express the oil; or mix a pint of olive or almond oil, with thirty drops of the essence of tuberose flowers. In this way also several of the above antique oils may be prepared. A red colour may be given to any of these oils by alkanet root, in the manner directed above for making the Russian Hair-oil.

Antique Oil *Verte.* Add a drachm of gum guaiac to a pound of olive-oil. Let it stand for some time, and then strain, adding any of the fragrant essences which you please.

Macassar Oil. This oil is much talked of, but is not better than many of the others. The following is given in some late works as the genuine receipt for this oil as prepared by several perfumers in London. Take a pound of olive-oil, coloured with alkanet root, and add to it a drachm of the oil of origanum. It may be remarked that olive-oil is an excellent basis for hair-oil, and it is also the most economical; for a thin, stale olive-oil, at ten shillings the gallon, will do equally well as a superior oil at fourteen shillings the gallon, because the powerful odour of the perfumes takes off or destroys any disagreeable smell peculiar to stale and thin olive-oil. When you have mixed your perfume with it, you must shake the bottle in which it is contained twice a day, for at least one week.

The use of these pomatums and hair-oils will, in some kinds of hair, assist in the important operation of curling, but in other cases will be disadvantageous. If the hair is soft and very fine, instead of washing and oiling it, it will be better to clean it with a brush dipped slightly in spirit of hartshorn, or to dress it with the following composition, which will give it both a fine gloss and strength to remain in the curl:

Curling Fluid. Cut into small pieces about two pounds of good common soap, and put it into three pints of spirit of wine or brandy, with eight ounces of potash, and melt the whole in a hot water-bath, stirring it the while with a glass rod or wooden spatula. After it is properly melted, leave it to settle, pour off the liquor clear, and perfume it with any fragrant essence you please.

Or, you may mix together equal parts of essence of violets, jasmine, orange-flowers, and ambrette, with half the quantity of vanilla and tuberose. With these, mix rose and orange-flower water, so as to form in all about three pints of liquid, in which dissolve, as in the first case, two pounds of good soap sliced and eight ounces of potash, and proceed as before. Add some drops of essence of amber, musk, vanilla, and neroli, to make it more fragrant. You will find this as good, if not superior to any of the articles sold under the name of curling fluids, and one-half cheaper.

——*The Duties of a Lady's Maid.*

Diversion 3.

Arguments against washing the Hair. The practice, which of late years appears to have gained ground, of washing the head with either warm or cold water, requires considerable judgement, as from it not unfrequently result head-ache, ear-ache, tooth-ache, and complaints of the eyes. Let the following observations of an experienced professional man operate, therefore, as a caution: "Beneath the paternal roof, this operation is frequently performed by inexperienced youth, from time to time, in secret. In some boarding-schools, on the contrary, every head is subjected to it by the regulations of the house: it is found to be a mode of cleansing them equally easy and expeditious. You afterwards hear complaints that the children are afflicted with tooth-ache, and that it is often necessary to draw their teeth. Instead of seeking elsewhere for the cause, nothing but this act of cleanliness is in some cases to blame. Look at those children whose heads are scarcely ever dry; their pallid faces will never be enlivened by the rich colour of adolescence, and the smiles of infancy will be speedily succeeded by the wrinkles of age. It is in vain to urge that the hair is well dressed. The water which remains is always sufficient to obstruct the perspiration, to keep the root continually wet, and the brain in a state of constant humidity, of which obstructed perspiration furnishes an abundant source. Those assuredly possessed great experience who transmitted to us this precept: 'Wash the hands often, the feet seldom, and the head never.'"

——*The Toilette of Health, Beauty, and Fashion.*

Arguments in favour of washing the Hair. Some persons have a strong prejudice against washing the hair, and imagine that it is productive of very serious evils. Were this prejudice confined to the ignorant and illiterate, I might pass it over without notice; but as it is put forth in books, and under the authority of professional men, it requires to be exposed and refuted, more particularly when they threaten those who wash their hair with "head-ache, ear-ache, tooth-ache, and complaints of the eyes" and not only so, but with premature old age and a shrivelled and wrinkled countenance.

On the contrary, I am of the opinion, and it is well supported by fact and experience, that nothing contributes more to prevent these very consequences than frequently washing the head with tepid water, that is, about milk-warm. When the hair is very long, or when much use is made of hair-oils and pomatums, I cannot imagine how the hair can be rendered comfortable without frequently washing it. I think it is a strong argument in favour of my opinion, that in taking the general cold bath, if the head is kept dry by a cap, head-ache and other bad consequences are almost certain to ensue. Nothing then can be more erroneous than that wetting the hair produces head-aches, catarrhs, and I know not how many evils.

I quote the following remarks from a French author as worthy of attention on this subject. Some ladies may say that their hair is too long to be conveniently washed; but as the most beautiful hair is the most difficult to keep clean, it is long hair which requires the more to be frequently washed with care. Water also is by far the best thing for giving a beautiful gloss to the hair, if care is taken to have it instantly dried and well combed, and brushed before the fire or in the sun. The same author thinks, that the inconveniences supposed to arise from the head being wetted are to be attributed to its being always kept dry, such as megrims and ear-aches, because the want of moisture in the hair prevents the comb or the brush from completely detaching the scales which form there, and closes the pores of the skin through which the perspiration ought to pass.

——*The Duties of a Lady's Maid.*

Diversion 4.

Depilatories. The depilatories in general are various, possessing different degrees of strength. The mildest are parsley water, acacia juice, and ivy-gum. It is asserted that nut-oil, with which many people rub the heads of children, prevents the hair from growing. The juice of the milk thistle mixed with oil is recommended by Dr. Turner to remove the hair which grows too low upon the forehead. It is also said that cherry-tree gum prevents the hair from growing.

Depilatory of Ants' Eggs. Take an ounce of ivy-gum, a drachm of ants' eggs, a drachm of gum-arabic, and a drachm of orpiment. Reduce these to a fine powder, and make it up into a liniment, with a sufficient quantity of vinegar. In pounding the materials, great precaution must be taken that the dust of the orpiment, which is a preparation of arsenic, is not inhaled.

——*The Toilette of Health, Beauty, and Fashion.*

Plucking and Shaving. Where the skin is strong and healthy, perhaps the best depilatory is the actual removal of the hairs, one by one, with the tweezers. I cannot indeed say that it is not painful; but it cannot surely be a question, that it is better to endure a little pain, than to run the hazard of the consequences likely to ensue from the use of nostrum depilatories. It is rarely indeed that any unpleasant circumstance has arisen from the use of the tweezers; and when accidents have occurred, it has always been more from the unhealthy state of the part operated upon, than from any other circumstance.

If the tweezers, however, are objected to, the razor is always a safe and effectual means of removing superfluous hair from every part of the body. To ladies who are troubled with superfluous hairs on the upper lip at a certain period of life, or in consequence of suppressions, or similar constitutional affections, I most strongly recommend the razor, as superior to all other means. It will seldom, in ordinary cases, be requisite to use it more than twice or thrice a week. But even if it should be necessary every second day, it will take but a few minutes; and it is surely preferable to undergo a little trouble of this kind, than to run the hazard of destroying the appearance of the skin by dangerous caustic applications. By a very little practice, it may be performed by the lady herself, and kept altogether secret—a circumstance which is sometimes important in such cases.

——*The Art of Preserving the Hair.*

Diversion 5.

Receipts for Dyes. When the hair has become grey, ladies are usually extremely anxious to conceal this mark of age, by having recourse to hair-dyes. It will be useful for you to know the composition of some of these, that you may be able to make them for use at a much cheaper rate than they can be purchased from perfumers. I can inform you, however, that all the advertised hair-dyes, under whatever name they may appear, such as "Grecian Water," "Vegetable Hair-dye," "Essence of Tyre," &c. are all nothing more than several ways of disguising the nitrate of silver, or lunar caustic, as it was formerly denominated, the same substance which is used for preparing permanent marking ink. You can, to a certainty, produce an immediate black colour upon every kind of hair, by dissolving it in water, and applying it carefully. You must take care, however, not to burn yourself with it, as it will eat through your skin like a piece of red-hot iron. It has the great disadvantage that the hair soon changes from black to purple. It has also been said, but I know not on what authority, that the use of it causes head-aches. At all events it will be better for you to make it for a few pence, than give away shillings and pounds to perfumers and patentees.

I have collected the following receipts for dyeing the hair; but as they may not all prove effectual, I recommend you to try them privately before committing yourself with your employers.

Composition for staining the Hair Black. Break to pieces a pound of gall-nuts. Boil them in olive-oil until they grow soft. Then dry them, and reduce them to a very fine powder, which incorporate with equal parts of powdered charcoal of willow and common salt, prepared and pulverized. Add a small quantity of lemon and orange-peel, dried and reduced to powder. Boil the whole in twelve pounds of water, until the sediment at the bottom of the vessel assumes the consistence of a black salve. With this anoint the hair, cover it with a cap until dry, and then comb it. This is an excellent composition for staining the hair black; it should be used once a week, which will prevent it from afterwards turning red.

Tinctures for staining the Hair Black. Boil an ounce of lead-ore, and a like quantity of ebony chips, for an hour, in a quart of clear water. Wash the hair in this tincture; and dip the comb into it before you use it. It turns the hair black; but this colour is rendered more lively, brilliant, and beautiful, by the addition of two drachms of camphor.

Or, boil on a slow fire, for half an hour, lemon-juice, vinegar, and pulverized litharge, of each equal parts. Wet the hair with this decoction, and in a short time it will become black.

Or, first wash your head, then dip your comb in oil of tartar, and comb your hair in the sun. Repeat this operation thrice a day, and in a week your hair will grow black. To give it an agreeable scent, anoint it with oil of benzoin.

Or, dissolve steel filings in good vinegar. With this vinegar, which will then resemble thick oil, wash your hair as often as you think fit, and it will make it black in a very short time.

Or, wash your head with lye made of the ashes of plants, in which a small quantity of alum has been dissolved. This wash prepares the hair to receive whatever tint you choose to give it. Then comb it with a leaden or horn comb, dipped in any matter which may impart a black colour, such as cedar oil mixed with liquid pitch, or myrtle oil beaten up for a considerable time in a leaden mortar.

To stain Light Hair a Chestnut-colour. First clean the hair with dry bran, or warm water in which alum has been dissolved. Then take two ounces of quicklime, which kill in the air, an ounce of litharge of gold, and half an ounce of lead-ore. Reduce the whole to powder, and sift it. Wet a small quantity of this powder with rose-water. Rub the hair with it, and let it dry again in the air, or dry it with cloths a little warm. This powder does not stain the skin, like the wash made of aquafortis and assaying silver.

It has been asserted that the hair may be stained black by impregnating it with lard, mixed with minium and lime. But in my opinion, this composition would produce only the chestnut-colour, of which I am here speaking.

The hair may likewise be turned black with different vegetable substances boiled in wine, with which the head is to be washed several times a day; but this operation ought to be continued for some time. The substances preferred for this purpose are: leaves of the mulberry, myrtle, fig, senna, raspberry, arbutus, and artichoke; the roots of the caper-tree; the bark of the walnut, sumach, skins of beans, gall-nuts, and cores of cypress. It is also necessary to make use of a leaden comb.

——*The Duties of a Lady's Maid.*

To dye the Hair Flaxen. Take a quart of lye prepared from the ashes of vine-twigs, and half an ounce each of bryony, celandine roots, and turmeric. Take two drachms each of saffron and lily-roots. Take a drachm each of flowers of mullein, yellow stechas, broom, and St. John's wort. Boil these together, and strain off the liquor clear. Frequently wash the hair with this fluid, and in a little time it will change it to a beautiful flaxen colour.

——*The Art of Beauty.*

Chapter II.
Preservation of the Teeth.

You must look after your teeth even more carefully than your hair, because teeth are as essential to health as to beauty. However good your health may be, if your teeth are dirty or decayed, your chewing is imperfect, your digestion is altered, and consequently your health is destroyed. Even before this inevitable result has effaced your charms, they lose all their value if a beautiful and good set of teeth does not enhance your bloom. What matter the freshness and grace of your features, of your mouth, if teeth covered by dirty tartar are revolting to see and smell? Do not deceive yourself; foul breath is almost always caused by dirty teeth, though it may commonly be attributed to the stomach or lungs. No doubt these causes exist, but very rarely, in an obscure way that only a physician can assess; whereas straightforward reasoning proves it is impossible that dirty teeth should not have a foul odour. When particles of food, and above all meat, lodge in the crevices, do they not smell fœtid when you remove them the next day? And when they remain constantly, and others accumulate incessantly, should the foulness of the mouth be attributed to another cause? Moreover, neglecting your teeth causes you to articulate badly, laugh with constraint, and expose yourself to intolerable pain.

The Formation of Tartar on the Teeth.

The great enemy of the whiteness and soundness of your teeth is the concretion called tartar, which the particles deposit around the teeth and on the edges of the gums. Tartar, which first resembles a yellowish slime, finishes by becoming a kind of bony crust which yellows the teeth, works them loose, and pushes back and destroys the gums. The essential thing is therefore to prevent its formation, and to remove, as they are deposited, particles which remain on the teeth.

These modes are extremely easy and cost little, because the best dentifrices are composed of simple, common substances; and if some high-priced salts are joined with them, the quantity is so small that the expense is always slight. It is only the pastes, powders, and liquors of the charlatans which are onerous.

Let us concern ourselves first with the proper measures to prevent the deposit of tartar. You must chew on both sides, and on all your teeth at once, because teeth deprived of the movement which is natural to them weaken, and become encrusted after some time. No doubt this prolonged inaction would eventually cause them to fall out. You should always rinse out your mouth when you have just eaten, to free your teeth from the deposits which the chewed particles have placed there. It is not enough to introduce water into your mouth and immediately expel it. You ought to repeatedly pass your tongue over both sides of each jaw, then reject the water. Next take in more and expel it at once, without moving your tongue.

If shreds of meat are still lodged in the crevices between your teeth, rinsing your mouth is insufficient, and a toothpick becomes necessary. If present or arrested decay has left a hole in a tooth, you must watch even more carefully that nothing remains in the hole. Fruit pips and the cores of hard pears frequently enter there. Though less susceptible to fœtidness than shreds of meat, these things must be very carefully extracted. But then you should not be satisfied with the ordinary manner of pushing a toothpick into the space between two teeth. It is advisable to open your mouth before a small mirror, to see where the pip is lodged, and remove it with a toothpick. By acting otherwise you might spend much time using this instrument without obtaining any result other than fatigue and bleeding gums.

All these operations must have their particular place, and I should not even need to recommend it. But the disgusting habit which has been established for some years, amongst persons of the better class, confirms my views. At the end of a meal, young ladies are seen rinsing their mouths at table, rubbing their teeth with the ends of their napkins, and spitting out onto their plates the water charged with impurities. It would be superfluous to describe such a practice, and to urge my amiable readers to abstain from it.

It is an equally excellent habit to rinse your mouth at night before retiring, and in the morning upon rising. The viscous particles of food being thus successively removed, you will have very little need to use the brush, still less to resort to a dentist, whose scraper in a clumsy hand may injure the enamel of your teeth, at the same time as it removes the tartar.

(See Div. 1.) Even when you are sure of dealing with a skilled dentist, always avoid the scraper, because it is impossible that its action should not injure your gums and weaken your teeth a little.

Water alone, however, is not enough to restore to your teeth the brilliance which the slime removes daily. You must also cleanse them with a dentifrice appropriate to the nature of your mouth, and which has recommendations other than the exaggerated praise of its dealers. You cannot be too much on guard against the multitude of powders, pastes, and dental elixirs extolled by the pompous and colourful prospectuses of charlatans.

Tooth-brushes from Marsh-mallow or Horse-radish Roots.

Pull up the roots of marsh-mallow, mallow, or horse-radish. Wash them and roast them well. Cut them into sticks, sloping both ends. Then boil them in water with pyrethrum root and cinnamon bark cut into little pieces. When they are well boiled and quite tender, remove them carefully, for fear of breaking them, and soak them for twenty-four hours in brandy. Dry them in the oven after you have baked and removed the bread. It is useless to colour them. When you want to use one, soak it in warm water, and rub your teeth with it.

Dentifrice Powder of M. Cadet de Gassicourt.

Mix together half an ounce of sifted sugar, two drachms of powdered grey quina, a drachm of insoluble cream of tartar, four drachms of extremely fine charcoal-powder, and twelve grains of cinnamon.

Each of these substances has a beneficial property, which the mixture increases. Quina strengthens the gums, sugar cleanses the teeth well by rubbing, and cream of tartar cleanses by its acidity. The antiseptic effects of charcoal are well known. Cinnamon gives flavour and contributes to the effect of the quina. However, these substances used separately would have greater or lesser disadvantages. Quina alone would yellow the enamel, cream of tartar would alter it in time, sugar would be insufficient, and charcoal would leave a blackish tinge on the edges of the gums; whereas the mixture not only neutralizes the bad effects, but doubles the good ones. This powder is especially suitable for persons whose gums are soft and bleed easily.

Another Powder for preserving the Teeth.

This receipt, though excellent, is intended more for preserving the teeth than the gums, though these organs preserve each other mutually. Persons whose gums are naturally firm may prefer it to the preceding powder. Those who are disposed to scurvy may also use it, provided that they rinse their mouth with water mixed with brandy in which quina has been dissolved (two drachms to a quart).

Take four drachms of powdered charcoal or burnt bread, and pass it through a silken sieve to render it extremely fine. Strain two drachms of ground sugar, and add two grains of sulphate of quinine and two grains of magnesia. Quinine is the essence of quina; it is extracted from the yellow bark.

Soap Solutions to whiten and preserve the Teeth.

Mix two parts of essence of purified toilet-soap with one part brandy, and a drachm of pulverized Spanish chamomile. Pour a finger of it into a glass, add a little water, dip the tooth-brush into this mixture, and rub your teeth.

You may also simply dissolve a little perfumed soap in water mixed with brandy, Cologne water, or spirit of scurvy-grass.

Preparation to strengthen the Teeth or check Caries.

This preparation is by Dr. Chaussier. Mix a pound of water, half a pound of spirit of wine, and half a drachm of salt of ammonia. Use this liquid to gargle, the dosage being a spoonful. Hold it in your mouth for a little while, then rinse. Keep the mixture for some time on teeth which are affected or threaten to become so.

To strengthen only, and to preserve the teeth which are healthy, dissolve a drachm of salt of ammonia in a pint of brandy. Pour a few drops of it into the water with which you rinse your mouth before cleansing your teeth, and after having done so.

Guaiac Brandy, to preserve the Teeth and Gums.

Take two ounces of crushed gum guaiac, four drachms of tincture of guaiac, and two ounces each of cloves, coriander, and cinnamon. Add the zest of a lemon. Let all these substances steep for a week in a quart of brandy, taking care to shake the bottle every day. At the end of this time, filter it through brown paper.

Dental Elixir.

This elixir, by M. Leroy-de-la-Faudignières, a Parisian dentist, merits its reputation. Here is the way to obtain it: take half a drachm of pyrethrum, six drops of essence of rosemary, four drops of bergamot, a drachm of nutmeg, and three ounces of brandy at twenty-six degrees (see Div. 2). After having crushed the substances which this preparation requires, let them steep in the brandy. At the end of a week, filter the liquor.

This excellent elixir is used by pouring a few drops into a glass of water with which you rinse your mouth in the morning, but only every two or three days.

Water to strengthen the Gums, especially when they are disposed to Scurvy.

Coarsely chop a pound of scurvy-grass, four ounces of water-cress, and four drachms of lemon zest. Crush an ounce of cloves and half a drachm of pyrethrum root, and infuse the whole in four quarts of good brandy for a week. Then distill it in a water-bath to obtain two quarts of spirituous liquor.

The Best Mode of cleansing the Teeth.

Every morning, before combing your hair, take river-water, which should be cool in summer and lukewarm in winter. Mix it with brandy or Dr. Chaussier's preparation. Substitute at will guaiac brandy, Cologne water, vulnerary balm-water, or the Dental Elixir of M. Leroy-de-la-Fandiguières, &c. But brandy, in some cases, is preferable to aromatic liquors.

Rinse your mouth several times with this aromatic water. Then take a piece of marsh-mallow root prepared for cleansing the teeth. Dip it into the aromatic water, and rub your teeth along their length, in order to remove all the slime around the little arch which your gums form above your teeth, carefully treating the arch at the same time. Rinse your mouth again. Soak a fine, very clean sponge in the aromatic water. Rub your teeth with it, not only on the outside, but on the inside of both jaws, especially in the front of the lower jaw, where tartar forms along this species of buttress. Also rub your upper jaw well, but very rapidly, because if the sponge rests on this part for a few moments, it may cause nausea. Lower your head well; this makes the operation easier. The large teeth also demand your attention. The more sunken they are, the more urgent it is to rub them. The ease with which the sponge penetrates to these teeth, without injuring your lips or gums, is one reason I prefer it to a brush. As it is impossible to rub along their length, the brush either imperfectly cleanses your teeth near the point where they are joined to your jaws, or it attacks your gums.

Every time that you have rubbed a part of your mouth, take out the sponge, rinse it in clear water, and re-soak it in the aromatic water. Finish by rubbing your tongue well. Then rinse your mouth, and the operation will be finished.

I prefer the sponge to the tongue-scraper, a long, flat instrument which is used to remove the slime which is attached principally to the middle of the tongue. This instrument is made of whale-bone, bone, tortoise-shell, or even silver or gold. The tongue-scraper is most suitable when your tongue is continually charged, but then you must not rely on it alone.

When by chance you feel a little inflammation in your gums, suspend the use of brandy or any other spirituous liquor for some days. Likewise abstain from any dentifrice powder in which quina may be found. A little finely-powdered burnt bread mixed with honey is the most suitable paste. Moreover, this paste may be used habitually, and if you add two grains of quinine (to half an ounce of powdered bread), you will have an excellent dentifrice.

The excellent habit of washing and rubbing your teeth every day with aromatic water is still insufficient to remove all the slime and preserve the flawlessness of the enamel. Every two, three, or four days (according to the degree of whiteness of your teeth), use one of the dentifrices recommended. For this, after you have rinsed your mouth with water flavoured with several drops of spirituous liquor, take a soft brush. Moisten it a little, touch the powder with it, and rub your teeth along their length. It would be better still to use a very soft little artist's brush, the bristles of which may be contained in the shaft of a feather. In this way you may delicately cleanse the arches near your gums and the spaces between your teeth. You may carry the powder or paste quite to the base of your jaws, and also cleanse the curved tops of the molars. The sponge, good as it is, is worthless when you use a dentifrice. After your teeth have been covered and rubbed with the damp powder, finish with the sponge as explained previously.

It is a very sound practice to clear your teeth with a toothpick before cleansing them, especially when you are not using a powdered dentifrice.

But even when you are washing with the aromatic water alone, the artist's brush is much better.

When your teeth are extremely thin and greyish, which betokens thinning and weakening of the enamel, avoid rubbing them, and above all use as little acid as possible. This condition is either natural, or results from the use of bad dentifrices, such as pumice, alum, and pure acids. Now nothing is possible but to use soft and absorbent substances such as finely-powdered gum-dragon, soft white wax, or potato-starch, mixed with well-pulverized sugar-candy.

Additional Means of preserving the Teeth.

I shall end these directions for preserving the teeth with several very important observations. When your teeth are uneven (this especially concerns the incisors in the upper jaw), they impede chewing and spoil the beautiful effect of the "dental arch," to use the language of dentists; you must always have them filed transversally. This operation is not painful, and does not loosen the teeth as is commonly feared. The only thing to be feared is a slight and passing irritation of the teeth, and even that is not experienced by every one. The teeth must also sometimes be filed lengthways when they are very crowded, and in some sort grown over each other. They retain tartar and so threaten to decay rapidly. But it is essential to spread them very little, because teeth with conspicuous gaps are ugly and nearly ridiculous. A person of my acquaintance likened such teeth to the keys of a hurdy-gurdy, and certainly with good reason.

The teeth also want to be filed when you have nicked them by the reprehensible habit of using them to bite off threads, which you should know well to avoid, as well as using pins, needles, or the point of a bodkin or a knife instead of a toothpick. Every one knows this, but what nearly every one forgets is that by doing so you destroy the grace and freshness of your gums and flatten the little conical points surrounding the base of your teeth, and consequently loosen the teeth. People equally forget that a pin may remove a bit of enamel and so open the way for the agony of caries, or deposit thereon noxious particles of verdigris. The habit of cracking fruit pits and hazel-nuts with your teeth exposes them to the misfortune of being broken, or the danger of being loosened.

Even more carefully avoid putting your teeth alternately in contact with substances which are too hot or too cold, such as a cold drink immediately after soup. I advise you to abstain from liquorice tablets, red-currant tablets, &c., which stain your teeth, unless it is in the morning before cleansing them, because rinsing your mouth after having eaten is insufficient to remove the yellow-brown stain with which these substances cover the enamel. Salty and viscous substances, all salty and smoked dishes, fermented cheeses, hard-boiled eggs, overly-tenderized venison, truffles and all kinds of mushrooms, beans, peas, chestnuts, vinegar, sharp wines, all kinds of acid fruits, jams, and sweets, especially *bon-bons glacé,* all contribute to producing tartar and accumulating it on your teeth. Furthermore, acids and sweets often encourage a disagreeable irritation. You need not deprive yourself of all these foods; only, after having eaten them, take particular care of your teeth, and cleanse them the same evening with dentifrice powder, or at least with aromatic water.

In case of illness, it is equally necessary and perhaps even more so, to keep your mouth meticulously clean. This is the means of getting rid of that thickness of the tongue, that fœtid and bloody coating, of which invalids constantly complain. Whenever you have taken a medicine or an emetic, rinse your mouth promptly, not only to rid yourself of an unpleasant taste, but to preserve your teeth as well. As soon as you have vomited, it is essential to free your teeth of the acidic and viscous matter which remains in your mouth after vomiting. It is urgent to rinse your mouth several times with lukewarm, slightly aromatic water. I recommend this above all to pregnant women who pay for the happiness of being mothers by constant vomiting.

When your gums are inflamed, you may have recourse to emollient gargles. Bathing your feet stops the swelling of gums engorged with blood. Generally all hygienic habits contribute to preserving the teeth. That of protecting your head from dampness has the most direct and effective results.

As soon as you perceive that one of your teeth is decaying, you must have a skilled dentist *décarier* it without delay. (See Div. 3.) This mode is far preferable to lead, which continually comes loose, rendering the tooth susceptible to suffering from the slightest breeze, and it does not always prevent a foul odour. You may also have the decayed part filed off if it is on a corner of the tooth, because you must try all means before consenting to extraction, even when this would not be visible. Nature does nothing useless, and if she has given us thirty-two teeth it is because they are absolutely necessary.

If the decay increases despite all your efforts, the tooth must be extracted, because it will spoil the neighbouring teeth. When the unhappy tooth is a large, invisible molar, you lose it only to gain an empty space, and then you must be very cautious in using the brush, for fear of loosening the teeth to the right and left of the space. As all the teeth hold each other, those deprived of part of their support are more suscep-tible than the others. When an incisor or a canine has been extracted, especially from the upper jaw, you will be obliged to replace it, because a tooth missing from the front of your jaw would alter the look of your face horribly. (Wearing an almost complete denture there seems impos-sible to me.) A toothless, bare, yellowed jaw is the most hideous object imaginable: I hope to have furnished the means of preventing such a misfortune. (See Div. 4.)

——*Manuel des dames.*

Diversion 1.

Davier in the original French was translated to "scraper," because *davier* means "forceps," which is an instrument for extracting teeth. The modern term is likely "scaler."

——Frances Grimble.

Diversion 2.

Measuring-glasses. In order to measure quantities of fluids, glasses graduated on their sides (see Fig. 1) will be found useful in all families and private laboratories. *A* represents a glass calculated to measure any quantity from two drachms to eight ounces. The glass in *B* measures from a drachm to two ounces. The one in *C* measures from half a drachm to an ounce. The one in *D* measures any quantity from five minims to a drachm.

——*The Alphabetical Receipt Book and Domestic Advisor.*

Diversion 3.

Decayed Teeth. The cause of decay in the teeth is still unknown, though it is conjectured that it may arise from taking too hot or too cold food and drink, or from the undue use of acids. Sugar and sweet things were, at one time, denounced as the common cause of bad teeth and tooth-ache, but this is now believed to be a vulgar error. Those who are in the habit of us-ing elixir of vitriol, will, if they are not careful to drink it through a quill or a glass tube, soon find their teeth much injured. Hollow teeth are likewise often caused by dentifrices and tooth-powders.

When tooth-ache evidently arises from a decayed or hollow tooth, and the patient is unwilling to have it extracted, the first thing to be done

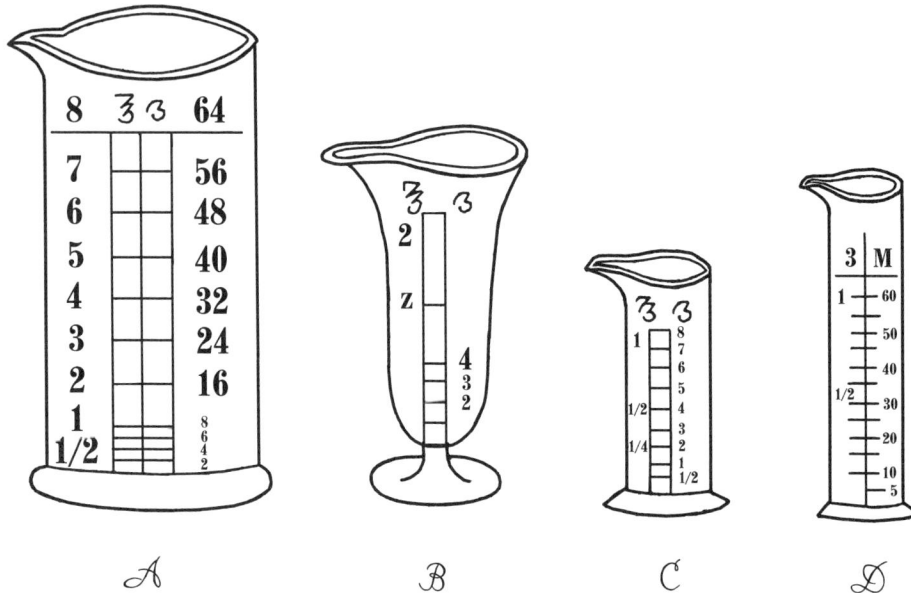

Figure 1. Four measuring-glasses.

is to ease the excruciating pain, which, as Burns says, bears the bell of all misery and rankest plagues. One of the most powerful remedies for this, is exciting some strong emotion of the mind, such as terror, hope, wonder, and the like. If you have faith in the remedy, the cure is certain. The notorious Valentine Greatrakes cured the tooth-ache by simply stroking the cheek; others, by blowing upon the patient; others, by a magnet held to the tooth; and any one who can obtain belief and confidence may cure it by saying, "Begone," or any other authoritative word.

When a patient is not sufficiently credulous to be cured by this kind of quackery, recourse may be had to opiates. A bit of opium, or some cotton-wool soaked in laudanum, may with this view be plugged into the hollow of the tooth. Camphor dissolved in oil of turpentine is also a favourite remedy, in the form of the following:

Lotion for the Tooth-ache. Put two drachms of camphor into an ounce of oil of turpentine, and let it dissolve; when it will be fit for use.

Cajeput oil is another valuable remedy for allaying the pain, when put into the hollow of the tooth. The most effectual, however, of all the remedies for destroying the sensibility of the nerve, is the putting of a red-hot wire into the hollow, which will destroy the nerve and prevent the return of the pain.

Pain in any other part of the body eases tooth-ache, chiefly as it would seem, by affecting the mind, and distracting or withdrawing attention. A box on the ear, a blow on the shin or on the elbow, has often given immediate relief. It is in this way that any thing which smarts the mouth relieves the pain, such as hot water, tobacco-smoke, or brandy held in the mouth, or what is still better, the:

Mucilage for the Tooth-ache. Take a drachm of the powdered leaves of pyrethrum, and a sufficient quantity of gum-arabic mucilage. Make a mass, and divide it into twelve portions. Take one into the mouth and let it lie until dissolved, as occasion requires. If an external application is preferred, the following liniment may be rubbed on the outside of the jaw.

Liniment for the Tooth-ache. Take an ounce of spirit of camphor, three drachms of liquid ammonia, and ten drops of essential oil of bergamot. Mix them in a phial for use.

A blister placed behind the ear, or burning the tip of the ear with a cloth dipped in boiling water, will often remove the pain entirely. The return of the pain, when the nerve is not destroyed, is best prevented by stopping the hollow of the tooth with melted sealing-wax, or with some metal, such as lead or gold. This, however, is best done by a dentist.

——*The Art of Beauty*.

Diversion 4.

False Teeth. The loss of teeth is not totally irreparable. Formerly they used to be transplanted from one individual to another; the practice, however, having been productive of serious consequences, caused it to be discontinued. Artificial teeth are now so naturally made, as to resemble the real ones so closely as almost to prevent detection; and if they do not completely satisfy the stomach, they at least leave nothing to be desired by the self-love of the fair, and perfectly fill up every unseemly gap. False teeth are commonly made of ivory; though latterly various compositions have been invented for the same purpose. To some of these any tint may be given; so that they have the advantage of matching perfectly in colour with the natural teeth, beside which they are to be placed—an advantage which ivory teeth do not afford.

——*The Toilette of Health, Beauty, and Fashion*.

Chapter III.
Preservation of the Complexion and the Skin.

In condemning, with reason, the use of paint and mineral substances, physicians all agree in acknowledging that the combination of hygienic methods and simple, sensible cosmetic care can effectively preserve and improve the skin. This experiment is proven daily. Indeed, the dull, flaccid, mealy skin of women who neglect themselves, the calloused and coarse skin of country-dwellers, is a completely different tissue from the soft, smooth, firm, fresh skin of a person who cares for herself properly. I shall describe in a few words how you may achieve this desirable result.

I shall begin by indicating the means of preservation, because it is especially true for the physique that it is better to prevent than to repair. Following this rule, protect yourself, as far as is possible without affectation, from the effects of the sun and strong winds, which dry and toughen the skin. Avoid smoke, and when by chance you find yourself exposed to it for a few moments, do not fail to wipe your neck and face with your handkerchief: it will be quite blackened from the vapour which was attached to your pores. Do the same when you are surrounded by dust. Habitually use a screen to prevent the fire from burning your face. When you feel a little moisture on your face, wipe that off too, but lightly, and by blotting with your handkerchief rather than by wiping it over your face. Try to cure yourself of the common enough habit of bringing your fingers to your face and idly scratching yourself, especially at night while undressing. Never stay out in the air after you have washed your face, neck, and arms. Furthermore, try to protect yourself from the bites of fleas, mosquitoes, and other insects.

It is necessary to strengthen the skin continually exposed to the air; it is also advisable to soften it. For strengthening, use water flavoured with spirituous liquors such as brandy, tincture of benzoin, or Cologne water. For softening, use milk, almond oil, cream diluted with water, cucumber pomatum, strawberry extract, lily-water, &c. (See Chapter IV for receipts.) All these things are beneficial and indispensable, though opposites. The nature of your skin will indicate which of these substances should predominate in your toilet. If your complexion is warm, if your skin is dry and easily irritated, emollients will be more necessary than spirituous liquors. If you are principally subject to chapping, blotches, and mealy skin, spirituous liquors will suit you better. However, in spite of these differences, I believe that the rules which I shall give are correct for all kinds of skin, and unite to the greatest advantage the benefits of spirituous liquors and emollients.

Because your skin has been exposed to the air all day, it must be softened at night; therefore, use emollients when going to bed. Take a very fine sponge, because a sponge, not forming creases, is far preferable to linen. Dip it in lukewarm water—cold water chaps the skin—and on the hottest days use water warmed by the sun. Wash your face and dry it, but in a particular manner. Take a very fine, well-worn towel, and apply it repeatedly to different places on your face, in order to absorb the moisture without rubbing. Then put a little cucumber pomatum on the palm of your hand, spread it out, and pass your palm over your face. This practice is excellent if you are subject to little heat pimples, and it is not at all disagreeable. You will not be in bed half an hour before you no longer feel this thin layer of pomatum. Yet if it appears awkward to you, or displeasing to your husband, you may use oil, almond-milk, common milk, and other substances which I listed earlier.

You may also commence by washing your face with lukewarm water to remove the dust which may be there, unless you prefer to use almond-milk for this first ablution. For all creamy liquors, it is urgent to use a little piece of worn toile or batiste, or the corner of a towel, because the liquors foul the toile considerably by soaking into it and making it odorous, and every night you must replace the piece of toile or corner of a handkerchief which you used the night before. For these reasons, never dip the sponge in any thing but clear water, or water flavoured with brandy, because this water is perfectly limpid. Less suitable is water flavoured with benzoin, Cologne water, or Ninon-de-l'Enclos water, because these last flavourings produce a slight milky deposit. Choosing therefore the piece of toile, soak it in almond-milk, rub your face lightly, then dry it as I have described. Then you may moisten the toile again, or even better a new piece. Squeeze it between your fingers to expel the liquor. When it is barely damp, shake it out and apply it on your face fully spread out; leave it there only a moment. This last operation imparts great freshness to the skin. In less than five or six minutes, the air will dissipate the slight dampness.

Act the same way for all other emollient liquors. It goes without saying that you must wash your neck and even your bosom at the same time as your face. I did not say so at the beginning, so that I would not be obliged to repeat it for all the directions.

The next morning, on rising, dry your face with a very white, very fine linen, in order to remove any thing which remains on your skin, both the almond-milk and the slight perspiration which accumulates during the night. Finish the series of tasks relative to your complexion and skin when you come to brushing your teeth, combing your hair, washing, &c.

Sprinkle several drops of brandy or benzoin in half a glass of water, and wash your face with it, following the same steps as the day before. Only, after having applied the dry linen, do not moisten it again for fear of rendering your skin too sensitive to the air. Make this ablution after cleansing your teeth, because any coloured powder which you use may cling to your lips and the edge of your chin. It must also be done before you comb your hair, because the dampness of the linen, and the movement necessary to wash your forehead, will disarrange your curls and deprive them of their firmness.

If you wish to remove some black points or scales from pimples, or take some of the measures in Chapter V regarding your eyebrows, lashes, ears, &c., you must start your toilet there. You may also employ veal or chicken broth with the greatest advantage; I have experienced their efficacy. But then it will be well to use them at night instead of the emollient mentioned. If you combine the use of this emollient and this kind of bouillon, your complexion will acquire an excessive shine, which is all the more disagreeable because people will not fail to attribute it to the use of paint.

Your hands also call for some special treatments, but these are less meticulous than the preceding. Almond paste or almond-milk may be advantageously employed to keep them white and soft. But I think that purified soap, lightly perfumed, agrees with them better, especially in winter, in that soap removes perfectly, with no need of prolonged rubbing, all the impurities which have crept into the pores, and which become tenacious with the effects of cold. It is chiefly necessary to dissolve the grease of pomatums and from your hair, which always sticks more or less to your fingers when you comb. You well know how to use soap. Therefore, I shall be contented with saying that when you have soaped and rinsed your hands, before drying them it is advisable to cover them anew with soap, rub your hands until it foams, and dry them without putting them back into the water. In this manner your skin is kept very white and extremely soft. To make it even more so, you may pass a linen moistened with benzoin water over your hands. All emollients are favourable to the hands; do not alternate them with spirituous liquors as you do for your face. However, in winter it is advantageous, especially for persons subject to chilblains, to wash their hands with water mixed with brandy, in order to strengthen the skin and prevent this obstinate and painful condition.

When you have an ink-spot on your fingers, soap it or shed a drop of vinegar on it. If you knock yourself, rub the place immediately with Cologne water, to avoid bleeding under the skin and the production of a bruise. In winter, continually wear silk gloves without finger-ends: these knitted gloves are narrow at each open end of the fingers, and do not hinder working in any way.

As for your finger-nails, rub the brush meant for them on a bar of soap. Then use it to brush your nails and remove all the dirt which may have accumulated. Soak the end of a very small sponge in a flask of essence of lemon, and wash your nails well with it: this cleans and strengthens them better than any thing.

I have said that it is necessary to wash your bosom both night and morning at the same time as your neck and face. But if you wish to maintain or to renew the firmness of your bosom, it is well to give it a kind of shower-bath. For this, take off your fichu, sit down, and put a large basin on your knees. Bend in such a manner that your bosom is over the basin; then with a large sponge which you hold slightly raised, pour water flavoured with benzoin or brandy over it. Dry yourself by applying warm linens, and finish with a light unction of fine, perfumed oil.

All this does not dispense with baths, the principal means of health and freshness. (See Div. 1.) Without them, whatever other care you may take of your person, your skin will never acquire all the perfection desirable. If your circumstances permit, bathe once a week in all seasons, and two or even three times in the hottest weather. Always have your bath a little cool. Remain there at least an hour and a half, rubbing yourself well, washing yourself with toilet-soap and a cake of almond paste. Then have the water drained from your tub. Rub yourself vigorously with soap dipped in benzoin water. Take off your wet bathing-gown; immediately throw on another very broad across the shoulders. Sit down in an arm-chair or on a chair covered with linens, and rub yourself with warm linens, not only until you are perfectly dry, but until the sensation of cold which follows your exit from the bath has entirely disappeared. If the confusion caused by an innate sense of modesty prevents you from taking these important steps, without which the bath is more hurtful than healthful, wrap yourself well in your bathing-gown; and if necessary, close your eyes until you have finished the operation.

If you have some part which is weak or sore, rub it with Cologne water immediately on quitting the bath. Lie down after finishing and rub yourself again with a large dry sponge wrapped in fine linen: this practice replaces the massage so strongly recommended as a hygienic measure.

——Manuel des dames.

Diversion 1.

Bathing. This, along with friction, is an essential part of beauty-training, for clearing the skin of its impurities, and giving transparency and freshness to the complexion. Whoever neglects it, therefore, cannot with justice complain of eruptions, and other disorders and affections of the skin. A large proportion of the refuse and worn materials of the body are carried off by exhalation from the skin, as well as from the lungs. I need scarcely tell you that if this refuse is in any way prevented from being carried off, or is in any way carried back into the system, it will produce derangement and disease—by obstructing perhaps the free flow of the blood, in the same way as mud and rubbish will obstruct the free flow of a stream of water. Now, with respect to the skin, the waste of the body passes in the form of vapour or moisture through innumerable small pores in it, and of course when these are in any way shut up or obstructed, one of the grand outlets of the body's waste is cut off. If it cannot find another passage, by the bowels or the lungs, it will remain and corrupt the mass of the blood, as the sediment called bee's-wing corrupts port wine. Even if it does, in the end, obtain an outlet by the lungs, the kidneys, or the bowels, it must first pass back again by the absorbents and the blood, and a disease may be produced before it can escape.

As these are indisputable facts, you will perceive at a glance that one of the most important effects of bathing is cleansing the skin, and freeing its pores from obstruction. The waste and refuse of the bones, the muscles, and the blood, which pass through the skin in the form of perspiration, are often arrested on the surface of the skin by dust and other impurities. The dust and the perspired moisture consequently unite, and form an incrustation on the skin thinner than India paper, and often, you must carefully remark, *invisible.* The pores of your skin may then be quite shut by a thin invisible crust of this sort, while you are altogether unaware of its existence, though it is the chief and perhaps the only cause of a sallow complexion, or unhealthy paleness, not to speak of the internal disorders it may occasion.

This is not all. When any thing goes wrong in any part of the body, Nature immediately sets up a self-correcting or counteractive process to restore things to their proper course; for example in the case of sneezing, to expel snuff from the nostrils, or of vomiting, to expel poison from the stomach. As soon, therefore, as a crust is formed by dust and perspiration on your skin, unless you remove it by washing, the absorbents instantly set about removing it, and carrying it back again into the mass of the blood, which will always produce more or less derangement, or bad health, and the complexion will accordingly suffer.

From this detail you will see the very great importance of bathing the whole body constantly and regularly, in order to keep the skin clean, and the pores open. This, however, must be taken with limitations; for you must by no means conclude that in order to clear the pores of the skin, you may indiscriminately use the warm or the cold bath, or any bath at all. The general principle is merely to cleanse the skin, and you may frequently do this more effectually, and more beneficially, by sponging and the flesh-brush, than by general bathing, either cold or warm. As bathing, however, always does cleanse the skin and clear the pores, it becomes of moment to take this into account.

I have not room here to enter upon the danger of indiscriminate cold bathing, particularly in the case of the nervous and debilitated, who are frequently made the victims of the cold bath, prescribed by medical men who are unaware of its injurious effects. I refer my readers, for a melancholy history of the fatal effects thus produced, to Dr. Beddoes' *Hygeia,* and to the *Oracle of Health,* where also directions are given for discovering when it is proper, and when improper.

The ingenuity of refinement, with the intention of improving upon baths of clear water, has devised various kinds of artificial baths, by adding aromatic herbs and other substances. Borax, when so added to a bath, is said to give a peculiar lustre to the skin, and for this purpose it is used in Egypt and the East.

The story of Æson becoming young from the medicated baths of Medea, seems to have been intended to teach the efficacy of warm bathing, in retarding the progress of old age. The words "relaxation" and "bracing," which are generally thought expressive of the effects of warm or cold bathing, are mechanical terms, properly applied to drums or strings; but are only metaphors when applied to the effects of cold or warm bathing on animal bodies. The immediate cause of old age seems to reside in the irritability of the finer parts, or vessels, of our system. Hence these cease to act, and collapse, or become horny or bony. The warm bath is peculiarly adapted to prevent these circumstances, by increasing irritability, and by moistening and softening the skin, and the extremities of the finer vessels which terminate in it. To those who are past the meridian of life, and have dry skins, and begin to be emaciated, the warm bath, for an hour twice a week, I believe to be eminently serviceable in retarding the advances of old age.

On this principle, when Dr. Franklin, the American philosopher, was in England many years ago, Dr. Darwin recommended to him the use of a warm bath twice a week, to prevent the too speedy access of old age, of which he then thought he felt the approach, and to relieve infirmities under which he actually laboured. It gave him considerable ease, in a disorder with which he was afflicted (the stone) and answered the other purposes for which he used it; for he died at an advanced age, having for many years been in the constant habit of using the tepid bath.

——*The Art of Beauty*.

Chapter IV.
Concerning Cosmetics.

Nothing is more opposed to the innocent and legitimate desire to please than the use of paints and most cosmetics. (See Div. 1.) Inspired by this desire, you should look to hygiene, the solicitude for cleanliness, and the means to an agreeable appearance in general, to please your husband in particular. When a woman strays into coquetry, her health is affected. Sometimes she uses the filthiest preparations, and far from endeavouring to please her husband, she only appears to him rendered pale and livid by paints. Too, she condemns him to disgust for the preparations with which she masks herself at night, in order to be more beautiful by day.

These condemnable efforts of vanity ruin the morals, the purse, and the health. I think it useless to insist on the first point. When the care she takes for her person ceases to have her husband as its object, it is already a prelude to infidelity. I shall also speak no further of the exorbitant expense of this multitude of whites to coat the skin, blacks to dye the hair, blues to trace the veins, reds to paint the cheeks, waters called "marvellous" and "miraculous" to render the eyes brilliant, crimsons to colour the lips, &c., &c. All the world knows that charlatans sell these preparations at the price of gold. I intend only to prove their danger and absurdity.

These detestable compositions have been divided into minor and major cosmetics. The minor cosmetics are: lime-water, vinegar and vegetable acids, camphorated applications, spirit of turpentine, and salt of tartar. As to the major cosmetics: calcined alum, salt of Saturn, spirit of nitre, white bismuth, white lead, litharge, coral, bismuth, Venetian talc, mercury, in short all the most deleterious substances compose their creams, powders, pastes, and essences. These poisonous substances may be communicated to the circulating fluids through the skin as well as the stomach. Once lead is introduced into the physical system, however small the quantity, it cannot be neutralized by medicine, and never fails to produce the most deplorable effects. Paralysis, contractions and convulsions of the limbs, total weakness, and the most excruciating colics are the common results.

In addition to these marked effects, the frequent external use of lead and mercury in cosmetics occasions cramps in all parts of the body, weakness and other nervous afflictions, catarrh, nervous consumption, consumption, spitting blood, dropsy, &c. Dr. Willich, an English physician, so expresses himself in the translation which the learned M. Itard made of his *Hygiène domestique*. All other men of science confirm these frightening results; and one of them, M. Mege, who has written a special work on this matter, cites several terrible deaths which had no other cause than the use of such cosmetics.

You may well think that freshness and beauty are incompatible with such illnesses. But yet, before they declare themselves, the colour is leaden and livid, and the skin is withered, wrinkled, and made hideous, by deleterious contact with these exorbitant compositions. When the layers of paint are removed, a woman has such an afflicted appearance that she redoubles them the next day, and so on, until she is laid up in a bed of pain.

To give an idea of the manner in which the makers of cosmetics operate, I shall cite a receipt chosen by chance from amongst a thousand. It consists of stirring a piece of calcined alum into an egg-white, then applying the resulting pulp to the skin to whiten it. Yet I know from my own experience that exactly the same mode is used to erode the leucomas which form on the eye.

I now come to the preparations which are merely ridiculous and disgusting: crushed egg-shells, chopped onions, sheep feet and guts, poultry cut into pieces, citronella, goat fat, chalk, animal excrements, &c. All this, distilled or simply cooked with every imaginable fruit and perfume, is seriously claimed to whiten and soften the skin and make it glow. Read the *Traité des odeurs,* by M. Dejean, and all the collections of receipts, and you will have proof that far from exaggerating, I am refraining from it.

Nowadays few women continually use all these compositions, but some are vexed by freckles, oily or mealy skin, pimples, or extreme pallor. Now and then the desire to remedy these, leads them to believe in the glowing promises of the prospectuses of certain perfumers and possessors of "wonderful secrets." Since they are determined to correct the faults of Nature with means other than those of hygiene and cleanliness, let me at least indicate to them innocent preparations which can do them no harm, and which will cost them ten times less than similar cosmetics decked out with pompous names, such as the famous "green rouge of Athens, recently discovered, which was used by Aspasia and Phryne." This is simply the following rouge.

True Vegetable Rouge, or Rose in a Cup.

Take the kind of red lac extracted from the safflower, which is sold cheaply under the name "rose in a cup." Dry, it is a greenish-bronze. Dissolve it in a glass of water, and pour it on talcum powder or on a piece of fine woollen. In this state it returns to a beautiful rose-colour. You may apply it to your cheeks without withering them, and if you have been careful in preparing the hue, the rouge will not be detected. For four or five sous, you will have the same rouge which costs eight francs when it is called green rouge.

Cream Pomatum for the Complexion.

When mentioning this and the next composition, I need not describe the manner of making them, but merely advise their use and list their properties. Cream pomatum is the only white which you may at all sensibly permit yourself. White wax, spermaceti, oil of sweet almonds, and rose-water are the basis of it. It conceals wrinkles and small-pox scars.

Pomatum for the Lips.

This is composed of almost the same ingredients as the above, excepting the spermaceti. Its beautiful vermilion colour is owing only to the great quantity of rose-water used in it. Consequently it can neither wither nor wrinkle the lips, as do pomatums with carmine or mineral substances.

Angel-water to firm and refresh the Skin.

Infuse myrtle flowers in water, then distill them, and you will obtain a perfumed water which will render your flesh firm and brilliant.

Rose Milk for preserving the Complexion.

Add an ounce of fine olive-oil and six drops of oil of tartar to a quart of rose-water. Decant the oil of tartar before adding it to the mixture.

Simple Almond-milk to make the Skin Fresh.

Here is another beneficial receipt, which is easy, cheap, and serves two ends. I beg my readers to make note of it.

Crush some peeled sweet almonds in a mortar, in proportion of twenty or thirty to a pint of water. Add a lump of sugar to prevent separation of the oil. When the almonds have been reduced to a very fine paste, mix it little by little into the water. Pass the whole through a flannel, and perfume with orange-flower water. To turn it into a drink, you have only to add another lump of sugar.

Lily-water for the Complexion.

It is said that the fragrant water drawn from lily-flowers by the warmth of the water-bath, and mixed with a little salt of tartar, is excellent for removing spots from the face and increasing the bloom of the complexion.

Cucumber Pomatum.

This pomatum, which I have so often recommended for all faults in the skin, is prepared thus: take a quantity of fine olive-oil proportionable to how much pomatum you want. Grate white cucumbers in a quantity equal to the oil. Put the whole in a dish or a silver tumbler, and place this vessel in a water-bath. Stir its contents continually with a silver soup-spoon, which replaces the pharmacist's spatula. Continue to stir the mixture for some time, but do not let it boil; then strain it through a cheese cloth. Repeat the process with the same oil up to six times, always keeping the heat of the water-bath below the boiling point.

This fine pomatum, white as snow, should be covered and used at once, because it turns rancid with time.

Preparation of Dr. Withering, to dispel Eruptions of the Skin.

Squeeze out the juice of a leek, mix it with an equal quantity of sweet milk or cream, and use it to wash the pimples, which will dry up and promptly go down without leaving spots.

Cosmetic Infusion of the Same Kind for the Skin.

Infuse horse-radish in milk, and wash your face every night in this simple mixture.

Strawberry Water to soften and whiten the Skin.

Take well-ripened strawberries, crush them well in a vessel, then press them through white linen. Mix the resulting liquid with milk and a little water. You must make this preparation every night because, especially in very hot weather, it swiftly turns sour.

Veal Broth to calm Reddened Skin.

Take a piece of veal twice the size of your thumb. Cook it in a *demi-tasse* of water, with neither herbs nor salt. When it is cooked, strain the liquid through white linen, and wash your face in it every night.

I especially recommend this mode to my readers; I used it formerly. It is the best of all cosmetics to calm irritated skin; but I do not advise its constant use, for fear that this may render the skin too shiny, which might be attributed to paint.

Oil of Bitter Almonds, to cure Sun-burn and Freckles.

Remove the yellow skins from some bitter almonds. Crush the almonds well, and press out the oil. Only a small amount should be prepared at a time, because it evaporates and easily turns rancid.

Athenian Water to efface Wrinkles.

Dissolve an ounce each of benzoin, incense, and gum-arabic in three quarts of brandy. Add half an ounce each of cloves and nutmeg, an ounce and a half each of pine-nuts and sweet almonds, and two grains each of amber and musk. (You would do well to dispense with these last two perfumes.) Crush it all and infuse it for two days, stirring it twice every day. Then add three cups of rose-water, and distill to obtain two and a half quarts.

Economical Paste to whiten the Hands.

Cook well the whitest and most mealy potatoes which you can find. Peel them, crush them well, and mix them with a little milk. This is just as good as almond paste.

Almond Paste with Brandy.

Take a pound of skinned sweet almonds and four ounces of pine-nuts. Crush them as fine as possible, then add two ounces of brandy. You may perfume this paste with essence of bergamot or jasmine.

Almond Paste with Egg-yolks.

Crush four ounces of sweet almonds in a very clean marble mortar. When they have been reduced to a paste, mix them with three fresh egg-yolks. Soak the mixture in a cup of milk. Cook it in a saucepan to the consistency of a paste, stirring continuously with a spatula. Store it in a tightly-closed pot.

Almond Paste with Honey.

This is made like the preceding, but with half an ounce of white honey added. It is chiefly used when putting on long gloves which lack suppleness. Your skin will be so soft that they will slip on without tearing.

Toilet-soap, called Lady Derby's Soap.

Take two ounces of blanched bitter almonds, an ounce and a quarter of tincture of benzoin, a pound of good plain white soap, and a piece of camphor the size of a walnut. Crush the almonds and the camphor in a separate mortar, until they are thoroughly mixed, then add the benzoin. When the mixing is accomplished, do your soap in the same manner. If it smells too much of camphor and benzoin, melt it on the fire again to weaken the odour. (See Div. 2.)

Soap with Honey, to whiten the Skin and dispel Sun-burn Marks.

Take four ounces of white Marseilles soap, as much of common honey, an ounce of benzoin, and half an ounce of storax. Mix every thing together in a marble mortar. When it has been well blended, shape it into little tablets.

Emollient Preparation for the Bath.

Take four ounces of blanched sweet almonds, a pound of elecampane, a pound of pine-nuts, four handfuls of flax-seed, an ounce of marsh-mallow root, and an ounce of lily-bulb. These must be crushed and reduced to a paste. Perfume it with storax or benzoin, and put it into three bags, to which you add a little wheat-flour. One bag should be larger than the others; put this at the bottom of the bath, to sit upon. The other two bags will serve to rub your body. (See Div. 3.)

——*Manuel des dames.*

Diversion 1.

The Use of Paints. Cosmetics really impart whiteness, freshness, suppleness, and brilliancy to the skin, when it is naturally deficient in these qualities. Consequently, they only assist Nature, and make amends for her defects; and it may be affirmed, that they are to beauty what medicine is to health. Paints are far from answering this description. They are not only incapable of embellishing the skin, but those who make use of paints are extremely fortunate when the paints do not contribute to increase their defects. Paints cannot give the skin the desired qualities; they only imitate them in a manner more or less coarse. In a word, they may be aptly denominated physical hypocrisy.

If paints are incapable of preventing or repairing the ravages of time, why are they used? For various reasons: in the first place, because they are sooner and more easily applied, because they produce a higher, more brilliant, and speedy effect. In the next, because in cases where cosmetics would be of no use (for instance, persons too plain or too old) paints afford a convenient resource, a last and only medium of disguising either the defects of the complexion or the ravages of time. In short, paint is the sheet anchor of the fair sex in these cases.

Ought people to use paint? Why not? When a person is young, and fresh, and handsome, to paint would be perfectly ridiculous; it would be wantonly spoiling the fairest gifts of Nature. But on the contrary, when an antique and venerable dowager covers her brown and shrivelled skin with a thick layer of white paint, heightened with a tint of vermilion, we are sincerely thankful to her; for then we can look at her at least without disgust. And are we not under obligations to her, for being at the pains to render herself in reality more ugly than she is, in order that she may appear less so?

These observations on paints are designed to allude more particularly to white. If ever paint were to be proscribed, I should plead for an exemption in favour of rouge, which may be rendered extremely innocent, and be applied with such art, as sometimes to give an expression to the countenance which it would not have without that auxiliary. How many charms has the delicate colour of modesty! And in an age when women blush so little, ought we not to value this innocent artifice? which is capable of now and then exhibiting to us at least the picture of modesty, and which in the absence of virtue, contrives at least to preserve her portrait.

The professed enemies of paints will perhaps take it amiss, that I here declare in favour of rouge; but I think it would be very wrong to include it in the same proscription as white. The latter is never becoming; but rouge, on the contrary, almost always looks well. At the same time, I only state my own sentiments on this subject, leaving my readers at liberty to think as they please.

It is not the present fashion to make so much use of red, as was done some years ago; at least, it is applied with more art and taste. With very few exceptions, ladies have absolutely renounced that glaring, fiery red with which our antiquated dames formerly masked their faces.

It is much to be wished that women would compose their rouge themselves. They would not then run the risk of using those dangerous reds, in which minerals are ingredients; of spoiling the skin, and exposing themselves to the inconveniences which result from the use of metallic paints. These dangerous reds are those compounded with red lead, or cinnabar, otherwise called vermilion, produced by sulphur and mercury. Vegetable reds therefore should alone be used, since they are attended with little danger, especially if they are used with moderation.

The vegetable substances which furnish rouge are red sandal-wood, alkanet root, cochineal, Brazil-wood, and especially safflower, which yields a very beautiful colour, when it is mixed with a sufficient quantity of talc. Some perfumers compose vegetable rouge, for which they take vinegar as the excipient. These reds are liable to injure the beauty of the skin; it is more advisable to mix them with oily or unctuous matter, and to form salves. For this purpose, you may employ balm of Mecca, butter of cacao, spermaceti, oil of behen, &c.

Carmine. Carmine is the highest and finest red colour there is. It comes chiefly from Germany, and is made from cochineal; it may therefore very safely be used. There are two or three sorts of this article. The finest, which is nearly double the price of the common kind, is in the end by far the cheapest. The difference between the two sorts will not easily be discerned by mere inspection; besides it is painful for the eyes, on account of the intensity of its colour, to look upon it even for a minute. Comparison will certainly point out a difference; but the most certain way of detecting adulteration, is to fill a very small silver thimble successively with each sort. The finest and best sort will not weigh above half or two-thirds of the worst, which is commonly adulterated with vermilion and red lead, both very heavy powders.

Portuguese Rouge. Of Portuguese dishes containing rouge for the face, there are two sorts. One of these is made in Portugal, and is rather scarce; the paint contained in the Portuguese dishes being of a fine pale pink hue, and very beautiful in its application to the face. The other sort is made in London, and is of a dirty, muddy, red colour; it passes very well, however, with those who never saw the genuine Portuguese dishes, or who wish to be cheaply beautified.

The most marked difference between these two sorts is that the true one from Portugal is confined in dishes which are rough on the outsides; whereas the dishes made here are glazed quite smooth.

Spanish Wool. Of this also there are several sorts; but that which is made here in London, by some of the Jews, is by far the best. That which comes from Spain is of a very dark red colour, whereas the former gives a bright pale red. When it is very good, the cakes, which ought to be the size and thickness of a crown-piece, shine and glisten, between a green and a gold-colour.

This kind of Spanish wool is always best, when made in dry and hot summer weather, for then it strikes the finest blooming colour; whereas what is made in wet winter weather, is of a coarse dirty colour, like the wool from Spain. It is therefore best always to buy it in the summer season.

Spanish Papers. These papers are of two sorts. They differ in nothing from the above; but the red colour, which in the latter tinges the wool, is here laid on paper; chiefly for the convenience of carrying in a pocket-book.

This coloured wool comes from China, in large round loose cakes, of the diameter of three inches. The finest of these give a most lovely and agreeable blush to the cheek; but it is seldom possible to pick more than three or four out of a parcel, which have a truly fine colour. As the cakes are loose, like carded wool, the voyage by sea and the exposure to air, even in opening them to show to a friend, carries off their fine colour.

Chinese Boxes of Colours. These boxes, which are beautifully painted and japanned, come from China. They contain each two dozen of papers, and in each paper are three smaller ones, viz., a small black paper for the eyebrows; a paper of the same size of a fine green colour, but which, when just arrived and fresh, makes a very fine red for the face; and lastly a paper containing about half an ounce of white powder (prepared from real pearl) for giving an alabaster colour to some parts of the face and neck.

As to the carmine, the French red, the genuine Portuguese dishes, the Chinese wool, and the green papers in the boxes of all colours, they are all preparations of cochineal. This is allowed to be of such sovereign service, even in the art of medicine, that the least harm need not be dreaded from its use, nor from any of its preparations, by those ladies who are accustomed to paint their faces, either from custom or from a desire to be thought beautiful and handsome.

The red powders above described are best put on by a fine camel's-hair pencil. The colours in the dishes, wools, and green papers are commonly laid on by the tip of the little finger, previously wetted. As all these have some gum used in their composition, they are apt to leave a shining appearance on the cheek, which too plainly shows that artificial beauty has been resorted to.

The Spanish wool, the papers, and the English-made Portuguese dishes are all made from a moss-like drug from Turkey called safflower, well known to scarlet dyers &c. But whether this drug, with its preparation, is equally innocent with those of the cochineal, is a subject which deserves further inquiry. These paints are all wetted previous to being used, and leave a shining appearance on the face, like the colours described, and from the same cause.

White Paints. White paints are extracted from minerals more or less pernicious, but always corrosive. They affect the eyes, which swell and inflame, and are rendered painful and watery. They change the texture of the skin, on which they produce pimples, and cause rheums. They attack the teeth, make them ache, destroy the enamel, and loosen them. They heat the mouth and throat, infecting and corrupting the saliva, and they penetrate through the pores of the skin, acting by degrees on the spongy substance of the lungs, and inducing diseases. Or in other cases, if the paint is composed of aluminous or calcareous substances, it stops the pores of the skin, which it tarnishes, and prevents the perspiration, which is of course carried to some other part, to the peril of the individual.

Metallic paints are extracted either from lead, tin, or bismuth. To the inconveniences just enumerated, I add this, of turning the skin black when it is exposed to the contact of sulphurous or phosphoric exhalations. Accordingly, those women who make use of them ought carefully to avoid going too near substances in a state of putrefaction, the vapours of sulphur, and liver of sulphur, and the exhalation of bruised garlic. I shall not give the way of composing the different metallic paints, but rather wish that these receipts were entirely lost. I shall only subjoin the process for making a cheap paint, which if not wholly free from inconvenience, is not accompanied by those dangers which always attend the use of whites prepared from bismuth, tin, or lead.

Talc White. Take a piece of the talc white known by the name of Briançon chalk; choose it of a pearl-grey colour, and rasp it gently with a piece of dog-skin; after this, sift it through a sieve of very fine silk. Put this powder into a pint of good distilled vinegar, in which leave it for a fortnight, taking care to shake the bottle or pot several times each day, except the last, on which it must not be disturbed. Pour off the vinegar, so as to leave the chalk behind in the bottle, into which pour very clear water which has been filtered.

Throw the whole into a clean pan, and stir the water well with a wooden spatula. Let the powder settle again to the bottom. Pour the water gently off, and wash the powder six or seven times, taking care always to make use of filtered water. When the powder is as soft and as white as you wish, dry it in a place where it is not exposed to the dust; sift it through a silken sieve, which will make it still finer. It may be either left in powder, or wetted and formed into cakes, like those sold by the perfumers. A pint of vinegar is sufficient to dissolve a pound of talc.

This white may be used in the same manner as carmine, dipping your finger, or a piece of paper, or what is preferable to either, a hare's foot prepared for the purpose, in ointment, and putting upon it about a grain of this white, which will not be removed even by perspiration. If the ointment with which it is applied is properly made, this white does no injury to the face. The same ingredients may be used for making rouge.

——*The Art of Beauty.*

Diversion 2.

Receipts for Perfumed Soaps. I shall now give you some receipts for preparing soaps which give the skin that whiteness and suppleness so desirable. They are very numerous, every perfumer having a particular way of making his own. I shall content myself with giving one or two processes.

Seraglio Soap. Take half a pound of orris, two ounces of benzoin, an ounce of storax, a like quantity of yellow sandal-wood, half a drachm of cinnamon, a few cloves, a little lemon zest, St. Lucia wood, and nutmeg. Well pulverize the whole. Take about half a pound of white soap, grate it, and put it to soak for four or five days in a pint and a half of brandy, with the powder. Knead up the whole with about a quart of orange-flower water. Make a paste of this soap, with a sufficient quantity of starch, and mould it into any size you please, adding egg-whites and gum-dragon, dissolved in some kind of scented water. If you wish to give it a stronger scent, mix with the paste a few grains of musk, some essential oil of lavender, bergamot, roses, carnations, jasmine, cinnamon, or in short any other matter the smell of which you may prefer.

Musk Soap. Take two ounces of marsh-mallow roots, cleansed and dried in the shade. Reduce them to powder. Add half an ounce of starch, and a like quantity of flour, three drachms of fresh pine-apple kernels, an ounce of orange pippins, an ounce of oil of tartar, an ounce of oil of sweet almonds, and a quarter of a drachm of musk. Reduce those articles which are to be pulverized to a very fine powder, and to each ounce of powder add half an ounce of orris.

Then steep four ounces of fresh marsh-mallow roots in orange-flower water. Let them stand a whole night, squeeze the whole well, and with the mucilage which comes from them, make a paste with the powder. Let this paste dry, and mould it into round balls. Make use of it, when necessary, when a little water must be poured over the hands. Nothing softens the skin more or makes the hands whiter.

——*The Duties of a Lady's Maid.*

Diversion 3.

Bath of Modesty. Take four ounces of peeled sweet almonds, a pound of pine-apple kernels, a pound of elecampane, ten handfuls of flax-seed, an ounce of marsh-mallow roots, and an ounce of white lily-roots. Pound all these until reduced to a paste, and tie it up in several small bags, which are to be thrown into a tepid bath, and pressed until the water becomes milky.

A more simple mode of preparing a bath of this kind is given by M. Jacques Louis Moreau de la Sarthe, in his *Histoire naturelle de la femme.* He says it is sufficient to throw into the bath enough almond paste to give the water a milky appearance.

——*The Art of Beauty.*

Chapter V.
Remedies for the Little Faults
which are injurious to Beauty.

Let us begin with pimples; there are several kinds. One is the round pimple, in which there is always a little seed resembling a hair bulb, and which to all appearances is also only an enlarged bulb, because the pores, especially on the chin, contain the roots of little invisible hairs. Others are the flat pimple, which encloses some drops of a very clear serous fluid; the live pimple, which contains a droplet of greenish serous fluid; and the composite pimple, which has a little mealy internal pellicle, a little seed, and a little serous fluid. All these pimples are caused by internal irritation. Consequently, the best modes of curing them and destroying their source are baths, refreshing herbal teas, walks, and repose. But you may also combat them externally, as I shall describe.

Remedies for Pimples.

Round Pimples. Just as soon as a lively burning, a light red spot, or a callus makes you suspect the presence of a round pimple, cover it at night with a little suet, cerate, or cucumber pomade. I believe that the first is best, in that it ripens the pimple more quickly. Next day, see in your mirror whether the red spot or callus presents a little white point, or touch it lightly to judge if the seed may be felt. It is important to make sure, because if the seed is unready to detach itself, the operation which I shall describe would be more hurtful than helpful, because it would damage the skin to no avail and increase the inflammation of the pimple. It is better to wait until a little after the maturity of the pimple, than to act before it. But when at last maturity is complete, gently press the pimple between your forefingers, without using your nails, and thus extract the seed. When it has come out, dip a very fine white linen in cold water, to which you have added a few drops of brandy or tincture of benzoin. Wash the pimple several times without rubbing.

After this do not concern yourself with it until a little scaly flake forms in place of the pimple; then lift it off delicately. You must not anticipate the moment when the flake is perfectly dry. The great desire which you have, with reason, to get rid of the pimple, may make you too hasty to tear off the flake. If it is still too adherent to the skin, the pimple bleeds and becomes worse than before. If, though detached from the epidermis, the flake is not completely dry, the part which it conceals, and whose vulnerability it protects, appears to be red-violet, and shows this disagreeable spot for a long time. In addition, the worn skin near the pimple is not slow to produce others. Round pimples when properly treated are ordinarily cured in four or five days. Hastened and badly peeled, they last twice or even thrice as long.

Flat Pimples. I have so named them to distinguish them from the preceding. They are a kind of inner burning with a partial eruption. You feel a very lively itching, a smarting followed by pain. Your skin reddens and swells, and the serous fluid collected under the epidermis gives it a disagreeable yellowish colour. The best remedy is to immediately apply a little piece of court plaster, and by the next day, or the day after at the latest, you are rid of it. When the plaster becomes hard, seems thickened and rounded, and when you feel something very hard underneath, as though the plaster may detach by itself, you may remove it, and with it the yellowish skin and the serous fluid which gives it this hue. This fluid, after it became dense, is what produced the hardness which you felt under the plaster.

Flat pimples are not always so easily cured; besides, many ladies are reluctant to wear black taffety patches. Then you must cover the pimple with cucumber pomade, or very white cerate. These mild substances soften the skin, and the serous fluid comes out in drops which succeed each other without interruption. Wipe them at need; sometimes it is necessary to press the skin about them a little with both forefingers to aid the emission of the serous fluid. When it has ceased to flow, wash the spot with a little benzoin water to strengthen your skin and reduce the inflammation; then end the treatment with cucumber pomade. By the next day a dry skin has formed, which may be removed that same evening.

Quick, or Living Pimples. These are revealed by a sharp pain and a deep red spot. Sometimes they do not form any excrescence or enlargement. They should be treated like round pimples, but only after the serous fluid is extracted. It is better to wash the place with a little marsh-mallow water than with brandy. Cucumber pomade, or any other emollient, may advantageously replace the marsh-mallow water.

Composite Pimples. These are only slightly painful and quite rare, but they have the great disadvantage of not being sufficiently distinctive; so that after having removed the first pellicle, you may think you have extracted the seed and the serous fluid, which are no longer found. You continue to press to bring up the main part, and cause a far more violent irritation. Other times you give up, and the imperfectly cured pimple continues to appear swollen; true, it is colourless and painless, but it always injures the smoothness of your skin, and produces black points or little pimples, of which I shall speak later. However disagreeable this expectation, it is better to resign yourself to seeing the pimple become a black point than to tease and tear it. Very often it flattens by itself, if it really has no seed, or if the seed disappears through absorption.

The pimples which hair brings out on the forehead are very easily removed by washing them with water mixed with benzoin or brandy. For some time it is necessary to spread your curls farther apart.

Black Points. You have seen that black points or little pimples arise from pimples which have seeds embedded in the pores. That is indeed one of their causes, but it is the least of them. Most often, without any pimples or swelling beforehand, all the pores on the chin, and especially the nose, are filled with black, dark grey, or even yellowish spots. Whatsoever their colour, they are a great nuisance. Your skin appears to be a miniature of those prison doors studded with nails, or seems sprinkled with coal-dust. There are sometimes protuberances; but this fresh defect carries a consolation, because the accursed pimples are easier to extract. Otherwise they prove themselves as tenacious as they are ugly.

The modes of prevention consist first of abstaining from paint and cosmetic pomades which, though made to whiten the skin, alter and check perspiration. The habits of covering your face with the bed-clothes while sleeping, wearing a mask, staying in rooms subject to smoke, and forgetting to carefully wipe dust and sweat from your face, are also amongst the most frequent causes of black points, and you see what you must do.

Let us now occupy ourselves with ways to remove them, when by misfortune they have taken root. I use this expression because it is very difficult to dislodge them. However, by taking a sponge or a very soft brush, and wetting it with essence of purified soap, you may, by frequent rubbing, hope that they will disappear by degrees. You may also, and preferably, dip a bar of toilet-soap in aromatic benzoin water, cover the black points well with it, then rub them with the soft brush until the soap is removed. Benzoin soap is most suitable. Then immediately wash with aromatic water. You must repeat this operation every morning. If despite this the black points persist, extract them by pressing with both forefingers, which will cause neither pain nor inflammation, and will produce at most a slight reddening for ten minutes. It will then be well to brush them and rub again with the sponge.

But black points, so troublesome to remove, easily return. Also, it is well now and again to gently press the part where they first appeared, and I am much mistaken if you will not see a multitude of little white seeds spurt out: sometimes round; sometimes like a thread, dry or swollen and slightly damp; and sometimes grey or black, at least on the upper part. If no sign warns you of their presence, if at the end of some time, the emission diminishes, you will know that the black points have been reabsorbed, and you will need only to use the moistened brush, without repeating the pressings.

Remedy for Mealy Skin.

Without having pimples, swelling, or eruptions, some persons see their complexions covered with little grainy pellicles, and the skin appears in some sort peeled: nothing is less attractive. (See Div. 1.) Happily you may easily remove the pellicles with aromatic waters such as Ninon-de-l'Enclos water, tincture of benzoin, brandy, or Cologne water.

Remedies for Chaps.

These remedies, all easy, and nearly all composed of very fresh animal fat and emollient substances, vary a little according to the location of the trouble. Thus chapped lips require rose pomade because of the colour. Chapped nostrils call for ordinary cerate; chapped fingers, butter mixed with cocoa (see Div. 2), or cerate mixed with beef marrow. The chaps which some persons experience in winter, on and around the knees, must be bathed with poppy-water and olive-oil. Very clean suet would be good, but it is difficult to ensure that it has not been in contact with any noxious thing, and then its disgusting odour must absolutely be rejected. Sprinkling barley-flour on the chaps quickly calms the pain. Honey-water is an even more powerful remedy for this painful inconvenience.

Remedy for Ruddiness.

A strong and persistent colour, sad omen of rosacea, requires first of all baths, a regime of vegetables and milk, and refreshing drinks. That is for the interior. As for the exterior: in the evening wash your face with milk, gently wipe it off without rubbing, then put on a very little cucumber pomade.

Modes of getting rid of Freckles.

Lily-water, balm of Mecca, rose milk, almond-milk, and tincture of benzoin may combat freckles. The last two recommended are the best. Here is what you must do: take care to wear a veil, carry a parasol, and wear a hat with a brim which shades your face, even when the freckles have already formed, in order to prevent them from darkening. Wash your face at night, because if you do it in the morning, you will make your skin tender, and even more susceptible to freckles. When you have washed your face with almond-milk or benzoin and dried it, pour a few drops of it on a dry linen and apply it to your face for some moments.

Remedy for Tanning.

The effect of full sunlight does not always produce freckles. There are people who never have them, even when taking no precautions, but every one is subject to tanning. It is easy to avoid it in the city; but when you live in the country, whether you busy yourself a little with country tasks, or only go for long walks, your skin is tanned; that is to say brown, flaking, and tough.

To alleviate this trouble, you must act as for freckles: the same remedies are suitable. Nonetheless there is a special, efficacious mode, though (it is well to say) a rather disgusting one. This remedy consists of washing your face with poultry blood. It is well known what a beautiful colour butchers have, and how good the vapour of blood is for the skin. Cream produces a somewhat lesser effect, but it does produce it, and I do not doubt that my readers may prefer it.

Blood and cream also dispel freckles.

Remedy for Scurf Patches.

When the patches show a cutaneous disorder or malady of the skin, you must consult a physician. When on the contrary they are rare, sudden, and produced by accident, it suffices to dissolve a few grains of white salt in lukewarm water or in your mouth, and wash them at once, without rubbing, with the salt-water or saliva.

Remedy for Wrinkles.

When the wrinkles are not caused by the irreparable ravages of time, but by sorrow or the bad habit of grimacing when smiling and speaking, you may hope to lessen them and efface them by degrees, by wearing compresses during the night. These are made of batiste, moistened with tincture of benzoin and veal broth cooked without herbs or salt.

Remedy for Mosquito-bites.

The repeated bites of these insects cause much burning and reddening of the skin, and must be numbered amongst the mishaps which alter beauty. It is well known that mosquitoes are drawn to certain persons whom they bite by preference. These persons have only to mix an infusion of the herb called unsavoury chamomile in the water with which they wash their face and arms. They will be shielded from the bites of the mosquitoes, who cannot bear the odour of this plant.

To lessen the inflammation of a mosquito-bite, it is advised to apply a little fuller's earth mixed with water. I have never tried this.

Remedy for Imperfections of the Eyebrows.

When your eyebrows are straw-coloured, cut them now and again, so that they darken in growing back. You run no risk, because the absence of this nearly white hair will not be remarked. (See Div. 3.)

When your eyebrows go only half-way over the eye-socket, rub them with soap moistened with brandy to make the hair grow. If they are too thin, the same practice is necessary.

If they are not sufficiently arched, raise them by directing the hair towards the top of your forehead. Above all, when you comb your hair, pass a little pomade over your eyebrows.

The worst flaw of this beautiful arch is to be covered with scurf, which makes the hair fall out. Take a sponge, and dip it in water to which you have added essence of toilet-soap and tincture of benzoin. Squeeze it out and wash your eyebrows well with it, being careful to close your eyes, so that the liquid will not get into them. If you prefer, rub your eyebrows with a tablet of perfumed soap dampened with aromatic benzoin water. Dry them, moisten your finger lightly with antique oil, and pass it over your eyebrows.

Modes of calming Redness and Inflammation of the Eyelids.

The shape, colour, and above all the expression of the eyes make up their principal beauty; but without the charm of the secondary attributes, that is, without the cleanliness of the eyelids, the strength, length, and bloom of the eyelashes, the most beautiful eye will be extremely defective. I emphasize this all the more because this kind of beauty is altogether voluntary, since it depends upon hygiene and cleanliness.

Take care to prevent inflammation of the eyelids by wearing a green veil in summer. In winter use a fire-screen of the same colour, because exposure to flame is as hurtful to the eyes as to the skin. Use proper lighting, do not read very fine print, and do not do meticulous work by lamp-light, such as embroidery, lace stitches, &c. Above all avoid working on red or black material. If despite these sensible precautions your eyes are red or inflamed, prepare a weak infusion of melilot, and bathe them at night before going to bed. This herb, which has a strong but agreeable odour, has also the property of reducing inflammation of the inside of the eye. From the next morning on you will feel relief, and at the end of three or four days at most, the cure will be complete. In the opposite case, the inflammation will persist from an internal cause, and it will become necessary to consult a physician.

Remedy for Little Foreign Bodies which get into the Eyes.

When some little foreign body has slipped into your eye, be careful not to rub it, but look at the ground for a long time. Open and close the eye rapidly.

Weakening of the Sight.

If your sight is temporarily weakened, bathe your eyes with cold water after dinner and when going to bed. Dr. Willich, an English physician whose work has been translated by M. Itard, recommends bathing the upper lip from time to time, because of its close link to the optic nerve. He also advises exposing the eyes, after dinner, to the steam of boiled coffee. He prefers using a dampened sponge, applied over the eyes, to bathing them in an eyecup or eyebath. Always keep your head thrown back, and while the sponge is on your eyes, open them gently and cautiously. Afterwards dry them at once with fine, very white batiste, without rubbing. After this, you must guard against bright lights and all kinds of strain.

Here is an excellent remedy to strengthen the sight: mix six grains of white copperas (sulphate of zinc, sold for two sous) and thirty-one grains of powdered orris-root. Cast them into a pint of river-water. Stop the bottle well, put it in a cool place, and use it after twenty-four hours.

Weakening of the sight almost always reddens the eyelids. It is also well to wash them with a very clean sponge moistened with melilot water. Your eye may remain closed while you apply the sponge.

Falling out of the Eyelashes.

When an eyelash chances to fall off and remains in the corner of the eye, it is necessary that some one near by remove it delicately, because it could infiltrate the pupil and cause you much suffering. That is the sole precaution to take, because this loss is nothing at all, if a lash falls only about once a fortnight in winter and once a week in summer. You must only avoid rubbing your eyes, because nothing is injured or falls out more easily than the eyelashes.

The total loss of the eyelashes gives the eyes a miserable and disgusting aspect, and is impossible to repair; therefore use all possible modes of preventing it. You already know that you must guard against rubbing your eyes with your fist. Furthermore, it is very useful to bathe your eyes with a little cold water, pure or flavoured with Cologne water or brandy. This is how you should proceed: close your eye tightly and pass around the edge the tip of a sponge moistened with the chosen liquid. Alternately raise and lower your eyelashes with the sponge. Then you may apply over them, as lightly as possible, a piece of slightly-warmed batiste: this practice will strengthen them. Some persons have been imprudent enough to rub the edges of their eyelids, devoid of lashes, with soap, and the soap infiltrates the eye and causes intolerable distress.

It is a very good habit to pass your forefinger, with an infinitely small amount of pomade spread on the end, delicately over your eyelashes. Do this every morning for your eyebrows as well.

If your lashes lack that agreeable wave which makes them first droop towards your cheek and then straighten towards your forehead, now and then you may, without affectation, pass your slanted forefinger over the upper lashes, and at length the lashes will curl up.

Their Waxy Matter.

Waxy matter on the eyelids is one of the most disgusting characteristics of ugliness and uncleanliness. It ordinarily arises from maladies of the eye, and then the care of a physician is indispensable; but extreme cleanliness is no less necessary. When you are subject to this misfortune, you should not only wash your eyelashes every morning and night, and every time you apply the recommended remedies, but also look in the mirror several times a day to see if new particles are forming. If so wash them off at once; you need only let a drop of water fall on the lashes from the tip of a finger. When you rise in the morning, if your eyelids are ordinarily stuck together, be very careful in making any effort to loosen them and in using your fingers there. Undoubtedly they are weakened, and you will break the lashes which the waxy matter has already worn away.

Without having waxy lashes, you may sometimes have two or three stuck together, without visible liquid. You must neither unglue them with your fingers, nor neglect this tendency. The little lotions already described will easily rid you of them.

The Droplets of White Matter which often appear in the Corner of the Eye.

This substance is never mentioned in advice relative to the toilet, and yet its presence strikes onlookers disagreeably. If it bulges, it inspires a certain disgust. The habit of washing the corners of your eyes prevents this. However, there are times when, without any discomfort to the eyes, the moisture is more often found. Therefore, now and then bring the tip of your forefinger very gently to the tear-duct and remove the droplet. This operation is very simple, yet I advise you to do it only when you are alone; otherwise it is advisable to replace your forefinger with your handkerchief. For a woman, disgust is like suspicion: she must dread its very shadow.

Remedies for Defects of the Ears.

The ears, to which ordinarily little attention is paid in scrutinizing a woman's beauty, contribute more than is believed to the charm of the whole. Ears which are small, pale, and flat, which stick out from the head, or which are long and hanging, disfigure a beautiful person, though no reason can be given. I shall provide a remedy.

For flat ears, avoid tightening your cap-strings over your ears. In the evening raise the under sides of your ears with a little cotton. When washing them on the outside, anoint the edges with fine oil to revive and encourage the skin which seems hardened.

Ears which stick out should be brought closer to your head at night and fixed with a broad tape. Every time that you put on a hat, flatten them by passing your hand over them. It is also well to do this from time to time during the day.

Ears which protrude are troublesome principally when you wear a hat, because they push it forwards ridiculously. Long, hanging ears, on the contrary, destroy all the charm of the coiffure *en cheveux*. At night, confine your ears in a piece of linen which you tighten slightly, then raise it to the sides of your cap.

When your ears exude a fœtid odour, every morning and evening insert an ear-pick wrapped in worn batiste, wash the outside well, and rub the edges with Cologne water, pure or diluted with a little water. Do not resort to overly strong perfumes, for fear of fatiguing your nerves.

Remedy for Thickening of the Neck.

The water in certain cities, such as Moulins, Clermont, &c., has the property of enlarging the front of the neck in some persons. The bad habit of wearing the collars of *fichus* and *guimpes* too tight contributes a great deal to this indisposition, and may even be its sole cause. Not only is all the grace of the neck obliterated by swelling; still more, if it increases it begins to resemble a goitre, and inspires the same disgust. I am certain that you may remedy this by wearing, during the night, a collar well thickened with cooking salt enclosed in taffety. This collar must not be too tight, or it may increase the indisposition.

Remedy for a Ropy Neck.

All ladies know this by the vulgar name of "cords," which a physician would not comprehend. The cords of the neck are the organs of articulation for breathing. The large muscles and those of the voice begin to protrude, and then the whiteness, roundness, and grace of the neck are lost. If this flaw is caused by leanness, you must refer to the article below on gaining weight.

If (as very often happens) it arises from the bad habit of raising your voice too much when speaking, from shouting, you must abstain from prolonged conversations, loud speech, and singing. The neck swells and the articulations show during passionate outbursts, of anger for example. Frequent movements of the neck also contribute to this condition. You see what you must do.

In addition, rub your neck with lightly-perfumed olive-oil every night. If all this does not suffice, it is well to always wear high-necked *fichus*.

The Mode of removing Pellicles and Scales from the Fingers.

However small the part you take in household tasks, the palms of your hands may be slightly callused. If you sew without a finger-stall to protect the forefinger of your left hand, it may be covered with little scales produced by repeated needle pricks. (See Div. 4.) Some persons have also little growths at the corners of the nails, owing to hang-nails which they had the imprudence to tear off. Cuts, burns, and chilblains leave disagreeable pellicles long after they are cured. Your penknife gashes the edge of your right thumb; the thread which you hold while sewing or embroidering cuts the fourth and little fingers of your right hand crossways.

It is easy to cure all the rough spots left by these little troubles. First wait until all the rough spots are perfectly dry, because otherwise you will make things much worse. Then take a piece of pumice-stone, which has already been used to rub other things, and especially hard objects, so that its surface is smooth and soft. All the little pellicles, scales, or growths will be effaced as you rub, without any painful sensation. It will be well to strengthen your skin by washing it before and after the rubbing with a little sponge or linen dipped in brandy. Cologne water may also be used.

The Mode of curing Hang-nails.

All negligence has some consequences, and not one single part of the body is exempt. Your nails, which may appear to require no care, have also a kind of hygiene, for want of which they become loose or cover themselves ridiculously. A host of causes daily attack the skin which borders the nails and lift it partially: these are called hang-nails. If you neglect them, they grow longer, detach themselves more and more from the nail, and become raw and very painful. Some persons, acting like savages, have the pernicious habit of tearing them, even (it must be said) with their teeth. When the edge of the nail is almost bare, the hang-nail extends beyond the first joint, and if by misfortune some dirt comes in contact with the finger so torn, it causes a felon. Even if this disastrous result does not occur, the afflicted nail will still suffer much, and lose its elegant form.

I believe it is needless to insist on the necessity of curing hang-nails, and I am going to give you the mode at once. As soon as you glimpse one, cut it with your scissors, and moisten it with a little brandy diluted with water. If it is a little enlarged, cover it with a piece of court plaster.

The Mode of ridding the Nails of the Skin which sometimes covers them.

As for the over skin which deforms the finger-nails, you must check it by using your thumb to push the skin on the edge of the nail as far as possible. The longer the nails are on the first joint, the more graceful they are. If you have neglected this measure, and as a result of chilblains or any other misfortune an over skin grows on your nails, push it down often, as much as you can without causing pain. You may dip your finger in water now and then, so that the over skin yields more readily.

Remedy for Warts.

Rubbing with woollen materials, and with corrosive substances such as aquafortis, are successfully used against these disgusting excrescences; but the first of these modes is excessively slow, and the second is dangerous. The following remedy has none of these disadvantages; I formerly tested its efficacy.

Take some yellow celandine, break off the stem close to the root, and rub the wart with the yellowish milky juice which flows from it. The wart will disappear after some time. If the wart is very large and old, it may be necessary to repeat the application several times.

It is said that the milk of tithymal and of the fig-tree commonly produce the same effect.

Corn Plaster of M. Laforest, Foot Surgeon.

This is taken from M. Nicholas Laurent Laforest's *L'art de soigner les pieds*. Take an ounce of pitch, such as is used in the navy, half an ounce of galbanum, and dissolve in vinegar a scruple of salt of ammonia. Add to this a drachm and a half of diachylon. Mix the whole well, apply it to a bit of leather, and cover the corn with it. When after some days you lift the plaster, the corn will follow.

Another Mode by Potash.

You may utterly destroy the corn by rubbing it every day with a little caustic solution of potash, until a soft and flexible skin forms in place of the corn.

Another Mode by Pumice-stone.

When a corn is new, or when it has been softened by soaking in warm water, you may wear it away and destroy it by rubbing it a long time with a pumice-stone. This substance thus does the office of a proper file.

Another Mode of curing Corns, with Ivy.

Take a leaf of creeping ivy, wash it well, and pass it over a flame to dispel impurities which might be on its surface. Soak it for several hours in vinegar, then apply it to the corn. Be careful to keep it there by means of a little strip of lamp-cotton, tightened and knotted in a manner which does not hamper the affected toe in any way. Some days after the corn turns yellow. Then it is dried out, and you may remove it with a penknife.

Another Cure, by means of Starched Muslin.

Two or three days in advance, soften the corn by rubbing it with a little suet. The last day, dry it well. Roll a strip of muslin over it round the affected toe; the muslin should be narrow, rather long and stiff, and recently starched. Do this several times. Leave the muslin in place until it comes apart and falls off. Very often the rubbing has completely worn away the corn, especially if it is not too old. You may finish the treatment by putting on another muslin bandage, or by using a pumice-stone.

Another Corn Plaster.

Mix equal parts of hemlock, vigo, and diachylon; make of them a kind of thick pulp, and place it on the corn. Cover it with a little circle of leather, and fasten it by tying it on with a narrow bandage. At the end of a week, or thereabouts, lift the plaster. The corn will be so much softened that you may cut it off without resistance or pain.

Remedy for Pain caused by Uncomfortable Shoes, or the Fatigue of the Dance.

When a shoe is too narrow, the folds of your stockings are too long, or the stitching in the toile sole rubs your foot, you may ease the pain at once by moistening a piece of white soap with brandy, and rubbing the affected place with it. Finish by washing it with pure brandy.

This operation also abates at once the burning on the soles of the feet when you have danced too much or walked too long. If the unpleasant sensation persists after the first rubbing, repeat it using a little brandy.

The Mode of dissipating the Coagulated Blood which collects under the Nails, following a Blow.

Crush some long plantain with a little salt, then apply this by forming a poultice over the nail. It is said that distilled scabiosa water also has the property of dissolving blood under the nails. For this you must often wash the bruised nail, and apply a compress soaked with this water.

Remedy for Broken or Very Weak Nails, especially those of the Feet.

Mix together an ounce of oil of bitter almonds, a drachm of oil of tartar, and a little lemon-juice. Wash the nails in this mixture often, and at night put a little compress on the toe-nails.

Regime to counter Leanness.

Total absence of rounding of the figure, yellowish skin, hollow and ringed eyes, drawn cheeks, a ridiculously sharp nose, a sunken mouth, a neck stretched and suffered to show all its articulations: these are the effects of the excessive leanness with which, whatever otherwise may be the regularity and beauty of your features, it is impossible not to be nearly hideous. Its most common causes are acute illness, profound sorrow, constant vigils for work or pleasure, or a natural inclination. Time, a calm spirit, and a wiser use of your moments cure the leanness which arises from the first causes, but the last requires special treatment.

As soon as you have determined to gain weight, you must distance yourself from all business projects, emotional agitation, and serious and prolonged thought. Above all, it is essential not to feel any care. In addition, take very little exercise and sleep for a long time, at least ten hours. On rising, take a cup of chocolate with salep of Persia mixed with two egg-yolks. Some hours later eat some white meat of poultry, lamb, very fat veal, or succulent beef. These meats must be roasted or grilled, so that their principal nutrients do not disappear. If you eat stews, they should be very lightly spiced, and enriched with coulis and meat juices.

Rice, potato-starch cooked in strong consommé, porridge mixed with cream, and almond-milk sugared lightly, but flavoured with a few drops of orange-flower water, are the things which you should take from time to time between your meals, which must be frequent.

It is essential to drink water, pure or reddened with a little wine, and to abstain from acid fruit, liqueurs, tea, and coffee. Only chocolate-covered chestnuts, custards, soft-boiled eggs, chocolate creams, and cream-cheese should vary the dishes.

Every day, immediately before the meal, take a bath, during which you should not move about at all. After a quarter of an hour, you may comfort yourself with a *consommé*. Quit the bath after another quarter of an hour, arrange yourself on a sopha, and take a cup of chocolate. Then sleep until the moment you sit down at table. It is well to chat and laugh during the meal to arouse your appetite and aid digestion. At twilight, always rest on a sopha or a bed, in a cool place, abandoning yourself to sweet idleness.

Regime to counter Excess Embonpoint.

If an excessively meagre figure is hideous, an enormously fat one is disgusting. It is nothing more than a heavy, shapeless mass, whose every movement is awkward, ludicrous, and often painful. Something of the coarse and crude is written all over these massive forms. The soul seems crushed, the eyes are dwarfed, the features are enveloped, and the fœtid odour of profuse sweat ends by arousing disgust.

To get rid of this wealth of fat, it is absolutely necessary to follow the course contrary to the preceding regime. (See Div. 5.) Take long walks, stay up late, eat little, talk, move about, and study a great deal. Take light foods which are sour, very spicy, sweetened, and flavoured. Abstain from meat, bread, starchy vegetables, broth, and milk. Preferable to any other things are dried fruits, salads, and preserves. Eat only two meals a day, and busy yourself immediately afterwards. Eat aromatic lozenges and spit often.

——*Manuel des dames.*

Diversion 1.

Small-pox and Vaccination. The greatest enemy to the beauty of the skin—the small-pox—was first checked in its career by the perseverance of Lady Mary Wortley Montague, in introducing inoculation; and subsequently, in a great degree, subdued and banished by the great discovery of Dr. Jenner. But the discovery of Dr. Jenner would have been quite superhuman—would have been an unearthly miracle—had it been free from all imperfection. There is no such thing in our poor world as perfection without a flaw. It is impossible, and whoever aims at it must be disappointed. But there are not wanting many, whose minds and feelings are so perverse and debased, that they fasten upon the slightest defect in our greatest and best discoveries, and multiply it, and magnify it in their diseased fancies, until like Satan in *Paradise Lost,* they make "the worse appear the better reason." In this light I am disposed to view the outcry and *mala fama* raised against vaccination, which like every thing of human contrivance, is confessedly imperfect. But its triumphs are gloriously emblazoned on the thousands of smooth faces now seen in our streets, which have, within the last twenty years, taken the place of those whose finest features and blooming complexions were marred by the small-pox. Look around you, and say whether you can now see, in the crowded street or the crowded assembly, an equal or any thing like an equal number of faces disfigured by small-pox, as might have been seen even ten years ago.

——*The Art of Beauty.*

Diversion 2.

Beurre mêle de cacao in the original French. However, possibly this is a mistake for butter of cacao, or butter mixed with butter of cacao.

——Frances Grimble.

Diversion 3.

To blacken the Eyelashes and Eyebrows. Rub them often with elder-berries. For the same purpose, some make use of burnt cork, or clove burned at the candle. Others employ black frankincense, resin, and mastic: this black, it is said, will not come off with perspiration.

Wash for blackening the Eyebrows. First wash with a decoction of galls. Then rub them with a brush dipped in a solution of green vitriol, and let them dry.

Black for the Eyebrows. Take an ounce of pitch, a like quantity of resin and of frankincense, and half an ounce of mastic. Throw them upon live charcoal, over which lay a plate to receive the smoke. A black soot will adhere to the plate; with this soot rub the eyelashes and eyebrows very delicately. This operation, if now and then repeated, will keep them perfectly black.

——*The Duties of a Lady's Maid.*

Diversion 4.

To calm Needle Pricks. Here is a little remedy which ladies will appreciate: while sewing, they often push the point of a needle under the left thumb-nail. The pain of this prick is really dreadful. To calm it, insert a little cucumber pomade under the nail; the pain will immediately cease.

——*Manuel des dames.*

Diversion 5.

Remedies for Corpulence. This is a disease which not unfrequently proves fatal, when it increases so much as to press upon the blood-vessels, and to prevent the free play of the lungs. It is always so far a disease as it exceeds the ordinary standard, the best test of which is, its attracting attention and calling forth remark.

The first thing to be ascertained, in order to discover a proper remedy, is the cause which has produced the affection. The most common causes are indolence and luxurious living, indulgence in sleep on a soft bed, and vacuity of mind, from having nothing to do or to think about. The ancients were well aware of this, when they described Minerva Pinguis as an indolent goddess; and Lord Chesterfield and Mr. Burke make a soft disposition and corpulence inseparable companions. Nothing will sooner reduce unwieldy corpulence, the deformity of a pot-belly, as it is called, or the squat porky shape of the body, than activity of both body and mind, particularly the latter, and short sleep on a hard mattress.

Besides this, Dr. Darwin recommends putting a proper bandage round the belly, so that it may be tightened and relaxed with ease, such as a tight belt or stays with a double row of buttons. This removes one principal cause of corpulence, which is the looseness of the skin. Tight drawers, supported by elastic braces over the shoulders, have also been found useful, by ladies who have a tendency to corpulence. The omission of one meal in the course of the day, such as supper, will be useful; as by decreasing the supply of food, the superfluous fat stored up under the skin will be drawn upon by the blood-vessels, to make up for the deficiency, and the fat will thus be reduced. The less drink or soup, the better; for drink, particularly malt liquor, is one very common cause of corpulence. Cream ought to be religiously abstained from, and all preparations from it; for nothing is more apt to produce corpulence. Dr. Darwin recommends salt, or salted meat, which has a tendency to carry off fat by perspiration. Soda water and soap have also been recommended, but upon no very certain evidence of their efficacy.

Contour of the Breasts. It may be important to remark, that the breasts are always the first part of the body which is affected by fat or emaciation; and my fair readers who are interested in the subject, will do well to follow the directions above given for corpulence and leanness, according as the circumstances may be. If leanness prevails, then will it be requisite, besides attending to rest, good temper, and good living, to have the bosom loosely clothed, so as to produce no pressure. Friction with the hand, or with a soft flesh-brush, for an hour or two every day, will also tend to develop their growth. Nothing will prevent this in a greater degree than the artificial padding usually worn to supply natural deficiency, with the exception perhaps of the artificial breasts, said to be made of India rubber, but which I only know by description.

When there is, on the other hand, too great a luxuriance of volume, the opposite modes must be pursued, the chief of which is bandaging. The newest mode of reducing the volume of the breasts is by means of an internal remedy of great power, and which was discovered, while it was given for wens and other enlargements, to act in a similar manner on the female breast. As so powerful a remedy may not be safe, however, in the hands of the inexperienced to be taken into the stomach, I shall prescribe it in the form directed by Dr. Ure, of Glasgow, in his *Chemical Dictionary;* and I shall call it:

Dr. Ure's Ointment for the Breasts. Take a drachm of iodide of zinc, and an ounce of prepared hog's lard. Make an ointment, and rub in daily on each breast, about the size of a nutmeg of the ointment; the regimen for reducing corpulence being attended to at the same time.

——*The Art of Beauty.*

Chapter VI.
Perfumes.

You ought to use perfumes with great discretion, and if you are delicate, it is absolutely necessary to abstain from them. Pallor, leanness, dark circles under the eyes, exhaustion, and nervous tremors are the common fruits of the exaggerated use of scents by persons whose nerves are more or less irritable. They end by suffering all these ills to no avail, because, according to the picturesque expression of Queen Marie Leczinska, "Perfumes are like grandeurs, those who wear them scarcely notice them." Far from pleasing, overly strong perfumes keep people at a distance. Many persons flee ladies who are ambergrised and musked like the plague. Besides, that denotes coquetry and pretentiousness.

But on the other hand, the total absence of perfume is an unnecessary deprivation, and sometimes even disadvantageous. It is well, in certain circumstances, to sprinkle a few drops of Cologne water on your shift, stockings, and handkerchief. Despite the greatest cleanliness, the human body is subject to so many disagreeable exhalations, general and particular, that you must not neglect these measures, especially when you have a husband who is very sensitive to odours. You may perfume your linen in the armoires, the pomatum for dressing your hair, the salve which guards your lips against chapping, the water for washing your face, and the almond pastes and soaps for cleansing your hands. But always use sweet, soft scents, such as iris, heliotrope, reseda, violet, rose, &c. Aromatic perfumes, such as carnation, cinnamon, and vanilla, must be employed rarely, in very small quantities, and softened by a mixture of weaker, fragrant scents such as lily, tuberose, and jasmine. The ambrosial perfumes (we owe this classification of scents to the celebrated Linnæus), such as amber and musk, must be entirely banished from your person and apartments.

I shall give directions for perfuming yourself in order to banish bad natural odours, make yourself agreeable, and achieve a neat toilet without affecting your health, disturbing delicate persons, or attracting the (to my mind) very unflattering appellations of *petite-maîtresse* and *merveilleuse*. (See Div. 1.)

The Mode of making Cologne Water.

It has not been so very long since the manufacture of the spirituous water called Cologne water was regarded as a great secret that must not even go beyond the family which had claimed the exclusive privilege. Little by little, additional manufacturers established in Cologne, and others elsewhere, succeeded in imitating it. They sent it into that city to distribute every where, when there was a need to make people believe it to be better because it came from the city which bore the name.

But since it was not difficult to see that the place cannot influence the product at all, and that any one any where is in a position to make excellent Cologne water, factories are now established in the principal cities of Germany, England, and France. And though every distiller pretends to be the manufacturer of "wonderful" and "true" Cologne water, which according to them is inimitable, and alone possesses all the qualities superior to all the others, it is no less true that the manner of making and the receipts of all of them are pretty nearly the same. Since I have no object but to be useful to the industrious, since I seek only to propagate all which may be economical and procure comfort for households, I do not fear to reveal a process which may prove advantageous to them, viz., making Cologne water.

Since Cologne water is nothing but spirit of wine of thirty degrees, into which fragrant essential oils are dissolved, it is only in the oils that it is possible to have several variations, or in their respective proportions, or in the proportions of the spirit of wine to the combined essences. The best is prepared with ninety-six parts of essence and nine hundred forty of spirit of wine, to a thousand parts of Cologne water. As for the essences, choose those of cinnamon, citron, lemon, cloves, bergamot, lavender, neroli, rosemary, &c. The mixing finished, let it stand for six, eight, or ten days at the most. Decant it when the liquid has clarified, or filter it through unsized paper. Some persons distill it in an alembic to store in great flasks, and then put it in the long phials found in commerce.

You will perceive, after what I have just said, how easy it would be for all housekeepers to make their supply of Cologne water for themselves. I must add that the more plants or substances used to make the essences aromatic, the more the Cologne water into which you put them will be pleasant and sweet smelling. To give it an extremely delicate scent, first filter the spirit of wine to be used through fresh and recently-gathered orange-leaves.

The quantities and proportions will be, for six pounds of spirit of wine at twenty-eight degrees by the Baumé hydrometer: an ounce and a drachm of essence of bergamot, six drops of essence of cinnamon, an hundred ninety-two drops of essence of lemon, ninety drops of essence of cloves, five hundred seventy-two drops of essence of lavender, an hundred forty-four drops of essence of neroli, forty drops of essence of rosemary, and three ounces of lemon-balm, called Carmelite water. Leave it all in contact with the spirit of wine for six, eight, or ten days, as I have indicated, and filter it to save and use as needed.

Another Mode.

"Eau admirable," or Cologne water is nothing but a solution of different fragrant oils in very pure spirit of wine of moderate strength. You will see what this famous secret amounts to, and what are the mysterious properties of this composition, so highly vaunted on the scrap of paper which is wrapped round the flasks.

Take a quart of rectified spirit of wine. Pour in an ounce of oil of bergamot, three drachms of essential oil of rosemary, half an ounce of essence of lemon, and a drachm of essence of lavender. When the mixing has been done, let it stand, and decant it when it is clear and limpid. If you wish to make a first-rate composition, filter the spirit of wine through fresh orange-flowers, of a weight of a quarter that of the spirit of wine. The odour will be infinitely sweeter.

A roll of Cologne water costs ten sous at most at the distiller or manufacturer.

A Simple and Easy Way of perfuming
Linens and Other Clothing.

Take some pieces of dried orris-root, such as are sold by pharmacies, and enclose them in your armoires and chests of drawers. They will generally disperse a slight odour of violets over all your clothing. If you wish the perfume to be stronger and more agreeable, insert a piece of the root between each fold of your shifts, night jackets, petticoats, &c. You may also slip it into the fluting which trims your *fichus*. Nothing is so mildly sweet and so healthful at the same time.

You may gather the petals of roses and carnations, and pieces of reseda, to use during the summer, and put these also in your drawers.

While drying there, they give off a sweet, balsamic odour. However, orris-root seems far preferable to me.

Fragrant Bags to perfume the Linen in Armoires and Ornaments in Boxes.

Gather some petals of roses, musky carnation, single hyacinth, lavender flowers, balsam leaves, and a few white horehound leaves. Suffer them to dry in the shade. When they are well dried, sprinkle them with powdered cloves and nutmeg. Enclose the whole in taffety bags, of what colour you please, and put the bags amongst your clothes.

Bags with Herbs *de Montpellier.*

This sachet is composed of the leaves of thyme, lavender, hyssop, verbena, Provence sage, rosemary, and basil, mixed with cloves and a crushed nutmeg. Put all these things in a piece of coloured toile, and place this bag on your night table, in your dressing-room, in your bath, &c.

Bags with Powdered Scent.

Take six ounces of orris-root, an ounce of dried orange-flowers, six ounces of dried rose-petals, six ounces of dried bergamot bark, six ounces of Portuguese orange zest, and two ounces of storax. Crush them well, pass them through a sieve, and make pretty taffety bags suitable for placing in your dressing-case and work-baskets, and on your fichus, gloves, and all delicate articles. (See Div. 2.)

Fragrant Pastilles to burn.

Take three ounces of benzoin, a drachm of dried orange zest, a drachm and a half of musk roses, a drachm of ambergris, a drachm and a half of red sandal-wood bark, and half an ounce of sugar. Pulverize all these things, and incorporate the very fine powder with the mucilage of gum-dragon mixed with rose-water or orange-flower water to make a paste. Divide this into little rounds, cones, hearts, or squares, and dry them in the sun or on a low fire.

When you wish to use one of these pastilles, set fire to it. Lay it on a stone table, or any other object which cannot suffer any damage. It sparkles as it burns and exudes an agreeable odour: this practice dispels bad air and purifies your apartments.

Pastilles formed from aromatic herbs, such as sage, tarragon, lavender, hyssop, and rosemary, dried and reduced to powder, and mixed with very strong vinegar, are excellent for purifying a sick-room. You may put them on the hearth shovel, after having lit the fire. Their tonic fumes, similar to those of burnt vinegar, are even more balsamic, and without occasioning the inconvenience of staining the floor, which vinegar sometimes does while boiling.

Flasks for the Mantel-piece.

Cologne water, Portugal water, Hungary water, or angel-water should be the sole contents of your flasks. (See Div. 3.)

Pocket Flasks.

As these have the aim of guarding you or others against foul odours, and combating faintness or nervous spasms, rose, bergamot, or lemon salt of vinegar; balsamic Cologne water; luce water; and even sulphuric ether, are the only things which you should choose for these flasks.

To perfume Handkerchiefs.

Use Cologne water, balm-water, angel-water, violet water, or imperial water.

To perfume Baths, General and Partial.

Use lavender-water, Cologne water, Portugal water, honey, or benzoin.
——*Manuel des dames, Manuel d'économie domestique.*

Diversion 1.

Mme. Celnart was also the author of the *Manuel du parfumeur,* and may have expected the readers of her other books to be familiar with it; hence the scantness of this chapter.
——Frances Grimble.

Diversion 2.

Perfume for Gloves. Take a drachm of ambergris and the like quantity of civet; add a quarter of an ounce of flour-butter. With these, well mixed, rub the gloves over gently with fine cotton wool, and press the perfume into them.

Another Mode. Take half an ounce of damask or rose scent, a drachm each of spirit of clove and mace, and a quarter of an ounce of frankincense. Mix them together, and lay them in papers, and when hard, press the gloves. They will take the scent in twenty-four hours, and hardly ever lose it.

——*The Alphabetical Receipt Book and Domestic Advisor.*

Diversion 3.

Hungary Water. Take a quantity of rosemary flowers. Put them into a glass retort, and pour in as much spirit of wine as the flowers can imbibe. Dilute the retort well, and let the flowers macerate well for six days; then distill it in a sand-heat.

Luce Water. Take two ounces of rectified spirit of wine, a drachm of oil of amber, two drachms of salt of tartar, two drachms of prepared powder of amber, and twenty drops of oil of nutmeg. Put them all into a bottle, and shake it well. Let it stand five hours, after which filter it, and always keep it by you; and when you would make luce water, put it into the strongest spirits of sal ammoniac.

Imperial Water. Put two ounces of cream of tartar into a jar, with the juice and zests of two lemons, and pour on it seven quarts of boiling water. When cold, clear it through a gauze sieve. Bottle it up, and the next day it may be used.

Lavender-water. Take a quart of highly-rectified spirit of wine, two ounces of essential oil of lavender, and five drachms of essence of amber-gris. Put it all into a bottle, and shake it until perfectly incorporated.

Or, put two pounds of lavender blossoms into half a gallon of water, and set them in a still over a slow fire. Distill it off gently until the water is all exhausted. Repeat the process a second time, then cork it closely down in bottles.

——*The Alphabetical Receipt Book and Domestic Advisor.*

Chapter VII.
Hygienic Habits.

Hygiene, which maintains health and encourages habits of order, cleanliness, and moderation, is therefore the only source of beauty. More than any thing else, this precious benefit preserves the freshness of a healthy body, and expresses the purity of the soul. Whatever there may be of regularity and charm in your features, you are not beautiful with a pallid complexion or hollow cheeks, any more than with a false smile, or a brazen, disdainful, or angry expression. Many things might be said about the relation of moral hygiene to beauty! But the plan of this book does not include them, and the hearts of my readers will supply what is lacking. Let me, therefore, confine myself to lessons in physical hygiene. Despite its extreme importance, this chapter will perhaps not be over-long, because hygiene is in some fashion discussed throughout Part I.

When you awaken, rub behind your ears with a piece of batiste or woollen material. This removes the sweat which has collected there during the night, and this practice is most beneficial. You may also dip your forefinger in a flask of Cologne water, and pass it all round the auricle.

You know that you must rinse your mouth when you arise. After that, you will do well to put into your mouth a pastille of marsh-mallow, jujube, or gum-arabic paste, or a little lump of barley-sugar or candy. All this may assist the expectoration which ordinarily takes place in the morning. Allow it to dissolve slowly.

When you have cleansed your teeth, it is well to breathe in cold water from a very clean sponge, as much as your nose will hold. Blow your nose and repeat several times. In winter use lukewarm water; when you have a slight cold, use a weak decoction of marsh-mallow roots. These aspirations are excellent for detaching the filth which sometimes lines the nostrils, and it is never necessary to remove it with your fingers. They refresh you, clear your head, and dissipate the dryness which dust or heat may cause in your nose. Marsh-mallow water, or any other emollient, facilitates blowing your nose, and I am persuaded that persons who take snuff by necessity would have been freed from that disagreeable subjection if they had followed the routine which I recommend.

Cut your nails straight, not with scissors, but with a small tool called the knife for cutting the nails. This very modern instrument is flat and sharp at one end; that is the knife. The other end resembles an ear-pick. This is used to cleanse the nails, and the blade forms a small file suitable for wearing away corns.

Inordinate sweating of the armpits stains the under portion of the sleeves and the corresponding part of the gown body. It gives white linen or cotton a yellowish colour and a most disagreeable stiffness. As for coloured materials, especially silk, the difficulty is far worse because sweat, which contains acids, completely destroys the colours. Furthermore, the material always so damp with acid puckers, corrodes, and tears at this place while the gown is still quite new. Your health also suffers from this annoying sweat, because once the sleeves of your shift and the under-arm areas of your stays and gown are soaked, they take a long time to dry in winter, become cold, and cause frequent colds and lively chest pains. What is more, it sometimes happens that this sweat exudes an extremely disagreeable odour, almost like the mephitic vapour of hemp soaking in water. This last case is happily quite rare, but sweat from the armpits incommodes three-quarters of all women.

Several modes are used to combat this inconvenience. Some persons furnish the under parts of the sleeves and the arm-holes of their silk gowns with white glove-leather, cotton wadding, or gummed taffety. In my experience each has its disadvantages. Glove-leather twists, hardens so as to hurt, and produces a rank odour, even when there is no sweat. Cotton wadding is uncomfortably warm, gummed taffety often rots, and when the sweat is of an acrid nature, it smells most unpleasant. Besides, all this serves only to prevent stains, and does nothing to counter the ills which the chest may suffer. I am going to provide a mode of preventing all the inconveniences of sweat at the same time. The simplicity of this mode should not seem unreliable to any but unthinking persons.

As you must guard against arresting the flow of sweat, whose purpose is to excrete hurtful fluids, cleanliness alone can contribute to freeing you from it. Every morning, wash under your arms with lukewarm water. Dry them thoroughly with a linen, which is warmed in winter. When you feel the first effects of sweat, slip a little square of fine linen or batiste over the sleeve gusset of your shift. This little piece, which may be called a removable gusset, should be about four inches in all directions. It is hemmed all round, and in the middle of one of the faces, you put a little piece of flat cord to tie the two gussets together when you want to wash them. You will do well to own a stock, in order to change when you feel them getting damp. In this manner, sweat does not penetrate to your gown, nor even to your stays. It does not remain in such a manner as to chill your skin, and its evaporation, thus encouraged, soon becomes less inconvenient. The contact with white linen, without being cold, sometimes suffices to stop it.

However, baths are also very beneficial for excessive sweat in the armpits, because by facilitating general perspiration they diminish that of this part. If these remedies are insufficient (which occurs only if the flow of sweat is extraordinary) you must wash under your arms again in the evening, and sprinkle them with powdered orris-root, which absorbs the sweat. This last practice is especially appropriate when there is an odour.

Sweating of the hands is very disagreeable, though less so, because it dirties all the work you do, and soils gloves horribly. You may again combat it with cleanliness, and by now and then sprinkling your hands with very dry powdered almond paste.

Sweating of the feet is almost always accompanied by an insupportable fœtid odour, and you must take the greatest precautions against it. Wash your feet with lukewarm water every morning and evening. Put on white stockings every day. Wear slippers of batiste or fine percale, in order to keep your feet from swelling, and renew them every morning. Have an inner sole of napped cotton in your shoe to absorb the sweat. Moisten this sole with Cologne water, lavender-water, mint brandy, &c. Change it frequently (see Chapter IX), and the fœtidness of your feet will first diminish and soon disappear. I do not advise an inner sole of gummed taffety, because this chills the foot too much. An excellent practice is to sprinkle your feet with powder of burnt alum. This powder absorbs the rank odour, and is no obstacle to perspiration. Those of my readers who have experienced this horrible exhalation, will find that these meticulous practices are not too dear a price for ending a veritable infirmity.

Never put your bare feet on the floor. Do not wear backless slippers, for fear of exposing your heels to the cold, and of making them appear larger than the rest of the foot. Constantly wear stockings on the hottest summer days, even in the morning. As custom and cleanliness demand that you wear them during the day, your legs are accustomed to them, and you would experience ill effects from taking them off temporarily. (See Div. 1.)

Never allow your feet to be damp and cold. To manage this, in winter wear cork soles, and especially articulated clogs when you go out. At home, do not keep on the shoes which you have worn outside, even when there is very little mud. The little which there is might produce moisture;

moreover the bottoms of your skirts, which fall over them, will be more or less soiled. Replace the white leather inner soles of your shoes with soles of flannel, or any other woollen material. Shoes so furnished are preferable to fur-lined slippers, which render your feet too sensible to the impression of cold.

Do not use *chaufferettes,* for many reasons. They carry blood to your head, redden your cheeks, and dry and wrinkle the skin of your lower limbs. Moreover, they often give forth a very disagreeable odour, and nothing is more vulgar or in worse taste. You may replace them with *chauffe-pieds à lampe,* which have none of these drawbacks; but when your stockings are warm enough, you should be satisfied with a rug or cushion under your feet.

Woollen stockings are healthful, and you may wear them over poor-quality stockings of very light cotton, in order to prevent the wool chafing you. Yet, as a lady cannot appear any where in this kind of stocking, and it is essential not to pass suddenly from heat to cold, it is better to wear silk, cotton, or even open-work stockings. But in the last case it is important to wear underneath, flesh-coloured silk stockings which give the appearance of a bare leg. You should equally fear having your bed warmed, but with your feet remaining cold. It is well, on retiring, to wrap them in a piece of linen or very warm woollen material.

Hygiene also requires you to keep your forearms warm; it is a means of avoiding chest pains. Flesh-coloured knitted sleeves, which take on the shape of the arms, are worn under sleeves of clear material, accommodating fashion and sense at the same time. Bracelets and cuffs must be very loose, in order not to hamper the circulation of your blood. When they are difficult to put on, be sure your arms will redden, look uncomfortable, lose all grace, and soon become quite painful.

Apropos of that, I cannot say too strongly how wrong ladies are to lace their stays too tightly. A deformed bosom, constrained movements, a stiff waist, reddened skin, a swollen neck, and insupportable discomfort, are the least drawbacks of this pernicious habit. The most painful maladies could result. (See Div. 2.) Chapter VIII gives directions for proper lacing.

According to M. Pierre Pelletan, steel busks merit censure, in that they collect electricity on the bosom and may cause internal irritation there and in the stomach. A whale-bone busk is insupportable because of its stiffness and its disposition to curl at both ends, which becomes truly agonizing if you cannot immediately reverse its direction. And how can that be done when you are visiting, taking a walk, or at a ball? A steel busk is an hundred times better, because the danger is completely prevented by covering it with gummed taffety. If despite the disadvantages of whale-bone busks, some of my readers would like to use them, they may soften and easily straighten these busks by heating them slightly.

After some time the whale-bones placed in the back of the stays take on the curves of your figure and are pushed into your flesh by the action of lacing, like an instrument of torture. When you perceive that they are no longer in a straight line, you must wear your stays wrong side out for a few days: this will be enough to straighten them. If the bones are too curved, take them out of their cases and turn them in the opposite direction, because otherwise the inside of the stays might cause you pain. Thin and delicate persons who are much troubled by whale-bones replace them with a kind of wide braid stiffened with wire. But when the whale-bones are straight and light they are preferable, because they prevent the stays from rising and creasing on the hips, which is extremely painful.

Whatever your desire to raise your bosom and give it conventional beauty, never make the gores at the top of your stays too short. (Chapter XIV gives directions for making stays.) That deforms the bosom to the point of keeping you from fulfilling the dear and sacred duty of nursing your children. While the compression might not have such a disastrous effect, it may furrow your bosom disagreeably with long, whitish streaks. The more fine and delicate your skin, the more it is exposed to these serious drawbacks.

I cannot recommend too strongly to a person whose breasts are too close together, that she place a pad of cotton wadding covered with white glove-leather inside her stays, at the upper end of the busk pocket. It is a means of preventing the painful rubbing continually produced by the two corners of the busk. I advise all ladies to put a similar pad at the lower end of the busk, the leather of which is first sewed over the end of the stays, and the part padded by the cotton placed at the end, and a little under the busk. This measure will prevent you from feeling the busk pressing on your thighs and injuring them every time you lower yourself to sit down.

A very elegant lady whom I once knew had the habit of placing two broad tapes on the straight-way of the stomach gores of her stays; the tapes were passed through a loop, also of tape, sewed to each of her stockings for this purpose. (See Chapter XIV.) These kinds of garters were intended to prevent the stays from working up on her hips; they held them so effectively that you could not do better. But that was not the only good result of this practice; it dispensed with ordinary garters, which are always hurtful to the circulation of the blood. If you adopt it, you ought to furnish all your stockings with loops to the right and left of the seam. At a pinch, one loop for each stocking will answer; but if when you put them on, you mistakenly put the loop on the inner side, you will be obliged to change the stockings about.

Your shifts should not be too ample, because then they produce folds under the stays, which are most annoying and mark your skin. For this reason, shifts should be made of very supple, very fine material. For some time, new linen shifts should be worn only in bed; percale has not this disadvantage. It is well known that linen shifts are proper for summer, and percale or fine calico ones for winter. It is a popular error to believe that cotton is injurious to the skin. In England, where the skin is so beautiful, and in the United States, they use no other material.

It is a very healthful practice to alternately wear a night shift and a day shift, because each is spread out in turn to evaporate sweat and all the emanations of your body, which otherwise would be reabsorbed by your pores. Decency also requires you to follow this mode, because then you are not obliged to examine yourself, to strip yourself almost naked in order to get rid of certain troublesome insects. Immediately after changing, you may search for them without difficulty in the shift you have just left off.

——*Manuel des dames.*

Diversion 1.

Clothing in regard to Health. It is evident that clothing ought to be accommodated to different ages, habits of life, climate, season, and state of health. With regard to the different periods of life, children should from their birth be habituated to light clothing, not only by day but by night; for nothing contributes more to form the constitution. Infants and children are less apt to have their perspiration checked than persons who are more advanced in life, and therefore less apt to catch cold. From the stage of childhood to the thirty-fifth year, the strength of the vital powers and a brisk circulation, tend very much to keep up an equal perspiration. But after that period, the force of the circulation being lessened, the clothing by day and the covering by night, should be gradually increased.

Climate and season of the year ought certainly to have clothing suited to them; but in England's unsteady climate, it is very difficult to accommodate them to the sudden changes. Upon the whole, however, after the age of thirty-five, it may be better to exceed rather than be deficient in clothing. If persons have been accustomed to warm clothing, there will always be hazard in sudden changes of any kind. Those who clothe and sleep warmly ought not to indulge in hot close rooms during the day, nor have fires in their bed-chambers. Those who have resided long in hot climates, when they come into this country, should rather exceed in their clothing.

With respect to the state of health, to persons of hale constitution and in high health, very warm clothing in the day or covering at night, would be very improper. Their vital powers being strong, and the circulation vigorous, the warmth and steady perspiration on the surface and extremities resist the impressions of cold or moisture, unless they are very violent.

Such persons, however, relying too much on the strength of their constitution, often expose themselves imprudently, and as the violence of the disease is in general in proportion to the vigour of their vital powers, so it is frequently rapid in its progress, and fatal in its termination. The grand rule is to regulate your clothing and covering so that when you expose yourself to the external air, the difference of the temperature of the air in both situations is such that you will not be susceptible of dangerous impressions under any inclemency of season when you go abroad. Persons in firm health ought to regulate the temperature within doors, so that it does not exceed 56 degrees of the thermometer in the winter, spring, and autumn; and in the summer, bring it as near to that as possible, by the admission of fresh air.

To render Cloth Water-proof according to the Manner of the Chinese. By the following very simple process for making cloth water-proof, it is asserted that the Chinese render not only the strongest cloths, but even the most open muslins, impenetrable to the heaviest showers of rain. Nor yet, it is said, will this composition fill up the interstices of the finest lawn, or in the slightest degree injure the most brilliant colours.

The composition to which these valuable qualities are imparted, is merely a solution of an ounce of white wax in a pint of spirit of turpentine. In a sufficient quantity of this mixture, made with these materials, immerse the articles intended to be rendered water-proof, and then hang them to dry in the open air, until they become perfectly dry.

This is all the process necessary for accomplishing so desirable a purpose, against which may perhaps be objected the expense and unpleasant scent of the turpentine spirit. This objection may be remedied by using equal parts of spirit of wine and oil of wormwood, a mixture of which is said to dissipate the smell of the turpentine; but the former, it is not to be denied, must necessarily be at the same time in some degree augmented.

Pliable Varnish for Umbrellas. Take any quantity of caoutchouc, for instance ten or twelve ounces. Cut it into small bits with a pair of scissors, and put a strong iron ladle (such as painters, plumbers, or glaziers melt their lead in) over a common pit-coal or other fire; which must be gentle, glowing, and without smoke. When the ladle is hot, put a single bit into it. If black smoke issues, it will presently flame and disappear, or it will evaporate without flame: the ladle is then too hot. When the ladle is less hot, put in a second bit, which will produce a white smoke; this white smoke will continue during the operation, and evaporate the caoutchouc. Therefore, lose no time, but put little bits in, a few at a time, until the whole are melted; it should be continually and gently stirred with an iron or brass spoon.

The instant the smoke changes from white to black, take off the ladle, or the whole will break out in a violent flame, or be spoiled, or lost. Care must be taken to add no water, a few drops only of which would, on account of its expansibility, make it boil over furiously, and with great noise. At this period of the process, put two pounds, or a quart of the best-drying oil into the melted caoutchouc, and stir it until hot, and pour the whole into a glazed vessel through a coarse gauze or wire sieve. When settled and clear, which will be in a few minutes, it is fit for use, either hot or cold.

The silk should always be stretched horizontally by pins, or tenter-hooks on frames (the longer they are the better) and the varnish poured on cold in hot weather, and hot in cold weather. It is perhaps best always to lay it on when cold. The art of laying it on properly consists of making no intestine motion in the varnish, which would create minute bubbles. Therefore, brushes of every kind are improper, as each bubble breaks in drying, and forms a small hole through which the air will transpire.

This varnish is pliant, unadhesive, and unalterable by weather.

——*The Alphabetical Receipt Book and Domestic Advisor.*

Diversion 2.

Stays. Besides the pressure on particular parts, and the injury consequent upon it, stiff stays act in the same manner as shoulder-braces, by preventing the natural and wholesome exercise of the muscles. A recent author (Dr. Dods) has well remarked, that it would be vain to attempt to dissuade ladies from the use of this pernicious article of dress; but however much they may disregard themselves, they ought certainly to reject for their children, whatever will be hurtful to them. Restraint, and particularly that of stays, is almost certain to distort the body during growth; whereas freedom of motion in all its members is the only certain preventive of deformity.

The unfettered Indian females, and even our own peasant girls in many parts of the country, are strangers to twists in the shape, and distortions of the spine; and clearly because they are unfettered by unnatural dress during their growth. They are happily unacquainted with the mechanical modes of producing deformity under the mistaken intention of preventing it. Unfortunately, the idea that the bodies of girls require support during their growth has by time and custom become so firmly rooted in the minds of most mothers, that no persuasion will influence them to give up the practice. The stays which are constructed with whale-bone or steel, must strongly prevent the natural bending of the body. A girl who has her body thus encased in such stiff materials, must suffer much injury from the forced position she is compelled to keep herself in, independent of the uneasiness she often manifests by shrugging and writhing her shoulders. I agree with Dr. Dods, that as the muscles of the spine are kept by stiff stays in a constant state of contraction, and never suffered to relax, they must become disorganized, and deformity of the spine will be produced. Instead of stays being a preventive of distortion, they evidently become a powerful assistant in its production.

It is an interesting fact that M. Portal, one of the most learned physicians of France, found the muscles of the back much larger, redder, and stronger in women who had not worn stays, than in those who had used them. He observes also, that where women who have worn stays from infancy, leave them off at a certain age for greater comfort, they are sure to become distorted; for the muscles have been so weakened by want of use, that when the artificial props are removed, they are no longer capable of supporting the body. We laugh at the folly of the Chinese ladies, who compress their feet until they are unable to walk, and at the Africans, who flatten their noses as an indispensable requisite of beauty. But we are still farther from Nature, when we imagine that the female chest is not so elegant as we can make it by the confinement of stays. Nature accordingly shows her resentment by rendering so many of our fashionable ladies, who thus encase themselves with steel or whale-bone, deformed either in the chest, the shoulders, or the spine.

Portal, however, allows of stays being occasionally worn by aged persons who are very feeble, and even by children; and he is supported in this by the great anatomist Winslow. If stays are worn, and it should be done with great caution, I must altogether prohibit the use of whale-bone or steel as decidedly injurious. The materials should all be elastic, so as to yield to every movement without compressing any part of the body. Dr. Dods recommends stays of fine white woollen stocking-web, doubled, and cut into forms; instead of whale-bone or steel, strips of jean are stitched closely down on both sides, in the places where the whale-bones are usually put. "These give," he says, "sufficient firmness, while the elastic web between them admits of the free motion of the body in all directions. The bosom part may be made as usual, entirely of jean, for the purpose of supporting the breasts." I should advise the addition of pieces of catgut, sewed within the strips of jean; or perhaps the newly-invented process of manufacturing India rubber may furnish something superior to any elastic material hitherto tried.

——*The Art of Beauty.*

Diversion 3.

Padding, Bandaging, &c. to improve the Shape. At Paris, they recommend for beautifying the breasts, the stays of Delacroix, which are light, flexible, firm, and elastic, and adapt themselves perfectly to the shape, so as not to compress nor injure any part. To do this are fitted such paddings as may be required to fill up any deficiency, which ought always to be of the lightest and most elastic materials.

The great danger incident to padding, wherever it may be applied, is precisely the same as that arising from tight bandages, for pressure will have the same injurious effect as tightness, and increase the evil which it is employed to remedy. For the stuff used in padding will press upon the parts under it, and prevent the circulation of the blood, which is so indispensable to supply nourishment for the daily waste of the body. If the blood is prevented from flowing freely and in a full current through the parts, they must pine and decrease for want of nourishment. The effect will be further increased by the waste of the parts immediately under a pad, by the augmented perspiration arising from a greater heat being occasioned by it than by the usual clothing. These are the inconveniences which you must endeavour to avoid in all your contrivances for remedying deficiencies of shape; and unless they are ingenious, considerable injury may sometimes be produced.

If your mistress is a married lady, it is of still greater importance to be careful in the use of padding and bandaging, as the consequence will be of a worse description than when the case is different. During pregnancy, tight-lacing and bandaging, in order to conceal it, or to render the shape as slender as possible, has been known to produce dangerous and fatal inflammations, and you ought to be aware of this, and endeavour to prevent it. It is a singular fact indeed, well ascertained by experience, that so far from reducing the size, tight-lacing and long stays actually increase it; those who dress loosely being uniformly observed to be less incommoded by extraordinary size than those who adopt the opposite plan; Nature, it seems, being determined to award the punishment of disappointment to those who infringe her laws.

——*The Duties of a Lady's Maid.*

Diversion 4.

Advice to Married Ladies. After being confined, it was formerly the practice, and in India is still carried to a most injurious length, to swathe the mother with tight belts and bandages; but this has recently, and so far very justly, been laid aside. The muscles, which have been for several months on the stretch, must unquestionably be relaxed; but so long as the lady is confined to bed, they can require no bandage to support them, as they have no weight to sustain and no effort to make. The case is very different when she begins to sit up, or to rise and move about. At this period, it will be highly necessary to have a binder, or a petticoat with a broad band, tied closely but not tightly, so as to support the weak parts until their usual strength is confirmed. This precaution is most necessary in women of relaxed habit, or who have a pale, bloated, and unnatural plumpness.

——*The Art of Beauty.*

Chapter VIII.
The Art of arranging the Hair, lacing the Stays, Dressing, &c.

Ladies whose pecuniary resources do not permit them to have a hair-dresser every day, or who have only one maid to arrange their hair, form the most numerous class. I could write this article on the art of dressing the hair for them alone, and it would still be very useful; but it should also be of service to wealthy persons. Suppose you will spend some time in the country with friends without being able to bring your maid; or on the day of a grand assembly, the hair-dresser fails to appear and your maid is much occupied. Instead of waiting, losing patience, and arriving too late at the assembly, you may do your part: to dress your hair yourself and enjoy the fruits of your success. (See Div. 1.)

Practical Directions for Hair-dressing.

In speaking of preserving the hair in Chapter I, I have already said that you should avoid using a curling-iron. I repeat this prohibition, but to comply you must arrange your curls in such a manner that they curl easily and for a long time. For this it is necessary that your hair be properly trimmed and curled with curl-papers. (See Div. 2.)

At about three inches from your forehead, part your hair from one ear to the other. Follow a straight line, and throw all the hair on each side of this crossways line to the back of your head, or over your face. Then make a new part through the middle of the first. This lengthways part starts in the middle of your forehead. Some persons place it to the side; I do not advise you to imitate them, because that is less elegant than affected. Next cut the hairs thus parted in the front. As they will be taken up by curling, leave them long enough so that when not curled they reach the middle of your cheek. Understand, however, that this measure is approximate, and that the hair which falls from the middle of your forehead, like that near your ears, is of a less exact length. Moreover, all the hairs are not of equal length. The front curls must be disposed in two rows. The upper row near the part requires that the hair be a little shorter, so that the curls are not confounded with those of the lower row; but this difference is scarcely discernable. It depends largely upon the manner of putting on the curl-papers and of curling.

Do not cut only your front hair, but also habitually trim the back hair. You "point" this; that is, take one lock between the thumb and forefinger of your left hand, and then, holding the scissors a little slanted in your right hand, trim the hairs obliquely, and so to speak one by one. In this manner, the end of each curl will slope off; whereas if cut straight across, the end would be heavy and would prevent the curl from holding.

When your front hair is thus trimmed on the right and left of the part to your forehead, put it in curl-papers in this fashion: cut some tolerably firm, thin paper into little pieces like the point of a *fichu*. Take the lock of hair closest to the lengthways part and the crossways part, draw it aside, smooth it well by passing it between your fingers, then roll it up to the roots in rings placed over each other. Hold it with your left hand, while your right hand reaches for one of the curl-papers and places it crossing slantways under the collected rings. The paper must touch the roots of the hairs. Fold it down to the left, then to the right over the rings, and finish by twisting the end firmly. A properly-placed curl-paper should give way only when you have untwisted the end.

This curl-paper placed, pass on to the next lock of hair, always dividing your hair evenly, so that you have about as much in the second lock as in the first. It is above all essential, in putting in the curl-papers for the upper row, to separate them well from the hair destined to form the curls of the lower row. The shortening of the curls of the first row, as I have said, depends much more upon the curl than the difference in length. It will be necessary to tighten the rings of the first row of curl-papers well, and to raise them to the roots, which you will not quite do for the second row.

Now that almost all the curl-papers are placed, let us take care of the love-lock, namely the little lock of hair which is found very near to the auricle of the ear. Formerly this was cut straight and brought back over the corner of the cheek; then it was cut into a point. At present it is made into a little curl or ringlet, onto which you put a curl-paper. This ringlet, though very pretty, is quite difficult to curl.

Usually the curl-papers are put in at night when you go to bed. Nonetheless, when you wish to dress your hair carefully to go out in the evening, you must put them in some hours before. You may avoid this difficulty by using a *tour roulé,* as described in Chapter I. If your hair is ruffled, that is some locks stick out disagreeably, affix the curl-papers to your forehead by means of a tolerably broad riband, which serves as a bandeau. In that case, the paper of which the curl-papers are made should be thin, to avoid causing a head-ache. Generally water-leaf paper, or any other unsized thin paper, is used.

The mass of hair thrown to the back demands much less care. Untangle and smooth it, always from front to back. Also comb yourself with your head much lowered. For this reason, avoid as much as possible combing yourself after you have been laced, because the pressure of your stays considerably increases the momentary congestion which this movement causes in your brain.

Pull your hair tightly, gathering it on the summit of your head. Hold it there firmly with your left hand; and if you wish to tie it, take with your right hand a black linen or silk cord about a third of an ell long. Lay one end to the right, as near as possible to your head, and hold this end between the third and fourth fingers of your left hand, at the same time as the other fingers of this hand firmly hold the hair. Then with your right hand, turn the cord from right to left, tightening it as much as possible, and finish by tying both ends over the front of your head. After that pass a comb through your hair to even it out.

I recommended in Chapter I that you be careful not to tangle your hair in the knot of the cord. Here I shall explain what I mentioned there on the possibility of dressing your hair *en cheveux,* when your hair, which has fallen out by accident and only partly grown back, can barely form an aigrette above the cord. Take a plait of hair matched to your own. At the end of this plait, where the hairs are sewed together, a black cord is fitted. Attach this cord under the tied hairs, so that you may finish your coiffure with the false plait as successfully as if you were working with your own hair.

Just as commonly, the hair is not tied: you gather it and hold it very firmly in your left hand, twist it with this same hand, and immediately place the comb on it to hold it. Then you make *nœuds d'Apollon,* or Apollo knots; so are called the large loops of hair on the summit of the head. This style has been in fashion for a long time; every one says that it will last, so I shall describe it in great detail. But first I shall say a few words on the coiffures which preceded it, so that in case they return, my readers will not find themselves at a loss. I shall, however, speak only of modern coiffures. (See Div. 3.) The powdered constructions and poufs of our grandmothers are quite unlikely to return, and besides it would be impossible to erect such an edifice by yourself.

Coiffure à Chou. So was called the flat chignon encircled by little plaits of hair formed on the summit of the head. When they have been tied, take a pad of black crape stuffed with cotton wadding or horse-hair. Attach it in front of the hair tied on the summit of your head with two black pins, which at the same time fasten the sides of the pad and the hair on which it rests. Then take from the right and left of the mass of hair, enough to make one or two small plaits, which you allow to fall over your shoulders for the time being. This operation achieved, pull your hair back over the pad, spread it gently, smoothing it with pomatum to make it very glossy, and fasten it with a black pin inserted crossways at the end of the pad. Then bring it back to the other end, to the point where the hair comes together. Attach the hair there again, and if it is long enough to come back over the pad yet another time, part it into two sections which you bring back over the edges or sides of the pad. A black pin holds the end. Then return to the little plaits, and wind them again and again round the pad, or rather the *chou*, because the pad covered with hair is so designated.

Coiffure à Cache-peigne. This coiffure much resembled the preceding one, only the *chou* was less flat, and on the side was placed a great quantity of ringlets, which by falling over the front partly concealed the comb, which accounts for the name of this coiffure. This fashion was very injurious to the natural hair, since the ringlets were necessarily made with a curling-iron; but ordinarily a *cache-peigne* matched to the hair was bought.

Couffure à Chinoise. This ludicrous style elevated the hair quite near the forehead. The hair was bound well and made into seven, or sometimes as many as sixteen or twenty little plaits, which were then crossed over each other by arranging them like so many arches more or less high. The first ones always exceeded the others by at least two inches. Happily this was somewhat hidden by a *cache-peigne*.

Coiffure en Couronne. A simple and graceful coiffure immediately succeeded the ridiculous Chinese style. The hair, tied a little to the back, nearly in the Grecian style, was all plaited at the same time. This large plait formed a coronet, which was joined by a riband bow to the point where the hair was tied. The comb was placed in the middle. Coronets were also made with twisted rather than plaited hair.

Coiffure en Chignon. This style came a little later. The hair was tied at about the summit of the head and well smoothed. A large comb was passed under it to raise it, then the comb was pushed down again. Thus covered, the comb produced a large chignon when the hair was thick.

Fashions for coiffures have also varied for the front of the hair. With the coiffure *à chou,* two tufts of crisp little curls were worn on the forehead. In the middle of these curls, a little above the lengthways part near the forehead, an aigrette was formed. This was a bunch of locks of hair formed into the shape of an aigrette, well frizzed, and with a multitude of little curls. The tufts of little curls on the forehead lasted a long time with the aigrettes. Soon came the fashion of adding long, narrow ringlets towards the ears; the ringlets have ended by adorning the entire forehead.

At the same time, a very pretty kind of coiffure was introduced for young persons. It consisted of dividing the hair so that the lengthways part on the forehead was placed very near to the left ear. The little hair which remained on the side served to make two ringlets. The rest, smooth and quite plain, crossed the forehead, was fastened behind the right ear, and terminated in a ringlet. There was no crossways part, or at least not always. The back of the hair was raised in a coronet or a *torsade.*

Coiffure *à la Ninon.* See Chapter I. This name was also applied to ringlets placed over the nape of the neck. When they were not long, they agreeably adorned the back of the neck, but long ringlets there were so pretentious that they were left to kept women.

Coiffure *à la Nœuds d'Apollon.* Now we have arrived at the current fashion. The hair being tied, comb and smooth it properly. Lift the hair to the left over the flat of your hand, which is held so that the little finger rests crossways on your head in front, and as near as possible to the tied portion. Pass the hair under the little finger, which holds it, and the first loop is made. Then, taking the comb in your right hand, push in the end to the left under the middle of the loop, and close to the hand which holds it and is now gently removed as the comb advances and takes its place. Your hand removed, raise the loop, pulling it slightly by the top, and smooth it with your palm. The hair is now falling from behind to the right. Repeat on this side what you have just done on the left. Hide the ends of the hair either by first attaching them to the middle of the comb with a black pin curved back, and pushing it under the loop to the left, or by withdrawing the comb a little and bringing the ends of hair under it.

When your hair is long, make a third loop between the other two. In this case, you fasten the hair under the middle of the comb with the curved black pin, then bring the end back behind the tied portion. Fasten it securely with several black pins. Medium-length hair which is sufficient for a loop may form this third one, while a false plait makes two others. After you have ended the second loop at the middle of the under side of the comb, bring back the short hairs tied at the back; these form the third loop.

Conceal the pins which hold this loop and the cord which ties the hair, with gauze riband bows, black or matched to your hair; but black seems to me more elegant, and it has the prettiest effect on blond hair. At home two bows ordinarily suffice, one at the back and the other between the two loops of hair. But when you wish to dress your hair to go out, put four or five in the middle, beside the hair loops. Flowers are placed in the same manner, in separate clusters. Later, when discussing curling, I shall explain how to arrange clusters of flowers on the forehead, and how to place garlands.

When you do not tie your hair to arrange the Apollo knots, proceed in the manner which I have just described; but push the comb deeper so that it retains the twist securely, and you must make it hold at the same time the twist and the two loops of hair.

Some ladies who wear false plaits make the Apollo knots separately on the comb, and then place it on their head. They fasten the cords of the plait to the middle of the comb, and finish as usual.

Let us return to the curl-papers. Sometimes you begin by opening them, striking them lightly with the back of the comb in order to detach the hair from the paper. This preliminary operation is especially the custom when the iron has been used. Undo all the curl-papers by untwisting them; mingle all the hair by combing it; follow its curves with the comb, which is inserted and removed rapidly, so as not to uncurl the hair. Next take a lock from the top, as if you meant to put on a curl-paper; then take a comb *à branche,* which is a comb with medium-fine teeth at one end, and at the other end a kind of long handle of the same material as the comb. Use the teeth to gently crimp the lock which is held by the end, between the third and fourth fingers of your left hand. The handle then serves to roll the crimped lock into a long curl, or rounded ringlet. Sometimes the handle is used only to lift the ringlets and put them in place when they are all curled, by means of the fourth finger of your left hand, which has replaced it in curling the ringlets. In either case, proceed to curl your hair as you did using curl-papers; that is, put the curls in two rows, but do not arrange one after the other. Begin with the upper lock next the forehead, but then pass immediately to the lower lock, also close to it on the forehead, and so on to the two sides. Some hair-dressers leave near the ear a lock much longer than the others, and after having made it into a ringlet they lay it crossways on the part made over the same, and consequently above the lengthways curls. The handle of the comb aids in this arrangement, which is pleasing; but you may dispense with it when you wish to put on a hat or a crowning garland.

When all the curls are finished, place to the right and left, near your ears, the combs *à papillottes*. These little combs, three or four inches long, are a very modern invention. They serve to lift the side of the curls to make them form a rounded tuft. These combs are made of tortoise-shell, brown or blond according to the colour of the hair. Persons whose curls lack substance raise their hair over the forehead with similar combs, but the back is seen through the curls, and nothing gives such an ugly effect.

Besides combs *à papillottes,* combs *du cou* have been invented even more recently, for placing at the back of the neck. These little combs are the same height as the first kind, are more or less wide, and are curved. They serve to lift the short hairs which are found under the long ones, towards the nape, and which greatly soil *fichus.* When the coiffure has been finished, comb this hair, which curls naturally. Pass it between your fingers, then insert the comb *du cou* so that the back of the comb is turned towards your nape. Then the little curls so contained cannot reach your neck, but fall back over the comb, and without affectation, agreeably adorn the back of your head.

I said earlier that flowers are put in the curls. It is done in this fashion: on the edge of the crossways part, or even under the end of the loop which should nearly touch the curls, attach a small bouquet similar to those which adorn the Apollo knots. There is no risk that the stem will be seen, because you may easily hide it in the midst of the leaves and curls, which you may stretch and bend at will. The attached flower is passed into the midst of the curls, or to put it more accurately, the curl-papers, because it is better to place it before curling your hair. The coloured buds come just to the edge of your eyebrow and mingle agreeably with the curls. Occasionally flowers are put on both sides, but usually only on the right side.

This year has just seen the arrival of a new style, which is very heavy and unbecoming; but nonetheless it must be mentioned. In place of the ringlets, there are two loops of hair similar to the Apollo knots. Nothing is so easy to make. It is the same mode as for chignons: comb the short hairs in the front well, and push the comb *à papillotes* at the ends underneath, as you do with the large comb which lifts the long hairs at the back. Place the little comb on the side, underneath, in such a manner that it cannot be seen. This fashion is proper only for *négligé.* For dress, place some ringlets to the left, and to the right an Apollo knot of this kind, but with some curls of hair falling over it. The new style also requires you to embellish this large loop with rows of little white pearls. This coiffure with great loops is called *à l'Anglaise.*

When you make your coiffure with gauze biases, dispose them in puffs between the Apollo knots and the loops of hair, by means of black pins which you push in so that they cannot be seen. Three-quarter *fichus* of cachemire gauze are also arranged in this fashion. The narrow border must be shown here and there. The garlands are positioned like a coronet on your forehead, under the curls, or round the Apollo knots, or like a helmet on the side, or even in a semicircle from one ear to the other. Feathers or gilt ornaments are disposed in the same way.

Concerning the Stays.

Let us now examine how you may lace yourself properly, and show off your waist without compressing curves, hampering movement, or injuring your circulation. (See also Chapter XIV.)

Before putting on your stays, begin by spreading out the folds of your shift well, so that they will not trouble you when you are laced. Next arrange the shoulder-straps on the edges of your shoulders; straighten them at the place where they join to the front, if the stays have already been put on. Pull down the stays by the stomach gores, so that they fit your hips well, without working up, and pull the busk by the bottom to prevent it from pressing too much on your bosom. All these adjustments are made while some one is lacing you.

Lacing is done as follows: the lace is always stopped on the right, at the bottom, by a long sliding loop. Begin at the bottom, avoiding tightening as you lace; moreover the lace should be at least two and a half ells long. (See Div. 4.) When all the eyelet-holes have been laced, the stays will be a little loose at the bottom, closer in the middle, and loose again towards the shoulders. It is done thus to render the waist slender, the shoulders broad, and the hips prominent. But in my opinion you should above all not be uncomfortable, and this manner of tightening the middle of the stays squeezes your stomach the most. However, it is well if the top and bottom of the stays are a little looser than the rest.

Next pull your shift, under the stays, not to the middle but to the right and left towards the sleeves, in order that nothing may appear above the edge of the stays. Then put on your petticoat. I have nothing to say about that, except that it is advisable to push the tape which forms the petticoat straps under the shoulder-straps of the stays, because when the straps fall over your arms they cause unbearable pain.

To put on your Gown.

If your gown is of transparent material, you must wear a chemisette. This is like a low-necked gown body in batiste or fine percale, with short sleeves, which fastens at the back. Luxury is exercised to such an extent on this little garment that it is embroidered all round, with very pretty designs adorned with lace, and each rather large point is adorned with Malines or Valenciennes lace. The sleeves are bordered by embroidered cuffs. Aside from these exaggerated ornaments, which may be replaced with a nice cotton tulle cut in points, chemisettes are very useful for hiding the case of the shift, the edge of the stays, and the top of your bosom. They dispense with trimming the neck of the shift as was done formerly. Apropos of that: I very strongly advise you to border your shift with a string-case through which a tape is passed, because otherwise you can scarcely have yourself laced without indecency. If you have very brown skin, wear a flesh-coloured *guimpe* under your clear gowns and *fichus*.

Take particular care when putting on your gown so as not to spoil your coiffure. To achieve this, bend your head low while your maid is holding the top of the gown open over your arms, and slip into it without touching your hair. When you have got into the gown, raise it a little so that it does not drag on the floor, and put on your *fichu*. Note well that I have let the gown precede the *fichu*, though that is contrary to the order of the garments, because it is important not to crumple the *collerette* of the *fichu*, which you are sure to do when getting into the gown if the *fichu* is already there. It is quite enough trouble to preserve your coiffure. However, if the *fichu* has a falling collar, you may put it on first. When your maid has fastened the top of the body, raise the collar so that it is not at all bothersome or creased. Enter a pin crossways in the middle of the waist-band on which your gown is mounted, so that the front does not work up.

Your belt demands attention only when it has riband loops: then it is important, for appearance and sturdiness, that it be placed properly. It must not crease round your waist; it must encircle your waist closely, but without visible strain on the riband; for that, it must be attached evenly. (To attain all this, some seamstresses make a crossways seam in the middle of the belt; this fixes a bias fold.) As for the bow, a pin is put first between the *coques* or loops, to attach them to the belt, and another pin is put in each loop to fix it delicately to the part of the gown body which is close to the belt.

Here is the final touch, so to speak, to give to your toilet: it is a *tournure,* which is a handkerchief which should be put by the end of the lace at the level of your belt. This raises the folds of your gown, and makes them drape agreeably. Since the folds of the skirt are extremely warm, in summer a *tournure* frees you from wearing more than one muslin petticoat, provided that the trimmings of your gown are slightly raised, the material is not transparent, and your shift is long. However, two petticoats of well-starched muslin give body to the gown, and you stay equally cool. In winter, when you wear two petticoats, you might perhaps dispense with the *tournure,* because you should take good care that the addition of the handkerchief is not perceptible. You might be suspected of wearing one of those devices of gummed toile, which form a species of arch which ridiculously thin or even more ridiculously flirtatious women wear behind to create an appearance of plumpness. That is of a kind with false hips, false bosoms, white paint, rouge, and all the pitiable arsenal of despicable coquetry.

To achieve a favourable appearance, pull your gown a little on the sides, smooth it down well over your hips by passing the back of your hand over it several times, and push the tips of your fingers into the folds at the back several times.

Small gauze *fichus* must be twisted, knotted, and one of the ends passed through your belt. I do not see that other clothing requires particular observations, excepting the shawl. The manner of arranging this is by no means a matter of indifference, because it gives a graceful and refined air if it is suitable, and entirely the opposite effect if not. Here is how to proceed: put on the shawl straight, so that the point falls behind to the middle of the body, and gather many folds about your neck; these folds form a roll. Place a pin on the front of each shoulder. Turn round and unroll the folds in the front to drape over your bosom up to the pins. Then arrange your *fichu* nicely above the shawl.

As for the hat, there is no fixed rule. Position it to suit your face, arranging the curls of your hair a little, according to what seems agreeable to you. Above all, avoid even the shadow of affectation. Even though fashion wills it, never place your hat to the side, nor too much towards the back or the front. Let your particular style be one of good taste. In our day there has been invented a kind of semicircle in whale-bone, with a little upright support, covered with black taffety, and finished with a bow of riband similar to the hat trimming. This is fitted to the back of the hat, on the inside at the base of the crown, to force the hat to tip forwards. This device is completely ridiculous, and you should never adopt it, nor any thing which resembles it. A lady's toilet should be as free as possible from all those frivolous accessories of which the evident result is to make her be regarded with pity.

The Choice and Care of the Foot-wear.

Foot-wear should always display a refined neatness. Stockings should be very white and fine; shoes should be closely fitted and well made; together they must perfectly delineate your foot and leg. But in this, as in all things, guard against sacrificing ease and health to elegance, because you expose yourself to the most unfortunate accidents by going directly counter to your purpose. (See Div. 5.) Open-work stockings in winter, which do not have flesh-coloured silk stockings underneath, may sometimes have very dangerous results on the natural order, and at all times on the lungs. Shoes which are too narrow and short cover your feet with corns and calluses, often cause your legs to swell, and render your walk constrained, hesitant, and ridiculous.

The details on foot-wear in Chapters VII and IX free me from expounding much now on this subject. But in what I do have to say, there is some advice which it is well to follow; amongst other things that of never, insofar as possible, wearing shoes of too light a colour, except with full dress. Then they must match the gown, because a light colour contributes to an appearance of large feet. Black or white shoes are the most refined. If you can spend on your foot-wear without being obliged to retrench on more necessary things, do not wear black leather shoes except to go out in winter, because small leather shoes always hurt dreadfully the first time you wear them, and if they are made in such a manner as not to cause pain, they soon enlarge and are distorted soon after. Prunella shoes are far preferable for elegance and convenience, but they wear out at least twice as fast. However, they may be re-covered, as may dancing shoes (see Chapter XVI). In this fashion, with a little skill, you may be shod elegantly and cheaply.

It is well to buy several pair of shoes at a time, by the dozen, for example. You will pay less for them, they will last longer because they will be thoroughly dried, and you may match them properly to your attire. As soon as the shoes are deformed, they must be renewed. You may have them made more or less open according to the shape of your feet. If your feet are small, narrow, and flat, your shoes should be open. In the contrary case, they should be more covered. Laced shoes with a rather large bow are always proper. Shoes which are not laced, without a bow, and with ribands which delineate the leg, are suitable for small feet. Besides, that is the prettiest kind of foot-wear.

The Foot-wear.

Black stockings in winter are in poor taste unless they are silk and worn with a black gown (whether you are in mourning or not). For these you may substitute black gaiters in order to combat cold and mud; but gaiters, though much in fashion, seem heavy and unbecoming to me. (See Div. 6.) However, I advise them in summer for persons whose feet perspire a great deal. The warmth of stockings is uncomfortable, and very often produces a foul odour which should be avoided by any means. I propose therefore that you wear slippers of fine toile, then gaiters of *écru* toile which go up your leg a little higher than ordinarily. In this way you may be cool and quite clean. If necessary, you may change your slippers twice a day. This, moreover, is a good economy in washing, because it is necessary to change your stockings every day, and the gaiters may serve at least a fortnight.

Boots do not appear to me to be very becoming foot-wear. You should wear them, I think, only when the bottom of your leg is too stout; they are a means of concealing this fault a little. But be careful never to tighten them too much, for your leg would swell. Even the colour should contribute to a more slender appearance. When your leg is too spindly, it is quite the opposite. When walking, raise your gown only a little above your ancle, and as the rest of the leg is not seen, it is supposed to be slender, and altogether well made. Only, it is necessary to take more precautions not to get filthy.

Observe that your stockings fit precisely. If they are too long, you are forced to turn the toe under the sole of your foot. That is extremely uncomfortable and contributes to enlargement. Besides, the stocking forms crossways creases on your instep, which take away all its grace and which soon cut. Stockings which are too short or narrow are also unbecoming and annoying. In the first place, they squeeze your toes and make them appear crooked; in the second, they wear on the skin of your instep, reddening it, and making criss-cross marks which may be seen through open-work stockings. Then the open-work material in its turn pulls excessively, becomes strained, and does not suffer the design to be seen. It is needless to add that stockings which do this continually wear out twice as fast as any others.

When your calf is very stout and your knee small, as sometimes happens, you should wear two pair of garters, one above the knee and the other below, so that the stockings are properly supported. Garters with slip-knots are very good for the first pair (see Chapter XX). I once knew an elegant lady who always gartered herself in this fashion.

——*Manuel des dames*.

Diversion 1.

The Dressing-room. It is necessary for a dressing-room to be more or less decorated with mirrors, and large enough so that three persons may be there at their ease. The hair-dresser is the one who has the most need of space, especially if the person has long hair. The dressing-room must be well lighted, without false light, with windows which do not directly face any others, and furnished with a fire-place for warmth and other purposes. The dressing-room should be situated in the part of the house which is most sheltered from cold, so that when you are not well clothed you cannot take cold; which often happens even though there is a fire in the fire-place. You must never expose yourself to draughts, which are always injurious to the health.

There are dressing-rooms which are more or less elegant. Some persons have their dressing-room hung with drap, to prevent dampness; others have many mirrors and toile hangings. It is advisable to have a carpet the size of the room, but an oil-cloth with designs may replace that ornament: this is entirely a matter of taste. It is essential to have a cheval mirror or a toilet-table. If you prefer the cheval mirror, it must be accompanied by a table where you place every thing which you may need. If you prefer the toilet-table, you do not need a separate table; put each object in the most suitable and convenient place.

If you are travelling, you must have a complete toilet-case; there are some which are more or less so. When travelling, leave the articles just as they are arranged in the case. When you are at home, place them on the table.

——*Art de se coiffer soi-même.*

Diversion 2.

Divers Operations of Hair-dressing. In Fig. 1, *A* shows how to hold the comb. *B* shows how to comb yourself. *C* shows how to put on the curl-papers. *D* shows how to pass the curling-iron over the curl-papers. *E* shows how to raise your hair. *F* shows how to put in the ornamental comb. *G* shows how to divide your hair. *H* shows how to frizz your hair. *I* shows how to form a loop and place a pin. *J* shows how to add flowers to your coiffure.

——*Art de se coiffer soi-même.*

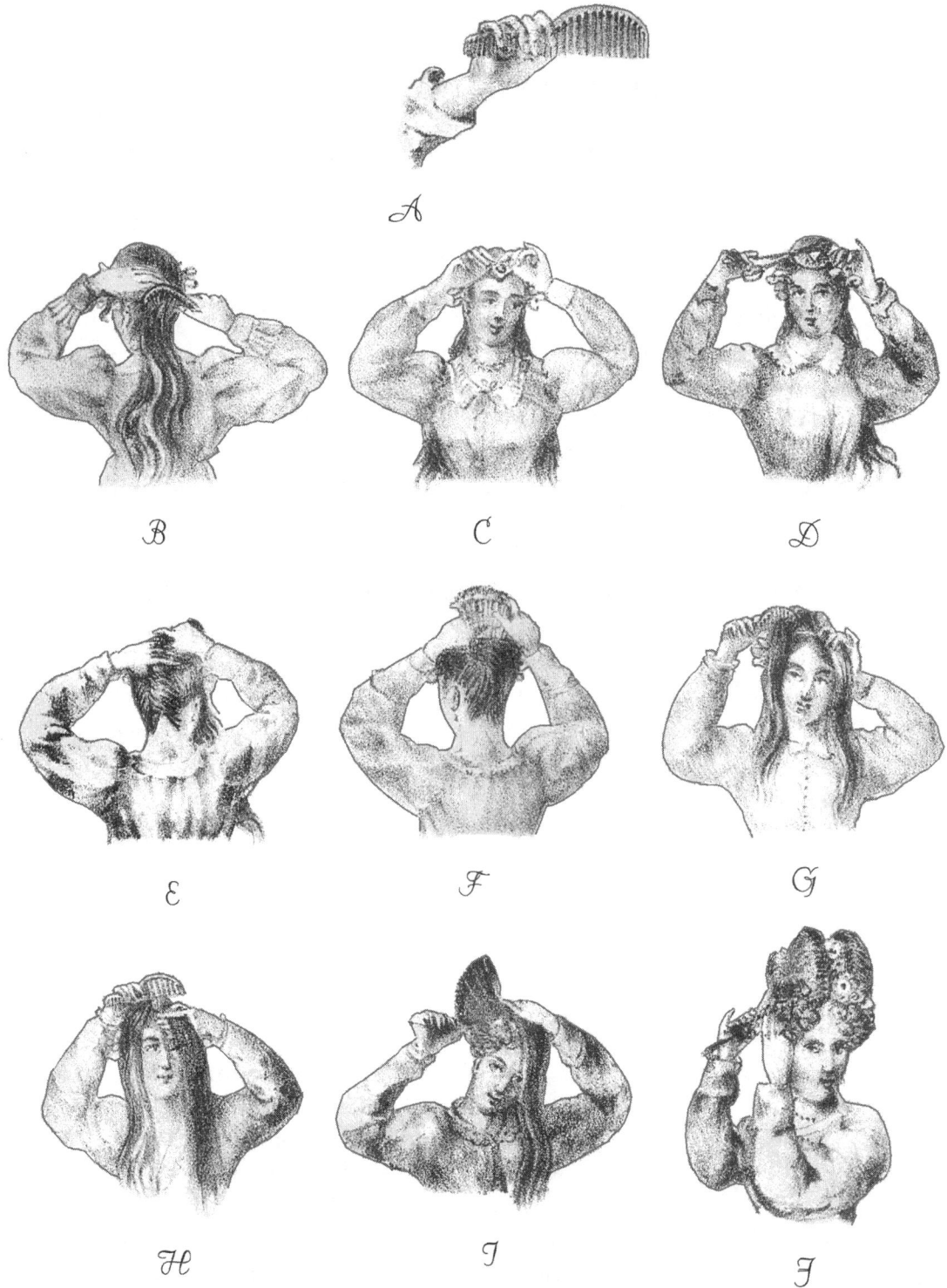

Figure 1. Illustrations of hair-dressing.

Diversion 3.

Fashions in Hair-dressing. For March 1824: balls and evening dress parties follow each other in gay succession, and beauty gains fresh attraction from elegant and tasteful costume. The matron who is yet young enough to share in the festive scene is distinguished by towering plumes, either nodding over the Highland cap, or drooping from the opera hat or costly turban; from the latter head-dress they fall gracefully over the left shoulder.

It is almost impossible to describe the many different ways which young ladies have of arranging their hair; what is becoming to the features and shape of the head seems most generally to prevail. If any one peculiar style is preferred, it is that of disposing the locks in numerous little ringlets. This is becoming to almost all *young* faces, but the lady of a certain age should never adopt it, as hers will be regarded as the "golden hair of Stella"—only "hers because she *bought* it!" Diadems, strings of pearls, and flowers should be lightly disposed amongst the ringlets above mentioned.

May 1824. Hair arranged in full curls, and adorned with bunches of grapes and very small down feathers, forms a favourite head-dress for the ball-room. However, very young ladies have their hair simply ornamented with flowers. Young married ladies add a bandeau of pearls or precious stones, which is bound across the forehead. Sometimes the married lady has a head-dress *à l'Inca,* viz., a bandeau of plain gold surmounted by flat feathers.

July 1824. Young ladies wear their own hair with wreaths of flowers, or sometimes the hair alone, very beautifully arranged in curls, braids, and bows, where the length and abundance of the tresses will admit. This does not look well on a short figure. Such should always have their hair prettily cropped and dressed in curls all over the head *à l'enfant;* and some very elegant, but not tall ladies have adopted this fashion.

November 1824. The hair continues to be arranged in large curls, in clusters on each side of the face, divided from the summit of the head by two small combs, exclusively adapted for that purpose. Very young ladies wear no other ornament. Young married women adorn their heads chiefly with flowers of a rich winter hue, intermixed with diadem combs or bandeaux of pearls, according to the style of dress they wish to observe and which etiquette demands. Plumage, either with diamonds in full dress, or with evening turbans and toques, seems confined now to the more matronly.

January 1827. Some young ladies, in spite of the predominance of large curls, have their hair arranged in a more becoming manner. The curls, it is true, are large, but they do not lie over the face in that wig-like way now so prevalent, but are relieved by two straight bands of hair on each temple. Above are large, but very light curls, with five large bows or puffs of hair, amongst which are placed Chinese roses.

The hair of the French ladies is now arranged in full curls on the temples, but not too large, and is very becomingly separated on the forehead. A large bow of hair on the summit of the head appears in the front. When young ladies wear their tresses disposed in this way, they ornament them with full-blown roses; yet these are often of the fancy kind, blue and yellow.

September 1827. Young ladies wear their hair parted on the forehead, with not quite so many curls on the temples as last month, but with very large ones brought together on the summit of the head. Not but what some clusters are yet preserved on each side of the face; but they are short at the ears, and an infinite number more on one side than on the other.

October 1827. Young ladies wear their hair well arranged, but not quite with the simplicity which prevailed last month. During the warmth of the summer months, the braids across the forehead were certainly the best. But now, when there is no fear of either heat or damp, the curls again appear in numerous clusters round the face. Some young ladies, who seem to place their chief pride in a fine head of hair, have such a multitude of small ringlets that they give to what is a natural charm, all the poodle-like appearance of a wig. The bows of hair are elevated on the summit of the head, and confined by a tortoise-shell comb.

November 1827. The hair is disposed in various ways; and the fair one seems as she ever ought to do, to study the effect given to her features. Regularity of a fine Roman contour of visage looks best in something of a dishevelled style, with ringlets depending over the ears, and a few gracefully shading the neck behind; while the longer tresses braided together, surround the summit of the head and are placed rather backwards. The round-faced beauty, whose charm is prettiness of countenance, appears to most advantage with full clusters of curls on each side of her face, short at the ears, and the longer tresses drawn up tight from the nape of the neck. When she is short of stature, however, she looks infinitely better with the hair tastefully cropped.

January 1829. The hair is arranged in various ways, though amongst the young it is disposed very much in the Vandyke style. Yet there are many ladies, especially of more mature age, who still persevere in patronizing the large curls next the face, though certainly these are less preposterous than formerly. They are often adorned by having puffs of coloured gauze or silver flowers mingled amongst them.

Young ladies wear their hair at the theatres and musical parties without any ornament, except sometimes a few bows of riband, or two or three strings of pearls. The hair is arranged according to what is most becoming to the features, in corkscrew ringlets, curls, or Madonna braids; and the plait which forms the Apollo knot is placed more forwards or backwards as may best agree with the length or shortness of the visage. A lady was remarked at the theatre with her hair arranged *à la Grecque,* with antique fillets of Greek blue and amber riband wound amongst the tresses at the back of the head.

February 1829. The hair is now arranged with the most beautiful diversity, so that it is not easy to say which is the decided fashion. Bows and puffs of hair, in general, adorn the summit of the head. Yet some young ladies compose the Apollo knot of braids or plaits, and twist them round and round until they form a kind of coronet on the back part of the head. One side of the face is ornamented with rich clusters of curls, the other with corkscrew ringlets, which fall as low as the throat. It is separated from the forehead by a Madonna band, which descends no lower than to the commencement of each temple, from whence the curls and ringlets begin. Bows of silver or coloured gauze riband are often mingled amongst the tresses, and flowers in greater profusion than have been seen for some time.

September 1829. The hair is arranged in ringlets or clustered curls next the face, as best accords with the fancy or features of the wearer. Plaited braids and bows adorn the summit of the head. A few flowers are interspersed with the tresses on particular occasions; but according to that simplicity of style usually observed in the country during the summer months, young ladies seldom add any ornament to the native beauty of a fine head of hair, well dressed.

Full-blown Provence roses are very favourite flowers on the hair of young persons. The Apollo knot on the back and summit of the head is formed of a plait wound twice round. Two puffs of hair surmount this ornament, above which are often placed pomegranate blossoms and poppies. At rural balls, young married ladies who wish to distinguish themselves from young single ladies, wear dress hats with two long white feathers. These, continually agitated by the dance, stand up towards the crown, where they often turn back. Hair arranged in bandeaux *à la Madonna* is now very much in vogue; and the hinder tresses are fastened up with a tortoise-shell comb with a very high gallery.

October 1829. The hair is dressed very high on the summit of the head; two bands of hair cross the forehead, and three loops approach very near the summit. A wreath formed of wheat-ears, corn poppies, and blue-flowers surrounds the head, with a small sheaf of corn on the summit. Chains *à la chevalière* are often wound round the head, and are at present a favourite ornament; they are of gold, enamel, or differently-coloured stones. Another accessory on a head-dress of hair is formed of green foliage and the winter cherry.

November 1829. Head-dresses of young females, consisting of their own hair, are arranged in various ways. Some wear it somewhat in the Madonna style, but not exactly, as the present way consists of parting the hair but very slightly on the forehead, and then forming it into two bands which are almost transparent, and these are so short that they terminate at the temples. The remainder is then carried upwards, and forms a bow on the summit of the head, where a braid closely plaited from the long hair behind winds round at the back of the bow, and finishes a coiffure very becoming to good features, a good complexion, and a youthful countenance. Other young ladies, equally moving in fashionable life, wear their hair almost concealing their faces, hanging down on each side in dishevelled ringlets—this is by no means unbecoming to seventeen. A young married lady was observed with her hair arranged in curls and bows in a truly elegant manner, and on the right side of her head was a full-blown Japanese rose, the glowing red of which well accorded with her ebon tresses.

——*Lady's Pocket Magazine.*

Diversion 4.

To unlace your Stays. To unlace yourself, pull the bottom loop of the lace, because by unlacing the stays from the top you would have too much lacing to pass back through each eyelet-hole. Besides, the tag would strike you, and might come loose. The bottom of the lace entails no such inconvenience.

——*Manuel des dames.*

Diversion 5.

Ill-fitting Shoes. Nearly nine-tenths of mankind are troubled with corns; a disease which is seldom or never occasioned but by straight shoes; and it may be added, that the remaining tenth do not envy their fellow-creatures for this modern improvement. The shoes formerly worn, but now out of fashion, showed people's good sense, and their attention to health and comfort. Those who wear small and short shoes are and ever will be exposed to many disappointments and inconveniences, by being deprived of both exercise and pleasure; independent of disposing them to gout and rheumatism and dropsy. Many persons, in fine, by wearing short and cramped shoes have been deprived of the use of their legs; and the pain of the more virulent species of corns, as well as that of the nails, when grown into the flesh from the same cause, is most excruciating.

——*The Toilette of Health, Beauty, and Fashion.*

Diversion 6.

To make Gaiters. For some time now, people have been wearing little gaiters which are very charming, but which cost extremely dear bought ready-made. Those made of canvas cost seven francs; and you may, by making them yourself, have three pair for that price, since only a quarter of an ell of canvas is required for each pair. The prettiest colour is dust-grey.

Taking the measures for gaiters and cutting them out by those measures is a very difficult thing to do. You will succeed much better and more easily by taking a paper pattern from a gaiter which you have unpicked; then it is much easier to remedy the defects.

Gaiters are composed of six pieces (see Fig. 2). All these pieces are cut along the straight-way; the selvages must be placed along the leg. The largest piece is the one which encircles the leg; it is slit in order to receive a gore. In A, cc', cc' shows the seam folds where the gore in two pieces is sewed. C shows only the half; to form the gore, the part shown by C must be doubled. C, c is the top of the gore, and d is the bottom; rs is the edge which will be sewed along cc' in A. C, e is the curve which contains the top of the foot; f is the end of the gore which falls onto the upper of the shoe; vx is the strip of leather which serves as the under strap. This leather must be very thick but flexible; ordinarily buffalo-hide is chosen.

To make Gaiters.

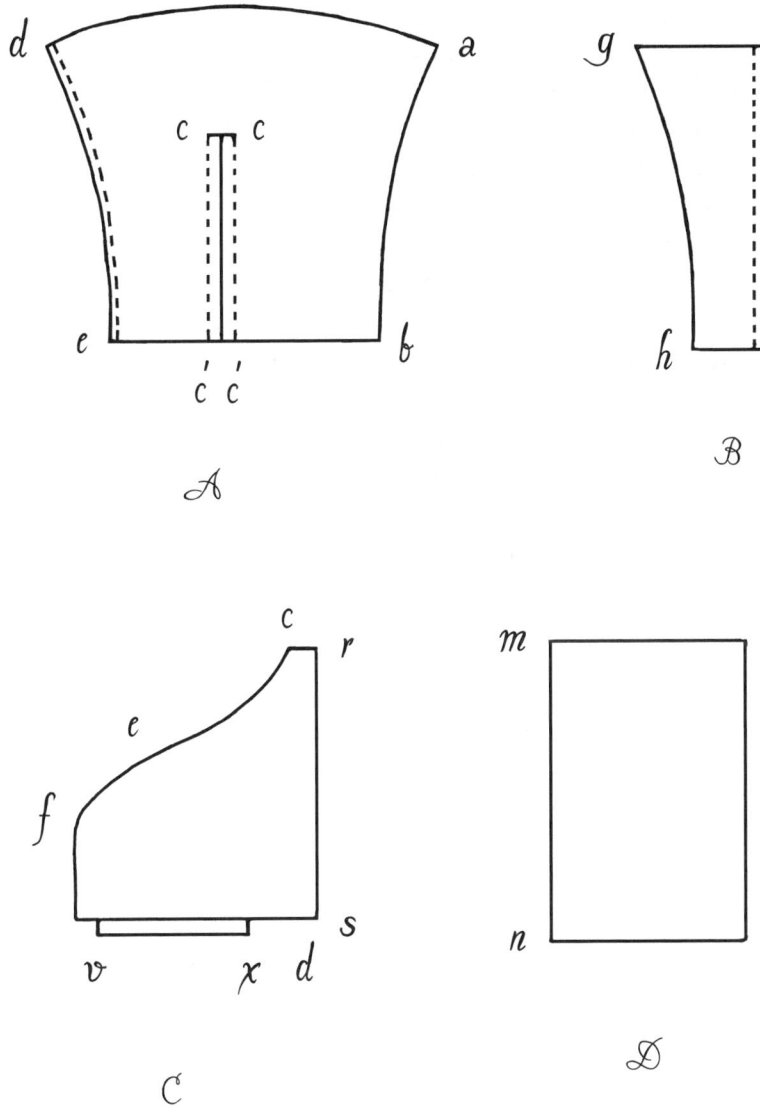

Figure 2. The parts of a gaiter.

In *B*, *gh* is the small band which is fixed along *ab* in *A*. They are sewed together with back-stitches made on the reverse side of the gaiter, like all the other seams. Pay attention that the widest ends of all the pieces are placed at the top of the gaiter. A piece of the same material is attached along *de*, only twice as wide as the strip shown by *B*; see *D*. This piece, called the tongue, serves as a loose lining for the two edges with eyelet-holes, in order to prevent the stocking from showing through the eyelet-holes.

Work all the seams of the gaiter from the inside. Since it is lined, make a narrow seam fold all round the gaiter, onto which you place the lining, which you fasten on top with side-stitches which go through to the right side of the gaiter. You may make there a row of prick-stitches spaced two lines from the side-stitches.

When these seams, as well as the edges, are finished, pierce the eyelet-holes the same way as for stays (see Chapter XIV). The eyelet-holes must be pierced very near to the edge and very close to each other; they must not be finished like those of stays. Take very little material on the needle, and make a fine *cordonnet*. Observe that the gaiter must be laced starting at the bottom.

When you have finished all of the above, place the under strap. Baste it very firmly, so that you may try it on to see if it is too large or small. Above all, try on the gaiters over the shoes which you will wear with them. The gaiters must look as if glued to the foot.

——*Art de faire les corsets, les guêtres, et les gants.*

Chapter IX.
Of the Order and Cleanliness which must preside over the Concerns of the Toilet.

I have too good an opinion of my readers to believe they will find this chapter too detailed and redundant. Doubtless most of the tasks which I shall describe are long-time habits for them, but amongst the great number of tasks, there may be some of which they are ignorant. By admitting the opposite possibility, I still do not fear to weary them, because order has such a charm of its own that they will enjoy reading about the routines which they follow every day. Even when it is otherwise, they will approve of my having included these lessons, thinking they may be useful. In any case, these directions will be perfectly suitable for their maids. (See Div. 1.)

To cleanse the Toilet Articles.

When you have just combed your hair, washed your face, &c., immediately take care of cleansing and arranging all the objects which you have used. Wash your sponges by immersing them in lukewarm water, and squeeze them out well between your hands. Then hang them from a nail in an inconspicuous corner of your dressing-room, by means of a cord which you have passed through each sponge. Despite daily washing, sponges acquire a blackish colour at the end of a certain length of service. Once a month, it is well to soak them for two or three hours in bleach diluted with water. Then wash them thoroughly and squeeze them in hot water to rid them of all the bleach, which might be injurious to your skin. You may also soap them.

Next set about cleansing your combs and hair-brushes. To this end, place the basin in which you wash your hands, on your knees or your toilet-table. Then take one of your combs and the small brush, and run the bristles of the brush between the teeth of the comb several times. Vigorously brush both sides of the comb. A more or less black and greasy powder will come out and fall into the basin. Some persons cleanse their combs over a towel; but the towel may be used only for this purpose and it needlessly multiplies the toilet linens, whereas the basin dries by itself. When the comb has been well cleansed with the brush, rub it with a piece of woollen material, in order to keep it as polished as if it were new. That done, pass the hair-brush several times over a towel or a dry sponge. Rub the back of it with the woollen material to maintain its varnish, then place the brush on the toilet-table, resting on its back. Plant the well-cleansed comb in it so that it does not exceed the end of the brush, if necessary extending beyond the roots towards the handle.

Cleanse all your combs like the first, and plant them thus in the brush, excepting the ivory fine comb, because the rice roots of which the brush is formed would be too coarse for its teeth and would spread them apart undesirably. You may store this comb apart in a little toile bag. Pushing the other combs into the brush is a very sound practice. It prevents them from being dropped and from broken teeth, and contributes further to de-greasing them, because the rice roots finish by taking off any filth which may have been left. It is better to put curved combs on a round brush, though when necessary they may very well be placed on an ordinary brush.

The small brush with which you cleanse the combs becomes soiled very quickly, so that after some time the greasy filth which it removes from the combs sticks to the bristles, fills up the spaces, and makes the brush stiff as a board. You may keep it from getting this soiled, but only by cleansing it in its turn with a rough box-wood comb. Each time that you comb through the bristles, wipe them with a linen cloth. Still, despite these measures, you will be obliged now and then to dismantle the brush and boil it in a strong solution of soap. I say that you dismantle the brush because it is, for this purpose, composed of two parts, the small handle and the block of bristles. These are joined together by a screw, and you have only to turn the little block of bristles to the left to detach it. You may then boil it, making it almost like new, then rejoin it to the handle by turning it to the right.

Now it remains only to rub the flasks, glasses, toothpicks, tweezers, and the knife for cutting your nails; in short all the little things which you have used. Put your curl-papers in a pasteboard box so as to be able to reuse them at night until they are worn out. Tightly close the boxes and packets which contain your cosmetics. (See Div. 2.) Carefully collect the black pins for your hair, and push them into their pincushions. Pass and repass the black cords which tie your hair through a linen, so that they do not become greasy. Fold or spread out towels, combing mantles, &c. to remove any dampness. Arrange all this in order on the toilet-table, then rub once or twice the glass in front of which you dress your hair, cleanse your teeth, &c. If you use a toothbrush, you will have sprayed forth a fine rain, coloured by the powder into which you dipped the end of the brush. Even when, as I strongly suggested in Chapter II, you replace the brush with a sponge, the vapour of your breath, the lukewarm water, and the particles of greasy dust released when you cleanse your combs, all require you to rub the inside of your toilet-table well. If you do not want to take all these little tasks upon yourself, charge your maid with them; but watch her work, for if some of these little steps are neglected, uncleanliness is introduced; and that is a crime in the toilet.

Directions for the Garments which you are putting on or taking off.

When you mean to dress, commence by taking out all the articles of attire which you want to put on, arranging them according to their kind upon the bed, or instead on a sopha. The petticoats and gown must be unfolded, spread out, and draped. Arrange the mantle in the same fashion. The shawl, which is always folded in a square in the armoire in order that the diagonal fold given while wearing it does not end by forming a worn streak on the bias, should receive this fold and be draped over one of the cushions or bed pillows.

Turn the stockings inside out, the feet inside the legs, and lay them near each other. Place the shoes near by, along with a shoe-horn. Spread the stays in the middle of the furniture, inside out, and bring the two backs together so that they appear right side out. The lace must be placed near by, arranged in loops, one over another, the way some knitters wind off their cotton.

Spread the *fichu* widthways and inside out on the furniture, in order not to crumple the *collerette* or other trimmings. The chemisette, spread out widthways like the stays, must be near by. If the belt has a bow, raise the loops and place it flat on the furniture. If it has a metal buckle, put the prongs through the eyelet-holes, taking care that the points are not turned to the back. Spread it out folded in half, putting the end opposite to the buckle on the furniture.

Place the cap towards the back of the furniture, being careful that nothing crushes its trimmings or riband bows. The handkerchief is brought out and either folded in a square opened so as to show the corners, as I shall explain later, or it may be unfolded and arranged in a cone *à tuyaux*, whether it is embroidered or not. I prefer the latter fashion, as much less pretentious. The bag is put near the handkerchief; it is needless to describe how if it is simple and untrimmed. If it is embellished with ruches, bows, points, or puffs, it is better to suspend it by the handle from the casement or the corner of a chair, after having delicately raised the trimmings. As for gloves, blow into them if they are new, and stretch out the fingers if they have already been worn.

Lift the hat from its box last, and place it on a wooden mushroom, which is used for nothing else. In putting the hat on this form, or in passing by it, you may knock the hat out of shape, or crumple the ruches and other trimmings. It is even advisable to take it delicately by a loop, or a riband end, to lift it from its box or form. If it must have a veil attached at the base of the crown, attach this before putting on the hat. If the veil has no drawing-strings, throw it over the hat when it is on your head. Jewels should remain in their box, from which you take them when you have need of them.

You thus arrange, or have arranged for you, the parts of your clothing when you dress finely. Ordinarily fewer tasks are necessary, but it is always done in much the same way. If the articles are not properly prepared according to their kind and the order in which you put them on, you risk creasing them and mislaying one or the other, which takes away much of their freshness, and causes you much impatience and wasted time.

As you remove your clothes, first spread them on the settee, the bed, or the chairs. Then see to folding them and replacing them in the armoires and chests of drawers, as I shall explain later. If you must wear these garments the next day, pile them on top of each other on the stuffed part of a chair. Here is the way to do it: fold the petticoats in quarters. The gown is folded in the same way, unless it is ornamented by flounces, rouleaux, or any other trimming which is starched or stands out, in which case you should spread it out, draping it over the back of a chair. Fold the shawl according to its size in halves or quarters, leaving the existing diagonal fold in place. The *fichu* is hung, unless it is a three-cornered one of linen or organdy. Roll up the stays, with the lace near by wound into a ball, or tied into bows forming long loops. The belt is folded or rolled up. Fold the stockings in half, one upon the other; place the garters on the stockings. The shoes are placed next each other on the floor by the edge of the chair, the strings collected inside so as not to trail and trip you up. In this fashion you will prevent all accidents which damage your things; your clothing is orderly and ready to hand and your bed-chamber, though differently arranged, is as tidy at night as during the day.

Your night-clothes should be arranged in the same order. Fold the night jacket in quarters, with the sleeves folded upon themselves, and the night shift in the same way; then the night-cap and *serre-tête* or bandeau, folded crossways, is placed upon the night jacket. If the weather, habit, or some indisposition makes you wear a double *fichu* of muslin over your night jacket or night shift, the *fichu* must be folded in a square and placed in front of the caps. It is better to take the trouble of folding and unfolding it night and morning, than to leave it in the diagonal fold, because a continual fold will before long produce a worn streak, and the streak will tear.

It is well to have near your night-clothes, but in a separate place, a square piece of linen, such as a handkerchief, or a little hand-towel with which you wipe your feet at night. This practice is above all indispensable for persons whose feet perspire. This foot cloth should be renewed often.

Even though your day-clothes are folded and arranged in good order at night, it is well to prepare them anew in the morning. Unfold them, and take the gown and petticoats to the open window to shake out the dust. If they are of merino or some other woollen material, you should brush them; if they have any creases, you should iron them. You may, however, be satisfied with spreading the petticoats out on a table, repeatedly passing your hand over the creases, and putting something heavy upon them, such as a large book. At the same time see if the clothing has any spots on it, and remove these at once, with the usual modes (see Chapter X). Examine the *agrafes*, cords, trimmings, and all the things which often need mending, and if there are a few stitches to take, proceed instantly. Also observe that the *fichu* and the cap are not crumpled, because if the fluting is mussed, you should goffer it. Moreover, clean and elegant ladies are in the habit of having their gowns (except those of silk or woollen), *fichus*, and caps ironed and goffered every time they put them on.

Shake out the stockings, and strike them several times gathered in your hand, the better to remove the dust. It is needless to take this trouble in summer, when you should change your stockings every day, but in autumn and winter it is indispensable. Persons who may wear their stockings for two days in summer must not fail, the second day, to cleanse them as I have just explained.

Shoes require particular tasks. Brush them every morning, even when you have not gone out the day before. The sole must be scraped with a knife, to remove the dirt which more or less always clings to it. Now and then it is proper to examine whether the strings and the binding of the shoe, principally that of the back of the heel and the corners over the toes, are in good shape. If they are not, take care of renewing them, as described in Chapter XVI. (All this advice is principally intended for maids, but I address it to ladies so that they may see it is followed.) The inner sole of the shoe equally demands your attention. When it is yellowed and almost shrivelled up, remove it and replace it with a white leather sole. The leather of the arms of your long gloves, which is still clean when the fingers are soiled, and which has seen hardly any use, will serve well for this. Fasten this new sole inside the shoe with a weak glue, putting very little inside the shoe. If your feet perspire a great deal, it will be necessary to change this sole often.

Then make sure that the pads of your stays are not soaked with sweat, and that the busk pocket is not rusty or torn; set about repairing them if they are. This examination need be done only about once a fortnight, according to the season and the amount of perspiration.

I believe that I have passed in review, in this second preparation of clothes for the day, all which may concern them. As for the morning clothes which you put on when you get up, on the day before place them on a chair close to your bed when your bed has been turned down. However common, they must be clean; they should have been put away neatly folded. When, after you have been combed, you put them away before dressing, take care that they are shaken at the window and refolded, unless you prefer to hang them in a small cabinet near the *porte-manteau*. It depends upon your arrangements.

Just as it is necessary to take hygienic precautions to avoid having to employ remedies, you should acquire the habit of cleansing and looking after your clothes, linen, and jewels every day, in order to avoid great mendings, cleansings, and repairs. Thus, by brushing your merino gowns daily, you do not need to beat them. By immediately removing any spots from your clothing, you avoid complicated modes, such as sulphuring, acids, essence of turpentine, &c., because simple soaping ordinarily suffices to efface recent spots. (See Chapter X.) You avoid the changes which these modes and substances more or less always inflict on the material, and save, at the same time, the expense of the scourer. By repairing the smallest hole, the slightest worn streak on your linen, you considerably delay the necessity of patching them. (See Chapter XVI.)

By frequently rubbing your jewels, you save the trouble of cleansing them with soap, or divers other substances which always deteriorate them a little. All you have to do is repeatedly wipe your jewels with a piece of fine clean white leather (that of the arms of long gloves when they are no longer wearable). If you wish to render them very brilliant, rub them from time to time with burnt paper.

Steel trinkets are preserved in the same way. To prevent them from rusting, be careful to rub your buckle, bracelets, chain, and above all the clasp of your bag when you have gone out in damp or rainy weather. If despite this precaution, these objects have some rusty spots, you may make these disappear either by passing a piece of tracing-paper over them, or by rubbing them with a little boiled olive-oil and soot.

Every time that you take off your watch, suspend it from the gilt hook in the corner of the mantelpiece, where it replaces the *porte-montre*. Yet as it often happens that the watch turns, and the glass may strike the wall, it is well to have one of the little supports recently invented to hold watches. This is a kind of box made of delicate wood, and about the shape of a very small *prie-dieu*. In the upper part, and on the square side, there is a little round hollow lined with velvet, to receive the watch and protect it from all harm.

Measures for preserving hats are limited to a few things. If the wind, or some knock or pressure has crumpled the ornaments or flowers, slightly raise them one at a time, delicately taking them with your fingertips; but flowers require a few more particulars. Tighten the petals by first gathering the flower in the rounded palm of your hand, then raise and round them. In this way you bring the spread-out petals together, and when you take away your hand, breathe lightly on the flower, which will resume its graceful form. If some petals refuse to straighten, grasp them with a small florist's pliers, or even toilet tweezers, and bring them close to the others; putting on them, if need be, an infinitesimal amount of glue or starch at the point where the petal is inserted. This is the mode used by flower-makers to give grace to flowers, and to straighten them in case of accident. If the leaves are loose, it will suffice to apply a little glue to the middle of the base of the leaf. Lacking this, use a bit of white or green sealing-wax, then press the leaf delicately onto its stalk. I have seen flower-makers mend them thus.

As to feathers, when you have just been out in the rain or fog, whether the feathers appear damp or not, you absolutely must put them as near as possible to the fire (the heat of the stove column or pipe is preferable, to avoid the risk of burning the feathers) in order to evaporate the moisture. As they are heated, open them out and put their little barbs right. Thanks to this precaution, you will very rarely be obliged to have your feathers curled, an operation which breaks them, and for several days gives them a stiff and common air.

If your shawls (especially those of *barège*) or veils have absorbed rain or only damp, when they are dry, iron them under some unsized paper. If you neglect this little task, they will appear rumpled and dull.

When your gloves are moist with either sweat or damp, take care not to roll them as usual, but on the contrary stretch them out well and enter a goffering-iron into each finger; it should not be particularly hot, in order to neither alter the colours nor wrinkle the leather. You will be wise to wait until the gloves are half dry. You may cleanse unglazed gloves very well by rubbing them with the crumb of stale bread, like drawings, then with very white linen. Cleansing is managed about the same way for glazed gloves, but it is less successful.

To tidy and put away Each Kind of Linen, Garment, and Ornament.

Let us now occupy ourselves with the properest way of arranging and preserving from all damage the different kinds of linen, clothing, and ornaments which make up a well-ordered wardrobe. The greater part of my directions for folding linen may appear to concern only laundresses; but it is always well to know the best means of keeping all in order, and not to put things away clumsily after you have unfolded them for repairs.

To fold and arrange day shifts: first fold the shift in half lengthways, next fold in at the same time the gores and the sleeves, then fold the shift in half again. The shift is then folded crossways, to bring the bottom hem onto the shoulder-pieces, and finally it is folded in half again. Thus your shift is folded in quarters in every direction. Night-dresses are folded lengthways in sixths, putting the sleeves between folds. Crossways they have four folds. When the night-dress has a falling collar, fold it in quarters and put it under the last fold. When it has a standing collar, let it exceed the folded parts.

The mode for night jackets is complicated. Fold the back lengthways in half, and put it between the two front pieces, so that the fold is even with the front edges. This operation exactly doubles the night jacket, putting all the parts one over the other. The sleeves are placed on each other, then redoubled in three nearly equal parts, commencing with the bottoms. Then fold the night jacket lengthways, bringing the under sides of the sleeves over the front. Lay the sleeves on the night jacket so that from the collar, where it touches their folds, they do not extend past the crossways half of the night jacket. Whether it is standing or falling, the collar, folded in quarters if it is broad, and in half if it is narrow, is folded back on the sleeves. The bottom part of the night jacket is brought up to the top to cover the whole, which makes a perfect square.

To fold petticoats, first make a fold on each side along the entire length of the front, starting a little forwards of the top of the side gore. The fold will be around seven or eight inches deep at the top, and wider at the bottom. Pass the points at the bottom under this fold, so that they are no longer visible, to form a smaller square. Then fold the back breadth into halves or thirds, according to the width, with the fold or folds parallel to the front folds. That done, fold the petticoat crossways in thirds, from the front side. Start by folding down the top in order to collect the drawing-strings and to hide the waist plaits in the middle of the folded petticoat, then fold up the bottom. The folded petticoat, of which you now see only the back, resembles a rectangle.

Handkerchiefs are ordinarily folded in the simplest way in the world; that is, a square folded in half, then in half again. But there is an additional task when the handkerchief is embroidered, and you wish to display this at the corners. This is the mode *lingères* use to display their wares: fold the handkerchief in half with the embroidery on the inside. Lay it crossways on a table. Fold back the corner on the left to the crossways fold, then the corner on the right. Then fold the handkerchief in half again with the folded corners to the outside. The result is that the handkerchief appears to be made of four embroidered squares. If you wish, the last fold may be made with the embroidered corners to the inside, so that the handkerchief looks like any other. Printed batiste handkerchiefs are folded in the same manner.

The kind of trimming on a gown, and the material of which it is made, determine the mode of arranging and folding it. If the trimmings stand out, or the material is inclined to crease, it must be hung in an armoire in your wardrobe. First put one sleeve and then the other on a kind of squared stick. This is about a foot and three inches long, rounded at the ends, and suspended at the middle by means of an iron hook. Hang this hook over a strong iron or wooden rod which goes across the inside of the armoire. Gowns which hang from this *porte-manteau* (for so these instruments are called), should not be hung too close together, so that the trimmings may be freely spread out, and the skirts may drape without being tightly packed. This mode is very sound, not only to preserve the lower trimmings, but even any which may be on the sleeves and the body. (See Div. 3.)

When gowns have flat trimmings, such as *entre-deux,* folds, bias bands, or piping, they may be arranged in a chest of drawers. Start with the back uppermost, and fold in the side gores and the points as for a petticoat. Fold both sides of the gown in towards the middle, so that the sides are even with the middle of the back. Then fold the skirt in half crossways, and fold back the body onto the top of the back skirt breadth, spreading well the plaits which form this breadth. By this process you see only the front of the body, which is partly hidden by the sleeves, which you bring back over it. Some persons fasten the sleeves together with a very small pin, as is done by fine laundresses, and fold them in half if they are long. The gown is in some sort folded in thirds, since the reversed body makes the third part. Some persons fold the gown in half, counting the body, which instead of turning onto the top of the back they spread out, like the sleeves, at the bottom of this breadth. That mode has this in its favour, that it is less likely to form creases; but it requires more space. You may, it is true, reduce this requirement by placing the bottom of one gown on the top of another in the same drawer.

Generally *fichus* with *collerettes* are arranged flat in the highest drawer of the chest of drawers, which is shallower than the others, or in flat boxes. The first requires that both parts of the front, next the arms, be folded flat over the back when the collar is standing. When the collar is falling, the *fichu* is folded in half if the collar is trimmed, or even in quarters if it is not, but always lengthways. Starched and goffered caps may be folded so that the back seems glued under the front, because both strings appear at the same time. This might be called a full-face fold. You may also use a profile fold, where the cap, doubled from the side, presents only a single string; whichever mode suits you.

It is important to explain how you may replace the numerous and awkward boxes which these articles require. As you may place only a single row in each box or drawer, and they must not be crowded, you will perceive that they require space. You may avoid proliferation of boxes by regularly using the travelling cases filled with tapes, stretched out and crossed, which form several levels, on each of which you may place *collerettes* and caps. Each level, supported by small brackets fitted to the sides of the case, lifts easily by means of tape loops placed on the two ends of the level. (Many of these cases have tapes permanently fixed, which means that the level is not removable. You must then place the *collerettes* lengthways, which is not convenient.) Because it is not a matter of packing up *fichus,* and since the cases are priced high, you yourself may easily place the tapes in this manner, in a great box for two hats. Night-caps are folded in half crossways, showing the strings, and hiding the drawing-strings between the folds.

As I said at the commencement of this chapter, shawls are always folded in a square, whatever their size. You may, and should, suspend cachemires from the *porte-manteau.*

Stockings are placed on top of each other and rolled, as every one knows. The rolls have two different faces, the part with the toe and that with the edges. You should profit by this arrangement to distinguish the stockings which are mended and ready to wear, from those which are not. All stockings in good condition should be laid with the edge on top, and those which require repair with the toe on top. In this way, when you are dressing you avoid the trouble of unrolling several pair of stockings before finding a good pair; and when you wish to mend them (see Chapter XVII), you see at a glance which you should choose. Also put a narrow cord or braid about three inches long on the edge of each stocking, near the end of the seam. Its purpose is to tie them together for washing, and thus preserve them from the scissor-cuts and tears which laundresses lavish on them while unpicking stitches (see Chapter X).

As for shoes, I have no advice, except that you should have several wooden lasts such as shoemakers use, in order to put them inside your shoes when wear or water has misshaped them. This is also the way to enlarge shoes which are too narrow, and prevent them from hurting you.

For belts with riband loops, it is well to hang them by a pin through the end of one of the loops. To do this, tightly stretch linen tapes crossways from one side of a box to the other. Fix the pin to the tapes; in this manner, the ends of the belt are not crumpled, and the loops puff out as they ought. If the belt is simply a piece of riband, roll it on one of those little wooden rolls, or one of the pasteboard strips formed into ovals, on which haberdashers and riband dealers ordinarily place them. As for every other article, adopt the habits of shop-keepers and workwomen as much as you can.

Following this principle, I advise my readers to hang the flowers which they wear in their hair as flower-makers hang up their bouquets, or the parts of bouquets as they finish them. They make a little hook at the end of the stem, and hook it onto a piece of string stretched crossways on the table where they are working. They do this to prevent the flowers from encountering any object, and likewise they put enough space between neighbouring flowers so that they cannot touch. Experience proves they are right to do so, because garlands and bouquets often wither more rapidly in boxes than in being used several times. Therefore, you will be wise to use stretched strings or round braids in the middle of a hat-box, and to hang your flowers as flower-makers do. This mode has yet another advantage: bouquets so hung have their flowers turned towards the bottom of the box; and the papers, linens, or gauzes which you place under the lid, to keep out dust, will neither alter nor rub against the delicate parts of the flowers. Garlands are also suspended by one end; feathers, whether single or bunched, must be hung likewise.

Parasols and umbrellas should be quite closed, with the folds layered slantways upon each other, but without any creases. If these articles have a metal ring, dispense with using it, because it will cut, or at least pull on the taffeta to no purpose. The sheath or long pocket into which you should always put the umbrella when you are not using it, will retain the folds sufficiently. Always open the umbrella promptly and let it dry, so that dampness does not quickly wear out the taffeta. Keep it clean and bright, cleansing the shaft, the foot, and the metal tips of the ribs with diatomaceous earth mixed with a little essence of turpentine if these parts are brass, and with Spanish white mixed with a little vinegar diluted with water, if they are of white copper.

Fans must be closed quite uniformly and arranged in their box. When you notice that some point of these delicate articles has come loose, re-glue it at once with a feather dipped in egg-white or a weak solution of gum-arabic.

I advise taking yet more precautions for preventing dust from penetrating to all the articles of which I have just spoken. It is not enough to have well-closed armoires, and drawers and boxes which shut tightly. Dust is so fine that it always finds a way to creep in. This is so true that in opening, after several days, the well-closed drawers of a chiffonier or any other piece of furniture, you will see that the inside is covered with a light coating of dust. Since drawers evidently do not stop dust, it is necessary to spread over the articles in them either a towel or better yet, a large piece of unsized paper, as better able to keep off the dust. In boxes, which close much less tightly than furniture, it is proper to use linen and paper at the same time, and many persons even put in several pieces of each; I believe that is an unnecessary precaution. This is what I do: I place tissue paper directly over the hats, *fichus,* &c. Then I spread a linen over the edge of the box. I close it tightly and cover it with a thick material. You may also place over the tissue paper some worn gauze veils or pieces of crape; in short, all kinds of light materials which do not wash.

Gowns hung on the *porte-manteau* require similar measures. Glue together several sheets of paper and spread them over the sleeves of the gowns: this part is most exposed, because the ends of the *porte-manteau* lift it and bring it close to the doors of the armoire. Next put an iron rod on the inside, as near as possible to the top of the armoire and close to the doors. Put a curtain, the full length and height of the armoire, on the rod. Fasten the curtain on the left side so that in opening it and closing it to the right, it does not all come off in your hand. It must entirely hide the gowns, and completely close the wardrobe. This curtain will keep out dust so well, and collect so much of it, that after some time it will become extremely dirty. Do not wait until then to renew it, lest in pulling it to remove the garments it protects, you shake dust onto them.

In the armoires or chests of drawers, arrange the linen in piles according to its kind, and match or sort it. That is, place the articles according to their relationship; for example, night jackets next to shifts, petticoats close to night jackets, and so forth. It is well to separate each dozen by a coloured tape which you hang over the twelfth article. Or you may begin by putting the first dozen shifts on the side where the shift is folded upon itself, and for the second dozen put the shifts on the side where the hem is united with the neck and the shoulder-pieces. Night jackets, petticoats, and every thing else may be disposed in the same fashion; but it seems to me that it is better to reserve this kind of placement to recognize the linen to be mended, or that which has just been washed, and should be used later. These habits are very useful for keeping order in your linens, without which they will soon be mixed up.

In view of the papers and the curtain with which you are furnishing your chests of drawers and armoires, you may, without any inconvenience, have much clean linen at the same time. But it is not the same for starched articles: the starch cuts them. You should not, however, leave your caps and *fichus* in the dirt, which wears them out and yellows them excessively. Take a middle course: wash *fichus* only when you want to use them, and rinse out those which are soiled, to wait without any risk until it is their turn to be washed. The mode of rinsing out is described in Chapter X.

Rinsing out equally prevents the trouble which you encounter with summer gowns during the winter. If you have them washed, however perfectly they are arranged and covered, they assume a yellow cast, and often you must wash them again in the spring without having worn them. If they are not washed, the dirt yellows them and wears them out still more. By rinsing them out, you have nothing to fear. Moreover, rinsed-out gowns leave more room for your other clothes, because you may fold them and put them in packets in a corner of the armoire. In addition the habit of rinsing out should be extended to all your linen, if you do not often send it to the laundress or if you do the washing at home. It is pleasant to find the linen all selected when you want to deliver it to the laundress, and to have all similar pieces sorted.

To preserve Furs.

The simplest modes are very often the best; this is especially true for the preservation of furs. Many persons lay them by with pepper, mint, essence of turpentine, camphor, sage, &c.; and moths almost always wreak destruction on the furs thus rendered foul smelling. While it might seem certain that moths fear these substances, you always have the unpleasantness of wearing for some time garments which are in good order, but which nonetheless constantly cause megrims.

I put nothing at all with my furs, and preserve them intact. It would be well if furriers followed my mode, because when you store furs with them they should return the furs without the slightest odour, and at short notice. (During the summer furriers store furs at a low price. You pay about five francs for a tippet, four for a trimming for a gown; but it is always better to save this money, since you can get the same result for free.) Besides, most of the advice I shall give on this matter follows the modes of furriers, in accordance with my plan of constantly imitating workmen; the rest records my experience.

Early in spring, beat the furs on the wrong side with a small stick, and comb them as usual; for it is well to pass a comb through them now and then, especially if the hair is long. If it is short, a slight brush is more suitable. Then wrap them in very white linen, or even simply put them into a chest of drawers, provided the chest is hermetically closed. Do not touch it until the season when moth eggs have been laid, and do not open the drawers which contain them at all, as long as you see little yellow-white moths flying to burn themselves on the candle: these are the moths which are the mortal enemies of furs. They lay their eggs on them, the eggs develop into larvæ, and they nourish themselves with the finest and most delicate part of the furs, the place where the hair is attached to the skin. (See Div. 4.) The moths have usually finished laying their eggs by about the middle of June. Then bring out the furs, and shake them out in the garden or only from a window; beat them and comb them.

This operation has the double advantage of keeping the pelt even and shining, and of showing you whether some eggs have slipped into the furs. Spread them out in full sunlight and leave them for twenty-four hours. When night arrives, shake them and arrange them well, because any moths which by chance have not yet laid their eggs will not fail, in the darkness, to deposit those eggs amongst your clothes. Though these insects are burned in looking for light, they are very fond of darkness, because ordinarily they lodge under the cushions of arm-chairs and sophas. That reminds me to tell you to be very careful not to spread out your furs in a room furnished with these, because nothing is more dangerous. Repeat the operation which I have just described every two or three weeks, and you will preserve your furs without the least alteration.

I would add to these directions concerning furs, that when they are damp you must not wipe them dry, but take care to shake them out immediately, and comb them gently when the hair is dry.

——*Manuel des dames.*

Diversion 1.

The Lady's Maid. The business of the lady's maid is extremely simple, and but little varied. She is generally to be near the person of her mistress; and to be properly qualified for her situation, her education should be superior to that of the ordinary class of women, particularly in needle-work, and the useful and ornamental branches of female acquirements. To be peculiarly neat and clean in her person and dress, is better than to be tawdry or attractive, as intrinsic merit is a much greater recommendation than extrinsic appearance. In temper she should be cheerful and submissive, studying her mistress's disposition, and conforming to it with alacrity. A soft and courteous demeanour will best entitle her to esteem and respect. In fine, her character should be remarkable for industry and moderation; her manners and deportment, for modesty and humility; and her dress, for neatness, simplicity, and frugality.

It will be her business to dress, re-dress, and undress her mistress. In this, she should learn to be perfectly *au fait* and expeditious, ever studying, as far as it depends upon herself, to manifest good taste, by suiting the ornaments and decoration of her mistress's dress to the complexion, habits, age, and general appearance of her person. Thus will she evince her own good sense, best serve her mistress, and gratify all those who are most interested in her mistress's welfare and happiness. She should always be punctual in her attendance, and assiduous in her attention. Hers will be the care of her mistress's wardrobe, and she should make it her *particular* care; appropriating to each article of dress its proper place, where it always may be found when wanted. It will be her business carefully to examine every part of her mistress's clothes, when taken off, and if they have sustained an injury, or acquired any spots or stains, immediately to cleanse and repair them; then fold them up neatly, and put them away.

Her first business, in the morning, will be to see that the house-maid has made the fire, and properly prepared her mistress's dressing-room. She then calls her mistress, informs her of the hour, and having laid out all her clothes, and carried her hot water to wash, she retires to her breakfast with the housekeeper and other principal servants. When her mistress's bell rings, she attends her in her dressing-room, combs her hair for the morning, and waits on her until dressed; after which, she folds and puts away her night-clothes, cleanses her combs and brushes, and adjusts her toilet-table. She then retires to her work-room, to be ready if wanted, and employs herself in making and altering gowns, millinery, &c.

About one o'clock the family generally takes their lunch, and the servants their dinner. After this, she is summoned to attend her mistress's toilet for dressing to go abroad. When her mistress is gone, she again adjusts her mistress's clothes, and every thing in the room, and lays out and prepares the several articles which may be required for her mistress's dinner or evening dress. She afterwards employs herself at needle-work in her own room, or in her other avocations, until her mistress returns to dress for dinner, perhaps about five, when she attends her for that purpose. Having done this, it may happen that no further attendance on her mistress's person will be required until she retires to bed. Meanwhile the lady's maid employs herself at needle-work, as in the morning, or else in the various occupations of getting up the fine linen, gauzes, muslins, cambrics, laces, &c.; washing silk stockings; taking the spots or stains out of silk, &c., &c. (In the absence of the housekeeper, she will be required to make tea and coffee for the drawing-room company.)

It is her business to see that the house-maid or chamber-maid empties the slops, keeps up the fires both in this and the bed-chamber (if wanted), and keeps the rooms in perfect order. Previous to her mistress's retiring for the night, she will have looked out her mistress's night-clothes, and aired them well. She will, not only now, but at all times when her mistress goes to dress, carry up hot water for washing, &c. When her mistress is gone to bed, she will carefully examine all her mistress's clothes, and do all that is necessary to be done to them, before she folds them away. If her mistress is aged, infirm, or unwell, she will sometimes be required to bring her work and sit with her, to administer her medicines, and sometimes to read to her. To qualify herself for this latter purpose, and to acquit herself with propriety, she will at her leisure practise reading aloud from the best authors; as it is important to acquire a proper style and manner of reading, in all the varieties of poetry or prose, ode or epistle, comedy or sermon. She should avoid alike the dull monotony of the school-girl, and the formal affectation of the pedant; but follow Nature as her guide, in all that appertains to emphasis, modulation, and delivery.

If acquainted with the superior branches of needle-work, she might afford her mistress much gratification in presenting her occasionally with such trifles as will be acceptable, and suitable ornaments for her person. This will evince her disposition to be grateful and to oblige; and this, combined with a feminine sweetness of temper, and suavity of manners, cannot fail to be her sure recommendation to the esteem of her mistress and others, through all the various circumstances of life.

In large families, where there are young ladies who require attendance, a young lady's maid is appointed to wait on all, or perhaps each lady has a maid. The duties of these are in all respects the same as the lady's maid; I therefore refer them to the directions given to her. As this situation is considered merely initiatory to a better, and is occupied generally by an upper house-maid, or a young woman on her outset in life, the salary is somewhat less than that of a well-qualified servant; and the perquisites, including that of her mistress's left-off clothes, are also reckoned at the same rate.

——*The Complete Servant.*

Diversion 2.

To store Pomatum. Cover the pomatum pot, or reverse it over the bottom of a drawer, so that the scent does not evaporate. In winter, be careful to keep it in a warm place, because the pomatum hardens, and putting it to the fire several times to soften it makes it lose its freshness. It is the same for oils.

——*Manuel des dames.*

Diversion 3.

To store Clothing. Mrs. L.—How shall I keep in tolerable order those parts of my wardrobe which belong to full dress? Full-trimmed gowns, white satin, and silks in general, very soon lose their fresh appearance.

Mrs. B.—Any mode, by which you can keep air, and consequently dirt, away from them, will answer for a short time; but all such things are of so perishable a nature, both in themselves, as well as from the evanescence of fashion, that the securest way is to have as few to preserve as possible.

White satin—and gauzes also, which change their colour almost as quickly—should be carefully wrapped up in light envelopes of paper. I have seen small closets nicely fitted up, in which to hang up gowns, and other parts of dress which would suffer if they were folded and laid within the narrow compass of a drawer or a wardrobe. These closets have wooden pegs arranged round them, and have muslin curtains drawn close round the whole, so as to render them impenetrable to sun or dust.

——*Domestic Duties.*

Diversion 4.

To increase the Value of Furs Tenfold, and beautify the Hair of Animals. This art consists of giving the hair of animals a metallic lustre to further increase the value of the most precious furs and to protect them from moths, and of similarly lustring the hair of live animals.

Take an ounce of fine silver at eleven deniers. Cut it up and dissolve it in aquafortis or nitric acid. Put this solution over hot ashes until it forms a film on the surface, then put it in the cellar to collect and remove the crystals so that you may use them at need. These are called lunar or silver crystals.

When you wish to lustre and glaze a fur in a lasting manner, dissolve a portion of these crystals in very clear water, and pass the solution over the hair with a sponge. When the fur dries it will be gilded or silvered, and assume a more brilliant aspect, according to its particular shade. The glaze is permanent, and insects will no longer attack the fur.

If you wish to likewise lustre and glaze a live animal, you also employ this mode. But you will perceive that when the animal sheds, the operation must be repeated.

——*Manuel complet d'économie domestique.*

Chapter X.
The Art of Laundering and Scouring.

Domestic economy consists largely of a set of practices which, meticulous and almost troublesome on their first introduction, become easy with practice and are very interesting in their results. One of the things to which this consideration most applies is maintaining linens, soiled as well as white. (See Div. 1.)

As it is well in households, especially farm households, to be able to perform the operations of the washhouse without resorting to laundresses, it is equally necessary to know the modes for scouring in order to avoid the errands, expenses, and delays attendant on the employment of a scourer. This is all the more useful since nearly all spots, which come off with the greatest ease when you proceed immediately after the mishap, become tenacious and sometimes hopeless when you allow some time to pass. Therefore, these directions would necessarily be incomplete if they did not include the modes of removing the spots which so often damage linens and clothing. I shall give the ones I use in daily practice, which are always completely successful.

The sorting of Linens.

The first operation of washing consists of sorting the linens, not only into three lots; viz., fine linen, coloured linen, and kitchen linen; but further to collect similar articles, in order to count them and put them into the tub together. (See Div. 2.) Thus you separate all the sheets, then the towels, shifts, &c. This operation is both very lengthy and very disagreeable, because you must handle the pieces several times and breathe the foul odour which is emitted by all the linen soiled for a long while. (See Div. 3.) Apart from that, you risk causing tears while untangling fine or slightly worn articles.

To avoid this disadvantage it is proper to have, for depositing soiled linen, poles arranged in an attic, or a large armoire or chest with compartments. Each shelf in the armoire, or each compartment, is to receive one kind of linen, which you deposit as it is left off. In this fashion the linen will be completely sorted, and you have only to count the contents of each compartment, or on each pole, when you want to put it in the wash.

The rinsing out of Linens.

You must have often been obliged to notice that linen worn two or three times, and consequently still clean, is thoroughly soiled after some time without it having been worn again. You see how linen discolours and deteriorates when it is left dirty for several months, while you wait until there is a sufficient quantity to do the wash. Therefore, well-run households practice rinsing out linen which has been left off, before putting it in the chest or on the poles.

This operation is exceedingly simple. It consists merely of soaking and washing the linen in clear water while rubbing it lightly. The water should be cold in summer and lukewarm in winter. Rinsing out removes the dirt before the material is thoroughly permeated, arrests its progress, and prepares the way for a good washing. For this reason, you may later wash the linen in a weak wash-liquor, dispensing with vigorous washing, or rubbing the linen energetically when soaping it; all things which break the threads and cost much labour. It is needless to say that you must always have a rope stretched near the chest of soiled linen, in order to dry it before putting it on the shelves or in the compartments.

To attach Pairs of Stockings, &c.

Before putting linens into the tub, attach pairs of stockings, slippers, and sleeves by sewing them together with a few stitches. The washing finished, you unstitch these articles. But this requires several scissor-cuts which may damage them greatly, especially the stockings, since one broken stitch of knitting pulls out others. Careful persons prevent this evil in part by connecting the stockings with long blanket-stitches, or over-cast stitches, or a *cordonnet* which they form by extending, by several lines, the first stitches taken onto the stockings, and sewing or blanket-stitching onto the stitches thus extended. The washing done, cut the *cordonnet* in the middle, and the separated parts remain on the stocking, which suffers no damage from the scissors; but it is then necessary to cut off these parts. It is true that there is little risk of cutting the edge of the stockings in removing them. However, if the thread which holds the stockings together is fine, the *cordonnet* is bound to break during washing; and if it is thick it might damage the edge of the articles which it unites, especially if they are delicate. Furthermore, it is always work to make the *cordonnet* on stockings and slippers, and disagreeable work too, because slippers have always an odour.

Therefore, I advise the habit which I have adopted, after becoming disgusted with the two modes about which I have just spoken. I take a piece of narrow tape or braid, either cotton or linen, about an eighth of an ell long, and sew it to a seam of each stocking. When the stockings are soiled, I tie both tapes together. The tape is passed under the garter when the stocking is put on.

You may do the same for gentlemen's toile slippers, but make the tape much shorter so that it is not awkward in the shoe. Women's night-caps are also fastened by one of these tapes. Avoid joining more than two or three caps at a time, because the tapes tangle, and you must cut them when the caps are put in press (which is described in the article on ironing linens).

Sew the rags from old linens into small bundles for bandages or other articles. Never make the bundles by bringing the pieces together and fixing them against each other. On the contrary, though you sew them securely, leave them loose enough that each piece may be turned over repeatedly. Without this precaution, the spots will come out very imperfectly. Also, to the same end, take care to unfold and shake each rag in succession.

Directions for the Wash-liquor.

People have always used wash-liquors to cleanse linen of all the substances which momentarily soil it, and especially greasy ones. It is indeed the best mode of removing greasy deposits, and rendering them soluble in water by transforming them into soap with the aid of an alkali. I shall describe it following the excellent work on washing which M. François René R. Curaudau published in 1806, and the article by M. Pierre-Jean Robiquet included in the third volume of the new *Dictionnaire technologique*.

Wash-liquor is, as every one knows, a solution of potash or soda, or rather of the water in which ashes have been boiled; in any case, water more or less charged with alkali. But the use of wash-liquor exacts several important precautions. It is very difficult, for example, to give wash-liquors a uniform degree of strength, and yet it is only too well proven that the strength has a very marked influence on the results. But how may you obtain such wash-liquors? Ashes are almost never of the same quality, and potash and soda are never sold in identical states of purity. Consequently, to obtain similar results it does not suffice to use the same quantity of water and the same amount of alkaline material. Chemists have several modes of estimating the strength of alkaline solutions. They use the hydrometer, which sometimes misleads them, or the alkalimeter, whose use is more reliable but more troublesome. But how can a household consult these delicate instruments?

You can only compensate for them with practice. When you put your fingers into a good wash-liquor, you will find it oily and greasy to the touch. Laundresses have the habit of saying that it is greasy, but this term is erroneous. (Housekeepers say that it is mild and better than soap.) It is necessary that the wash-liquor have some affinity to greasy substances. But in that state, having become more caustic, it combines with greasy substances which are on the surface of the skin, even attacks the epidermis, eats into it, and transforms it into soap; and it is elementary that your fingers seem to glide over each other as if they had been coated with oil. But whatever may be the cause of this phenomenon, you will perceive by how easy it is to take advantage of it, that one practiced hand can become an excellent alkalimeter, and that the different degrees of oiliness of the wash-liquor provide the mode of estimating its strength.

You may augment the causticity of the wash-liquor with lime. Here is the reason: the potash contained in the ashes, and commercial potash and soda, are always combined with enough carbonic acid to markedly diminish their strength. If you mix a little lime into the water, and mix it with the ashes, soda, or potash, the lime will combine with the carbonic acid, neutralize it, and the salt will precipitate at the bottom of the vessel.

Many persons have an unconquerable repugnance to the use of lime. They are persuaded that this earth burns the fibres, and do not imagine that it has, in this case, functions in addition to removing materials which would otherwise partially neutralize the alkali. All this results in the need of less ash, soda, or potash. And if, in spite of this economical reduction, the wash-liquor is too strong, it will suffice for softening it to increase the water until it is no stronger than proper.

Nonetheless, it is necessary not to neglect a precaution recommended by the most experienced laundresses. This is not to allow the lime to mix with the linen; not because the liquor would become too corrosive, but because the gritty particles, more or less coarse, would deposit by degrees on the materials contained in the tub, and would wear on them during the operations which they will be submitted to later on. The lime acts mechanically in this case as a hard substance: ashes would have the same disadvantage.

To make the wash-liquor for an hundred pounds of dry and very soiled linen, it is generally necessary to use six and three-fifths gallons of water and six pounds, nine and a half ounces of washing soda; or instead, two and three-quarter pounds of Russian potash; or instead again, eight pounds, thirteen ounces of unrefined soda. But you will perceive that the strength must be subordinated to the degree of sturdiness of the linen, and the greater or lesser quantity of impurities with which it is charged.

Once the linen has been sorted and attached, as explained above, deposit it in layers into the tub, always putting the finest and least soiled at the bottom. Pour in water with each layer of linen so that it becomes saturated, and let it soak cold for a day before starting the washing. (See Div. 4.) Some persons are in the habit of rinsing out the linen immediately before putting it into the tub. They think linen thus scrubbed will come clean easier. Curaudeau criticizes both of these modes, with good reason. Linen soaked with water does not easily allow the wash-liquor to penetrate, since its place is already taken. The portion which does reach the fibres is diluted by the water already there, and consequently almost inactive. You see, therefore, how the practice of rinsing out the linen when leaving it off facilitates washing while saving water, trouble, and time.

For applying wash-liquor to the linen, whether it has been rinsed out or not, you use a great tub which is placed upon a kind of wooden tripod. The tub is pierced on its lower side by a hole, which you plug simply with a handful of straw folded over itself. Arrange the linen on the inside, piece by piece, as uniformly as possible and leaving no empty space, taking care to compress it forcefully. Without all this the wash-liquor would not distribute evenly; that is why this is called placing the wash-liquor. Take care not to fill the tub completely because the linen will puff up, and you would then be obliged to raise the tub, that is, to fit a wide hoop the size of the tub at the top round the ashes (see below). When the wash-liquor is good, the water, of a chestnut-brown colour, foams like soap.

Cover the whole with a heavy toile, which hangs over the side of the tub. Onto this toile, put a quantity of ashes proportionable to the mass of linen which you want to wash. Fold the edges of the toile over to form a kind of roll all round the ashes, which you support in several places by forcing flattened wedges of soft wood here and there between the toile and the tub.

Then pour, every now and then, a certain quantity of hot water through the ashes with which the linen has previously been covered. The potassium carbonate, dissolved by the liquid, filters successively through all the layers of linen, and finishes by collecting in the lower part, from where it drains with the aid of the above-mentioned opening into a tub placed below the opening. Take the drained liquid, and pour it into a boiler placed over a fire. When it is properly hot pour it back through the ashes; and so on for about a day. This process is called pouring the wash-liquor. Towards the end of it, many persons put over the ashes the linen whose colour would not withstand the prolonged action of the wash-liquor, and which they judge too soiled to be merely soaped.

The following day, or when you judge the operation completed (this depends upon the quantity of linen), remove the cloth with the ashes, take the linen from the tub, and then soap it using clear running water.

Such is the summary of this well-known operation, but I must add several important observations. First, instead of putting the ashes on top of the linen, it is better to make the wash-liquor separately: there is less risk of staining. Put your ashes in a small tub, the bottom of which has an opening covered by a little bundle of straw, through which the liquor may pass. This opening is again closed by a stopper of cork or wood. Cover the ashes with straw, then carefully pour in the hot water. When it floats, unplug the opening. As the water runs out, add more before the ashes have time to coagulate. But avoid using so much water that the wash-liquor becomes too weak; it is better to have to increase it. Use it in the ordinary way, and it suffices to cover the linen with a tolerably thick sheet, which retains all the impurities which the wash-liquor may contain.

When you use potash or soda, which is now most common at Paris, it suffices to dissolve these salts in lukewarm or cold water.

Linen washes badly when you use too high a temperature. It is preferable go from a mild heat, to the temperature of boiling water, by carefully managed gradations. Without this, the impurities which still remain in the linen are found, so to speak, coagulated and set in the material, which then acquires a tawny shade, often uneven. When the heat acts all at once on the spots, the linen is scalded and the spots no longer disappear. On the contrary, when the temperature is graduated, the material swells by degrees and allows penetration more easily.

It is a great disadvantage to use wash-liquors which are too strong, and it is equally so to use ones which are too weak. In the first case they eat into and spot the material. In the second, they are insufficient to attack and dissolve the dirt, and the linen is odorous and unhealthy when taken out.

It is urgent to thoroughly examine the ashes which will be placed upon the tub. They sometimes contain fruit peels, nails, and other foreign substances which badly stain the linen. Kitchen ashes are especially subject to this disadvantage.

Finally, I must not neglect to say that when you wash fine linens, in practice it is generally enough to soak them, first in a mildly soapy water until they are thoroughly impregnated with it, then put them again into the tub to be washed in the ordinary manner.

The rubbing and beating which linen is submitted to during soaping and washing, is unquestionably one of the things most detrimental to its durability. Therefore, you must avoid these as much as possible for very fine linen. To obviate this disadvantage, several machines have been invented, but none of them may be usefully applied to household washing.

The Art of making your own Soap by the American Mode.

Soap may be made with all solids and liquids, as well as with resins, which appear in a greasy, oily, or resinous state. The best soaps are those obtained from fatty substances which have much consistency, such as greases, fats, &c. It is the same for certain resins and olive-oil; and generally all those which congeal when cold, furnish excellent soap as well. It is hard, firm, and dry. But those made with oils which cold does not congeal, such as those from colza (rape seed), give a half-liquid soap: this is green soap or black soap. (See Div. 5.)

To make soap, such an essential article nowadays in a household, you must combine the greases, oils, or resins with an alkali. The ones most commonly used are soda or potash, with quicklime added to increase the causticity. You may also make wash-liquor from ordinary wood-ashes, adding some quicklime and a small portion of sea-salt, in order to make it more active.

In the United States of America, every household makes the soap needed for its use, and makes it with refuse materials which seem to be scorned every where else. I shall describe the American mode first. You will perceive, as experience confirms, that while the large-scale manufacture of soap is a considerable branch of commerce for all peoples, it must also be an important one in domestic economy.

In all of North America, since the beginning of colonization, the isolation of families in the midst of forests, the absolute remoteness from all workshops and manufactories, have forced the colonists to make for themselves a multitude of articles of the first necessity. Every family has become self-sufficient, and amongst other articles of daily consumption, each of them has come to make soap.

For this purpose, throughout the year they gradually collect all the bones as the meat is consumed. They throw the bones into the corner of a dry place, and leave them there to dry. They likewise accumulate all greases which are rancid or unsuitable for use, candle-ends, and in short all greasy and resinous substances from the household which cannot serve for nourishment.

When the day destined for making soap has arrived, they take the bones one by one, put them on a block, and holding them upright, reduce them to more or less fine pieces and splinters with a chopping-knife. These are put with the pieces of grease or fat, in order to pass the whole like a wash-liquor into the boiler. This wash-liquor may be weak, or more or less concentrated.

A New Way to apply Wash-liquor, after the Preceding Mode.

Put on the fire your boiler half filled with the bone fragments and grease or fat. Soak the whole in rather weak wash-liquor. Cook it over a low fire, and as the liquor evaporates, add more concentrated wash-liquor; the absorption of the wash-liquor will take a long time. After there is no more left, the greasy, oily, or resinous materials are saturated, and saponification is done. Nothing more is required but to lift out the bony pieces with a skimmer, and to continue gently cooking the soap as indicated by its greater or lesser degree of consistency. You may then remove it from the fire; fill vessels, little casks, or moulds; and put it away to use as needed. It is necessary to put it in a dry place because soap naturally absorbs damp, and you use double the amount when it is soft.

In this way you may employ refuse materials from your household, and using only bones and grease, make the best of soaps, which will have the most consistency and dryness. If the greases or the contents of the bones are extremely rancid and have a disagreeable odour, at the end of cooking you may correct this by putting into the boiler an ounce of essence of turpentine, to thirty pounds of soap.

The Experiment of washing with Steam.

This mode of washing has, as of yet, been adopted by only a small number of institutions, despite its incontestable advantages over the mode generally used. I think people will read the details of the following experiment with interest, since its success leaves the partisans of the old routine without rejoinder.

The experiment was made on eighteen hundred pounds of very soiled dry linen. The linen consisted of sheets, table-cloths, napkins, shifts, and towels. It was simply rinsed out the day before in water from a cistern, then drained. No soap was used for the rinsing-out; that was particularly insisted upon.

The linen was then soaked in wash-liquor prepared with American potash, but without the addition of soap. Forty-five pounds of potash were used for the wash-liquor, which provided two and a half pounds for each hundred pounds of linen. However, as each kind of linen was more or less impregnated with greasy and dirty substances, it was important in making the choice to separately give each kind of linen a wash-liquor whose strength was in proportion to its requirements. The quantity of water used to prepare the wash-liquor was equivalent to about two-thirds the weight of the dry linen.

The linen was put into the tub, starting at eleven o'clock in the morning. The towels were put in the bottom of the tub, then the table-cloths and napkins, and finally the shifts and sheets. This was finished around half past noon. The fire was lit immediately, and kept up until it was assured that the heat carried to the linen was distributed uniformly, and that it was an hundred seventy-six degrees. At nine o'clock, it was recognized that the operation had been continued long enough; then the fire was stopped. Only two hundred and fourteen pounds of wood had been burned, estimated to cost four francs, fifty centimes. This expense could have been partly recovered if the embers had been pulled out. However, at nine o'clock the following morning they were collected for thirty-five centimes. On the morning of the third and final day, the linen was put into a tub for washing. Never did a wash-liquor wash better, nor render the linen whiter.

The results of this experiment were first, that it should be continued. Second, that linen washed by this mode is infinitely whiter and easier to wash than by the old mode. Third, that the vermin which are found often enough in hospitals, and which the action of ordinary wash-liquor does not ordinarily destroy (as has been remarked by all directors of hospitals) are completely destroyed by the heat of an hundred seventy-six degrees which is assuredly given to the linen. Finally, that the economy in fuel and soap is two-thirds.

It is well to remark that the sheets submitted to the wash-liquor for the first time were much whiter than similar ones compared to them, which had already been subjected to the action of ordinary wash-liquor three times. This observation proves that unbleached linen will become white faster by this mode, than linen subjected to the ordinary one.

According to the information recorded in the institutions where this operation was carried out with the greatest economy, the same quantity of linen would have required forty-five pounds of potash, five pounds of soap, and six hundred pounds of wood. How many other institutions find that their expenses even exceed this last! With this experiment, the expense in raw materials was forty-five pounds of potash, a pound and a half of soap, and two hundred fourteen pounds of wood. Concerning labour, it cannot be precisely determined which mode is most economical. Only experience will make this known.

The Experiment of washing with Potatoes.

As my intention is to give directions for the most useful and least expensive modes, I can do nothing better than to popularize, as much as I can, the attempts of M. Cadet de Vaux to obtain better washing by means of the most common vegetable. Philanthropy recommends it as much as economy. How many poor people rarely wash their linen because they cannot afford soap! Besides, by increasing the use of potatoes in ordinary times, a greater quantity is assured in times of scarcity.

The trials by the inestimable scientist to whom this process is owing are so simple that it will suffice for me, to present all the requisite notions, to give an extract from a lecture by M. Héricart de Thury, concerning an experiment made on the linen of the Paris hospitals, in the presence of the administration and the prefect of the Seine.

The linen was thrown into a tub to soak for half an hour. The rinsings-out lasted half an hour at the most. After this operation, all the linen was thrown into a boiler of warm water. It was retrieved, piece by piece, to be rubbed in turn on the top and the bottom in the manner of soaping, with potatoes which were three-quarters cooked. (It often happened that this was done badly, for want of having achieved this condition. You nonetheless understand that the degree of cooking is approximate.) After all the pieces were well rubbed, rolled, and wrung out, they were thrown back into the boiler of warn water, and boiled for half an hour. The linen was rubbed again, beaten, rolled, turned, and pressed in all directions. It was next immersed in the boiler for several more minutes, then rinsed twice in a great deal of water. Immediately afterwards, all the linen was put in press. Thanks to this measure, the spread-out linen dried promptly, and all the operations together took only two and a half hours.

The results of this experiment were that the linens were perfectly cleansed, scoured, and whitened. They did not retain any odour, not even the kitchen linens, which commonly do so despite the most vigorous washing. The blankets and napkins of infants, which in ordinary washing always retain a yellow or greenish tint in the middle, were completely cleansed and stripped of all colour.

The other advantages of this mode over the ones in use are evident. The entire wash gives hardly more trouble than a simple soaping. It suffices to have a pot of potatoes and a boiler full of water near by. You are no longer obliged to spend precious time on the wash, to pass a whole day pouring water into a tub, and another day scrubbing. Neither soda, potash, nor soap is used. Perhaps the water might serve for hogs, and become a means of fertilizing potatoes.

Do not be horrified to see linen placed over the fire in a boiler: the heat is really no higher there than in a tub. As long as the boiler contains water, there is no fear of burning the linen. This is a natural law proven in the most complete manner. It is no less demonstrated by experience; for in several regions and notably the Upper Auvergne, the boiler serves as the tub. Moreover, you know that dyers boil the materials which they dye, and that many Parisian laundresses finish soaping by boiling the linen in a weak solution of soap and indigo.

I advise familiarizing yourself with this mode by using it first for small washes, for which it is especially well suited. By rendering the same more convenient, you might dispense with great washes.

Furthermore, a new way to use potatoes in washing has recently been proposed. After having washed and scrubbed them with a brush, grate them and let the pulp drop into water, as if you wished to extract the starch. Pass the whole through a sieve. When the starch has collected on the bottom as a white precipitate, carefully pour off the mucilaginous liquor, and keep it for use. The articles to cleanse are spread out on a table covered with thick linen, and you rub them lightly several times with this liquor. Then wash them and let them dry. This mode, proposed for cleansing delicate silken, woollen, and cotton materials, seems likely to produce the best results. I have no doubt that it merits the prize awarded by the Society for Encouragement in London to its inventor Mr. Morris. (See Div. 6.)

The Mode of washing with Rice.

M. Sebastien Lenormand, whom it is so often necessary to consult on technological matters, reports this mode of cleansing the calicoes which are used to furnish beds and windows. You will perceive that it may be applied to every other material of this kind.

This mode generally succeeds when the material is not very soiled. Take two pounds, three and a quarter ounces of rice. Boil it in two gallons, a cup and three-quarters of water until it is softened, that is to say until it becomes slightly mucilaginous. Pour the whole into a tub. When the liquor has cooled off enough that you can hold your hand in it, immerse the calicoes, and wash them as you would do with soapy water. Then take the same quantity of water and rice. After boiling, filter to separate the rice from the liquid, and use the new liquid to wash the calicoes until they are well cleansed. Then rinse them in the water in which the rice was boiled, smooth them with your hand, and spread them out to dry. If you wish them to be lustrous, rub them with a sleeking stone.

This mode starches calicoes properly, and preserves their gloss and beauty so well that they appear altogether new.

The Mode of washing with Soapwort.

It is well known that botanists have found in a class of plants (named for the genus of *saponaria*) an alkali similar to that of soap. Soapwort is the one in which the soapy property is strongest. In the country and all the places where this flower abounds, it would be most economical to use it for washing. It is especially good for thick materials of bleached woollen, such as serge, burat, blankets, &c., which this plant renders as white as soap does, and much softer to the touch.

Its use is as simple as can be. It suffices to make a strong decoction of the leaves and flowers, and thoroughly wash the material in it. You may, if you wish, alternate; that is first immerse the articles in water with soap, then in water with soapwort. Since it is necessary to do three soapings on heavy woollen materials, you may easily practice this combination. But it is necessary to finish the operation with the soapwort water, as this is cleaner and imparts suppleness.

The Best Mode of Soaping.

Perhaps you will be surprised to see me discuss such a familiar operation. However, I do not pretend to provide an explanation, but to propose several practices to render it both more effective and easier.

Instead of rubbing the linen with a tablet of soap as laundresses do, it is better to first make a solution of soap in water, cutting it into thin slices. Then immerse the linen in this soap solution and wash it in the customary manner. The linen will be cleansed uniformly all over, which is never the case when you rub it with soap. A goodly portion of the undissolved soap lodges in the interstices of the cotton. It does not always come out with washing, and consequently keeps these parts of the material from appearing quite clean. If the soap is instead thoroughly dissolved in the water, it uniformly removes all the dirt from the linen. That is how scourers work.

Repeated soapings, and the necessity of rinsing, blueing, and drying the linen, require you to wring it often to squeeze out the water. When you must wash only pieces of small or middling size, such as caps, napkins, or shifts, you may wring them out easily with your hands. But when the pieces are large, such as table-cloths, sheets, or even gowns, you are obliged to use two persons, or to wring out only partially. When at least two persons are required, doing it alone is often impossible, or at best very awkward. For example, while you wring the middle of a gown after having wrung the bottom, the water you squeeze out falls back over the bottom; and the rest, the body and sleeves, drags on the floor or falls into the water, because you cannot grasp every thing at once. Besides, when you wring heavy linen for a long time, you suffer from a most painful feeling in the palms of your hands, and often from calluses. The difficulty is much greater still if you must wring blankets, curtains, or woollen materials. Hardly any water is expelled, which first hampers the divers operations of washing, and then requires a vast deal of time for drying.

Why not remedy so much fatigue and difficulty by adopting the wringing-out practice of scourers and dyers? Nothing is more simple or convenient. They have only two instruments (see Div. 7). The first is an iron hook securely fastened to the wall at the height of support. The second is a cylindrical stick of hard, very smooth wood, a little shorter than half an ell. The workman folds the material into three or four parts, and hangs one end on the hook, passing the hook between the doubled material. At the opposite end, near himself, he passes the stick, and easily wrings as much as he wishes, without trouble, fatigue, or awkwardness. A tub placed below the hook catches the water expelled from the material. It is very easy to procure these instruments for yourself. If need be, you may re-place the hook with the first peg which comes to hand, and the stick with a rolling-pin or any other smooth, rounded stick.

The Best Mode of Blueing.

It remains only for me to discuss the ways in which you may vary the use of indigo, which is applied after soaping the linen. Some persons apply blue with a lump of indigo securely wrapped in a piece of thick linen or woollen. Others use blue as a liquid, called chemic blue.

People differ as well in the application of blue. Most commonly, when the linen is well rinsed and removed from the soapy water, it is immersed in water in which indigo is dissolved. But at Paris it is done differently. The linen is left in the last change of soapy water. In a tureen full of water, put soap cut into very thin slices, several drops of blue, and a little very white tallow, thinly sliced from the square end of an unused candle. When the blue is in a lump, put it in first to prevent the bag which holds it from encountering the soap and tallow. Throw the linen into the water thus pre-pared, cover the tureen, and put it over the fire to subject it to a thorough boiling. Then remove it and allow it to cool until you can hold your hand in the water. Rub the linen, and repeatedly turn it over well. Rinse it in clear water and let it dry.

This washing mode is usually excellent, and the shade of blue is the best. But if you boil the linen before soaping has perfectly removed the dirt, it will be fixed in the fibres by the effect of the heat, and nothing can detach it.

To Compose Chemic or Liquid Blue.

Take a pound, and an ounce and a half of good sulphuric acid, and pour it onto an ounce of good flora indigo, well pulverized and sifted. Stir the liquor well, then add a fourteenth of an ounce of good potash. It will in-stantly produce a violent effervescence and a more perfect dissolution of the indigo. As soon as the effervescence ceases, pour the liquor into a tightly-stoppered flask. It may be used twenty-four hours after its prepara-tion. Take care not to increase the quantity of potash indicated, because it will dull the colour.

When you wish to use liquid blue, dilute it with a greater or lesser quantity of warm water, according to the shade you desire.

The Mode of M. Estève of Flushing for making Balls of Celestial Blue, called English Blue.

Take a pound of good indigo, crushed and sifted. Dissolve it in three pounds of good sulphuric acid. Add a pound of powdered chalk, finely sifted, and stir it. The effervescence occasioned by the acid and the chalk having ceased, indicating a perfect saturation, add six pounds of powdered and sifted starch, and four pounds of very finely-powdered white marble, to thicken it to a paste. Stir the whole to mix it well. To perfect it, grind it between two stones, gradually adding a quantity of ox-blood, which you mix according to the intensity of the colour which you mean to give your blue.

Having obtained a soft paste which is smooth to the touch, and perceiving no imperfection in the mixture, make it into balls and suffer them to dry in the air.

The Mode of Mr. William Story for the Same Composition.

Take a great earthen vessel or an iron boiler; for the latter it is unnecessary to use iron filings as an ingredient. Take a pound of the finest indigo. Reduce it to powder, and cast about three pounds of sulphuric acid into the vessel. Stir the mixture, and let it stand twenty-four hours at the most.

Then dissolve ten pounds of good potash in a quart of water, and add a quart of this strong solution of potash to the preceding mixture. Mix the whole well. Add a pound of the best blue mottled soap, cut up small, and mix well. Continue to add the potash solution until the mixture appears in the form of a dry powder. Then pour in a pint of clear water and mix it again. After that continue to add the potash solution, stirring constantly, until it is all used up. Then carefully mix in half a pound of finely-powdered alum, which has been passed through a sieve.

After standing for three days, this composition will be ready to use. It will have the consistency of a paste. Form it into balls and let them dry in the air, as for the mode of M. Estève.

To make ironing Linens easier, with a Handsome Result.

To begin with, do not allow your linen to dry completely or so that it will crease. Remove it from being spread out while it is still a little damp. Fold it into several parts according to the size of the piece, for example a towel in half, and a shift in quarters. To do this best, spread the articles on a table. Pass and repass your hands thoroughly over the top each time you fold, then sort them into piles. This operation is called putting the linen in press.

I shall not describe ironing, which every one understands. (See Div. 8.) I shall say only that if the flat-iron refuses to glide quickly, you ought to rub it lightly with a little rubbing wax enclosed in a toile bag. Some persons replace the wax with tallow or some other grease, but these give off a foul odour. This step is especially necessary when you iron starched linen. (See Div. 9.)

You may, in certain cases, advantageously substitute thick rice-water for starch. The gum which rice imparts to muslins is less stiff, but it renders them more clear and glossy. Rice-starch is also easier to iron. If you wish the starch to neither thicken the material nor hinder the flat-iron, add several drops of white vinegar, and allow starched articles to dry a little before handing them over for ironing.

Preparation for restoring Scorched or Almost Burned Linen.

Put in a pint of vinegar, two ounces of fuller's earth, an ounce of chicken droppings, half an ounce of tablet soap, and the juice of two onions. Boil until the whole has thickened. Pour some of the mixture onto all of the damaged parts. If they are not entirely burned, nor the threads consumed, after letting the top dry, and a good washing or two, the damaged spots will appear as white and in as good a condition as the rest of the article.

To wash Calico or Gingham Gowns to look like new.

Instead of rubbing the material with tablet soap, as is done by all laundresses, prepare a strong solution of soap, immerse the gown in it, then wash it in the ordinary manner. Two advantages result from this mode. First, the material is spared rubbing with hard soap, which wears it accordingly. Second, it is evenly cleansed all over, which is never the case when you rub with soap. Frequently, coloured cotton materials fade, especially calicoes printed with reds or greens. You may nonetheless preserve them by adding to the rinsing water several drops of acid, be it lemon-juice, citric acid, vinegar, or sulphuric acid. Some persons let calicoes soak in hard water before washing them, or in water into which some hay has been put.

Scourers ordinarily cleanse calicoes by washing them in a great quantity of lukewarm soapy water. Then they mix some wheat-flour and starch into the water. They beat it well and bring the water to an oily consistency. Next they beat the calicoes in this liquor. They spread them out so that they are quite smooth, suffer them to dry, and rub them with a sleeking stone. My readers may easily imitate this process. (See Div. 10.)

To wash Nankeen when it is Soiled, so that it does not lose its Colour.

Put the nankeen to soak twenty-four hours in cool water into which you have put a good handful of salt. Then wash it without soap in hot wash-liquor. Do not wring it. You may also wash it in water in which you have boiled some hay.

To wash Unbleached Materials.

The straw-coloured tint of unbleached material, such as muslin, and the batiste used to make bonnets, gloves, parasols, &c., is preserved by washing them in a decoction of hay, tea, and principally in a preparation of bullock's gall.

To soap White Silks, Gauzes, Silk Tulle, Ribands, &c.

Dissolve a sufficient quantity of white soap in boiling water. Add a little gum-water, and several drops of brandy or Cologne water when the water has cooled a little. In it soak the silk material which you wish to wash. Rub it as little as possible, and wash it by crushing it and squeezing it often in your hand, which you immediately re-open, to expel all the liquid without wringing the silk, which would pull the threads.

If necessary, repeat this operation in a second or even a third soapy water; you may only put the gum-water and the Cologne water into the third bath. Rinse in lukewarm water, then in cold water. If you wash sturdy material, such as taffety, brush it with a soft brush after it has dried, always in the same direction. (See Div. 11.) If you are working on gauze, dispense with this: but all these articles equally require sulphuring.

Sulphuring.

This operation is used to impart a beautiful bluish white to all materials of white silk or woollen. Here is how to proceed: hang your well-washed and dried materials about six feet up in a small room without a fire-place, whose windows close tightly, and whose door has no cracks and closes hermetically. Place a stove full of burning coals slightly away from the windows. Put a plate of sheet iron supporting several pieces of crushed sulphur on the stove. Leave the room and close the door tightly. The melted sulphur will ignite slightly and convert into sulphurous acid gas, which acts upon the silks.

It is impossible to specify the quantity of sulphur to use; that depends upon the thickness of the materials and the size of the room. You will perceive that it is necessary to burn more sulphur for woollen than for silk. But since the sulphurous acid gas would eventually damage the tissue, it is useful to arrange an opening in the door, covered by glass, through which you may determine the moment when the articles have become quite white. Then halt the operation.

If it is merely a matter of treating a little material (such as a few veils or pair of stockings) nothing prevents doing the sulphuring under an inverted box with the articles hung inside, which you then place over the burning sulphur. It is necessary to be careful so that nothing burns. It is well to lift the box from time to time, to observe the progress of the sulphuring. You may instead make two facing holes on opposite sides of the box, and fit them with glass. Howsoever you do it, you must carefully avoid breathing the suffocating and deleterious sulphur vapour.

The Mode of cleansing Black Silk Materials.

Dilute some bullock's gall with enough boiling water to render it tolerably warm. Soak a clean sponge in the mixture, rub the material on both sides, and squeeze it between your hands to drain it. Then wash it in river-water until the water runs perfectly clear, and squeeze it again. Dry it on a frame in the open air. Rub it on the wrong side with fish-glue, then brush it immediately. (See Div. 12.)

If the black colour has become reddened or dull, it is necessary to revive it. After having cleansed and rinsed it as I have just explained, immerse the piece of silk in river-water into which you have put five or six drops of sulphuric acid, enough for the water to become slightly acid, but not excessively, or it will burn the material. Squeeze the material between your hands for five minutes, then rinse it carefully for a long time in a great quantity of clear water. Finish in the ordinary manner.

If the colour has altered too much, you must re-dye the material. But this term should not frighten you: the operation is so simple that any one may easily execute it. Suppose you are dyeing a gown. Fill a small boiler with enough water to immerse the gown. In the water, boil an ounce and three-quarters to two ounces of logwood, cut into very thin little pieces, for half an hour. Keep the gown there for another half-hour while heating it slightly; then hang it above the boiler to drain. Powder a piece of iron sulphate or green copperas half an inch in size, and throw the powder into the thick liquor. When it has dissolved, add enough water so that there is as much in the boiler as at the beginning. Again boil the gown gently for half an hour, occasionally stirring with a stick. Then wash it in several waters. Let it dry, and put on the finish.

These divers processes give silks the appearance of new material.

The Mode of cleansing Silks dyed Other than Black.

Soap these the same as white silks, and rinse them in lukewarm water. (See Div. 13.) But as it often happens that the colours are not fast, and discharge in the water, you must work with great rapidity. It is not that it is always impossible to revive the colours. On the contrary, several modes are described below.

Modes of reviving Colours.

When the colours of silk or woollen materials are not fast, and as often happens, discharge in soapy water, you must promptly set about reviving the colours. Immerse materials of brilliant yellow, *lavallière*, or crimson in river-water, to which you have added a few drops of sulphuric acid to render it mildly sour. Then wash them well in clear water, and press them between your hands. Spread a thick toile over a table, place your materials flat on it, roll the whole together, and wring forcefully. For rose, crimson-pink, and flesh-colour, substitute lemon-juice or vinegar for the sulphuric acid. The mode is the same for scarlet materials, provided that you put into the water, instead of acid, a little of the solution which dyers call scarlet composition. As for olive-green, use water into which you have thrown several drops of a solution composed of blue copperas or copper sulphate in a little water.

For blues the mode is more difficult; and I advise you, before undertaking the scouring of such a material, to always begin by testing a small sample, in order to judge whether you should proceed. Soaping indeed fades blues obtained by dissolving indigo in sulphuric acid, called liquid blue, and the more brilliant blues given by Prussian blue or iron prussiate. For the latter, the damage is irreparable. But for the former, you may remedy it very well by re-tinting the material after soaping, be it with balls of blue, or with liquid blue diluted with water. It is the contrary with other blues, which alkalis enhance, far from destroying them. These are the blues for which cudbear has been used, this being the most common way to dye deep blues, royal blues, and purples. You may recognize that cudbear has been used, because the colour is subject to reddening. In order to revive it, add a small quantity of good white potash to the soap solution. The brightness of the material and of the colour may be enhanced by again adding a small quantity of potash to the preparation of fish-glue which will be used for finishing.

I shall end this article with some important observations. With the exception of the blues from cudbear, soft soap is preferable to hard soap for cleansing all dyed materials, because it is much less active. It would be still better to use potato water following the washing mode proposed by Mr. Morris. Since alkalis, however weak, always act a little upon colours, you must work as rapidly as possible. If you are not using one of the modes which I just described to revive the colour, it is useful to check the action of the alkali by throwing the material into hard water immediately after soaping. (Water which does not dissolve soap is called hard water. All the water from Paris wells has this property.) If you do not have such water at hand, it is easy to obtain by throwing a little sulphuric acid into soft water; but avoid making it markedly sour.

When black has reddened or dulled, you may revive it after cleansing the material. You will perceive how valuable this resource is for garments, aprons, and above all for stockings. After all the dirtiness of the black material has disappeared, boil in a boiler for about half an hour, an ounce and three-quarters, or two ounces and an eighth, of logwood, cut into pieces and enclosed in a bag of clear toile. Soak the material well in slightly warm water. Wring it by means of the hook and stick as hard as you can, and plunge it into the boiler, where it must boil a good half-hour. Remove it, and add to the bath a piece of green copperas (ferrous sulphate) as big as a hazel-nut. Allow it a moment to dissolve, stir the bath with a stick, re-immerse the material, and boil it for another half-hour.

The Way to partially replace the Glaze of Materials spotted by Water.

All gummed or calendered materials are spotted when water falls on the surface, because it removes the gloss and the glaze. (See Div. 14.) You may re-glaze dyed woollen or cotton materials by ironing them damp with a very hot flat-iron while they are stretched and pinned to a table padded with drap. Pin either on the edges or the seams nearest the spot, so as not to damage the material. Delicately moisten the unglazed spot with the end of a sponge, then pass the point of an iron lightly over the moistened area. Since the heat of the iron might damage the colour, put a doubled paper on the iron, excepting the part reserved for ironing the spot. If the spot is very small, you may heat the end of an iron for goffering *collerettes,* and place it upright on the moistened spot. This is much less awkward.

If the material is silk, after removing the spots, gum it as I have indicated for replacing the finish.

The Mode of raising the Nap of Velvets.

When the rain or some other mishap has crumpled and flattened the nap of velvet, use the following mode to raise it. Put a copper plate over a grill furnished with embers. Cover the plate with a damp toile, and spread the wrong side of the velvet over it; then delicately raise the pile with a soft brush. The steam which the heat releases from the damp toile renders this operation very easy.

You may replace the plate with a flat-iron supported flat between two bricks, and the brush with a new fine-toothed ivory comb: you must rub the comb against the nap. When you have removed the grease-spots from the top of velvet, it is always necessary to finish with this operation.

To wash Woollen Materials or Merino Shawls.

It is needless to say that you use the same mode as for washing gowns of the same material. You must unpick them beforehand, and remove the stitches, so that the calender does not catch on the material. You will perceive that removing them after calendering would crumple the material disagreeably.

First observe the colour of the shawl, in order to proceed according to the principles given for washing coloured silk materials. You must always resort to soaping, but this is more or less strong according to the fastness of the colour, save for using a stronger soap solution when the material is more soiled. All chemists who have written on the subject of scouring, say to rinse woollen materials several times in clear water to remove the soap. Laundresses, on the contrary, leave the soap in the material, especially for knitted woollen petticoats.

The cleansing of white shawls has much in common with that of white silks. As to washing, spread the material on a wash-board to brush it as you soap. Finishing it is another thing; you send the shawl to be calendered. This operation is an extremely good bargain. A shawl is calendered for four, six, or eight sous, according to its size. A gown costs proportionably.

If a calenderer is not available, or if you do not wish to send the shawl to one, you may substitute as follows. On a card-table, successively attach all the pieces of a merino gown, or a shawl along its entire length. Stretch it evenly in all directions, as explained for veils. These pieces of material must be half damp. When they are well stretched, take a very hot flat-iron and pass it evenly over the entire article attached, so that the ironing finishes drying it. It is essential not to rest the iron longer in one place than another, for the place where it stays longer will turn darker than the rest of the article.

If the shawl has spots, remove them beforehand according to the modes given below. It is also necessary, before soaping it, to mark all the most soiled parts with a piece of soap. It is true that you may discover these parts after soaping by examining them against daylight. But it is always well to mark them, because it is possible to encounter spots which are not seen when the material is wet, but which reappear when it is dry. You ought also to remove the dust from a shawl or gown before putting it in water.

To wash Lace, and Linen or Cotton Tulles, to look like new.

All these articles are washed like white silks, except that you add neither honey nor brandy to the soap liquor, in which you squeeze them without rubbing them. (See Div. 15.) Before putting them into the water, inspect them thoroughly for breaks in the net. Mend these immediately, because a hole greatly enlarges during the washing, and especially during the stretching of this light tissue. If you have *fichus*, collars, veils, or in general more or less large pieces of tulle, use a card-table for spreading them out in all directions, and attach them to it with pins. If there are three-piece caps, or others which have the shape of the head, you may put the cap of a *serre-tête* made of lined green drap, onto one of the plaster heads used by milliners. Then put the cap on top and fasten it all round with lace pins. It is essential that the drap *serre-tête* be firmly secured to the plaster head.

Another tool is necessary for stretching laces, but it is simple. Take a large kerchief, or instead one of the large sieves for bolting flour, removing the clear toile which forms the bottom. Pad the square well on top with cotton wadding or light hay. In short, do every thing proper for use as a pincushion. Cover the whole with green drap.

Spread the lace over the middle of the square and attach it securely while stretching it. Stick lace pins into the heading and the footing, but in very different ways. For the footing or selvage, embed the pins lengthways, as you insert a needle to take a running stitch. For the heading or *picot*, thrust one pin perpendicularly through each loop of the *picot*. To this end, raise the threads of each loop narrowed by washing. Stick a pin there, turn it round, and insert it as if you were really making the *picot*. Tulle *entre-deux* requires pins embedded along both sides as for a footing.

This preparation completed, pass over the lace a fine, clean sponge dampened with lightly-gummed water, as explained below. When tulle veils, *fichus*, or caps have *picots* sewed on, proceed as for the *picots* of laces. It is essential to hold the edges very straight and smooth.

Finishing.

Dissolve a very small quantity of very white fish-glue or gum-dragon in some water. Soak up this solution with a fine sponge, then rub the material on the wrong side. Take a frame of suitable size, on which a piece of green serge is tightly stretched. In the absence of this stretcher, you may use an old card-table. Stretch the woollen or silk material tightly over the frame, while fastening it with closely-spaced pins. Brush it again in this position and let it dry quickly. For this it is necessary to put it in the sun or a heated room.

The finishing of gauzes differs a little. As soon as they are rinsed, they are arranged on a stretcher, as I have explained. Then you wet the sponge in the glue solution. Move the sponge evenly over the surface of the gauze, being watchful not to re-apply it on spots where it has already passed.

The Mode of preparing Fish-glue.

Fish-glue is sold in tablets. Take one, and strike it with a hammer on a block of solid wood. It is well to first wrap the tablet in linen or paper, because thin pieces will flake off and fly here and there. Cut the flakes into little pieces. Soak them in river-water, in the proportion of three and a sixth ounces of water to a third of an ounce of glue, for five to six hours. Dissolve in a water-bath, then pass the solution through a toile to filter out all impurities. Add a little hot water to it. You may use this glue immediately; it thickens in cooling and takes on the aspect of transparent jelly.

To have Fish-glue ready to use at Any Time.

After having thus prepared the fish-glue jelly, and immediately after having passed it through the toile, evaporate half the water in the water-bath. Add as much spirit of wine as the remaining liquid. Pour this solution into the small flat bottles of green glass, found at chemist's shops, called *figues* or *figuettes*. Cover the opening with paper stretched and tied round the neck with thread, to counter evaporation. When the liquid is cooled it becomes a jelly; immediately stop the mouth with linen. This glue keeps indefinitely.

When you wish to use some, put one of these phials into your pocket or *fichu*. The heat of your body is enough to liquefy it in a few minutes, and you may use it immediately to finish materials, and even to glue small objects. This glue is extremely strong.

To wash Black Lace Veils and Black Blonds.

To cleanse these different articles, wash them in warm water mixed with bullock's gall. Rinse them in cold water until the odour of the gall has disappeared. Squeeze out the water thoroughly without wringing, then stiffen the lace.

To do this, dissolve a little fish-glue in boiling water. Soak the veils or blonds in this lightly-gummed water, then press them between your hands. Spread and stretch them as explained for white laces. You may also use a sponge to bathe them in the gum-water.

The Mode of cleansing Gold and Silver Lace.

Sew the lace in a piece of linen, and boil it in a quart of water and two ounces of soap. Then wash and rinse it, always holding it spread between your hands for fear of crumpling it. Spread it on a card-table to dry. (See Div. 16.)

The Mode of cleansing Embroidery in general.

Embroidery is cleansed by a very simple mode which may always be used, particularly for silver embroidery, which strong odours blacken easily.

(See Div. 17.) Heat the crumb of some stale bread in a very clean casserole. While it is thoroughly hot, distribute it over the embroidery. Rub it with the palm of your hand, and spread it so that it is every where on the work. Cover the whole with several toiles. When it has cooled, turn the work over and beat the wrong side with a stick. Nothing more remains but to brush the embroidery gently. Take care to coat it on the wrong side with gum, or starch evenly smoothed on.

The Mode of cleansing Silk Stockings.

First wash your silk stockings in lukewarm water infused with white soap to remove the filth. (See Div. 18.) Rinse them in clear water, and rub them well in fresh, lukewarm soapy water. Then make a third rather strong soapy water, just as hot as your hand can bear. Put in a little blue wrapped in a flannel bag, just until the water becomes sufficiently blue. Wash the stockings in it; remove them and wring them. Let them dry so that they remain a little damp. Warm them in burning sulphur, after which put them over two wooden forms, taking care to put the fronts or sides face to face. Finish by smoothing them with a glaze.

Blonds and gauzes are washed in the same way, except that you put a little gum in the water before heating it.

To cleanse Ribands.

Ribands are washed like silk materials according to their colour. They must be glazed very lightly with fish-glue, by spreading the glue over the riband with a sponge, or even with water. Do not attach ribands to a tenter to dry. Put a sheet of white paper on a card-table, put the riband on the sheet of paper, then another sheet on the riband. Then take a very hot flat-iron, and pass it over the second sheet of paper. As you iron the riband thus covered, another person must pull it in a straight line: it should come out highly glazed.

To whiten Unbleached Toiles.

Commence by soaking the toiles for five to six hours in a cold wash-liquor prepared in the following way. In twenty quarts of river-water or well-water—it is unimportant whether it is soft or selenious—thin down eight to ten pounds of cow-dung, and four to five pounds of sheep-dung or goat-dung. Mix about a pound of sea-salt into the vat of wash-liquor. When the toiles are very brown, such as nankeens and all those made of cotton with russet wool, sharpen the wash-liquor by throwing in two or three handfuls of well-pulverized quicklime after the toiles have been sufficiently soaked that they are saturated with water. The lime, because of its alkaline and astringent quality, strengthens the fibres, develops the salts contained in the dung, and fixes them to the toiles. The wash-liquor bath must be applied in open air, exposed to the strongest rays of the sun. Remove the toiles from the bath, and spread them over the ground to dry in the sun. Before they become completely dry, shake them to detach the largest parts of the dung. Wring them when they are half dry to remove all dampness.

Then prepare to give the toiles their second bath. This consists of soaking them in another wash-liquor composed of a kind of marly and alkaline earth (such as grey or red clay, mixed with a small quantity of soda, or with about a fifth of quicklime and of sea-salt). For fifty quarts of water, dilute ten to twelve pounds of this earth after having reduced it to a powder. For muslin, soak the material while rubbing it with your hands. If the toiles are strong, trample them with your feet. This work completed, soak fine toiles, such as muslin, organdy, and dorea, for five to six hours. Soak strong toiles, such as percale, madapolame, cassas, materials of European courtrai, Holland toiles, and even the beautiful French batiste, for eight to ten hours.

Immediately after having removed the toiles and drained off the moisture by wringing them sufficiently, spread them in the sun to dry them to a proper point, that is, so that they are slightly damp. In this state they are already bleached. It only remains to pass them to the steam-bath to impart the brilliant whiteness of which they are susceptible, and which all toiles should have.

To give the steam-bath, arrange the pieces of toile, loosely tied up, over the opening of a great tub placed on a permanently installed stove. The tub contains a wash-liquor similar to the second bath, with the addition of a small quantity of banana-leaf ashes or sea-salt, and some quicklime. The tub must be two-thirds full and the mixture ready to start boiling. With the pieces tied, twist them into the shape of a cone or concave pyramid, so that each upper round is placed securely over the one underneath and allows the steam to circulate freely. Maintain the boiling with a moderate fire for three to four hours for muslin, and for five to six hours for strong toiles. The steam, carried by the heat, penetrates every fold and passes into every fibre, and absorbs the different alkaline salts, acids, and the most elusive lixivia of the cow-dung, &c., which compose the two baths which I have already described. It detaches and drives out the odours and the filth attached to the material, lightens its russet and grey colour, and gives it a beautiful milk-white; and even an agreeable, healthful, and beneficial odour.

When the toiles have cooled a little, hasten to rinse them in several waters, or in a pond, or better in a running stream, while beating them against a very smooth rock or an equally smooth piece of wood, broad and long. Do not use beetles because they break the tissue. Confine yourself to turning the pieces alternately by grasping now one end, then the other. Wring them to force all the moisture out. Then dry them in the sun, spread on the ground, or better on the masonry terraces constructed for this purpose at the great bleaching establishments.

That is all there is to the task of bleaching toiles. (See Div. 19.) From this moment the warp and weft threads have finished changing. They do not shorten any more, and the pieces will not draw or shrink any more in either length or width. That is a novel benefit of this mode of cleansing toiles. It is now only a matter of perfecting your work by sizing the toiles; that is, applying a dressing which enhances their whiteness and brightness.

To size Toiles.

Daily experience proves to us that toiles of European manufacture, batiste as well as muslin, do not have that pleasing finish noticeable in India goods. This is due to the difference in the sizing used. In India, all toiles are sized with rice-water. In Europe, they are sized with starch. Rice, which is soft and does not turn at all yellow, leaves all the suppleness in the toiles and increases their whiteness, which they always preserve. Starch is dryer, rougher, and has a more or less grey or russet colour, which gives the material a yellowish appearance and a harshness to the touch. Though rice may be dearer than starch, the cost of sizing is not increased, because it is only a matter of using the water in which it has cooked, which would not prevent the rice from being eaten.

To determine the Manner
in which Toiles have been whitened.

To determine if toile has been whitened with lime, wet some place on it, and suffer it to dry. If the boundary between the wetted place and the rest of the material is reddish, you will have certain proof that the whitening was done with lime, and consequently you have been deceived.

There is yet another way, which consists of putting a sample of the toile which you wish to test in a glass, and pouring over it several spoonfuls of good vinegar or hydrochloric acid diluted with water. If the toile contains lime, the acid will cause an effervescence and rather considerable bubbling, accompanied by a slight noise. But if the toile does not contain lime, immersing the toile in the acid produces no effect.

To scour with Sand and Bullock's Gall.

Here is the mode which scourers generally use to cleanse woollen materials of every colour, especially thick ones, such as carpets, arm-chairs, *bergères*, carriage linings, horse-blankets, &c. Never neglect to first beat carpets and all other materials soiled with dust.

After having marked all the places where there are spots with soap or chalk, soak a firm brush in warm bullock's gall, and rub all the spots. When they are no longer apparent, rinse the material in cold water and suffer it to dry. This operation completed, take fine sand, such as that sold by grocers under the name *sablon*. Dampen it a little, then sprinkle the material while it lies flat on an inclined table, which you must have for scouring so that the dirty water runs off more easily. Strike it with a hard brush in order to penetrate the dust well, then rub with a stiff brush. When the sand comes out, it carries all the dirt with it.

When these materials are embroidered, whether in wool or silk, you must work very quickly, and rinse in hard water as I have already advised.

The Mode of purifying Bullock's Gall.

I think that for scouring, prepared bullock's gall is preferable to every other substance, especially for difficult cleansing. This animal matter combines very well with greasy matters. According to M. Chaptal, it scarcely alters colours. Perhaps you have been discouraged from frequent use of it merely by its foul odour, its greenish colour, and its ease of putrefaction; but you may make these disadvantages disappear entirely by purifying it. There is thus no reason for not using it routinely.

Here is the way to purify bullock's gall, as found in an excellent work titled *Manuel du teinturier et du dégraisseur*, by M. Jean René Denis Riffault des Hêtres. To about a quart and two ounces of fresh bullock's gall, boiled and skimmed, add an ounce of finely-powdered alum. Leave the liquor on the fire until the combination is perfect. When it has cooled, pour it into a bottle and cork it loosely. Then take a similar quantity of bullock's gall, likewise boiled and skimmed. Add an ounce of common salt, and leave it on the fire until it has all combined. Then put it in a bottle and cork it loosely.

When you have left the gall in a room where a moderate temperature prevails, for about three months, it deposits a thick sediment and clarifies. But since it still contains much yellow-coloured matter which would make the colours turn, decant each of these above-mentioned liquors, or filter them well and mix them together in equal parts. The yellow-coloured matter which the mixture still contains coagulates immediately, precipitates, and leaves the bullock's gall perfectly purified and colourless. If you wish, at the end you may filter it through a paper filter.

This preparation keeps without deterioration, clarifies with aging, never exudes any disagreeable odour, and does not lose any of its useful qualities.

The Mode of scouring Woollens.

First soak the woollen in lukewarm water, the temperature of milk as it is just drawn. Leave it there for an hour, then remove and drain it. For a pound of woollen, dissolve an ounce and a half of soap in about a pint of boiling water, which you then pour into five pots of water, hot enough that you can hold your hand in it only with difficulty. Put the woollen prepared by the first bath into this second bath, and allow it to soak for half an hour. Make a third bath like the preceding one, but entirely with boiling water, and soak the woollen for the same interval of time. To avoid fulling it, you must merely soak the woollen in the bath without agitating it. Remove it at the end of the prescribed time. Rinse it in cold water, then allow it to dry.

To cleanse Garments of Blue, Black, or Dark Brown Drap.

After beating the garment well, mark all the spots which cover it with a piece of white soap. Then wet these marks with bullock's gall mixed with an equal quantity of water. Mix enough for the collar, the ends of the sleeves, the openings of the pockets, the under-arms, and the revers, because these parts are ordinarily more soiled than the rest of the garment. Rub well between your hands until the greasy tinge has disappeared. If you wish to avoid crumpling the collar and revers, be content to apply a light coat of clay diluted with water, or fuller's earth, which at Paris is sold by tinsmiths.

That done, mix some bullock's gall with eight times as much water. Using a brush, moisten the garment with this water, rubbing vigorously along the direction of the nap. This will suffice if you use purified bullock's gall. But if you use ordinary bullock's gall, you must completely wash the garment in clear water to get rid of the bad odour. In that case wait until the garment is nearly dry to lay down the nap with the brush. For drying, pass into the sleeves a half-hoop or a stick, suspended by a cord in the middle. If the garment has lost its nap in several places and shows the ground, when it is damp rub it vigorously with the heads of the plant commonly known as fuller's teasel, until the nap is raised. (See Div. 20.)

After a garment has been well beaten, it is necessary to restore a deep colour. Even with brushing, in summer this is quite difficult, because the dust has penetrated too thoroughly. Finishing with olive-oil is the surest and easiest way to render the colour more brilliant, especially if the drap is blue, black, or green. When the garment is quite dry, take a drop of good olive-oil in your hand. Coat a brush with it, and use this to lightly rub the entire garment. If you take care not to use too much oil, and if you distribute it evenly over the whole surface of the drap, it will look like new. You must be very attentive and skilful in order not to make spots.

The Art of removing Spots.

Spots are divided into two kinds: spots which do not alter the colour, and spots which alter or destroy it. The first include spots from simple greases, such as oil, tallow, broth, milk, butter, pomatum, wax, divers fats, and resin; and those from greasy mixtures, such as sauces and oil-paints.

This first class is followed by all the spots caused by iron in its different states: ink, rust, and dirty oil. A third class includes vegetable spots: wine, tea, syrup, jam, grape jelly, coffee, chocolate, divers fruits, cider, beer, and tobacco. Sanguine spots are not included in any of these categories, but are no fewer in number than the simple spots.

The second kind of spots, which alter or destroy the colour, includes vinegar, lemon-juice or orange-juice, melon, red currant, sorrel, fresh or old urine, &c. Besides these, several spots in the preceding class alter the colour of the material when it is fugitive.

Spots from Simple Grease, Tallow, Broth, &c.

When these spots are on linen or cotton material, you may content yourself with dry-soaping the spot, then rubbing it. Next pour on several drops of warm water, continually rubbing until the spot has disappeared. Finish by washing. This mode is especially effective when the spot is recent.

On woollen or silk, when the spot has just formed, you may remove it by means of mild heat. To this end, place a piece of tissue paper over the spot. Then apply a warm iron on top, just to melt the greasy substance, which is absorbed by the paper. If the iron is too hot, the grease will be more firmly fixed in the material. Keep changing the position of the paper. This mode is especially suitable for tallow, or congealed wax which forms a lump on the material.

When the grease has penetrated farther into the material, take a soup-spoon made of silver, copper, or iron which is not tin-plated. Place a burning coal on it. Then move it around over the spot, which you have covered with unsized paper, water-leaf paper, or tissue paper.

You may employ fuller's earth, chalk, or clay even more successfully. Take some clay or fuller's earth, very soft to the touch and not mixed with sand. Reduce it to a very fine powder. Cover the spot with it, cover this with water-leaf paper, and pass a moderately warm flat-iron over it: the grease will be absorbed by the clay. White chalk or Paris white is used on white satin and other white silk materials. This mode has the advantage of not removing the finish, and does not alter the colour.

If all this is unsuccessful, use spirit of turpentine which is very fresh; otherwise it will make a new spot. When this essence is mixed with spirit of wine, its effect is infallible. Pour several drops upon the spot and rub until it is removed.

All the spots of resinous substances, such as resin, pitch, tar, and turpentine, may be removed with spirit of wine, Hungary water, or good Cologne water. Pour several drops of these substances on the spot and rub.

To easily prepare Essence of Soap.

Grease-spots of every kind are removed by soaping, if you act against them immediately, or with the substances described in the previous article. But there are many others which you may also use in preference to them. Besides, even if the spot is fresh, it is not very proper to soap silk, for fear of dulling a large portion of the material in washing, which often makes the remedy worse than the ill. Furthermore, if you spot your gown body or sleeves, it is most annoying, and sometimes impossible, to instantly undress to remove the spot. Therefore, it would be a genuine service to provide a way to remove the spot at once, without damaging the material and without the need to take off any garments. Essence of soap, of which I shall give the receipt after M. Sebastien Lenormand, fulfills all these conditions.

Cast ten and a half ounces of good white Marseilles soap, cut into thin slices, into a quart, one and seven-eighths ounces of spirit of wine. Add two ounces of potash. Dissolve the whole, be it with the warmth of the sun, a water-bath, or a low fire, stirring the mixture from time to time. The dissolution complete, let the liquor rest. Then draw it off clear, or filter it. Save it in well-stopped bottles.

Here is its use: take a small sponge, which you squeeze in a way which allows only a small pointed end under your fingers, or replace it with a little cotton wadding. Soak up a little of the essence with one of these articles, rub the spot, and you will see it disappear. But immediately take the precaution of covering the spot with brick-clay reduced to powder, or fine ashes passed through a silken sieve. If you neglect this, the entire portion moistened by the essence will develop a discolouration, which workmen call a ring. All liquid substances for removing spots are used in the same way, whether essence of turpentine, of lavender, of lemon, &c.

When the spot is not very spread out, you may dispense with replacing the finish removed with the spot. Otherwise, moisten the material with lukewarm water into which you have dissolved some very white gum-dragon. Then stretch it on a card-table, fixing the pins at the seams in order not to mar the material.

To remove Grease-spots from All Kinds of Materials without wetting.

This mode has the advantage over the preceding one of not soaking the material, but it requires a few more steps. Start by taking five or six burning coals about the size of a walnut. Wrap them in a well-moistened piece of linen, which you have squeezed hard in your hand to expel the excess water. Spread the stained material over a table, on which you have previously placed a very clean towel folded in quarters. Then take the linen which contains the coals by all four corners, and put it on the spot. Alternately lift and rest it very lightly on the spot ten or twelve times in succession: the spot will entirely disappear. As you place and remove the linen you will see a little vapour rise, which will have the odour of the spot.

Grease-spots.

To remove these spots, you may use a dilute solution of pure potash, but you must proceed cautiously so as not to damage the material. Wax-spots are removed with spirit of turpentine or sulphuric ether. Paint spots are removed in the same way.

There is a mode of removing grease-spots from silk which may be usefully applied to other cases. Spirit of wine, or alcohol, which does not act immediately upon grease, removes greasy substances when the volatile oil called essence of lemon is dissolved in it. To apply this liquor, moisten the spot with it, then rub it with a sponge or linen while the material is damp. Spirit of turpentine, which forms the basis of all liquors for removing spots, could perhaps be substituted for the essence of lemon.

Spots from Grease contained in Dirty Oil, Sauces, Oil-paints, Ointments, &c.

Dirty oil and similar substances are easily removed by putting raw egg-yolk on the spot, letting it thoroughly penetrate the material, then soaping and rinsing. Oil-paints and ointments yield to cold purified bullock's gall, or to fresh spirit of turpentine, pure or combined with spirit of wine.

It is essential to treat these spots—and all others—as soon as you notice them, before they have thoroughly penetrated the tissue. They will be much less trouble to remove, and you will not have to wear out the material with rubbing. It is very true that the spots which are most stubborn when they are old, commonly yield to a simple soaping when they are new.

You may remove all these spots with essence of soap and Dupleix's "Essence Vestimentale," which is nothing but a combination of essential oil of turpentine, lavender oil, and lemon oil; but it is important that all these substances be fresh.

Ink, Mud, Rust, and Dirty Oil Spots.

This mode is excellent for removing ink-spots from white material, but first try it on a sample. Fill a tin spoon with river-water, and add about a pinch of salt of sorrel. Hold the spoon over the fire until the salt is entirely dissolved. Pour the boiling water on the spot, which will instantly disappear without rubbing. If the spot resists, repeat the operation.

On calicoes or printed toiles, where the colour would be removed by the above mixture, rub the ink with sorrel leaves, then soap. For this to succeed the spot must be recent. Oxalic acid also removes ink-spots.

For mud spots on silk, when the mud has been picked off and is not very thick, it is only necessary to rub the material with woollen. The brush which is ordinarily used will ruin the gloss, whereas the woollen will enhance it. When the mud is very dark, it is mixed with iron particles. It is similar to ink-spots and requires to be removed the same way. But as it is less tenacious, salt of sorrel put on the spot and moistened with warm water should succeed.

When newly made, these spots may yield to simple soaping. Very fine cream of tarter removes mud from silk, but it must be used with great caution so as not to worsen the spot: it is well to first try it on a sample. Moisten this substance, leave it moist on the spot for a moment, then rub it well. Soap well after the application, in order to remove all the cream of tarter.

Rust spots are only removed completely by a solution of salt of sorrel in a tin spoon, or lemon-juice, or in the following manner; which, however, has the disadvantage of greatly soiling the material. Moreover, it is only used on white cotton or linen. Take a warm flat-iron. Use your left hand to rest the wrong side of the stained part of the material on top of it, then rub the material with a thick slice of lemon. Soap, and the spot will no longer appear.

Dirty oil, which I have already discussed, belongs equally in this class since it is composed of grease and iron.

The Mode of M. Rue, to remove Ink, Rust, and Other Spots.

For two ounces of well-pulverized tarter crystals, add an ounce of pulverized alum. Mix it all to use in the same manner as true salt of sorrel. Take care not to use copper or iron utensils, but instead a marble mortar and a wooden pestle.

This mode does not entirely remove ink-spots from silk; a certain dirty grey colour remains round the spot. Here is the way to make it disappear: sprinkle a pinch of fixed alkaline salt over the spot. Wet it with a little water, rub lightly, put on a little green soap where you sprinkled the first composition, and rub again. In this way, with a little water now and then, you remove the soap. Then rinse, and the spot will entirely disappear.

Aquafortis is also successfully used to remove ink-spots from linen. A drop or two is enough to accomplish this without damaging the linen. It is necessary to moisten the spot with water beforehand, and rinse it in water as well.

Vegetable Spots.

When on white material, spots from strawberries, cherries, red currents, beer, cider, or perry yield to warm soaping if they are recent.

Spots from wine, mulberries, black currents, liqueurs, and dyer's weed yield only to soaping followed by sulphur fumigation. To do this form a cone, wide or narrow according to the size of the spot. Ignite the sulphur with several matches passed into the pointed end of the cone, then invert the cone over the spot. In this way the sulphurous gas removes it completely.

For coffee spots, it is sometimes necessary to repeat the operation three times, according to the age of the spot. Chocolate spots are treated like coffee spots, but yield much more quickly. Coffee and chocolate with milk yield to soaping. Tobacco also yields simply. Absinthe spots are removed by sulphur alkali, that is, potassium sulphide. Blood-spots disappear with soaping: on silk and woollen it is sometimes necessary to sulphur them.

To remove fruit and wine spots, use liquid oxygenated muriatic acid, or oxygenated muriate of potash or of lime, to which you add a little sulphuric acid. Let the stained spot soak in one of these solutions until the spot disappears. But you may only apply these reagents to white materials, since the uncombined oxygenated acid destroys all printed and dyed colours.

Persons who do not have the equipment needed to saturate water with gaseous oxygenated muriatic acid may use this mode: put about a spoonful of muriatic acid (spirit of salt) in a coffee-cup, and add about a full coffee-spoon of powdered manganese. Put this earth into a larger vessel filled with hot water. Moisten the stained spot, and expose it to the fumes which are released from the cup. After a certain time the spot will disappear.

Soap for removing Spots.

Nothing is more convenient and economical than to have a substance always ready to remove spots which happen to form. A well-run household should always have it on hand. On these two points, the soap whose receipt I shall provide leaves nothing to be desired. As it is well known that simple soaping removes, wholly or in part, recent spots of every possible kind, greasy or vegetable, simple or compound, it may be said that this soap will act effectively upon all of them, even on the oldest. It is sometimes necessary to employ it following a light sulphuring (as described earlier) for wine, fruit, and coffee spots; but only when these things have aged on the material a good deal. Here is how you should make this soap:

Take a pound of Marseilles soap, six egg-yolks (which are well known to be effective against grease) and half a spoonful of crushed salt. Blend it all with a sufficient quantity of purified bullock's gall. Form cakes of it, and put them to dry in the shade. To use it, moisten the stained material with clear water, and rub it on both sides with the soap. Then wash, and the spot will be removed.

If you prefer, you may rub the spot while dry with this soap. Then pour on several drops of water and rub the material, then again pour on a drop or two of water. The spot will disappear.

Water for removing Spots.

M. Garin, battalion chief, was kind enough to pass on this receipt for a water which soldiers use to remove spots from materials. To make it, put into a glazed earthenware tureen a *bouteille* of lukewarm water, in which has been dissolved a little white soap and an ounce of powdered soda of Alicante. The dissolution finished, add two spoonfuls of bullock's gall and several drops of essential oil of lavender, or another aromatic plant. When you have mixed it thoroughly, pass it through a linen for sealing in a bottle.

To use it, put several drops on the spot; the quantity must be in proportion to its extent. Rub with a small brush. Then wash it all with ordinary water, slightly warm, in order to entirely remove the liquor, which could alter the tissue if it were to dry on the drap.

Spots which alter or destroy the Colour.

These spots are almost hopeless: here, however, are several measures. Spots from the smoke or liquid from a stove require first a warm soaping, salt of sorrel, spirit of turpentine, then finally oxalic acid.

Ammonia or volatile alkali, slightly diluted with water, removes fresh urine spots. Wash the stained place with this solution, then soap immediately afterwards, to keep it from altering the material. Oxalic acid, applied in the same manner, removes old urine spots and those caused by dried sweat. When one of these measures is insufficient, employ them successively, beginning with the volatile alkali. Lemon-juice may also be used.

When you have spilled acid on drap or dyed material, immediately put volatile alkali or several drops of strong soap solution on it. By this means you may sometimes prevent damage.

You may restore the colour removed from silks by acids, by passing a solution of potash through the material, alone or mixed with soap: the latter mode is preferable.

To repair Spots which have altered or destroyed the Colour.

When the colour of a material has been completely destroyed by vegetable acids, such as orange-juice or lemon-juice, vinegar, currants, &c., mineral acids, or fresh or old urine, and it is impossible to revive it with the modes indicated previously, you should apply a tint locally. This easy mode is excellent and sound for materials which are not washed. As for the others, you must renew the colour with every washing, but you will see that this is not a very troublesome obligation.

Take a pastel crayon matched to the removed colour (you may always find these crayons at shops which sell artist's paints). Dilute it with a matched liquid colour, such as liquid blue for blue crayon, scarlet composition for red crayon, and so on. Take a little water and dissolve some starch in it, or better still some gum, and mix this solution well with your little preparation.

That done, take a fine paint-brush. Soak the tip in the colour, and put it on the spot as delicately as possible, while pulling the material tight. Take care that this operation does not produce a ring, which would be a fresh and more disagreeable spot. To avoid this, in addition to applying the paint-brush delicately, use only as much water as is indispensable for liquidity.

As soon as the coloured water is applied, cover it with fine sand, powdered clay, or fine ashes; in short a soft powder of any kind, so that the colour does not spread beyond the places where you desire to apply it. Then expose the material to the greatest heat, so that the colour penetrates the tissue thoroughly. If the material is woollen, put it a little above a boiling pot, and allow it to thus be impregnated with steam for about an hour. Let it dry, then brush it. If the colour stands out, wash gently. It will be impossible to detect the repaired spot.

——*Manuel d'économie domestique, Manuel des dames, Manuel des demoiselles.*

Diversion 1.

The Washhouse. Mrs. L.—What a serious expense is washing in a family! I am desirous of ascertaining the least expensive way of having it *well done*.

Mrs. B.—I am glad to hear you lay an emphasis on the words *well done*. Bad washing can never be at a cheap rate; however little you may fancy you pay for it, it is still too dear. It will ruin your clothes and linen, which will not serve half the time they might have done with a good clean washing, and a proper getting-up.

Mrs. L.—Is it better to have the washing done at home, or send it out to a laundress?

Mrs. B.—Our grandmothers would be surprised at that question, and particularly with modern management in respect to washing, could they see it. In their day a family washing was a matter of deep interest. The clouds and the weather-glass were examined, and all the usual domestic arrangements were made subservient to the happy accomplishment of this grand event. A wash was a season of toil and anxiety both to mistress and maiden, and I believe of dismay and discomfiture to every other member of the family. Its advantages, however, were great, though not in proportion to the inconveniences endured. The whiteness of the linen, and the superior clear-starching and ironing of those days, are not by any means equalled in modern washing; nor can our economists boast of any mode by which it can be done at so comparatively trifling an expense. But the presence and scrutiny of the mistress or housekeeper were essential to the good progress of the work, as well as to prevent any waste of provisions.

The present habits, both of the heads of families and of their servants, render the old-fashioned monthly wash out of the question, in these days; and if that were not the case, I doubt whether, taking every thing into consideration, it would be desirable to revive the custom. To keep a laundry-maid, and to send the linen out weekly to a laundress, are the two modes of management now generally adopted. The expediency of the first plan depends upon the size of a family, and the conveniences which the house may afford for this arrangement. When the family is large enough to employ the whole time of a laundry-maid in washing, getting up, and assisting to repair the linens, I am inclined to think it a desirable plan to be adopted. It *almost* ensures good washing, and the proper airing of the linen. The inconveniences are, the danger of extravagance in soap, candles, and coals, which would render it very expensive. The laundry also is often a place of resort and gossip for the other servants of the family, which is an evil difficult to prevent, unless a very strict observation is kept up on the part of the mistress.

It is perhaps the most convenient and least troublesome plan to send out your washing to a laundress, though if your family is large, the expense is immense; each article being separately charged makes the whole amount to a considerable sum weekly. The expense may in some degree be diminished, by stipulating that the smaller articles, such as pocket-handkerchiefs, neckcloths, and the like, be charged by the dozen, instead of each article being separately charged. Some good managers get their washing done by contract; and this, when you can ensure its being well done, is a pleasant plan, because you ascertain the exact sum your washing will cost you during the year. But it often happens that the laundress does not discharge her part of the contract very conscientiously, but sends home the linen miserably got up and badly aired. When this happens, you cannot consider such washing as cheaply performed.

Mrs. L.—I am looking out for a good laundry-maid; what ought I to require from her?

Mrs. B.—I would certainly advise you to procure one who has been accustomed to the business of the laundry, as that is not a department which you yourself can superintend; nor can a housekeeper do it to any great extent, without neglecting some of her other avocations. Your eyes will quickly tell you if she washes the linen clean, and gets up fine muslin tolerably well. If this should not be the case, you must certainly notice it directly, or the colour of your linen will be injured.

One thing you must remember, is that your laundry should have every convenience to facilitate the work. The washhouse should be well supplied with soft water, boilers, and tubs. A washing-machine saves labour, but I believe that the clothes are not so well washed as by hand; and some imagine that it wears out the linen, and tears it. In the laundry there should be a good stove (for the double purpose of heating the irons and airing the linen) and also a mangle.

Besides the essential articles of soap, blue, and starch, the laundry-maid should always have a supply of salt of lemon, citrate of potash, and bleaching liquor, with which to remove ink-spots, iron-moulds, or other spots from the linen before it is washed.

Some laundry-maids are so careless as to tear the linen in stirring it while boiling, making use of any rough stick they can find; and also sometimes to permit the water in the copper to get very low, by which means the linen is liable to be scorched by the fire. Such negligence should always be reproved. Soap is an article very easily wasted by a careless servant; and it requires some vigilance, either in the housekeeper or in the mistress of the family, to prevent it. When the quantity used weekly has been ascertained, it should be weighed out for each washing; nor should the laundry-maid be permitted to exceed it, without some apparent reason being given for the additional consumption.

Small coal and cinders will serve as fuel for stoves and coppers, after they are well lighted. Horse-hair lines for hanging out the linen should be taken down when not in constant use, and before they are again put up they should be wiped very clean.

——Domestic Duties.

The Laundry-maid. She washes all the household and other linen belonging to her employers, and is assisted generally by the house-maids; or the house-maids, kitchen-maids, and scullery-maids wash for themselves. All the men-servants find their own washing, excepting the footmen's aprons and jackets. The foul linen is given out to her on Monday morning, and returned clean on Friday night or Saturday morning.

——The Complete Servant.

Diversion 2.

The Mode of marking Linens. The following composition is much employed in England. It does not damage the linens, and is not effaced by wash-liquor.

Moisten the place where you wish to write the characters with a solution of an ounce of potash in two ounces of water. Let it dry. Then write with a solution of three drachms of silver nitrate, six drachms of distilled verdigris, and half an ounce of gum-arabic, in two ounces of distilled water.

To obtain a Black Liquor for marking Linens in a Strong and Lasting Manner. This preparation consists of two liquors, one containing the mordant, and the other containing ink of a dark brown colour. Be careful to stir it well before using it, because it settles when it stands.

First impregnate the place which you wish to mark with the mordant, and let it dry on the linen. Next rub the place which has been moistened with a sleeker. Then, with an ordinary pen which has been dipped into the well-stirred ink, write the names and letters you desire on the place thus prepared. No wash-liquor or chemical process effaces this ink, which when well dried is a very beautiful black.

Preparation of the Mordant. Dissolve two and an eighth ounces of white glue, and as much fish-glue, in three ounces of alcohol and as much distilled water. It will be dissolved in the space of two days. Use a water-bath, and take care to stir these two kinds of glue now and then. After the whole are dissolved, filter it through a flannel to catch all the mucilaginous parts. The liquor, filtered and kept in a well-stopped bottle, will be ready to use as desired.

Preparation of the Ink. Dissolve the desired quantity of silver coins in nitric acid (aquafortis). This solution will be sapphire-blue because of the copper contained in the coins. To separate the copper from the silver, add to the solution twelve times its weight in distilled water, or failing that rain-water, and suspend a strip of copper in it. As the strip dissolves, the pure silver will precipitate in the form of a white powder. When precipitation has ceased, decant the liquor. Swill down the powder by pouring a great deal of water on it, until this water is no longer tinted blue, but remains perfectly limpid. When well made the residue or powder will be perfectly pure silver.

If the residue weighs an ounce, dissolve as much Senegal gum and a pound and twelve ounces of white glue, in two and an eighth ounces of distilled water. Mix this solution with two pounds, eight ounces of well-calcined lamp-black in a lidded crucible. To make this mixture well, you must grind it in a glass mortar. This operation done, pour the silver on top, diluting it with eight times its weight in distilled water. Stir the whole well with a spatula, and the ink is made.

Application of this Ink for printing *Toile d'Orange* and Other Materials. You will readily understand that this ink may be advantageously employed for printing toiles with a white, yellow, pink, or other light-coloured ground. The preparation of the materials which you wish to print only requires soaking them in a solution of parchment or fish-glue. After they have dried, smooth them with a glass sleeker. Thicken the ink with a large quantity of gum-senegal and apply it to the materials in the ordinary manner, with wooden or metal blocks. Three or four days after this operation, wash the materials in a great deal of water, then in soapy water, and they will appear a more beautiful black.

——*Manuel d'économie domestique.*

Diversion 3.

Contagion. When fevers are prevalent, or any complaints, even common colds, it is of much importance that the dirty linen of the sick should be washed in separate waters by itself, for a degree of infectious taint will attach and communicate to all linen washed with the linen of the sick. Particular directions, therefore, should be given by all considerate persons to their laundresses on this subject.

——*The Alphabetical Receipt Book and Domestic Advisor.*

Diversion 4.

The Wash-water. Do not wash with any kind of water, unless it has stood two or three days, for when newly taken in, it is always thick and muddy. If it is from a stream where there is a muddy bottom, it will be better to let it stand four days.

——*The Female Instructor.*

Diversion 5.

The Choice of Soap. Newly-made soap always spoils the linen. Therefore make choice of the oldest you can get, as it will be of much more service, and make the clothes look better.

——*The Female Instructor.*

Diversion 6.

Probably the Society for the Encouragement of Arts, Manufactures, and Commerce; now the Royal Society of Arts.

——Frances Grimble.

Diversion 7.

Utensils for the Art of Dyeing. All the utensils necessary are a copper, a frame, a horse, a tub, and a doll; the latter are represented in Fig. 1. *A* shows the wall in which the peg is put. *B* shows the tub, and *C* the doll. *D* is a blanket being wrung, and *E* the short stick used to wring it.

The horse is to put your goods upon when they come from the dye, and resembles a carpenter's stool, about four feet long, and four feet high, supported upon four legs. The goods, when taken from the copper or boiler, may be thrown across this to drain, though any other contrivance may do as well; and instead of a copper boiler, any tin or brass boiler will do, so that there is room to stir and handle over the goods. (By handling over is meant passing the goods through your hand end to end, to make the colour communicate equally through the piece.) Many dyers carry on a large trade in one room, and with only one copper, which will contain from ten to fifteen gallons. Instead of a frame for finishing silks on, they may be pinned out, as a clear-starcher pins out muslin, &c.; and ribands are finished by drawing the flat-iron on the wrong side, between pressed paper.

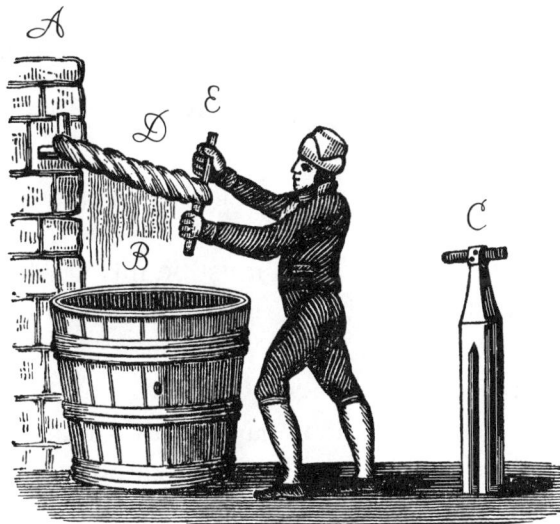

Figure 1. A workman wringing out a blanket.

The doll, or maid, is used for beating blankets, counterpanes, &c. in the tub, in order to cleanse them. For purchasing this doll or getting it made, it is necessary to observe that the upper part, or the shoulders, should measure a circumference of twenty-one inches. The four feet are made square; each foot measures seven inches round. The doll is twenty inches long from the fork to the extremity of the feet; from the fork to the top is sixteen inches, making the height of it altogether three feet.

The tub is two feet and a half in height; the diameter of the top about two feet, and that of the bottom fourteen inches. It has also a false bottom, in order that the under part of the tub may be level with the floor on which it stands, this being more solid to beat on; for if it were not so, the bottom would soon be beaten out.

——*The Family Dyer and Scourer*.

Diversion 8.

Ironing. If you use flat-irons, be sure to rub them smooth against a mat, until they are very bright, and then rub them with a smooth flannel, which must be done every time they come to the fire. It will be better for the linen, that you use the flat-iron as hot as you can; only take care to try the iron on a rag, lest it damage the linen. Sprinkle a few drops of water upon the linen before you begin to iron, always taking care to put more water to the fine than the coarse. The water makes it more pliable in ironing, and more stiff afterwards.

——*The Female Instructor.*

Diversion 9.

To make Starch. Peel and grate a quantity of potatoes. Put the pulp into a coarse cloth between two boards, and press it into a dry cake. The juice thus pressed out of the potatoes must be mixed with an equal quantity of water. In an hour's time it will deposit a fine sediment, which may be used as starch.

To make Starch from Horse Chestnuts. Take off the outward green prickly husks. Then either by hand, with a knife or other tool, or else with a mill adapted for the purpose, very carefully pare off the brown rind, being particular not to leave the smallest speck, and to entirely eradicate the sprout or growth. Next take the nuts, and rasp, grate, or grind them fine into water, either by hand, or with a mill adapted for the purpose. The pulp which is thereby formed in this water must be washed as clean as possible through a coarse horse-hair sieve, then again through a finer sieve, and again through a still finer, constantly adding clear water to prevent any starch adhering to the pulp.

The last process is to put it with a large quantity of water, about four gallons to a pound of starch, through a fine gauze, muslin, or lawn, so as to entirely clear it of all bran or other impurities. As soon as it settles, pour off the water. Then mix it up with clear water, repeating this operation until it no longer imparts any green, yellow, or other colour to the water. Drain it off until nearly dry, and set it to bake either in the usual mode of baking starch, or else spread out before a brisk fire, being very attentive to stir it frequently to prevent its burning; that is, turning to a paste or jelly which on being dried, turns hard like horn. The whole process should be conducted as quickly as possible.

——*The Alphabetical Receipt Book and Domestic Advisor.*

The Best Mode of making and using Starch. Take such a quantity of starch as you think proportionable to the things you have to use it for, just moisten it with a little water, and then mix a small quantity of powder-blue with it. Then put it into about half a pint of water, and stir it well together. Have about a quart of water boiling on the fire, and when your starch and blue is sufficiently stirred up, put it into the water as it boils. Let it boil for about a quarter of an hour, and be sure to keep it stirring all the while. The more it is stirred the stiffer it will be, and your linen will look the better. You should always boil your starch in a copper vessel, because it requires a deal of boiling. Tin is very apt to make it burn too.

Those things you would have most stiffened must be dipped in first. You must not rub the starch too strong; you may weaken it by the addition of a little water. Before you use it, be sure to let it be well strained.

There are various things which different persons mix with their starch, such as alum, gum-arabic, and tallow; but if you do put any thing in, let it be a little isinglass, for that is by far the best. About an ounce, to a quarter of a pound of starch, will be sufficient.

——*The Female Instructor.*

Diversion 10.

To wash Fine Muslins. Let the muslins be folded in quarters, and put into clear water, not very hot; otherwise they are apt to be yellow. When you have strained the water through a fine cloth, take a piece of the finest soap, and beat it to a lather with a stick turned very smooth; for if the stick is of soft wood, or has any flaws about it, some splinters will be apt to remain in the water. Then put in the muslins, and wash them one by one. Next let them lie in the water for the dirt to soak out. When you take them out, wash them in milk-warm water, and squeeze them as hard as possible, lest any of the dirt should be left in. Then shake them, and lay them into an earthen dish.

Let them lie there until you have made a second lather in the same manner as the first, only the water must be hotter, but not boiling; otherwise it will injure them. Put a little water to as much powder-blue as is necessary, and then pour it into the scalding water, stirring it about until it appears blue. Make a lather in the same manner as before, and when you have put in your muslins, cover them over with a fine clean cloth. It will be better that they stand all night in the water. In the morning wash the blue clean out; then lay them in cold pump-water until you starch them.

To rinse Muslins before you starch them. Take a cup of powder-blue, and mix it with some pump-water in a clean pan. When you have shaken it about for some time it is properly mixed; then put to it a cup more of cold pump-water. Squeeze your muslins through it one by one, never putting more than one in at a time. Otherwise you will be apt to spoil them by giving them a yellowish colour. If the remains of the blue settle upon them, rub them in the water with your hand very slightly. But if any of them appear yellow, you must put more blue to the water, as the only mode of making them change their colour. When you have rinsed them clean, squeeze them as hard as they can bear without hurting them, because unless the water is quite out they will never take the starch so well. Let your hands be very dry when you pull the muslins out. Then lay them on a fine dry cloth, by which you will be able to see whether any wet is left in them.

To starch Fine Muslins. Take a clean skillet, and put in it a pint of pump-water, mixed with a quarter of a pound of starch, and keep it over a slow fire until it is lukewarm. Keep stirring it until it boils, then take it off. When it has stood about a minute, pour it into a clean earthen dish, and cover it up with a Delft plate until it is cold. Then mix a handful of it with half as much blue.

Take your muslin, and spread it out double, so as to lay the starch upon it, but do not let it be too thick. Lay the starch first over the one side and then the other; but do not let the muslin be opened out, because the starch will soak through sufficiently to answer the end. Lay it on the finest muslins first, and afterwards on the thicker ones. The starch which is laid upon the fine ones will serve to do the others, and most sorts of coarser clothes made of muslin may be done with the same starch.

When you have done starching the muslins, lay them in a clean earthen dish, and keep pressing them until the starch begins to stick to your hands. Then wring it out of them. When you have wiped them with a clean dry cloth, open them out and rub them gently.

To clap Muslins before they are ironed. After you have opened them, rub them through your hands, and then clap them together, holding them by the ends in your hands until they are hard. But if you perceive any wet or starch upon your hands, then wash them, and keep them as dry as possible, otherwise the muslin will never look well. You must pull them with your hands both ways, which is the best mode which can be used to prevent fraying. When they are dry enough, spread them out and hold them between you and the light, by which you will see whether any of the starch remains in them. If any thing shines, it is starch, and you must rub the muslins again with your hands. If none is left, they will fly asunder when you clap them; but they must be clapped as fast as possible, lest they become too soft, and lose their colour. It is also necessary to observe, that they must not be clapped singly, otherwise they will fray and tear. Always keep two or three in your hand, and the colour will be much better.

The Proper Mode of ironing Muslins. When you have clapped the muslins and dried them as well as you can, pull them out double on a very smooth board, laying about five or six on each other. Then heat your flat-iron, and put it into the box. When the box is properly heated, take that which is lowest, because it will be drier than the others. By this mode you will not only prevent them from fraying, but also make them look extremely well. Plain muslins must be done upon a very soft and clean woollen cloth. Coarse ones may be done on a cloth which is more damp than the other, or upon the under side of that first used.

To starch Lawns. Lawns must be washed and rinsed in the same manner as muslins, and the starch must be as thin as possible. When you have dipped them in it, take them out and squeeze them hard, in order to force out the wet. Then dry them with a fine cloth. Take care to clap them properly between your hands, otherwise they will be apt to receive damage. When you have folded them up, put them into a clean pan, but do not touch them with any wet, otherwise they will not look so well. Let the cloth upon which you iron them be clean and smooth. Take great care that the flat-iron is not too hot, because it spoils the colours, and gives them a yellowish appearance. The starch must be made for the purpose, for that used for muslin will not be proper, but rather do the lawns an injury.

——*The Female Instructor.*

Diversion 11.

The Mode of cleansing White Satins. French chalk must be strewed over them, and then well brushed off with a hard brush. Should the satin not be sufficiently cleansed by the first dusting, it may be done a second time, and it will both cleanse and beautify the satin. The more the satin is brushed the better.

——*The Family Dyer and Scourer.*

Diversion 12.

To wash Black Silks. Warm a little small beer, and mix it with ink. Then wash the silk in it, and it will have a fine black colour.

——*The Female Instructor.*

Diversion 13.

To cleanse Silks of All Kinds. After you have thoroughly taken out the spots, take about a peck of bran, and dry it well by the fire. Then spread your clothes on a convenient place, and rub them well with the bran while it is warm. After this shake it well off, and rub them with a piece of clean, soft, dry material.

If your silks are flowered, take the crumb of a stale three-penny loaf, mix with it about a quarter of an ounce of powder-blue, and crumble them well together. Rub it gently over the silk with your hands, and then with a piece of clean material, as for plain silks.

——*The Female Instructor.*

Diversion 14.

To keep Silks from staining in washing. Warm some rain-water in a saucepan until it is pretty hot. Then put into it some Castile soap, and dissolve it well. Take it off the fire, and when it is almost cold sprinkle into it a small quantity of fuller's earth; then scour your silks with it. Do not let them be on heaps, but spread them, and clap them between dry cloths, and they will be as fresh as when new.

——*The Female Instructor.*

Diversion 15.

To wash Lace. Take your lace and soap it well with soft soap. Then take a piece of plain deal board, sew a piece of material on it very tightly, and roll your lace very smooth round it. Sew another piece of material over it, and put it into a clean boiler of water, and set it on the fire until the water is scalding hot. Shake out the lace, put it into a pan, and pour the water on it. Then rest one end of the board on the dresser or table. With the other rub it well with a hard brush, dipping it at the same time into water, and pressing your hand downwards with the brush to squeeze out the soap and dirt. You must repeat this in a second kettle of water, pressing it with the brush as before. When you have got the dirt all out, take some clear water, put some blue into it, and let it boil well. After this make some good starch, give the lace a gentle boil in it, and then squeeze it well out. Hang the board up until the lace is thoroughly dry, and then take off the material. Put the lace between some clean sheets of paper, and lay a heavy weight on it all night. Take off the weight in the morning, and your lace will look as well as when it was new.

——The Female Instructor.

Diversion 16.

To cleanse Gold and Silver Lace, Stuffs, &c. Take a three-penny stale loaf, and rub the crumb of it well between your hands until it is quite fine. Put about a quarter of an ounce of powder-blue to it, and mix the whole well together. Lay it plentifully on the gold and silver. Rub it well with your hands, and it will soon become bright. When this is done, take a piece of clean flannel and dust the crumbs well off. Take a piece of crimson velvet, rub it gently, and the lace will look as well as when new.

——The Female Instructor.

To cleanse Gold and Silver Lace. Take the gall of an ox, and of a pike. Mix them well together in clear water, and rub the gold or silver with the mixture. It will soon recover its former lustre.

To cleanse Gold Lace. Gold lace is easily cleansed and restored to its original brightness, by rubbing it with a soft brush dipped in burnt rock alum, sifted to a very fine powder.

——The Alphabetical Receipt Book and Domestic Advisor.

Diversion 17.

To wash Gold or Silver Work on Linen, or Any Other Stuff, to look like new. Take a pound of ox-gall, three ounces each of honey and soap, and three ounces of orris-root in fine powder. Mix the whole in a glass vessel into a paste, and expose it to the sun for ten days. Then make a decoction of bran, and strain it clear. Afterwards plaster over the places you wish to cleanse with your bitter paste, and wash the paste off with bran-water until it is no longer tinged. Wipe the places you have washed with a clean linen cloth, and cover them with a clean napkin. Dry them in the sun, iron and glaze, and the work will look as well as when new.

——The Alphabetical Receipt Book and Domestic Advisor.

Diversion 18.

To wash Thread and Cotton Stockings. Both these must have two lathers and a boil, and the water must be well blued. When this is done, wash them out of the boil. Then fold them up very smooth without rinsing, and press them under a weight for about half an hour. Hang them up. When they are thoroughly dry, roll them up without ironing, and they will look as well as when new.

Worsted stockings must be washed in two cool lathers until they are quite clean, but do not put any soap on them. When you have done this, rinse them well, hang them up, and as soon as they are dry, fold them up for use.

——*The Female Instructor.*

Diversion 19.

The Best Mode of whitening Any Kind of Material. First, let your material be well washed. Then spread it on the grass, and sprinkle it with alum water. Let it continue in this situation for three or four days. Wash it again with soap and fuller's earth, and use it as before; by which mode it will not only grow white, but swell in its substance.

To make Linen White that is turned Yellow. Take two quarts of milk, heat it over the fire, and scrape into it half a pound of tablet soap. When the soap is thoroughly dissolved, put the linens in. When they have boiled for some time, take them out, put them into a lather of hot water, and wash them out.

——*The Female Instructor.*

Diversion 20.

To prevent Scarlet Cloth from being stained Black. All corrosive, vitriolic, or salt liquors stain this colour, such as the dirt of the streets, the droppings of horses, &c. As these generally contain a vitriolic property, especially in large cities, when any spots of this nature appear upon your return home, wash them out in a little hard spring-water, into which a dust of tartar has been thrown. It will extract the filth, and leave no manner of stain.

For cleansing Scarlet Cloth. Ladies' pelisses, mantles, habits, &c. of this colour should be taken to pieces, that they may be ironed; and so should all garments which require finishing, except gentlemen's clothes. Even these should be taken to pieces when they are worn, that they may be turned.

There are various modes of cleansing scarlet, each dyer considering his own the best. However, the way in which I have best succeeded is the only one in which a dirty scarlet cloth may be cleansed. For a woman's mantle, dissolve half a pound of the best white soap; but as the quantity of soap depends upon the state of the garment, two ounces will frequently do. I have used a whole pound for such a sized garment. If any black-looking spots appear, rub your dry soap on them; in the meanwhile have your other soap sliced and dissolving. When the mantle is spotted all over with the soap, take hot water and a brush, and brush it off. If it is very filthy, some part of the spots will still remain. In that case you must immerse the whole garment into your solution at rather under a hand heat, and rub lustily such parts as are most stained. Have ready prepared a second liquor of white soap, as at first, only somewhat hotter. Wring it strongly from the first soap liquor. You will find, soon after you get it in this second liquor, that the colour will begin to discharge: that is, it will spend itself in the liquor. This must be your signal to dispatch it hastily.

If this second liquor does not effectually cleanse your article, you will know that the garment has been too hard worn, and requires what is called dipping, or re-dyeing. As soon, however, as the colour begins to give, wring it out, and immerse it in a pan or pail of warm water, to extract what soap remains in it. Wring it out of this, and immerse it in a pan of cold spring-water, in which a table-spoonful of solution of tin has been previously mixed. This solution generally turns the water a milky white. Let your garment remain in it, now and then handling it, ten minutes. Hang it to dry in the shade, which is best, or in a warm room, if the colour is much worn. If not, hang it any where, and let it be cold pressed.

I have cleansed some hundreds of these mantles, &c. Many of them looked equal to new, and some, which had been overloaded with the dye, looked better than when new.

Another Mode. When these things are not much soiled, which generally happens if worn in country places; or if the colour inclines to what is termed a fire-coloured scarlet, which is more tenacious, having less body of cochineal, and more spirits, and is often falsified with young fustic, turmeric, &c., the goods will require a milder mode to extract the dirt, without prejudice to the colour; therefore act as follows.

Take a quarter of a peck of wheat-bran. Pour boiling water on it through a hair-sieve. When the bran-water comes down to a hand heat, immerse your cloth. Rub it well now and then; and holding it up to the light, look to it, to see where the spots are. In the meanwhile prepare a second liquor like the former, adding to it nearly a quarter of an ounce of white or crude tartar. Wring the cloth out from the first bran liquor, and put in this. If the colour is not saddened, which may be known by wringing one end of it tight, and blowing strongly on it, which will show the colour it will be when dry, it is finished. But if it is saddened, or darkened, a clean liquor must be made of cold spring-water, to which add a drop or two of solution of tin. Let it remain in this liquor ten minutes; then wring it, and hang it to dry.

The Mode of dipping Scarlet Cloth. The mode of dipping scarlet cloth, after it has been thoroughly cleansed with soap, and rinsed in warm water, is as follows. When the spring-water in your copper (or boiler, or tin kettle, or whatever your convenience may be) boils, put in a quarter of a pound of young fustic, or what is known better by the name of Zante fustic, a drachm of pounded and sifted cochineal, and an equal quantity of cream of tartar and cochineal. When these have boiled for five or six minutes, cool down your copper by adding a pint or two of cold spring-water, and a table-spoonful of solution of tin. Then stir the mixture, put in your cloth, and boil it for ten minutes. When dry, send it to be cold pressed.

A Cheaper Mode. But not so good as the foregoing, which I never knew to fail, is as follows. Heat your copper to a hand heat. Add two ounces of the best crap-madder, and a like quantity of turmeric, if required; but for a deep red, turmeric must be omitted. When these have simmered ten minutes, and the madder begins to give out its dye, then put in your goods, and simmer them ten minutes, or longer if required. The Irish dyers, instead of solution of tin, use a few drops of oil of vitriol, so as to make the liquor taste tart. Handle the goods through this for two or three minutes. Then take them out, rinse them in cold spring-water, and hang them up to dry. Care must be taken, when madder is used for reds, not to let the water boil, because this drug as well as safflower affords two colours, the one red, the other brown: madder, on being boiled, gives out the brown. This mode will not answer for fire-coloured scarlet, but will do for bright-coloured reds, when the colour requires to be saddened.

——*The Family Dyer and Scourer.*

Chapter XI.
Of the Choice of Clothing.

❦❦❦❦

Propriety requires that your clothing be in keeping with the different hours of the day, and your different occupations, as well as your fortune, profession, age, and shape; the latter subjects being addressed in Chapter XII.

Night Clothing.

A clean and tidy woman should constantly look to the good order of her night-clothes: they should differ from day-clothes only in the number of garments and their weight. Let those who do not know the pleasure of an exquisite cleanliness, or who do not think of the awakening of their spouse, use darkness as an excuse. To a delicate conscience, "That is not seen" is an additional reason for a well-ordered toilet. Therefore, to make this chapter as useful and as complete as possible, I shall indicate the best kinds of night-clothes.

In summer wear a night-cap without strings, because they keep the neck too warm. This cap should be prettily trimmed in two rows. (See Chapter XX.) Replace your ordinary shift with a night-dress, which will serve at the same time as shift and night jacket. This garment unites all that is most convenient in a shirt and a shift. Up to the sleeves, it is a shift, but the rest is the top of a shirt: long sleeves, collar, shoulder-pieces, lengthways slit down the middle of the front, all is like a shirt; only the sleeves are not so wide, especially round the cuff, which should be trimmed. The collar is either turned down or standing, like that of a *fichu,* and is trimmed in the same way (see Chapter XX). Finally, the front slit is fastened with three buttons placed at an equal distance apart. Unlike all other button-holes, these are made lengthways on the hem, so you are not obliged to make the hem very wide, which would be absolutely necessary if the button-holes were cross-ways. If it is a little too hot, and you find that your night-dress outlines your shape too closely, you may wear a muslin *fichu.* This *fichu* should be a square of four quarters of middling-quality muslin, which you fold like a shawl.

When the night is extremely hot, you may wear a day shift; you should put on the muslin *fichu*. But when it is cold, a night jacket should replace the *fichu:* it must always be of white material, trimmed or embroidered, with a turned-down or standing collar. (See Chapter XV.) The first kind wears out much less quickly, but has the inconvenience of crumpling much in bed. If the night jacket does not guard sufficiently against the cold, add a muslin shawl if you like, but never a coloured shawl.

Neither do I like any better the scarfs which many women wear on their heads at night. These turbans, poised on a ruche or trimming, half gauze and half lace, are indeed elegant and very becoming. But nothing is prettier, to my mind, than a woman completely clad in white in her bed; this is the picture of freshness and modesty. If I have condemned coloured *fichus* and scarfs, you will understand that I forbid as well any night jacket made of calico, gingham, &c. (See Div. 1.) Night-clothes of this kind are in the worst taste. You may have white night jackets lined for winter.

In winter wear a *serre-tête,* and over it a cap with strings. The *serre-tête* should be trimmed in the front with a narrow tulle cut in points or embroidery cut likewise; whichever becomes you best. The string-case which was once used, and which is still sometimes used at the back of the *serre-tête,* has the disadvantage of producing an awkward, ugly bulge when the strings are tightened. It is well to replace it thus: terminate the two parts of the *serre-tête* in points rather like those of the pointed gores of a pair of stays, but reversed. Hem both parts thus cut out, and sew to the end of each a linen tape about half an inch wide, and three-quarters of an ell long, so that it goes round your head. It ties at the point where it began. The ends of the *serre-tête* cross each other without causing any bulging, making themselves felt, or becoming disarranged during the night. Moreover, if they are rather elegantly trimmed, they may serve as a bandeau.

The bandeau is indispensable in a night head-dress which is at all tidy, unless it is replaced by the *serre-tête.* It serves to hide your curl-papers, and fills the space which they make between your forehead and the trimming of the night-cap; it agrees charmingly with both. The bandeau is a band about an eighth of an ell high, and about a third of an ell wide. It is made of percale or batiste, and hemmed all round with a hem of middle width, stitched with back-stitches on the front of the bandeau, which is trimmed with pointed tulle, or an unplaited narrow lace. You may embroider in place of this decoration, but that is much less becoming. In the middle of the sides of the bandeau, sew a tape like that used on the *serre-tête.*

Morning Clothing.

It would be quite impractical and almost ridiculous to dress in the morning as you are obliged to dress for the rest of the day. On awakening, put on garments which are very simple and even common, but always clean, because under no circumstances should a woman dispense with order and cleanliness. Put on slippers which do not have a tight foot; but slippers properly speaking are not worn-out shoes. Always wear half-stays or a morning belt; I shall discuss those in Chapter XIV. Without them your clothes will be loose on your body, ill-fitting, and look untidy. When it is very hot you may wear a white petticoat and a similar night jacket. When these articles are very white, embroidered, and of fine material, this is a very nice costume. But it is necessary to renew it often, and since in every situation it is wise to economize, I advise you to have a redingote of calico for summer, and of common merino for winter. (See Chapter XV and Div. 2.) In hot weather you may remove your night-cap on quitting your bed, provided that, following my previous directions, your hair is properly plaited; because, I again repeat, never must any sign of disorder or carelessness be seen for an instant in persons of our sex. If you have the excellent habit of helping with the first household tasks of the day, you must retain your night head-dress at all times, in order to prevent dust from dulling your hair. Do not forget to wear gloves to preserve your hands from stains, scratches, and calluses.

Heat also permits you to wrap yourself in a dressing-gown with sleeves, but even though you are wearing only a long shift underneath, do not leave off your half-stays. The dressing-gown must be very wide in order to have an ample crossing in the front. It goes without saying that it must be trimmed, at least the collar. This too is a very graceful garment, and I advise you to have several shorter ones of batiste or fine percale; they will be very useful when you have to make a grand toilet. When you must put on your finery in the evening, you cannot remain all that time in a night jacket. Dressing several times is extremely tiresome; on the other hand a fine gown is excessively awkward, and would run a thousand risks if you put it on before the moment you go out. A pretty dressing-gown, very fine, very white, and highly trimmed, takes care of all that. You lace yourself, put on your slip and the dressing-gown, and when it is time to dress, you may manage quietly without being obliged to hurry, and without having wasted time in undressing repeatedly.

The combing mantles you throw over your shoulders in order to dress your hair are quite different from these. They should be of linen or calico, with no sleeves or trimming.

Clothing for Ordinary Days.

When at home, you should always be dressed neatly and respectably enough to go out or visit your friends without having to put on any thing except your gloves, shawl, and hat; but dress without any affectation. (See Div. 3.) If your clothing is over-trimmed or appears to hamper daily occupations, it might perhaps be even more ridiculous than if it were too common. Wear pretty prunella shoes; very white cotton stockings; a gown of gingham, a beautiful calico, or merino according to the season, suitably trimmed; a belt without riband loops; a *collerette* or *fichu de lingère;* a very neat coiffure *en cheveux;* and finally, if you have a great deal to do, a black silk apron. Such is the costume which is proper for a woman in her home. Gowns of silk, muslin, and other such materials, unless you have a very considerable fortune, bespeak vanity and indolence. In my opinion a young woman's attire should be a constant testimony of modesty, order, and industry.

I recommend a black apron especially to my readers who have the good fortune to be mothers, save that it is taken off for a ceremonious visit. Not only does the apron preserve the gown, but it is very becoming to the figure, above all for persons inclined to embonpoint. Taffety, black levantine, and even the very beautiful bombasine are the only materials which should be used for these aprons. It is well to cut them gored, or at least to form a bias which conforms well to the shape of the hips, on the right and left of the front breadth (see Chapter XVI). All kinds of pockets should be rejected. When the apron is fastened with hooks, the belt is placed over it. When the apron is fastened in the front with long ribands, the belt is placed under it; this is very pretty. An apron with a body is proper only for children, and straps are only for lady's maids.

A small *fichu* crossed *en sautoir*, of gauze or silk according to the fashion, and a shawl of three quarters, are proper for the home, whereas a scarf or a long pelerine would be reprehensible. If in winter you wear a shawl at home, it should not exceed four quarters, because nothing is more cumbersome. Moreover, it is better to dress warmly under your gown (though without enlarging and encumbering your waist) than to wear a shawl habitually. That veils your bosom, hampers movement, and renders you more susceptible to colds.

When you are accustomed to a coiffure *en cheveux,* you need not have any other head-dress during the whole winter. (See Chapter VIII.) This gives a very agreeable youthful air; only too soon you must have recourse to caps. If you are obliged to cover your head, the velvet berets now worn are preferable to any other head-dress. You should wear a black beret, without odd ornaments and unaccompanied by the tulle ruches used by some ladies. In this, as in all things, over-dressing and affectation ought to be carefully avoided.

Négligé.

Let us pass to the description of a pretty *négligé:* a bonnet of silk, light-coloured riband, or woollen or muslin gauze; a percale redingote, trimmed all round with embroidered and fluted muslin, or with Vandyked embroidery on the material, or a band of unplaited pointed tulle; a pelerine next the gown; a barège shawl thrown carelessly over your shoulders; or even a gingham gown cut redingote style, with or without trimmings: these are for summer. For winter, wear an untrimmed *douillette* of dark-coloured taffety, fastened in the front from top to bottom with bows of similar riband placed at equal distances; a merino redingote, bordered on only one edge by a strip of silk similar to the gown; and a square shawl of merino or wadded silk with large palm-leaves, an ell or five quarters in size. The head-dress is always a bonnet, but of a tolerably deep colour. (See Div. 4.)

Demi-négligé.

Before luxury had reached the appalling point seen nowadays, the *demi-négligé* which I am about to describe would have passed for a perfect toilet, and when I have listed the articles which compose it, you will not be surprised. Indeed, beautiful percale gowns trimmed with muslin rouleaux, tulle *entre-deux,* and embroidered flounces; muslin or lawn redingotes lined with taffety; merino or taffety gowns, suitably embellished; and printed muslins, coloured bombasine, and many other fancy materials, are garments which are not precisely suitable for a *demi-négligé,* all the more that amongst the percale gowns with embroidered flounces there are often those worth eight hundred francs. Such gowns are worn with *fichus;* turned-down collars of cotton tulle; collars trimmed with ruches of the same tulle; pelerines of muslin gauze or embroidered muslin; shawls of barège, *crêpe de chine,* or wadded silk; tippets of divers furs; hats of Leghorn straw (unless they are only trimmed with great white plumes, because then they are hats for toilet); hats matching the costume; hats of Swiss or cotton material; and hats of *gros de Naples,* satin, velvet, &c. It is true that the style and the ornaments count for more than the materials, but it is nonetheless true that a *demi-négligé* seems to form a complete toilet if need be.

It would be ridiculous to wear precious gems with a *négligé* or *demi-négligé.* You should wear absolutely nothing round your neck save for the black or brown ribands, about half an inch wide, which serve to suspend watches; or steel or gold chains with these useful jewels likewise hung at the end; or lorgnettes or *pince-nez* (double lorgnettes with supports) which are worn of necessity, and which you should never wear otherwise. Some persons wear their watch on their belt, passed through a chain only about half a foot long, but composed of a multitude of rows. This custom is impractical and pretentious. It is in better taste not to make the watch conspicuous, and this is so well founded that when the style of body permits the watch to be concealed underneath it, you should never fail to do so. Since we are discussing this jewel, I shall say that nothing is more childish and ludicrous than the custom of wearing a quantity of gold trinkets, representing a thousand objects such as children's toys, animals, comic figures, &c. Excepting the watch-key, which may be more or less rich and varied, and if you wish, a seal of precious stone, all this paraphernalia should be disdained.

The little flasks which were suspended from the neck like watches were an agreeable and pretty fashion, but those overly tiny flasks were not very serviceable. We therefore need not much regret that their use has been left off. Pocket flasks, especially those held by a second metal stopper, by means of a hinge, are far preferable. I advise my readers to always carry them filled with salt of vinegar, balsamic Cologne water, or any other balsamic liquid, to be prepared for any accidents which might happen, and to render service when there is occasion. (See Chapter VI and Div. 5.)

The purses suspended on the side which are carried for *demi-négligé* seem to merit the same reproach as watches placed in the same fashion. As in the kind of costume under discussion it is customary to carry a bag, decorated more or less according to the degree of elegance of the *demi-négligé,* it is incomparably better to put your purse in your bag. Especially at Paris, it is much safer. Many ladies adopt for *demi-négligé* a custom of the grand toilet, of carrying their purse in their hand, over the handkerchief. Since fashion has brought back long purses, closed with drawing-strings or moveable rings, these ladies twist them round a finger. I cannot refrain from finding this affected.

I have said that some differences in the style of articles, though similar, class them as either *demi-négligé* or the toilet properly speaking. Here are some examples: veils of white, black, or green gauze; and half-veils of tulle and even blond, with a drawing-string, are *demi-négligé*. Veils embroidered all round, and thrown over the hat, are toilet. (See Chapter XX.) Open-work cotton stockings are still *demi-négligé;* open-work white silk stockings are the contrary. Black ones may be classed with cotton stockings. Gauze caps *de modiste* are *demi-négligé;* berets which resemble them are toilet. Spencers of the richest materials—*reibs,* satin, and velvet—are always *demi-négligé*. Blouse gowns with plaits on the front breadth are ordinarily ranked in this last class.

The Manner of dressing for an Ordinary Walk.

It appears that I have few observations to make on this subject, after what I have previously said: that you ought to look tidy enough at home to be able to go out unexpectedly. But to go out is not to promenade, and the latter pursuit usually requires you to be a little more elaborately dressed. (See Div. 6.)

For morning walks, is it true, a *négligé* or *demi-négligé* suffices. For walks on summer evenings, gowns of muslin, figured silks, and *gros de Naples* are worn. Merino, levantine, and other beautiful silk materials are worn on winter afternoons. Many fashionables even wear assembly toilets on these promenades: white weeping willow plumes, and gowns of satin, velvet, &c. I do not believe they should be imitated. A simple, graceful toilet is more proper for a promenade than showy clothing.

The Manner of dressing for a Morning Repast.

If this is a lunch with a friend, see the article on *négligé*. If a little ceremony creeps in, adopt a *demi-négligé*. If the meal is considered an early dinner, you must dress as if for dinner.

The Manner of dressing for an Evening Repast.

This depends upon the number of guests and the formality of the meal. (See Div. 7.) A small dinner accords very well with a trimmed *demi-négligé,* or the costume adopted for promenades. But if it is a matter of a grand, and in parenthesis, tiresome gathering, your hair should be carefully dressed *en cheveux*, with numerous riband loops or gauze biases; or you might wear a fancy beret with or without feathers, or even a toque *de salon*. The gown must be of *gros de Naples, côte-pali,* barège, India muslin, poplin, satin, or velvet, according to the season. The *fichu* should be a *somnambule* of tulle, or black or white blond; a scarf of the same material; or an extremely elegant *fichu-pelerine.* (See Chapter XX.) These are matched to the gowns described above. You may also have a rather low neck. It goes without saying that ornaments of divers precious gems are the complement to these toilets.

For an Assembly Properly Speaking.

For an evening of play, a punch, a tea, or a concert, the ensemble is similar, but even richer than for a dinner. (See Div. 8.) If you appear in white, let it be India muslin, trimmed or with a gold border or embroidered flounces; a tulle gown, with lustreless festooned flounces; or a cotton gauze gown embroidered in coloured wool. All these gowns are worn with satin slips. If it is winter, wear silk gowns (*bourré,* poplin, *reibs,* velvet, or *crêpe de chine*) trimmed with blond lace or elegant furs, such as miniver, golden fox, marten, or chinchilla. A coiffure *en cheveux* would appear mean. Berets of blond, with flowers or marabouts; toques of coloured velvet, with gold or steel ornaments; toques with grand plumes; turbans with bunches of bird-of-paradise feathers; hats with flowers of the greatest elegance, which must often be renewed; cachemire shawls; and satin or drap-cachemire mantles: this gives an idea of the costume required for these ruinous assemblies.

The Manner of dressing for a Ball.

All that your toilet has of grace, lightness, and freshness should shine, preferably with luxuriance, for this gay assembly. (See Div. 9.) If sometimes you wish to display signs of opulence, let these be jewels, and not gold and silver flowers or embroideries. All this tinselly apparel is in bad taste. As the degree of elegance varies much in ball dress, I shall divide it into three kinds: the simple toilet, the demi-toilet, and the grand toilet.

The Simple Toilet. White or black prunella shoes; open-work cotton stockings; white taffety slip; muslin gauze gown, trimmed with a wide riband in puffs, or three satin ribands; simple sleeves and body, the latter a little low; belt with loops or *agrafes* the colour of the trimming; hair *en cheveux* ornamented with riband bows or a few flowers; ear-rings and necklace of black or white jet, pink paste, or the glass pearls called English; white gloves; and a scarf of barège or grenadine gauze, matched to the principal colour, which is ordinarily rose or celestial blue: such is this pretty toilet. As the gown is always a little lower-necked than usual, the scarf, or any equivalent *fichu,* is put on in the interval between quadrilles, and left off while dancing.

The Demi-toilet. Silk shoes, either black or matched to the colour of the costume; open-work silk stockings; and white satin slip. White or coloured crape gown, trimmed with several rows of similar ruches or *bouillons* of mingled crape and satin. The satin is cut into leaves; rolled into *torsades;* or disposed in Vandykes, rosettes, or draperies, beneath which the gauze or crape puffs out in large *bouillons;* sometimes a bunch of mixed or similar flowers holds the trimming over the knee. (See Chapter XV.) Draped body; embellished sleeves; and an ordinary belt or *fichu à la duchesse,* of riband or satin matched to the gown, either untrimmed, or bordered by tulle or gauze. The scarf is of cachemire barège, embroidered cotton tulle, or a three-cornered *fichu* or *somnambule* of similar tulle. Coiffure with flowers or matching gauze biases; a *parure* of false pearls with a clasp of brilliants, steel, coral, or turquoises according to the colour of the trimmings; and a bouquet matching the belt or another part of the costume.

The Grand Toilet. White satin shoes; very beautiful open-work silk stockings; satin slip trimmed with white satin riband; gown of *gaze de laine* figured like a veil, plain cotton tulle, plain silk tulle, or tulle with leaves of satin-stitch embroidery in steel or silver; blond trimmings held by flowers, or pearl or steel ornaments; trimmings formed of several garlands of flowers held by a bouquet over the knee (in this case, the hem of the gown is hidden by a riband *à bouillons* or by a riband of the slip); and a *fichu à la duchesse* trimmed with blond, or a body decorated with blond draperies held on the shoulders by ornaments similar to the trimmings—flowers excepted, because nothing is in worse taste than flowers on the shoulders, as I have seen on some ladies. Bouquet on the side; coiffure with pearls, marabout feathers mixed with flowers, or ornaments similar to the trimmings; a *parure* of amethysts, rubies, topazes, chrysolites, or diamonds; and a scarf or shawl of white silk blond. That is the maximum of the ball toilet. Ribands and white bouquets accord with this sumptuous finery.

I do not pretend to have detailed all kinds of ball toilets; the task would be impossible. I wish only to give my readers an idea of the ensembles suitable to the occasion, which you choose from according to your fortune, or the degree of elegance of the assembly. For an unceremonious evening dance, a lawn or organdy gown with folds or flounces suffices, especially for very young persons. A barège or *côte-pali* gown with *gaze de laine* sleeves also does very well. It would be ridiculous to display, at a modest assembly, the luxury of the third toilet described above. I have also not spoken of the turbans or the high toques which ladies often wear at these assemblies, because I shall treat of them in the article on the differences in the toilet between married women and young ladies.

Nonetheless, I shall not yet quit the subject. I must say that formerly (a very recent formerly) people wore satin bodies *à la Marie Stuart,* of the same colour as the trimming, with gauze or white crape skirts. A short time before that, the slip received the trimming, ordinarily a sixth of an ell high; and the gown, shortened so that it did not fall round the trimming, formed a species of tunic, of which the edge, trimmed with a riband similar to that which hid the hem of the slip, completed the trimming.

Though I have advised you to reject any thing which seems tawdry for a ball toilet, I must say that nothing is at the same time richer and more elegant for trimming the head-dress than silver ears of grain, either alone or mixed with other things. *Lamé* is also an exception. But all embroidery with spangles, and all ribands decorated with tinsel or similar flowers and leaves, seem to me more suitable for an opera ballet than a society ball.

I shall finish with some reflections on the decency which ought to prevail in a ball toilet. Immodesty in such garments is almost received usage, and if people reveal themselves a little less at present, it is solely because the mode dictates it. Let not so deplorable a motive sway my dear readers. Whether fashion requires it or not, their *décolletage* should not extend more than about an inch below the neck and the base of the shoulders. If, as formerly, it is *de rigueur* that the gown leaves part of the back and the bosom uncovered, as did the bodies *à l'enfant,* you will do perfectly to cut your gowns only to the middle of your shoulder-blades, to the beginning of your bosom, and to wear a clinging *fichu* with no trimming. (See Chapter XX.) Your necklace falling over the edge of the *fichu* will conceal it, and from a little distance it will scarcely be perceived. The art of pleasing properly understood will gain perhaps as much as decency, because this light tissue of tulle or gauze whitens your skin, beautifies it, and conceals the sweat and redness which, nearly always in dancing, finish by streaking your neck and shoulders. Moreover, the attraction of modesty, woman's most powerful charm, will make this simple *fichu* the most beautiful part of your clothing. But if your chief end is to use modesty for calculated coquetry—if your neck is too low, or if you wear a *fichu* too spread apart or transparent—you will lose both the attraction of modesty and the elegance of fashion.

I shall add only that a dancer should never carry a bag. She must have a very beautiful embroidered handkerchief and a fan suited to the luxuriance of her toilet. It is customary to put several pair of bracelets over long gloves: this odd fashion would look much better if the gown were simple. Half-long gloves are much more becoming to the figure than long ones; but then you must have pretty arms, or at least pretty forearms. Now people dance with great gigot sleeves of *gaze de laine*. Nothing could be uglier, and unless you have red arms and goose-flesh, do not force yourself to follow such an unbecoming fashion. Wear short sleeves, and trim the border or cuff with a rouleau of riband matched to the trimming; and below the riband, tulle folded double, or pointed if this is a simple or a demi-toilet, or blond lace if it is a grand toilet.

Differences in the Toilet between Married Women and Young Ladies.

Their age, their position in society, the protection of their husbands, and the valuable things which they received at the time of marriage, explain why married women are more splendidly dressed than unmarried girls. A graceful simplicity composes the entire toilet of the latter, especially when they are very young; because when they reach a certain age without having changed their state, they make amends by dressing more like married women. It should be said in passing that this ensures they always remain single. Be that as it may, let us note the differences.

Very beautiful hats of Leghorn straw, plumes *de salon,* likewise marabouts, *esprits,* toques *d'assemblée,* fancy berets, and great tulle and blond veils embroidered all round and thrown over the hat, are the privilege of married women. Any other head-dress is in the domain of young ladies, but principally the large uncut straw hats trimmed with white ribands. (See Chapter XXI.)

Real or false cachemires, especially those of six quarters, and great shawls of black or white blond, or even of tulle, cannot be more out of place for young ladies. The same must be said of tulle, blond, and cachemire scarfs.

Gowns of satin, velvet, *crêpe de Chine,* plain or embroidered tulle, India muslin, and matching trimmings would be criticized, with reason, in the costume of a young lady. "What will she have after marriage?" would be a general and very natural question.

Finally, ornaments of fine pearls, brilliants, or costly precious gems are strictly forbidden. Black or white jet, false pearls, corals, turquoises, and steel ornaments are permitted.

The Manner of wearing Mourning properly.

To the young, the macerations which constituted mourning amongst nearly all the peoples of antiquity, would scarcely seem more severe to elegant Parisian ladies than the necessity of renouncing for some time a variety of colours and ornaments at spectacles and balls. Therefore, they cut this cruel privation as short as possible. The mourning of a widow, ordinarily fixed at two years in the provinces, is only thirteen months at Paris. Mourning for the loss of a father, mother, grandfather, grandmother, godfather, or godmother, commonly a year, is no more than half that. Mourning for an uncle, aunt, brother, or sister was once six months; now three months seems sufficient. Mourning for a first cousin is not obligatory, but through respect or friendship, it may be worn for six weeks or a month.

Mourning has three different stages: full mourning, second mourning, and half-mourning. (See also Div. 10 and Chapter XXX.) For full mourning, you may wear an untrimmed bombasine or merino gown; a black shawl without any border; a black crape *fichu;* an extremely simple crape cap or bonnet; a crape veil; black gloves and shoes; and no jewellery—unless it is of blued steel, and then only the belt buckle. Widows do not curl or even show their hair during the whole full mourning.

For second mourning, you may wear a trimmed silk gown; a *gaze de laine fichu;* a similar hat, or even one of silk and velvet; and a little later, pearls and white stones. For half-mourning, wear materials of black and white mixed. For example, a gown of gingham, Madras, or grey and light lapis which imitates grey; a white gown and belt, and a *fichu* of black ribands; scarfs and shawls of the same colour; grey silk hats; and white hats with black flowers, or even grey flowers strewn over lapis. Half-mourning usually lasts half as long as full mourning.

Finally, at the end of mourning, you may wish, without breaking it off, to go to an assembly or appear at a ball. Then wear a white silk gauze gown, trimmed with white satin, with silver ears of grain, or white flowers without leaves, such as tuberoses. These are costumes for half-mourning. Half-mourning ends with brilliants or pearls; but ordinarily you wear what is called an iron *parure* for mourning. Plaques of blued steel, representing antique heads or cameos in relief, compose the comb, necklace, and bracelets. These *parures* are made in Prussia and are extremely elegant. (See Div. 11.)

——*Manuel des dames.*

Diversion 1.

The Trade of the Linen-draper. The linen-draper sells materials which are made of flax and hemp, such as Irish linens, Russia towelling, cambrics, &c., and also shawls, printed calicoes, muslin, &c., &c. In London this business is, in the number of its articles, much more circumscribed than it is in the country. In the country linen-drapers frequently combine their trade with that of a silk-mercer, whereas in London the two trades are wholly distinct.

The linen-draper is now comprehended under two, or at most three distinct branches. The linen merchant is a person whose more immediate province is to import articles of linen manufacture from foreign countries, such as Irish materials from Ireland; a variety of materials made of hemp and flax from Russia; ticklenburgs, &c., from Germany; and nankeens, calicoes, muslins, &c. from the East Indies. The wholesale linen-draper is a person whose business it is to purchase linens from the merchant, and muslins, calicoes, printed cottons, &c. from the different manufacturers, and to sell them to the retail linen-drapers throughout the kingdom, as well as frequently for exportation.

The most striking part, however, is the retail linen-draper. There is no trade in England in which more efforts are made to captivate the public, and more especially the ladies, by a display of goods; and in London this display is carried to a most costly and sumptuous extent. (See the frontispiece to Part II.) In most of the principal streets of the metropolis, shawls, muslins, pieces for ladies' gowns, and a variety of other goods, are shown with the assistance of mirrors, and at night by chandeliers, aided by the brilliancy which the gas-lights afford, in a way almost as dazzling to a stranger as many of those poetical fictions of which we read in the *Arabian Nights.*

Calico. In the East Indies they paint all their calicoes with a pencil. Here the pattern is first drawn on paper the whole breadth of the material intended to be printed. The workman then divides the pattern into several parts according to its size, each part being about eight inches wide by twelve inches long. Each distinct part or pattern thus divided is cut out upon wooden blocks. The material to be printed is extended upon a table, and the types being covered with the proper colours, are laid on, and the impression is left upon the material. Great care must be taken that the parts join accurately, and that there is no interstice or vacancy left.

The manner of printing with wooden blocks is easy and expeditious, if there are only two colours, such as green and blue, or black on a white ground. Then the block requires only to be dipped in the printing-ink and impressed on the material. If more colours are used, they are laid on with a brush or brushes, and the impressions made as before with the hand. When the whole piece is printed, the material is washed and bleached, to take away any accidental stains it may have acquired in the operation. It is then dried, calendered, and laid up in folds fit for the shop.

The application of engraving on copper has given birth to a new and important branch of calico-printing. The machines are of two kinds: the flat press, and the rolling or cylinder press. These machines surpass the ordinary mode of block-printing, not only in neatness, accuracy, and precision, but still more in the economy and art with which the labour is performed. The flat press, in its original form, was merely a modification, considerably enlarged, of the press for ornamental prints and engravings; to which was added a contrivance for joining with accuracy, the numerous and successive impressions necessary to cover a piece of material. It was confined at first to one colour, but later improvements have extended it to two or even three. The single-colour presses are, however, principally in use.

—*The Book of English Trades.*

Diversion 2.

Costumes for Morning Wear. For March 1824: white is very little worn, and merely appears as a cambric wrapping-gown for the breakfast-table. The modish fair one speedily divests herself of this, and passes the remainder of the morning in a gown made of slight wash-silk, coloured bombasine, or dark chintz. The gowns are well made, with the bodies very simply trimmed, and the waists of a moderate length. The skirt, though yet rather too long, is shorter than last month.

August 1824. Printed muslins are yet worn in town for the breakfast-table. But the *négligé* dress for the morning, in preparation for the different watering-places, is a white muslin or cambric pelisse-robe; this pelisse is made with a pelerine cape.

June 1829. White gowns of cambric, made high, and slightly embroidered, with sleeves *à la Mameluke,* are much worn as breakfast gowns.

——*Ladies' Pocket Magazine.*

Diversion 3.

Costumes for Home Wear. For April 1824: Fig. 1 shows a lavender-coloured gown of *gros de Naples,* with one rouleau of silk next the hem, above which are two rows of lotus-leaves edged with pink. A belt of the same material as the gown buckles on one side with a silver buckle. The gown is finished next the throat by a *collerette* of muslin trimmed with lace. The head-dress is a cornette of fine lace, lined with lavender satin, and crowned with a bouquet of roses. Coral necklace, black satin slippers, and sea-green gloves.

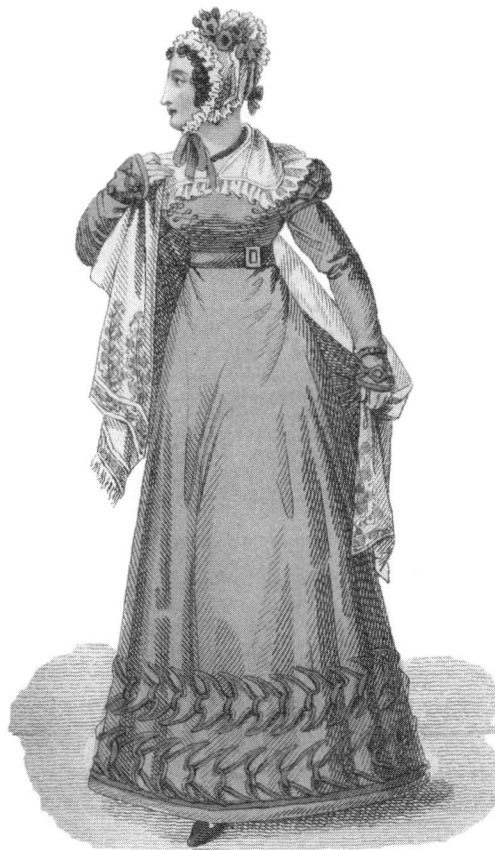

Figure 1. Home dress.

May 1824. When the day is destined to retirement at home, she puts on a silk gown of rather a sombre colour, made high, with a pelerine cape, and handsomely ornamented across the body with Brandenburghs, and three narrow flounces round the border. This is now the correct number when the gown is flounced; but the trimmings at the borders of gowns are now all light.

June 1824. A favourite in-door costume is a high gown of light-coloured *gros de Naples,* with a double square collar falling over the throat. This is of fine India muslin, beautifully embroidered, and edged round with narrow Mechlin lace. The body of the gown is ornamented *en chevrons.* Rows of trimming representing thick foliage are often placed on the borders of silk gowns. If the gown is high, sometimes a pelerine collar lies over the neck, but is not wide enough to fall over the shoulders. Printed muslins are preferred to white in dishabille; and dark silks of a slight texture for morning gowns.

July 1824. High gowns are much worn for in-door costume. The bodies form a heart in the front and at the back, by means of plaits which begin from the bottom of the waist, and spread out as they attain the shoulders.

October 1824. The blouse form is still the reigning fashion for gowns. It certainly is a convenient gown for a Parisian lady who is indisposed, because it is well known that when a Frenchwoman is sick she never wears stays of any kind. A wrapping morning gown would discover this; but the blouse, which always looks clumsy and inelegant, does not show any particular omission or defect. But these favourite gowns are made of silk or muslin, beautifully embroidered in colours, and the richest materials of the toilet.

December 1824. White canezou-spencers are much worn over coloured silk gowns for in-door costume.

March 1827. Pelisse-robe of *gros de Naples,* of a lavender-grey, with satin Vandyke trimmings. It fastens down the front with rosettes, the same as the gown. The body is *en gerbe,* partially high, with a narrow double falling collar, trimmed round with satin Vandykes, and fastening in the front with a rosette. Antique points at the wrists, and next the hand a gold bracelet clasped by a cameo head. Over the silk collar of this dress falls a *collerette* of India muslin, trimmed with a quilling of fine lace. The cap is of yellow crape, with pointed borders edged with black, and ornamented with black and yellow riband; the strings of which float loose.

Pelisses of *gros de Naples* have made their appearance, and seem to gain favour rapidly. They are worn as gowns in the house over a very richly-embroidered cambric or muslin petticoat.

April 1827. Coloured gowns for afternoon home costume have long white crape sleeves. The morning gowns are very elegant; they are much in the pelisse-robe style, and are trimmed in various ways. They have a pelerine cape, are made only partially high, and fasten down the front with rosettes of riband. The materials are merinos, slight silks, and sometimes coloured cambrics.

May 1827. Printed muslins and chintzes prevail in home costume, with coloured lawns of bright and beautiful tints. These articles are much improved in their texture, the stripes and chequers having a rich and satin-like appearance.

June 1827. Gowns of fine cambric, of camel's-hair brown or other unobtrusive colours, are preferred in home costume to the chintzes so much patronized last summer; the latter now being confined only to morning dress. These cambric gowns are, however, rendered expensive by a superb wide border of shawl-work, of the most variegated and brilliant colours. The sleeves are ornamented at the shoulders and wrists with this shawl bordering. The gown is made half-high, and the body is tight to the shape. Over the shoulders is worn a *collerette* pelerine, double, of richly-embroidered muslin.

August 1827. The new summer gowns are of light materials, amongst which coloured muslins form a very favourite gown. When these gowns are all of one colour, they are admirable, as well adapted to the weather. But beautiful as are the printed muslins, and often infinitely higher in price than silk gowns, they never will look dignified on any woman, however noble her appearance and station in life. The fawn and the plain rose-coloured muslins, when tastefully made and with long white sleeves, look well on young persons, and they are at present more in favour than the costly printed muslins devoted to the morning drive, or the early walk by the sea-shore. These are hastily thrown aside by the fair wearer as soon as she reaches her elegant home, where if she finishes the day without company, she prefers the *plain,* elegant muslin; for the white gowns are so very splendid with lace and embroidery that they are seldom worn in home costume.

September 1827. A gown of pink muslin, with a full puckering of the same at the border of the skirt; over which is a row of embroidery in white shining cotton. The body is made high and partially *en gerbe,* and surmounted at the throat by a full ruff of lace. The sleeves are *à la Marie,* with slightly puckered mancherons. The cap is of tulle, with yellow gauze ribands, edged with cherry-colour.

December 1827. In home costume, when a gown is of chintz, an India muslin *fichu-pelerine,* superbly embroidered, is worn over the gown. When the gown is of *gros de Naples,* a pelerine of the same, trimmed round with a pinked ruche, with the ends drawn through the belt, is generally adopted.

January 1829. Poplin gowns, both plain and figured, are much in request. The plain, being the real Irish tabinets, are reckoned the most genteel, and are worn in every style of dress. The figured, often of British manufacture, are confined to home costume.

August 1829. Gowns of batiste striped in various colours are much worn in home costume, as are printed muslins. Many of these are of the most beautiful patterns of various colours, on a white or very light-coloured ground. These gowns have generally a very wide hem round the border, over which are two bias folds set separately at an equal distance. The body is *en gerbe* in the front, and plain at the back.

October 1829. Dark chintzes of beautiful patterns are much worn as morning dishabille, or as retired home costume.

French home gown consisting of a pelisse-robe of lilac *gros de Naples.* The body is made quite plain, with sleeves *à l'imbecile,* confined at the wrist by a tight cuff, surmounted by a very full triple quilling of white lace. A French ruff of lace encircles the neck just below the throat. A rich blond cap is worn with this gown, with a wide border turned back, and ornamented next the hair with branches of roses and green leaves, and the flowers of a shrub of the frutrix kind, known by the name of fox-tails. Strings of rose-colour float loose.

Gowns of brown or grey, and other such retired colours, are worn for demi-toilet and for home costume.

November 1829. When the weather is mild, the favourite home costume is a petticoat of coloured *gros de Naples* with a canezou-spencer of muslin. But this will shortly give place to the more appropriate gown of fine merino, made partially low, with a handsome pelerine of embroidered tulle or very fine muslin trimmed with lace.

December 1829. Merino gowns for home costume are very much in favour. Though the fine double merino is certainly expensive, yet its purchase is advisable, since it appears like a very fine and light cloth, not discovering the twill, which in other merinos always imparts the idea of a stuff gown.

One charming merino gown is of a bright geranium. It is bordered by two wide bias folds, each headed by narrow black velvet. The body is made partially low, *à l'enfant,* and the sleeves are of a very moderate width, finished at the wrists by a wide cuff of black velvet, fastened with jet buttons. Other merino gowns, of myrtle green and slate-colour, are ornamented in much the same manner.

Two home gowns of *gros de Naples,* of the latter colours, appeared lately on two very elegant young women of fashion. They were trimmed round the border of the skirt with two narrow flounces. The bodies were made quite high and fitting tight to the shape, with sleeves *à l'Amadis.* An India muslin collar, trimmed at the edge with fine lace, finished these tasteful gowns.

——*Ladies' Pocket Magazine.*

Diversion 4.

Fashions for *Néglige*. For October 1824: Fig. 2 shows a morning visiting gown of fine jaconet muslin, finished next the shoe with one narrow full flounce. Over this flounce is a very rich border of two rows of embossed leaves, set on in bias, each row separated by a wide insertion lace of a handsome pattern, and the whole surmounted by a row of the same lace. This gown is made partially high, with the body very plain, and finished at the bottom of the waist in the canezou style, where it is confined by a brown and pink striped riband. It is worn with a large pilgrim hat of Leghorn, simply ornamented, and tied with riband the same as the belt; a superb white lace veil is also adopted. Over the long sleeves are worn two bracelets of hair or wrought gold. The slippers are white kid, and the gloves yellow.

August 1827. The sleeves are *en gigot,* but so well stiffened at the wide part next the shoulder with buckram, that there is nothing to be feared from the pressure of a shawl, &c.

October 1827. Fig. 3 shows a morning visiting gown of sea-green *gros de Naples,* with two wide flounces. The body is made plain with long sleeves. An elegant *fichu-pelerine* is worn with this gown, with a standing collar, finished by a triple frill of lace and left open at the throat. The ends of the *fichu* are short, and but just appear beneath the belt, through which

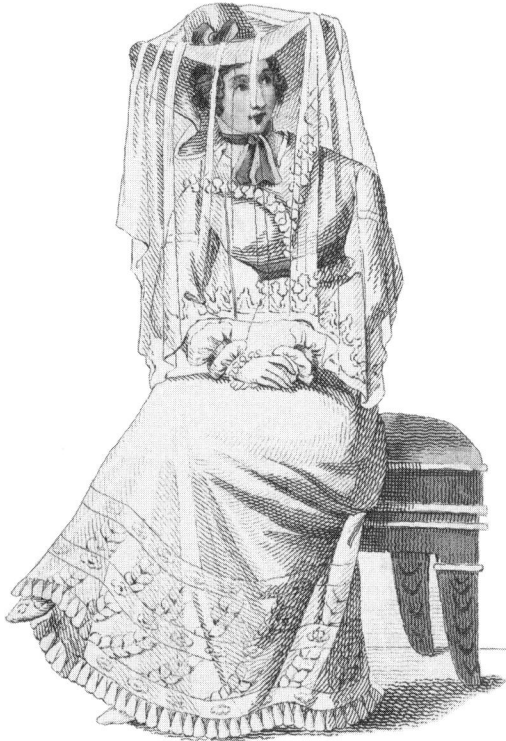

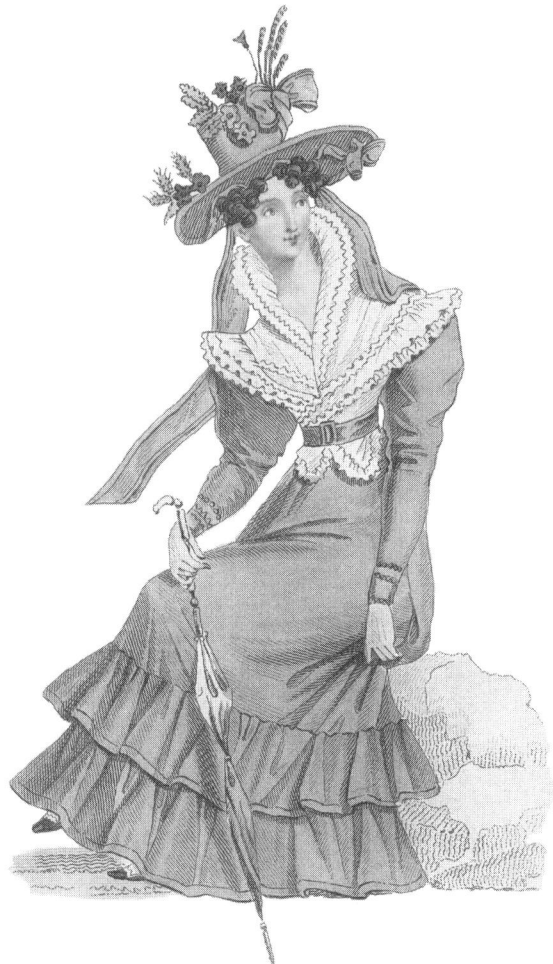

Figure 2. Morning visiting dress.   **Figure 3. Morning visiting dress.**

they are drawn. This *fichu* is of fine India muslin, trimmed with lace. A blue crape hat is ornamented with yellow roses and blue gauze riband, the strings of which float loose.

June 1829. The frightful stiffening at the top of the present enormously wide sleeves is now, we are pleased to say, entirely laid aside by every woman who has the least pretensions to good taste. These sleeves, called *à la Mameluke,* now fall down from the shoulders in all their amplitude; and on a fine figure they do not appear ungraceful.

August 1829. As the sleeves *à l'Amadis* are equally in fashion with those *à l'imbecile,* ladies who are fond of moderation in their compliance with fashion wisely prefer the former. These too are extremely wide from the top of the arm to the elbow. But at the smaller part, next the wrist, they almost fit closely, and so do not appear so preposterous as those *à l'imbecile,* and are less *gauche* than the sleeves *à la Mameluke.*

December 1829. In order to have some medium between the sleeves *à l'Amadis* and those called *à l'imbecile,* the mantua-makers confine the fulness of the latter half-way up the arm by four narrow bands. So that the fluted plaits caused by this confinement may preserve all their first form, the sleeve is lined with stiffened gauze; the top part of the sleeve then falls in all its amplitude over the elbow. Ruffles are still worn at the wrists; they are of fine lawn edged with Valenciennes.

——*Ladies' Pocket Magazine.*

Diversion 5.

To open a Blocked Flask. It is necessary at this time to describe a mode of opening a flask whose stopper obstinately resists. Ordinarily, the harder you try to open it, the more it sticks. To make it yield in a few moments, it is enough to strike the neck of the flask lengthways with the ring at the end of a key. These repeated light blows loosen the stopper, which then comes out when you pull. For lack of this simple remedy, you might otherwise be forced to abandon flasks blocked in this manner.

——*Manuel des dames.*

Diversion 6.

Walking and Carriage Costumes. For January 1824: pelisses chiefly of *gros de Naples,* and cachemire shawls, rich as to colour and pattern, form the most prevailing envelopes for the carriage and the promenade. The style of make and the manner of trimming these pelisses are various. Some of them are of the robe make, and discover a handsome petticoat of embroidered muslin underneath; these are confined to the carriage, and to mild weather. They are generally of striped silk, and are lined throughout with sarcenet coloured to suit the stripe. The more comfortable out-door pelisse is of some striking colour, and is made in the close German fashion, and richly trimmed with fur.

The newest out-door dress is a pelisse of a new kind, called the Prussian pelisse; it is of velvet or plush silk. It has two enormous capes which touch the elbow; these are temporary, and are made to put on and off at pleasure. Pinked silk is still used in the trimming of silk pelisses. Mantles are more in favour than pelisses. They are generally of black satin lined with blue, fire-colour, or pink. They are tied with ribands striped the colour of the lining, on black.

February 1824. The new pelisses are made without collars, and very plain. They are chiefly of *gros de Naples,* lined with a rich twilled sarcenet; and as they are of dark colours, this lining is white. Wide and warm cloaks, either of the Spanish or French kind, are however preferred, particularly for the carriage. Pelerines, either of ermine, sable, or some other valuable fur, still continue fashionable. Braiding is again much in use for spencers and pelisses; of the former but few have made their appearance. The half-boots and shoes are generally of the same colour as the spencer or pelisse.

March 1824. Fig. 4 shows a walking dress consisting of a pelisse of *gros de Naples,* the colour *café à la crème.* It is elegantly ornamented down the front of the skirt with a satin rouleau in diamonds, on each side

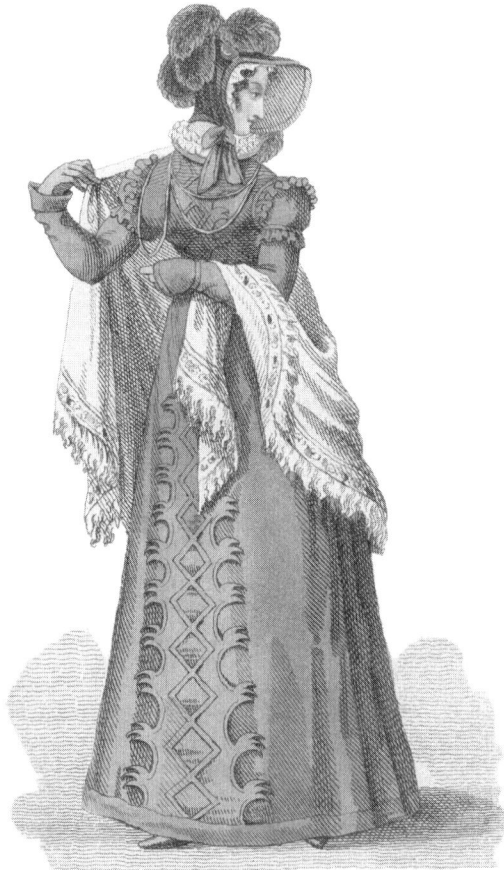

Figure 4. Walking dress.

of which are ornaments representing sea-weed. The sleeves are trimmed at the top with epaulette plaitings, with one row of plaiting round the thick part of the arm, forming a mancheron. The body is trimmed in the front to correspond with the skirt. The pelisse is finished at the throat by a round collar, and a double frill of embroidered muslin. When the weather is cold, a white cachemire shawl with a coloured border is thrown over the pelisse. The bonnet is of black vevet, with a plume of feathers and one full-blown rose. Half-boots of plum-coloured kid, and lemon-coloured kid gloves.

High gowns of merino are often worn at the promenades in lieu of a pelisse. They are of grey-lilac, Nile-water green, or some other light colour, and look well. They have a narrow velvet collar, over which falls a muslin collar trimmed round with plaited lace. Cachemire mantles of Parma-violet colour, richly braided, with pelerine capes, and folded round the form with taste and elegance, are much in favour with women of distinction.

June 1824. So devoted are our tasteful belles to the brilliant spring tints, that white is adopted with regret, and nothing makes it tolerated but the beautiful spencers which have lately made their appearance, and promise to be very general as the summer advances. At present, however, spencers come on but slowly, because it is impossible to wear any other dress with them than a fine white cambric or India muslin, elegantly embroidered. When the weather is chill, a close enveloping pelisse is preferred, of blue, palm-leaf green, or canary-yellow *gros de Naples*. At other times a cachemire shawl, thrown over a gown of any colour, is the more favoured out-door covering. The ground of these shawls is generally lead-colour, with a superb variegated border. Riding habits are of dark blue fine cloth. A plain black equestrian hat, rather small, is worn with them, and sometimes a green veil when the weather is sultry.

Pelerines which fasten behind are again in favour; some of the new spencers fasten likewise.

July 1824. A fashionable out-door covering is a white half-handkerchief called the *fichu à la neige;* it is of muslin, and cut in points round the border. A few muslin pelisses have made their appearance since the weather became warmer; they have a double pelerine cape. Square shawls of black and of white lace also promise to be much in favour this summer. Scarf-shawls of dark-coloured silk, or of marsh-mallow-blossom colour, with the ends striped with yellow satin, are in great esteem. Spencers are made with drawn bodies, have loose sleeves, and are by no means the smart elegant dress they were heretofore.

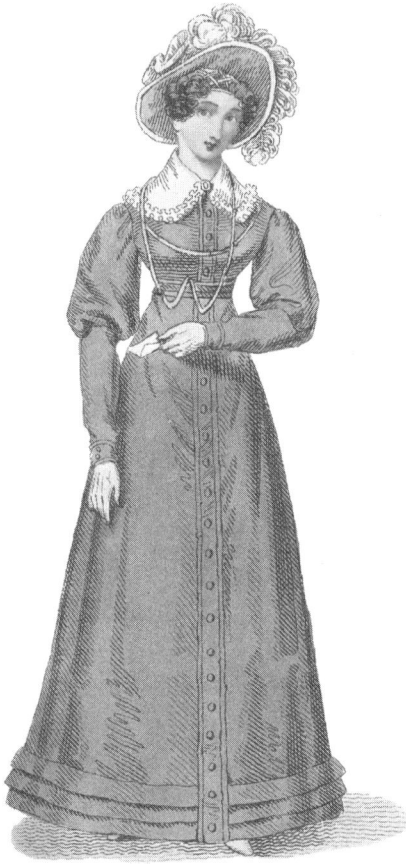

Figure 5. Carriage dress.   **Figure 6. Carriage dress.**

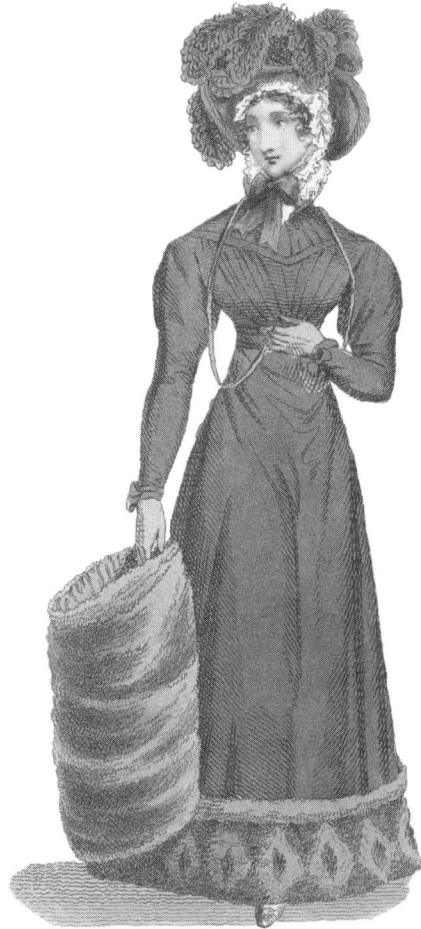

August 1824. Fig. 5 shows a carriage dress consisting of a sky-blue pelisse of *gros de Naples,* buttoning close down the front from the throat to the shoe. Three bias folds finish the border at the bottom. The sleeves are made in the French style, close to the arm from the wrist to the elbow, and then are carried up to the shoulder full, *à l'évêque.* The falling collar is of fine muslin, edged with Mechlin lace. The hat is of white figured *gros de Naples,* placed very backwards, lined with pink, and crowned with handsome white plumes. On the hair, under the hat, are seen white blond and small white flowers. Yellow kid half-boots and gloves; gold neck-chain and eye-glass.

Cachemire scarfs are thrown over the shoulders in easy negligence, over a high gown of white or light-coloured silk. The fulness of the skirts of some pelisses is brought very forward: though this style is highly patronized it spoils the figure. The collars of the pelisses are pointed in the Chinese fashion, with pagoda-bell tassels depending from each point, as they again turn down from the stiffened collar. Other pelisses have collars with battlement indentings. Some have no collar, but have that want supplied by a falling tucker, or a full French ruff ornamented with coloured ribands. This ruff, however, requires a collar partially standing up, as then it fills the hollow space at the back part of the throat, and is becoming to every face, imparting a softness to the features.

October 1824. High gowns of a dark but cheerful colour, with a shawl of Chinese or Cyprus crape, mark the declining year. Though summer-like in appearance, these shawls are very warm owing to the peculiar way in which they cling to the form, particularly the Cyprus crape; they are charming articles for *demi-saison* wear. *Fichus* of striped silk, or white and light-coloured silk, with very large figures on them of a conspicuous tint, are still worn over white gowns when the weather is warm. The canezou-spencer is another summer covering yet retained, when the sunny day will permit so cool an article of out-door costume.

December 1824. Fig. 6 shows a carriage dress consisting of a blouse pelisse of a fine vermilion-coloured *gros de Naples*, with a border of light sable beautifully shaded in diamonds, and a muff of the same. The collar terminates in a point before and is edged with a satin rouleau. The village hat is of black velvet, lined with pink and ornamented with a superb plume of black feathers. A lace cornette is worn underneath. Plum-coloured kid slippers, and yellow gloves.

Wrapping cloaks are indeed in high and general estimation, both for the carriage and the promenade. They are certainly more fitted for the former, and have a truly elegant appearance. They are convenient, and easier thrown aside on entering the house than a pelisse. But for walking, nothing can be more smart or comfortable than this last-mentioned envelope, especially when fastened close, as now, from the throat to the bottom of the skirt. They have generally a pelerine cape which takes on and off, when a lady, on a very cold day, prefers wearing a pelerine mantelet of fur. This warm material bids fair to be as much the mode as it was last winter. The skins most in favour are those of the Arctic fox, the lynx, light sable, and grey squirrel. The first-mentioned of these furs is seldom used except in long tippets; in pelerines or in short tippets the ermine bears a decided preference. The pelisses are chiefly of *gros de Naples*. The sleeves are wide, and when they are surmounted by mancherons, they are in the Persian style; indeed no other could be worn with the capacious sleeves now so much the rage.

January 1827. Rich cachemire shawls, mantles, and pelisses press upon the sight in various succession. The first of these articles is confined to the morning call, or early evening visit; when the mildness of the weather, such as was experienced about the middle of December, rendered such an envelope sufficient, which could be left open or wrapped close over the form at pleasure. The mantles have received an improvement which adds much to the warmth and comfort they impart; they have a kind of pelerine waistcoat underneath, which buttons close down the chest. A large pelerine cape, with a falling collar the same colour as the lining, finishes these cloaks. Those of scarlet with large black chequers prevail much, but they are now getting too common to be admired by ladies belonging to the higher classes. Fur mantelets are worn, as last winter, over high gowns.

March 1827. Spencers are partially worn by the young. But these are chiefly adopted during the first of the morning, when a handsome gown of *gros de Naples* is thus made a *robe aux deux fins*. When the spencer is laid aside it becomes a low gown, cut away at the shoulders, with short sleeves. The same gown serves for demi-toilet, with the spencer, and only the addition of a handsome shawl for the promenade. Fur tippets *en pelerine* are much worn over high gowns, and even over pelisses, when the weather is very chill.

April 1827. Mantles and pelisses of beautiful spring colours, now form the favourite envelopes for the carriage and promenade. The mantles are very plain; the pelisses exhibit much fancy in their different modes of trimming, and all have pelerine capes. These are finished in the same manner as the sides and border of the skirt, either by *dents de loups*, bias folds, or sharp Spanish points, for all these trimmings are equally fashionable. Most of the pelisses fasten down the front of the skirt with rosettes; though some ladies prefer a plain piece of silk underneath, which fastens imperceptibly, and appears as if the pelisse discovered a small portion of a petticoat of the same material. Coloured silk scarfs, tied carelessly over a pelisse or a high gown, have now succeeded to the fur tippets and thick shawls of various kinds.

June 1827. Fig. 7 shows a walking dress consisting of a high gown of slate-coloured *gros de Naples,* with two narrow flounces in festoons. The body is plain, and the sleeves have antique points at the wrists, of fine lace. The collar is *à la chevalière,* edged with lace. A lace cornette is worn under a Leghorn bonnet, bound and trimmed with ethereal blue satin and white blond. Half-boots of the palest shade of straw-colour, in kid.

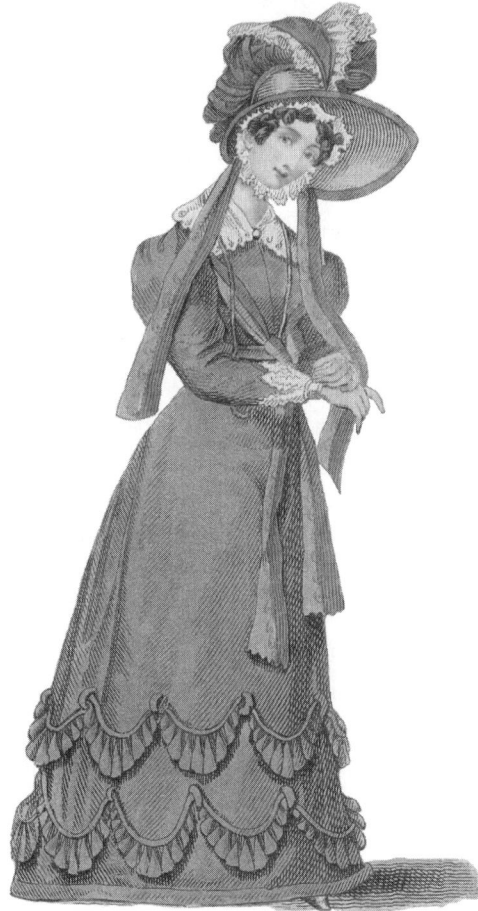

Figure 7. Walking dress.

For walking costume, when a gown is made high, and of *gros de Naples,* a pelerine with long ends is the favourite out-door appendage. The ends are drawn through the belt, and the pelerine is trimmed round with a narrow ruche, pinked in scollops. Muslin spencers worn with coloured *gros de Naples* petticoats promise to be very general this summer. The spencers are only partially high; and a *sautoir* is usually tied across the throat. But many ladies wear a *fichu-pelerine* of soft India muslin embroidered and edged also with lace; the ends are drawn through the belt, which is of the same colour as the petticoat.

August 1827. Walking Dress. The gown is of fawn-coloured muslin, with two flounces embroidered at the edges in black, and headed by full *cordon-rouleaux.* The sleeves are *en gigot,* and the canezou-spencer is of muslin trimmed with lace, confined round the waist by a belt of spring green, fastened with a square silver buckle. The hat is of chequered green silk, ornamented with Portugal laurel and white sarcenet. The parasol is of spring green.

Scarf-shawls and large handkerchief-shawls, either of beautifully coloured and figured gauze, or of Chinese crape, are much in favour for out-door costume; but the mantilla-canezou and the canezou-spencer are very prevalent. They are of embroidered tulle or muslin, and whether over a white or a coloured gown, they have a genteel and unique appearance. Elegantly-made silk spencers are also increasing in favour, and with a white muslin gown they form a beautiful promenade costume for the young. Pelisses and pelisse-robes are still patronized by our matrons, and in no dress do they appear to more advantage. The make and the style of the trimming is very simple; but their fine summer colours are most lovely. Indeed, many young ladies wear those of delicate tints, such as celestial blue, lilac, or pink.

Muslin pelisses are very much in favour. They are ornamented with half-a-dozen gold buckles wrought like that which confines the belt; these buckles are placed at about six inches' distance from each other. Next in favour are white crape pelisses, lined with coloured sarcenet; but these are only fit for the carriage or the public promenade. The canezous are very elegantly made, and are much improved by being made across the bosom *à la Circassienne*. The back is formed in the shape of a heart; the sides and front are trimmed with lace.

September 1827. Pelerines of the same colour and material as the gown form a favourite out-door costume. They are generally surmounted at the throat by a full frill of tulle. The new pelisses are of sarcenet, which is certainly more appropriate to the summer than either *gros de Naples* or levantine. Their colours are light, chaste, and beautiful; the reverse of the green sage leaf, the green of the date leaf, and lavender-grey are amongst the most attractive hues. They are made in a tasteful style, lightly trimmed, and without any *outré* affectation of extreme plainness.

November 1827. Riding habits are much worn in the country, not only as an equestrian, but as a promenade costume. They are of fine cloth, of a beautiful Maccassa brown, and are made in a charming style, most becoming and appropriate to this kind of dress. This has a high collar, and small smart lappels turned back from the front, displaying an elegant waist-coat with small buttons from the throat, which is encircled by a cravat. The beaver hat is of a charming shape, with a band and rosette in the front.

December 1827. Scarf-shawls of real cachemire are much in request; they have a plain ground, and the ends are bordered by large palm-leaves. Some pelisses are of *gros de Naples,* and many are of levantine. They are fastened down the front either with straps and buttons, or with rosettes of riband. The new cloaks are elegant, but few persons look well with them tied down at the bottom of the waist, as they are worn at present; it requires shoulders of uncommon beauty. The cloak being of necessity full there, it gives a roundness to the back, and answers no purpose whatever as to warmth. All these cloaks should be wide, and well wrapped round the form *à l'assassin.*

Many of the silk and satin pelisses button down the front from the waist to the feet; when for the carriage or public walks the buttons are of jet. Seven buttons are placed up the small part of each arm, in a row from the wrist.

January 1829. Nothing is reckoned more genteel for the out-door costume for young persons than a merino gown made partially high, with a pelerine-tippet of lynx or black fox. Another favourite dress of this kind is of a beautiful cinnamon brown, and over this is a tippet of grey American squirrel, with a muff of the same. Black satin pelisses are very fashionable. They are made very plain, but fasten down the front of the skirt with bows of black and of rose-coloured ribands, intermingled. Cloaks are as much in favour as they have been for these two months past. They have often a black pelerine worn with them in place of a hood; this is of velvet, and some ladies have velvet capes the colour of the cloak, particularly if it is red.

Witzchoura pelisses lined with fur, and a very wide fur round the border, promise to be much in favour this winter. The sleeves are wide enough to answer the purpose of a muff, and such is the use made of them at present.

March 1829. Fig. 8 shows a carriage costume consisting of a high gown of mignonette-leaf green satin, with a wide hem round the border, headed by three rouleaux set close together. The body is made plain, and over it is a square pelerine, cleft at each shoulder and forming a stomacher in the front, with a row of buttons down the centre. The sleeves are *à la Marie,* confined only once, near the wrist, forming there a bouffant close to the hand, terminated by a wide gold bracelet. The throat is surmounted by a ruff of light, clear net, *bouilonnée.* The black velvet hat is fastened under the chin with a string of plaited tulle, and the hat is ornamented under the brim with pink satin riband; two elegant black feathers

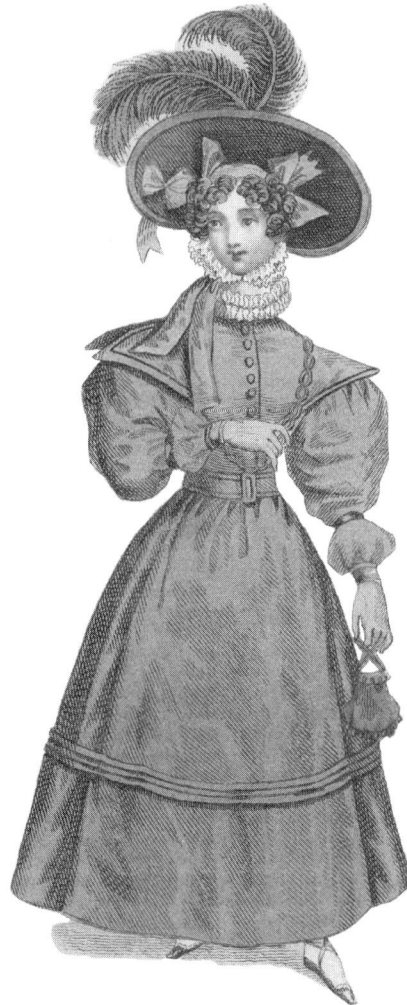

Figure 8. Carriage costume.

are placed at the front of the hat. A bag of celestial blue velvet is carried with this dress.

Pelisses are made very plain, and are most admired when of velvet or satin. For morning walks many have appeared of fine merino trimmed with fur; they have pelerines, or sometimes long tippets, of the same skin which ornaments the pelisse. The few cloaks which are worn are very elegant; but they visibly decline for the promenade, on genteel ladies, who use them exclusively for the carriage, the evening party, or the theatre. Some of these are of the fine cloth called European cachemire, and are ornamented all round the cape, cuffs, and collar in an elegant pattern of silk embroidery.

Many ladies, when the weather is chill, wear cloaks of fine cloth chequered with black on scarlet. Pelisses, however, are most fashionable, and these are of satin or velvet. The sleeves are immensely wide at the top; they are *à la Marie,* and are confined at the elbow and at the wrist by two bands, set very near together, the fulness between forming a bouffant. Short mantles, called cloaks *à la Witzchoura,* are thrown over gowns on quitting a ball-room; they are lined throughout with fur.

May 1829. The newest pelisses are of satin, and have the backs and the bodies entirely square; they are plaited very full in the skirt, all round the waist; the sleeves are very wide, and the cuffs very narrow. Many ladies wear their *chatelaines* at the promenades, but it is reckoned most elegant to have them turned round the belt. When a gown of silk or satin is worn as an out-door walking costume, it is usual to have a pelerine of the same, trimmed round with fringe, particularly if the gown is so ornamented. Sometimes these pelerines are triple, and the fringe has then a very rich effect.

June 1829. Pelisses of *gros de Naples,* in colours light and delicate but not glaring, seem much in favour for out-door costume, as are shawls of the most flexible cachemire, and scarfs of spring-coloured light silks, beautifully variegated. Very large muslin pelerine-tippets, forming almost a little mantelet, are much in favour, and increase in requisition as the summer weather advances. They are either embroidered exquisitely in feather-stitch, or trimmed round with a very fine wide lace.

A gown of *gros de Naples* with a matching pelerine often constitutes the favourite out-door covering in the public walks; these pelerines are fastened over the bosom with a gold pin called *à la Sévigné.* The chief novelty in out-door dress is a canezou of white muslin, embroidered in different colours to correspond with the gown of *gros de Naples* or coloured muslin which may be worn with it. *Fichu-canezous* of coloured *gros de Naples* are worn over white gowns. Some of the riding dresses have only a cloth petticoat, with the jacket consisting of a white muslin canezou-spencer.

July 1829. Nothing can be more plain and simple than the style of costume now adopted by ladies of real elegance in the morning, or for the retired rural walk. A high silk gown, with an apron of the same colour and material, both the gown and apron made as plain as possible, is the present order of the day. A pelisse either of *gros de Naples* or poplin, made quite plain, is much in favour for walking. Some of these are made as pelisse-robes and are left open in the front over a petticoat of embroidered muslin.

August 1829. Fig. 9 shows a walking gown of amber-coloured *gros de Naples,* with a very wide hem round the border of the skirt, surmounted by two narrow flounces, the upper one falling over the lower so as to conceal the half of it. The body is made only partially high, with a tulle *fichu* worn underneath. The tucker part is surrounded by a triple frill of *gros de Naples*. A blue silk scarf, with a wide violet-coloured fringe at the

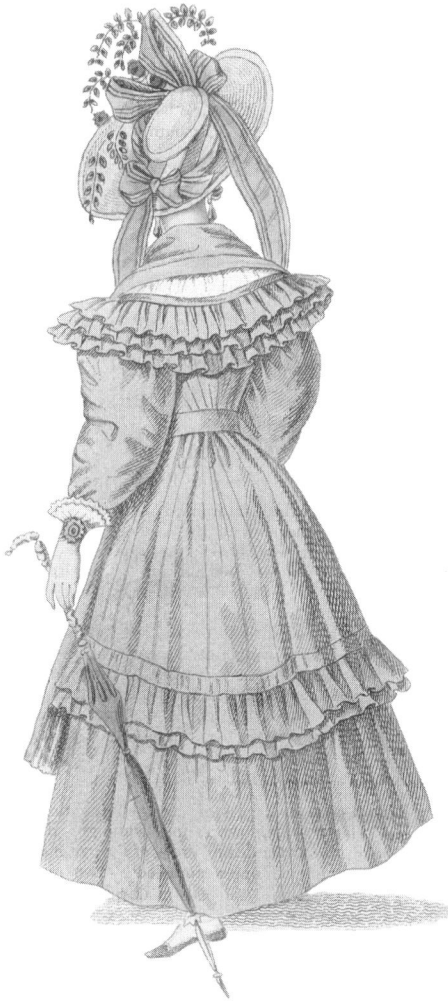

Figure 9. Walking dress.   **Figure 10. Walking dress.**

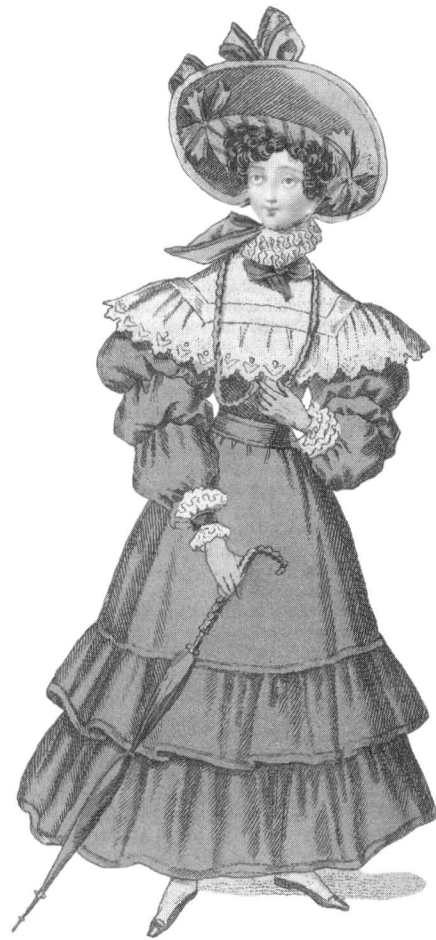

ends, is tied at the throat. The body of the gown is made *en gerbe.* The sleeves are *à l'imbecile* with embroidered muslin cuffs, with a lace ruffle next the arm, and confined at the wrists by wide gold bracelets, clasped by a large garnet set round with pearls. Leghorn hat, elegantly ornamented with branches of foliage and pink riband.

The pelisses are made chiefly in the wrapping style, with the body *à la Circassienne;* but pelisses are not very much worn. Shawls of Chinese and of Cyprus crape are infinitely more in request. The former set beautifully to the form, keep out the chill air, yet never appear too warm for the short summers of England's uncertain climate. The Cyprus crape shawls are very pretty; but they are so easily imitated that they have become extremely common. A few muslin pelisses have appeared at Tunbridge and other places of fashionable resort, but they are by no means general. The weather was cold during the commencement of July, and the fashionable pedestrian thus enveloped was compelled to add a shawl of Chinese crape, forming thereby a very pretty costume.

September 1829. A favourite out-door covering is a pelerine of black velvet, or one the same as the gown, if the gown is of *gros de Naples.* These graceful auxiliaries are of an entirely new form compared to those worn last autumn. They are pointed at the termination behind, and from thence carried up on each side, in a gradual direction. The ends in the front, which are confined under the belt, reach nearly to the feet. The pelerine, when of black velvet, is lined throughout with bright rose-coloured, cherry-coloured, or rock-geranium sarcenet.

For young persons, nothing is more fashionable for the promenade than a petticoat of levantine or *gros de Naples,* with a white muslin spencer with very full sleeves. Silk pelisses are now becoming more general.

Scarfs are very much worn in out-door costume, and also at the public spectacles. For out-doors they are of silk or cachemire, according to the temperature of the weather; for spectacles they are generally of gauze, and either of white or cherry-colour. The pelisses are chiefly of the wrapping kind; and when of muslin or cambric are trimmed round with a double frill laid on in very small plaits. A pelerine of the same material and style of ornament, is generally worn with this kind of pelisse; but the trimming is edged with narrow lace.

October 1829. Fig. 10 shows a walking gown of stone-coloured *gros de Naples,* bordered by two flounces. The body is plain, with sleeves *à la Marie.* A muslin pelerine is worn with this dress, trimmed round with wide lace, and surmounted at the throat by a full ruff of lace. The hat is of pink *gros de Naples,* trimmed with riband of the same colour.

Cachemire shawls are favourite envelopes in promenade costume. The newest are in chequered patterns, the chequers formed of numerous hair-stripes; some of these shawls have been sent to Paris from Pekin in China. Pelisses of organdy and of jaconet muslin are yet worn. The sleeves are immensely large, and are opened all the way down the arm, and closed again by a double row of gold buttons. The belt, the cuffs, and the ruff round the throat, are all fastened with double buttons. For the morning walks, both at Paris and in the country, ladies who follow the extremes of fashion wear pelisses *à la maîtresse,* of jaconet muslin with a blue, pink, or chamois-coloured ground, with a cambric petticoat. These pelisses have a double falling *fichu* collar; one of these collars is laid in a great number of small plaits, the other in flutings.

November 1829. Cloaks have already become very general, and are expected to be much in favour this winter; those which have appeared at present are of *gros de Naples.* The new pelisses are made in the long tunic style. Two bias folds surround the border next the shoe, and the tunic is formed by two similar folds on each side; the pelisse fastens imperceptibly under one of these sides. The sleeves are chiefly *à l'imbecile.* These pelisses of the tunic kind are made without cape or collar; a pelerine of fine India muslin, richly embroidered, or one of tulle trimmed with lace, being always worn with them. On pelisses merely intended for the morning promenade, a square cape is generally added, of the same material as the pelisse.

Pelisses of India cachemire are also much admired. The colour is that of the shawls of this kind, in general a cream-colour, trimmed with narrow bordering of different colours in shawl-patterns. These latter pelisses are lined throughout with white *gros de Naples,* discovering a petticoat of the same silk. The newest wadded silk and satin pelisses have the sleeves much tighter at the small part of the arm than heretofore. Five bias folds are carried from the wrist up to the bend of the arm, and have a very graceful effect.

December 1829. Some of the new pelisses fasten on the shoulder, by means of hooks concealed by the part which folds over, which prevents the sleeves of the gown underneath being rumpled in drawing the pelisse over them. Black velvet pelerines are much in favour at the Tuileries, and are trimmed with fringe. Within these ten days past several spencers have appeared at the promenades. Some were of black velvet, with a coloured silk petticoat; others were of blue or green *gros de Chine,* and were worn with a white petticoat; the bodies were *à la Sévigné.*

——*Ladies' Pocket Magazine.*

Diversion 7.

Dinner-party Dress. Mrs. L.—It is not usual, I believe, for a lady to be in full dress when she entertains a party at dinner.

Mrs. B.—The dress of a lady at dinner-parties, should be plainer at home than abroad; otherwise a reflection might be implied on such of her guests whose dress is inferior. But in evening parties the lady of the house is generally full dressed.

——*Domestic Duties.*

September 1827. A gown of pale pink crape, ornamented with a wide border of narrow blond *en carreaux.* The body is in the Circassian-wrap style, embroidered at the edge where it folds over the bosom, in a pattern of vine-leaves two shades darker than the colour of the gown. The long sleeves are of white gauze, with mancherons formed of points in pink crape edged round with narrow blond. The bracelets are gold, clasped by a brooch formed of a cluster of fine garnets. The hat is of transparent white crape, surmounted by a plume of white feathers; it has very long strings, looped, of wide white gauze riband.

November 1827. A gown of white muslin with three flounces, embroidered at the edges; the upper one surmounted by a row of delicate foliage in embroidery. The body is made slightly *en gerbe.* The sleeves are long and full, and clasped at the wrists by two bracelets. The lower one is of wide gold lace, fastened with a cameo; the upper one is formed of two rows of gold beads, fastened with an antique head in *alto relievo.* This gown is made partially low, with a wide collar *à la paladin,* edged round with Vandyked points; above the row of points is a tulle ruche. Round the waist is a wide belt of scarlet and green striped riband. The hat is of white chip, ornamented with sarcenet and bird-of-paradise plumes.

April 1829. A gown of corn-flower blue gauze, with black satin spots, and two flounces of the same round the border. The body is plain, and the tucker part surmounted by a collar *en paladin* edged with narrow blond; the sleeves are very short and full. The hair is arranged in full curls round the face, and ornamented with puffs of blue and pink gauze ribands in long loops. The ear-rings are of wrought gold.

——*Ladies' Pocket Magazine.*

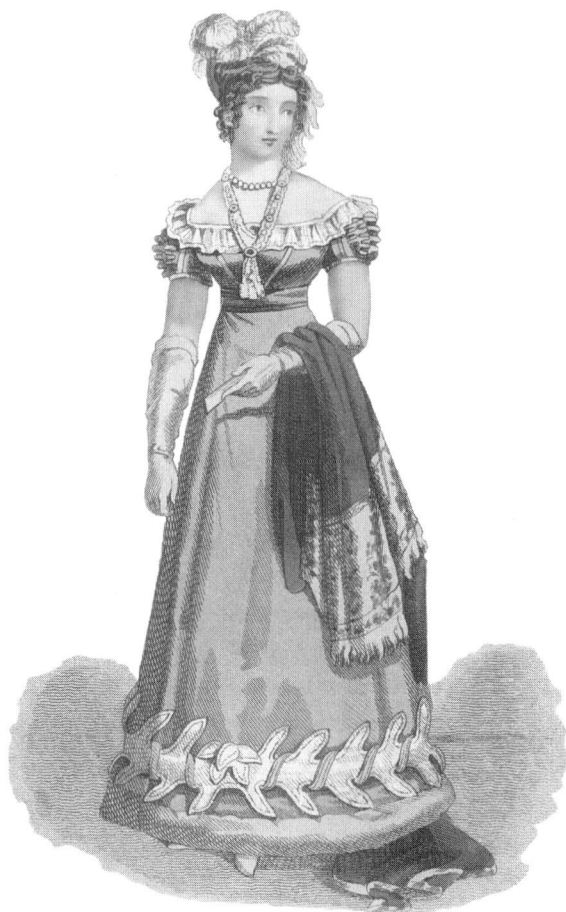

Figure 11. Full evening dress.

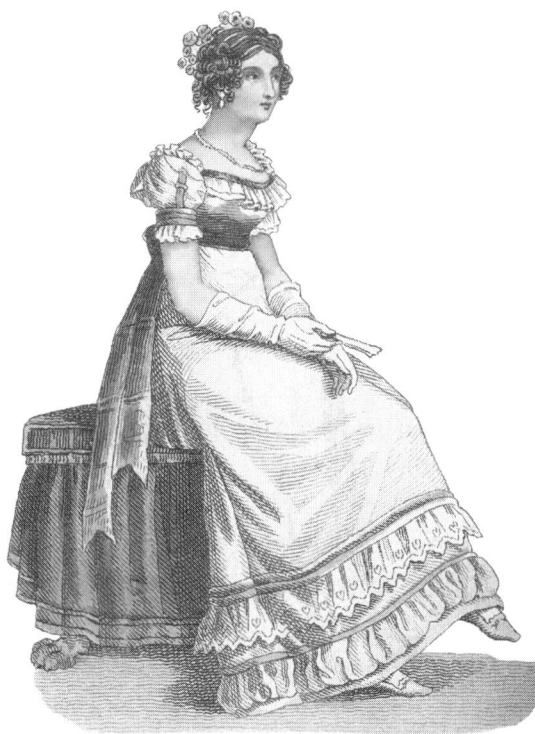

Figure 12. Private-concert dress.

Diversion 8.

Costumes for Assemblies, Concerts, &c. For January 1824: Fig. 11 shows the most approved full-dress costume for evening parties. It consists of a soft satin gown, of a celestial blue colour, ornamented with white satin and beading, a foliage trimming of which is laid on the border of the skirt, entwined with silk *cordon*. A very full wadded rouleau of white satin is placed next the hem, which it entirely conceals. The body is very simply made, being ornamented only with two narrow rouleaux of white satin, forming a stomacher. The sleeves are very short, and are trimmed with puffings of white satin. The body is ornamented with a falling tucker of blond. A toque turban of scarlet and yellow gauze is placed very backwards, the front part entirely concealed by short white ostrich feathers. Necklace and ear-rings of large pearls, with an Arabian necklace of small pearls. Shoes of white satin, and white kid gloves.

May 1824. Fig. 12 shows a private-concert dress. The gown is of tulle over blush-coloured satin, with two wide flounces of blond, each headed by pink satin rouleaux. The body is of white satin, with a falling tucker of blond; the belt is pink and has long ends. The hair is parted from the forehead *à la Madonna,* and terminates on each side of the face with flowing ringlets like the portraits painted by Vandyke, and crowned with small bouquets of flowers. Pearl ear-rings, white satin shoes, and white kid gloves.

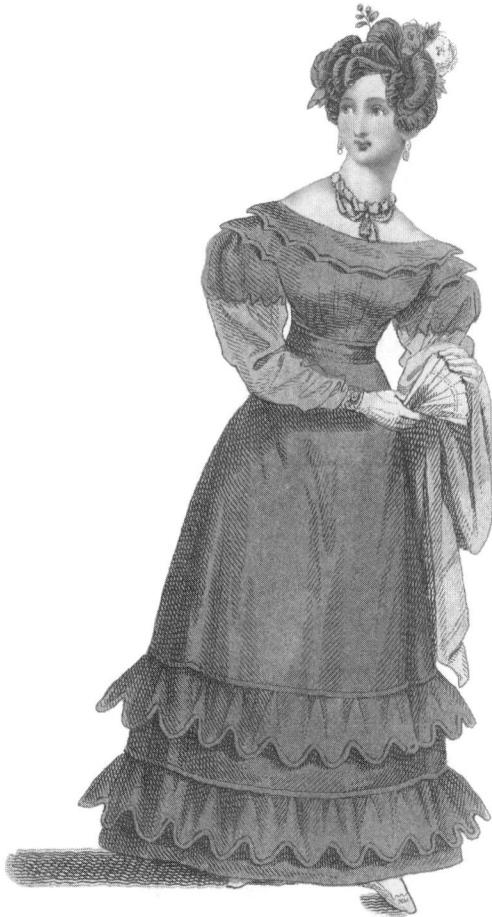

Figure 13. Evening dress.   Figure 14. Opera dress.

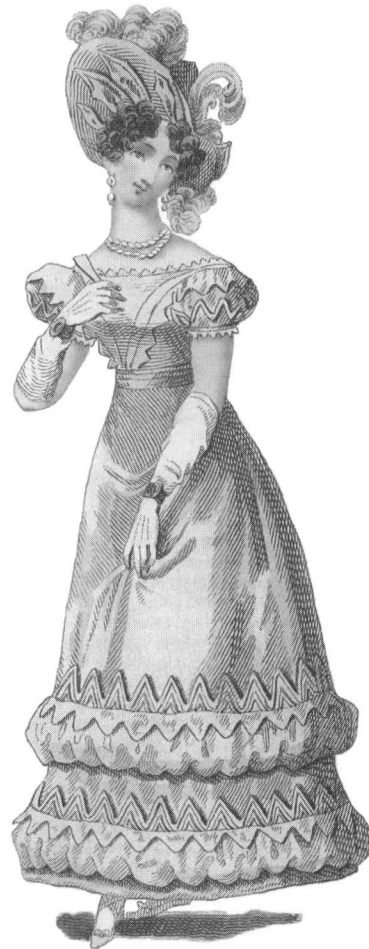

An extremely elegant gown for a full-dress evening party is of white levantine, the border ornamented with three wreaths of lilacs separated by two puckerings of tulle. The body is made with a stomacher, and the tops of the short sleeves are ornamented with a small sprig of lilac. A *fichu* of fine lace is worn under the gown; the present correct fashion of shielding the bosom promises to render this elegant little covering more universal. Some of these *fichus* are of blond; their make is antique, and they form a modest ornament, concealing the part from the bosom to the throat, without disguising it.

January 1827. The evening gown in Fig. 13 is of rose-coloured *gros de Naples*, with two scolloped flounces bound round with satin. The body is plain with a narrow scolloped cape and gigot sleeves. The hair is arranged in large curls, with white and red roses; pear-pearl ear-rings; necklace *à la négligé*, of turquoises, gold, and pearls.

Velvet gowns, either black or crimson, increase in favour for married ladies at evening parties. Evening gowns of *gros de Naples* or satin are generally of light colours, though black gowns are much worn this winter. A favourite way of trimming *gros de Naples* gowns is with two flounces, delicately pinked in scollops, and falling one over the other; the upper one is surmounted by a ruche of a novel description, and beautifully executed. Short sleeves now prevail in full dress, as is usual in winter; though most of the velvet gowns have long tulle sleeves. Young ladies at balls and evening parties wear gowns of coloured barège or crape, and sometimes of tulle. The bodies are in the Castilian style, with drapery and blond; the borders are trimmed either with two or three headed flounces, or with the same number of ruches entwined with satin rouleaux.

April 1827. The opera gown in Fig. 14 is of soft white satin, bordered by two rows of tulle *bouillonnée,* surmounted by points of white satin falling over the tulle, and points formed of three rows of rich silk *cordon* standing upwards on the dress. The body is in the Anglo-Greek style; the stomacher, or robing part is formed of *cordon,* and disposed so as to answer the ornament on the border. The short sleeves are of tulle over satin, and finished at the shoulders and round the arm by Vandyke points. The dress hat is of blue crape, much elevated on one side, under which part of the brim are blue satin leaves. Blue feathers playing in various directions ornament the hat. Ear-rings, necklace, and bracelets of turquoises.

June 1827. Evening gowns are in coloured tulle, and the bodies are in drapery across the bosom. The sleeves are short, and are always ornamented in a manner analogous to the skirt. This trimming depends entirely upon fancy. Sometimes it consists in *bouillons* ornamented with satin; sometimes it is flounces, ruches, or bias folds, headed by a tulle quilling.

January 1829. The gowns are very much cut away at the shoulders, and are rather awkwardly square across the bosom, which if a little more seen, and the shoulders less, especially in evening costume, would have a much more attractive appearance. Tulle gowns with satin bodies are worn at balls and full-dress evening parties. Merinos are much in favour for demi-toilet. The silk gowns are still made in that grotesque fashion of being plaited equally full all round the waist.

Some gowns of coloured satin have long sleeves of white *crêpe aérophane,* the style being *à la Mameluke,* or *à la Marie.* Those of Ispahan satin cross in drapery over the bosom, and are trimmed with a double falling tucker of blond, which forms a pelerine over the back and shoulders.

February 1829. Many of the most elegant and approved gowns are of coloured satin, and the body laces behind. With these, when worn only in demi-toilet, is a pelerine of the same colour and material as the gown. It is trimmed at the collar, which is left open, with a frill of wide white blond; a very wide hem surrounds the border, in bias. A black velvet belt, pointed in the front, is often worn with these gowns, particularly when the gown is of a light colour. Ball gowns are often trimmed with blond or tulle ruches. All these gowns have been for some time made truly appropriate to dancing, by the simplicity of their border trimming; many borders now consist of wide satin riband set in rows at equal distances. Black velvet gowns ornamented with pearls form an elegant evening costume for married ladies.

March 1829. The opera gown in Fig. 15 is of lilac *gros de Naples,* with one wide flounce, edged with a slight pattern of black embroidery; the body is *en gerbe.* The long white crape sleeves are *en gigot,* over which are cleft mancherons of lilac silk. An ornament *en fleurs de lys* of the same material is placed on the outside of the wrist; and a very wide gold bracelet confines the sleeve next the hand. The Spanish toque is of ponceau velvet striped with black, and ornamented with gold bows and tassels. The gold ear-rings are *en girandole,* and the necklace is formed of twisted rows of pearls, fastened in the front with a brooch of wrought gold. A white swan's-down long tippet is thrown over this dress.

The short sleeves are of immense width, and are called *en beret;* the fulness round the arm is gathered in by a tight band. Gowns of Navarin

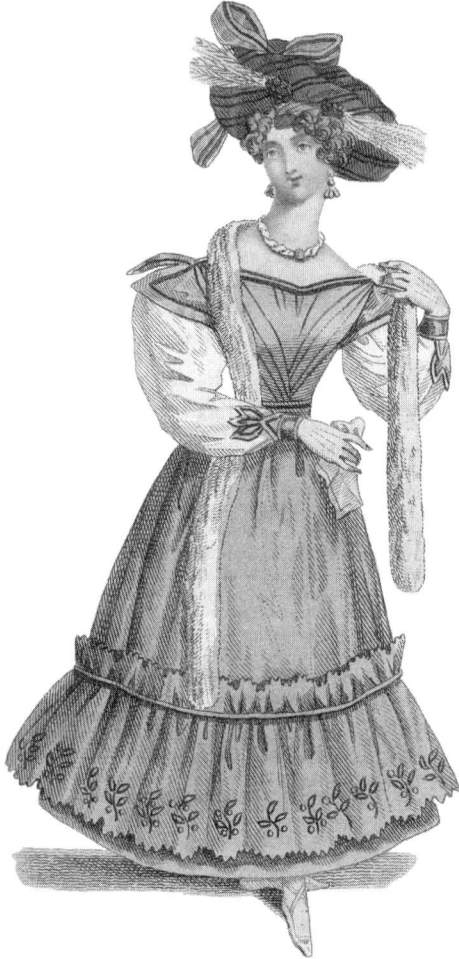

Figure 15. Opera dress.   **Figure 16. Evening dress.**

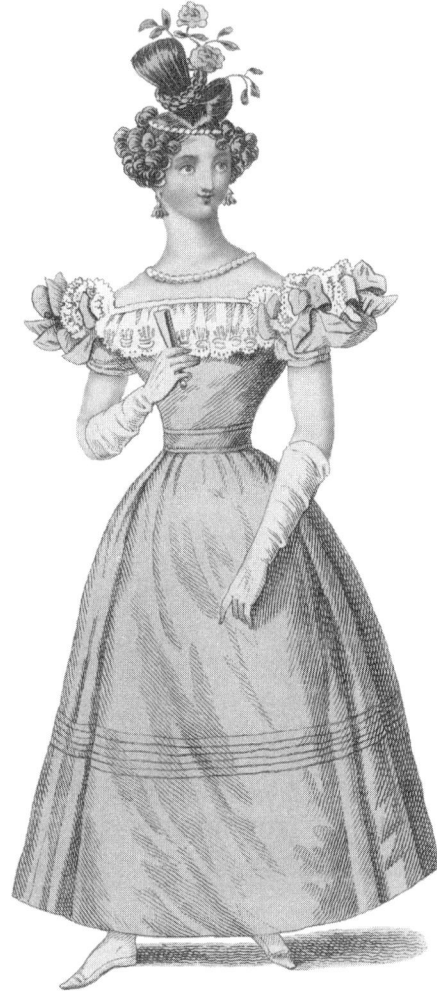

blue crape, with sleeves of the above description, are favourite costumes at public concerts; they are bordered by a wide bias fold, surmounted by three satin rouleaux. A young married lady appeared at one of these concerts with pantaloons of muslin, richly embroidered, which were discovered under a very short gown of silver-grey poplin.

April 1829. Many young ladies wear coloured muslin gowns, which amongst the French ladies always seem like harbingers of spring. The newest muslins of this kind are generally of rose-colour, with two very wide stripes of two shades. They are bordered by one very deep flounce, cut in bias, with a heading to it, which is also in bias, and falls over the flounce.

The bodies of these gowns are *à la Vierge,* trimmed round the neck with a wide falling tucker of white blond; the short sleeves are covered with long white sleeves. This is a favourite dress at public concerts; as is a dress of Navarin blue crape, with two flounces embroidered at the edges, and short sleeves. All gowns for demi-toilet are now made with pocket-holes, and pockets are worn.

May 1829. Fig. 16 shows an evening gown of pink crape, with a wide hem round the border, headed by three narrow satin rouleaux of the same colour. The body is quite plain, with a double falling tucker of blond; the sleeves are short and very full. The hair is arranged in full curls on each side of the face, and in bows on the summit of the head, on which are placed full-blown roses. The ear-rings and necklace are of fine Oriental pearls.

Norwich crape and poplins are much in request for afternoon home costume, the colours light or bright. Many of these have short sleeves, and are worn for receiving friendly evening parties. They are generally ornamented round the border of the skirt with three bias folds.

June 1829. White gowns of every description, and adapted to every time of day and every style of dress, are fast coming into favour. For evening and dinner-party gowns, those of slight summer satins and *gros de Naples* are preferred; those which are coloured have long sleeves of white gauze. The belt, when fastened round the waist, without ends, is generally confined by a buckle of precious stones set in gold.

July 1829. There are very few gowns now which are made high, or even partially so; they are all cut down very low at the back, and the shoulders are entirely discovered. Whether chintzes, printed calicoes, or muslins, materials which were formerly only used for dishabille, are all cut away at the back and shoulders the same as in full dress. For the manner in which a body is made, there is no decided fashion. The gowns are all made very short in the skirt, and plaited equally full all round the waist.

White gowns, both organdy and muslin, are much in request. Very clear muslin of steam yellow is an admired article for evening *parure,* as is clear white muslin, trimmed with fringe formed of white cotton *cordon.* Above this fringe is a wreath of embroidery worked on the gown, and above that a letting-in of lace. The gowns for evening parties, and on particular nights at the theatres, are of coloured crape or gauze. Some are of white crape embroidered or painted in different colours; they have fringes of suitable colours over the wide hem at the border. Gowns of blue crape embroidered in straw-colour have a very pretty effect.

September 1829. At the last fête at Tivoli, one lady appeared in a gown, the sleeves of which hung down from the shoulder to the bend of the arm, and then ended *à l'Amadis.* The opening of these new kind of sleeves, which are named *engageantes,* was trimmed round with fringe with a net heading. A fringe of the same kind bordered the body. The gown was of organdy, of a very bright rose-colour. Embroidered white muslin gowns are now very prevalent for evening costume. The designs are often diamond chequers, with a small bouquet in each diamond.

October 1829. Gowns still continue to be made very short and very full; the skirts are plaited evenly all round the waist. In spite of the chill weather, white gowns predominate much, both in town and in the country. The embroidery on the flounces and borders of these gowns is superb. The flounces are worked in diamonds or chains of open-work, and have the appearance of rich lace. Wide borders admirably executed in satin-stitch, or the lighter feather-stitch, render these expensive gowns fit for the evening party as well as for demi-toilet.

The French ladies are so fond of the clear printed muslins which they call *fragoletta,* that they wear them at concerts and other assemblies. These have white or very light-coloured grounds, figured over in a pattern of green leaves and wood strawberries. A canezou-pelerine of splendidly embroidered tulle is worn on the above occasions with these gowns; and a braid of red, white, and green marks out the edge of the hem as high as the knee.

November 1829. The sleeves are yet extremely large. At a card-party, a few evenings ago, we saw one lady hold up the sleeves of her friend, while she dealt the cards, fearful of the safety of the wax-lights. Some satin gowns have, however, appeared with the sleeves *à l'Amadis;* and even these are not so wide at the top as these sleeves are in general. They are surmounted by a mancheron slashed *à l'Espagnole,* and the slashes filled in with white satin. Other mancherons on satin gowns are puckered of the same material and colour as the gown, and are ornamented with rings of white satin formed of several very narrow rouleaux. This is not new, but it is a fashion revived of about two years back; it has now become a novelty which seems much admired.

December 1829. Fig. 17 shows an evening gown of apricot-coloured India taffety, with a very wide flounce of white blond at the border in a Vandyke pattern, headed by a rouleau of white satin in scollops. At the point of each scollop is a rich tufted ornament composed of white silk. The body is *à la Sévigné.* The sleeves are long and of white *crêpe lisse;* they are

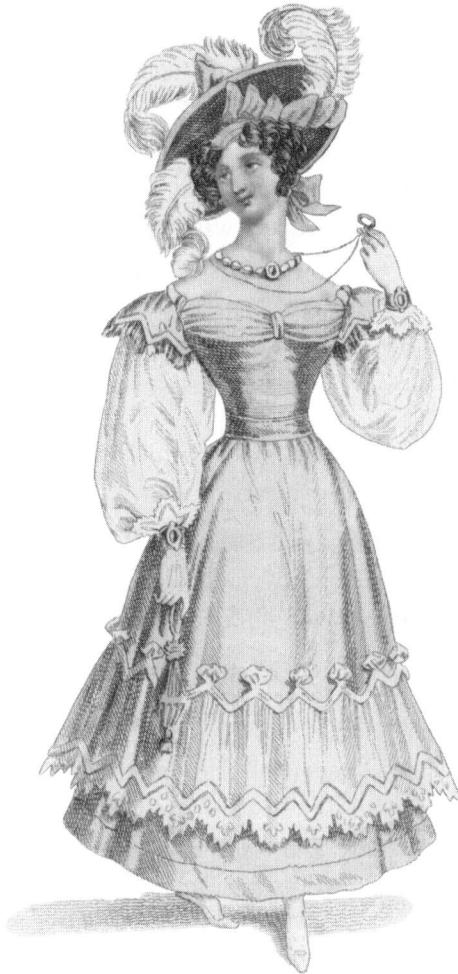

Figure 17. Evening dress.   **Figure 18. Ball dress.**

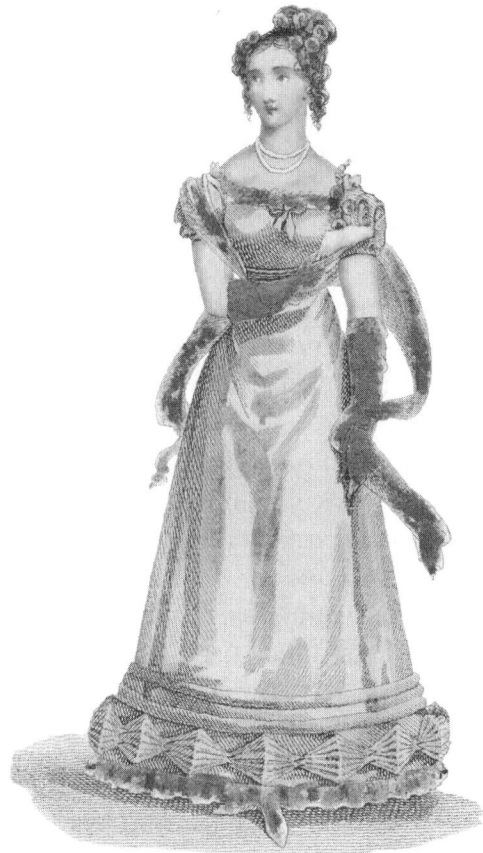

à l'imbecile, with Vandyke mancherons of the same material as the gown, edged with fringe of the same colour. Antique English points of blond finish the sleeves at the wrist, below which, confining it next the hand, are wide bracelets of black velvet, with a large emerald or a red carnelian set in gold filigree. The head-dress is a black velvet beret ornamented with pink riband under the brim; one white feather is also placed beneath it on the right side; over the brim is an elegant plumage of white ostrich feathers.

——Ladies' Pocket Magazine.

Diversion 9.

Costumes for the Ball. For February 1824: Fig. 18 shows a round gown of pale yellow satin, ornamented at the border with a row of diamonds *à l'antique;* each diamond or lozenge is separated by a double lotus-leaf. A large full-wadded rouleau is placed over the hem, of the same material as the gown. The body is made plain, with a handsome tucker of fine blond. The sleeves are short, and ornamented with antique diamonds to answer those on the border of the gown. Over the shoulders is gracefully disposed a white lace scarf of fine and light texture. The hair is formed in numerous ringlets, with an Apollo knot on the summit of the head.

March 1824. For ball gowns, gauzes of the most rich and curious patterns, and both plain and figured tulle, over white or light-coloured satin, form the chief materials. They are festooned, are fancifully drawn up on one side, and fold over the body and part of the skirt with all the Asiatic grace of those worn by the beauties of the East. Flowers and blond form the favourite trimming on these superb ball gowns. The hair is generally ornamented with flowers; and the ear-rings, necklace, and cross should be of pearls.

At evening parties it is customary to wear three different bracelets on each wrist, and three different kinds of necklace at the same time. The first bracelet is very narrow, the second wider, and the third nearly twice the width of the second. The necklaces have the same distinction, except that the third is very long, and on it are suspended a small opera-glass and other trinkets.

May 1824. Some of the gowns are cut low at the back and high in the front, and others *vice versa.* At the most select balls the young ladies are dressed either in white or in rose-colour. The bodies cross over the bosom, in full drapery; the belt is of satin riband, with a small bow and long ends. White gowns ornamented with myrtle and poppies are much in favour at private balls. Drawn bodies *en blouse* are still the rage.

September 1824. Ball gowns are of coloured muslin for the rural scene, where the costume of the dancers is never more than demi-toilet. The most approved colours for these gowns are Evelina blue and rose.

January 1827. Tulle gowns over white satin are much admired for the ball and evening party; as is yellow crape trimmed with satin rosettes, and sleeves slashed after the Spanish fashion. Spotted barège, of lively colours, is also a favourite material for dancing costume: the body is *à la Sévigné.* These gowns are trimmed at the border in various ways, but the most prevalent is with either flounces or ruches.

March 1827. Fig. 19 shows a ball gown of tulle over pink satin, with *bouillons* of *crêpe lisse* at the border, surmounted by ornaments of white satin, in points, which fall partially over the *bouillons;* these pointed puffs are edged round with pink. In the front are two ornaments proceeding from the border of white satin riband, each terminating in a bow as high as the knee, and a bunch of the blue hedge-flower called forget-me-not. These ornaments are carried in bias across the front of the skirt. The body is in the Gallo-Greek style, and discovers a white crape fluted stomacher, trimmed on each side with blond. The sleeves are short and full, and headed by the same kind of oblong puffs which

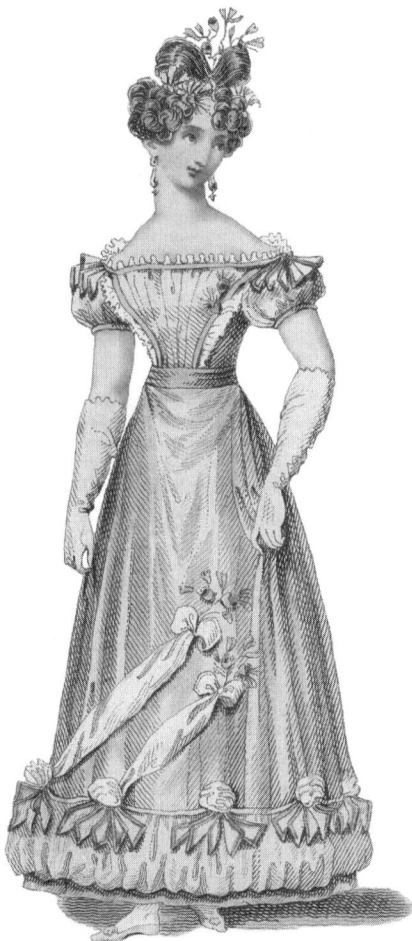

Figure 19. Ball dress.

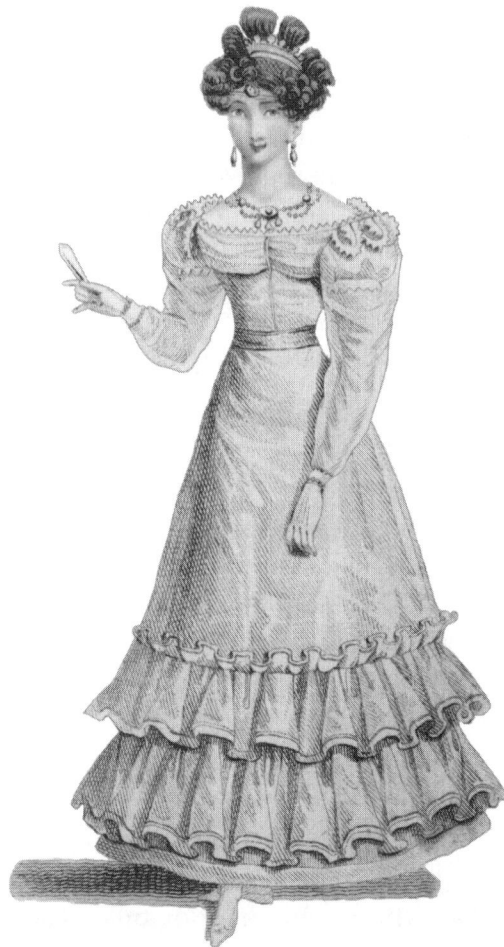

Figure 20. Ball dress.

adorn the bouillon on the skirt. The hair is ornamented with bouquets of pearls, and on the summit of the head is a group of forget-me-nots. Pear-pearl ear-rings.

April 1827. Coloured gauze with satin stripes is a material much in favour for the evening dress of young ladies. Gowns of this kind are generally trimmed at the border with two wide flounces; the body is made to fit the shape, and trimmed round the bosom with blond. White gauze or tulle gowns are the most prevalent in the ball-room. They are trimmed with two rows of *bouillons,* intermingled slightly with flowers, or ears of corn. The bodies of these gowns are generally satin, and often coloured; they are often finished in front of the bosom *à la Sévigné.* Coloured crape gowns are often seen with long sleeves of white tulle or *crêpe lissé.* An elegant scarf or pelerine of blond is thrown over the shoulders.

June 1827. Fig. 20 shows a ball gown of white Japanese gauze over white satin, with two wide flounces bound with white satin. The body is *à la Sévigné;* the sleeves are *en gigot,* with foliage ornaments on the shoulders, trimmed round with blond. The hair is arranged in curls and bows, with a beautiful regal coronet-ornament across the front, formed of pearls. Pear-pearl ear-rings, and a necklace of pearls, set *à l'antique;* in the center a cameo set round with pearls, from which ornament depend three valuable pear-pearls.

White tulle gowns, over *gros de Naples* slips, are worn at balls in preference to white satin. But the balls in town, of any consequence, will soon end; and those for the rural scene are generally marked by more simplicity.

August 1827. Fig. 21 shows a summer ball gown of blue gauze over satin, elegantly embroidered on the two flounces which border it, with black floss-silk. Above each flounce is a row of the same exquisite embroidery in branches of small leaves. The body is made slightly *en gerbe,* with a tucker of fine blond. The sleeves are short and full, with a small pointed ornament at the shoulder, edged round with embroidery. The hair is arranged in curls and bows, with full-blown Provence roses. The necklace is of pearls, and the ear-rings are of gold filigree. Wide gold jointed bracelets are worn over the gloves.

November 1827. As there are but few balls at present where much dress is required, the sleeves are often long and of transparent material, either white *crêpe lisse* or tulle. The gown itself is generally of coloured crape, slightly ornamented round the border with ruches, satin rouleaux, and sometimes a few flowers. The body is finished in the front with *fichu*

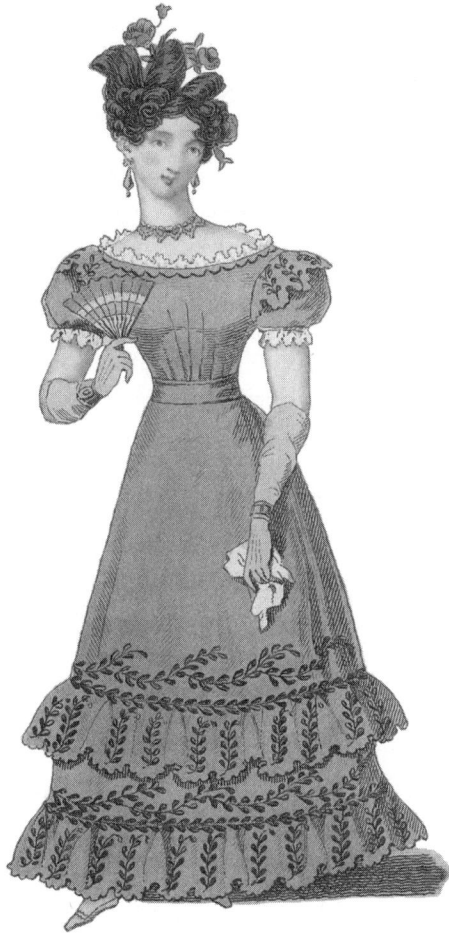

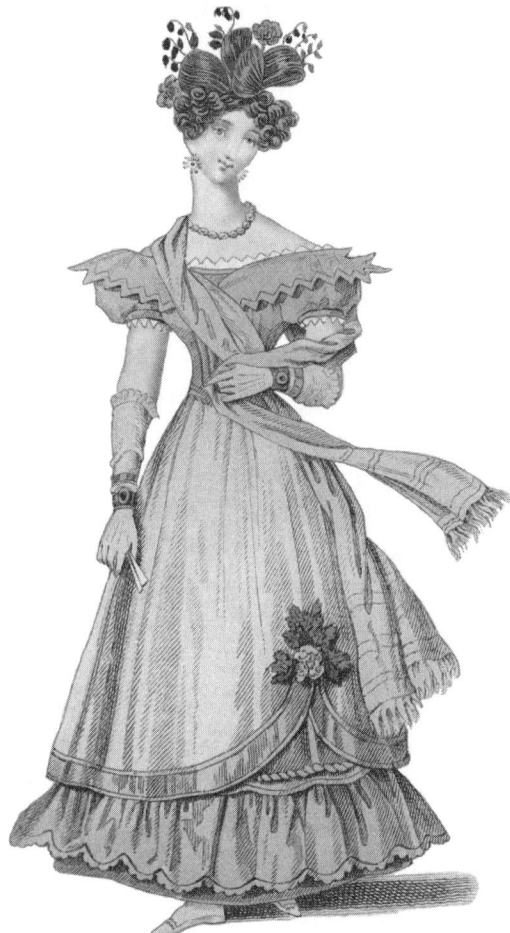

Figure 21. Summer ball dress. **Figure 22. Ball dress.**

robings of three rows of blond, one above the other set on full. These ornaments have a much better effect on evening or dinner gowns, than on those for balls, which cannot be too light.

December 1827. The ball gown in Fig. 22 has a pink satin slip, bordered by one wide flounce. Over this is a tunic-petticoat of white *crêpe lisse*, edged round with pink satin, and caught up in the front by a bouquet formed of one very large full-blown Provence rose and its green leaves. The body is of pink satin, cut low, with a collar-cape in points, and short, full sleeves. Gold bracelets are worn over the gloves; that next the wrist is clasped by a ruby set round with pearls; above this is a double chain brace-let of gold. The necklace and ear-rings are of large pearls; the ear-rings are set in the form of a star. The hair is arranged in curls and bows, sur-mounted by yellow China asters and barberries.

February 1829. Ball gowns are chiefly of crape, with a wide hem as high as the knee. The body is *à l'Edith.* Short sleeves, which discover a narrow ruffle of very fine lace, are supposed to belong to the shift. Gowns of coloured crape are often bordered by a very wide bias fold, headed by satin quillings in very large plaits. Above these are sometimes placed bouquets of various flowers, which descend in three ribands from the waist; amongst the flowers imitating those of the garden, are min-gled a few of gold and silver. For grand balls there are gowns of tulle or of *gaze brillantine,* ornamented with gold or silver. Gowns of coloured gauze, on these splendid occasions, arc also trimmed in the same man-ner. Some ladies at such balls have their gowns made *à la Diane,* that is with the body so cut as to entirely cover the right shoulder; on the left side it seems falling off, and leaves the shoulder nearly bare. Wide flounces of white blond on coloured satin gowns are very prevalent. In full dress these are sometimes set on in festoons, caught up by rosettes of pearls; the mancherons at the top of the sleeves are then ornamented with the same rosettes.

March 1829. Gowns of tulle or crape, either white or coloured, for the ball-room are worn over satin slips, and the favourite trimming on the border is composed of satin rouleaux of the same colour. These gowns have short sleeves of tulle over those of white satin. The gowns are all very much cut away at the shoulders.

August 1829. The rural ball gown in Fig. 23 is of white gauze, with wide satin stripes of celestial blue, over a slip of white *gros de Naples.* Two bias folds surround the border of the gauze gown, set on rather full; the upper one is surmounted by two satin rouleaux placed close together. The body is made quite plain, and fitting tight to the shape, with a double falling tucker of very wide blond. The sleeves are short, with a very wide blond frill next the elbow, where the edge of it almost touches. The hair is adorned with bows of blue riband. The ear-rings and necklace are of pearls.

For the balls which have been given this summer, the most admired gowns are of white organdy worked in different colours, and of very fine India muslin embroidered in feather-stitch. The belts worn with these gowns are of beautiful workmanship.

A lady was seen in the public walks in a pelisse, which she retained as a dress at a rural ball. It was of lilac poplin, ornamented with *pattes* placed on a satin bias, which concealed where the skirt was supposed to fasten in the front; these ornaments were edged round with a narrow blond. On each hip were large plaits, and ascending as high as the knees were two satin rouleaux, and two blond flounces separated by two satin rouleaux. The belt was pointed, and embroidered in white silk on a lilac satin ground.

September 1829. Gowns of muslin, generally clear and trimmed with lace, and those of coloured crape or gauze over white satin slips, are most prevalent at balls in the country. For the most part the gowns are made square across the bosom with a drapery *à la Sévigné,* and are cut very low at the shoulders. At dress parties, many ladies partially cover this nude appearance with an elegant pelerine of blond, with a frill border of very

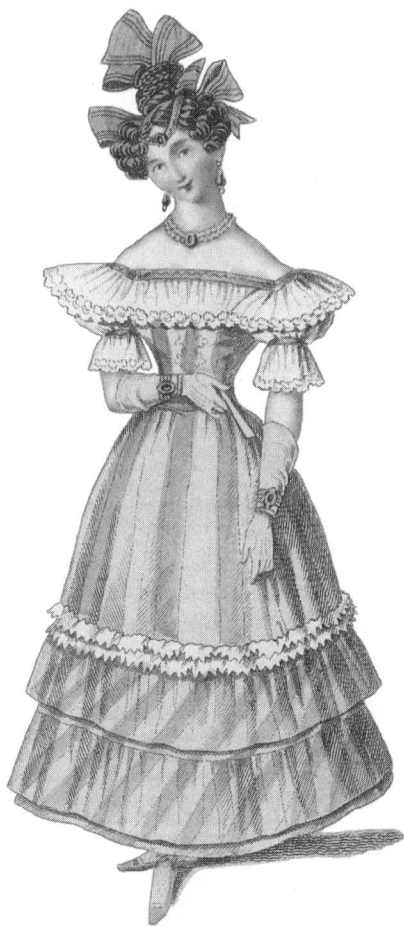

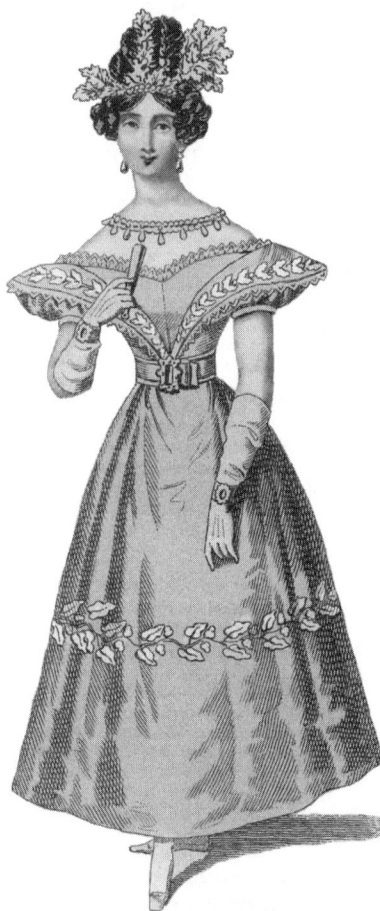

Figure 23. Rural ball dress.   Figure 24. Ball dress.

handsome Vandyked blond. The petticoats are still worn short, and the skirts of the gowns are set on very full round the waist. The favourite long sleeves are yet *à l'imbecile;* and at the top are frill mancherons.

November 1829. The ball gown in Fig. 24 is of celestial blue crape, over a satin slip of the same colour. A wide hem surrounds the border, headed by a beautiful wreath of leaves, worked in raised embroidery of white floss-silk. The body is made plain, with an ornament from the back and shoulders, descending to and forming on each side of the bosom, *fichu* robings, which gradually diminishing, are lost in a point under the belt. These ornaments are embroidered at the edge, to correspond with the work over the hem at the edge of the skirt. The sleeves are short and full, and the belt fastens in the front with a pearl buckle. A very narrow tucker of blond surrounds the bosom.

The hair is parted on the forehead, and arranged in curls on each side of the face. The bows of hair on the summit of the head are formed of three loops—one large, the next smaller, and the third, which is on the right side, very small. This is a pleasing novelty, and diminishes the elevation so long prevalent on the summit of the head. A very beautiful bandeau-ornament of foliage, formed of pearls, crosses the forehead; and on the left side, amongst the bows, is a branch of the same valuable articles. The ear-rings are of pear-pearls, and the necklace is formed of two rows of very large pearls, the lower row set round with pear-pearls.

——*Ladies' Pocket Magazine.*

Diversion 10.

Court Mourning. For November 1824: in a mourning for seven months, three of which are devoted to close mourning, there is but little novelty to be obtained as to French fashions; for the mourning is at present very general. In general or ordinary costume, ladies of rank wear bonnets of *gros de Naples* trimmed with crape; and sometimes these are tied down with a small half-handkerchief of the same material. Yet many French ladies wear white crape bonnets trimmed with black. The blouse gowns of slight black silk have very wide sleeves; the pelisses are trimmed with bias folds of crape. Women of some fashion, but who do not belong to the court, often wear white gowns with black hats, belts, veils, and trimmings. Black cloth gowns are very fashionable; the cloth is very fine, and black crape is introduced as trimming. Toques and turbans are of black crape, ornamented with drooping feathers. Fans are of crape or of black glazed paper. In home costume, many ladies wear gowns chequered or striped, with black on grey or on lavender.

December 1824. A mourning ordered for seven months cannot yet be supposed to have ended; but as people do not mourn for ever, great innovations have been made by the French ladies, always best pleased with gaiety in manner and attire. Silk gowns of the lightest pearl-grey have now almost universally succeeded to black. These are trimmed with black tulle quillings, and the long sleeves are of crape the colour of the gown. Gowns for full dress are trimmed with jet beads and five flounces of blond, a row of beads separating each flounce. When the gown is of black silk, all the ornaments, and the hat, cap, or turban, are now invariably white. The jewellery is of pearls or wrought gold.

Some ladies have been seen with ponceau ribands entwined in their hair, and in white gowns ornamented with black. Three blond flounces form a favourite trimming on all silk gowns. Black velvet toques ornamented with pearls are reckoned the most elegant evening head-dress. Young ladies who have fair hair have it arranged in very full curls, and ornament it with a simple bandeau of jet, or a few Spanish bows of black riband. Sometimes a carriage dress is seen completely white—a white satin hat ornamented with white roses, and a white silk pelisse. Nothing discovers mourning but an eye-glass suspended from a string of jet beads, and a pair of long jet ear-rings. Mantles of light colours, ornamented round with black braiding, are seen at the theatres.

Blue and black are favourite mixtures. The greatest innovation was seen at a dress party a few evenings ago. This was a gown of a very bright summer-coloured gauze, ornamented with black flowers; the flowers in the lady's hair, which was dark, were of various colours. At present the favourite colours mingled with black are lavender, lilac, ponceau, light blue, and fire-colour.

February 1827. For walking, a pelisse of black *gros de Naples.* A quilling of this material, set on in *dents de loup,* depends from each shoulder, forming a stomacher, which is brought to a point under the belt. The same trimming is carried down the front of the skirt, and round the border next the feet. The sleeves are full, and plain at the wrists, except the ornament of jet bracelets, with a black cameo head on gold. The pelisse is surmounted at the throat by a ruff of wide-hemmed muslin. The bonnet is of black *gros de Naples,* with white crape points under the lining, ornamented on the crown with black chequered velvet and bows of love-riband.

A dinner gown is of black Italian net over black sarcenet, trimmed with separate ruches, in bias. The body is trimmed in the same manner, with the ruches lengthways. The sarcenet short sleeves are trimmed similarly, and to these are attached long sleeves of white transparent crape, with wide-hemmed antique points at the wrists. These are fastened next the hand with jet bracelets, with a cameo head on gold. Ear-rings and necklace of jet, and Turkish turban of white crape.

During the greater part of the month of January, the gloom of solemn black cast a cloud over female attire, divesting it of all its gaiety. Yet we now look forward to the period of its cessation, and much relief and brightness has already taken place, and a style of fancy begins to prevail in the general mourning. We now not only behold the black mantle lined with coloured sarcenet, but even coloured mantles begin to appear, especially on entering or quitting the theatres. However, during the first part of the mourning, the favourite walking costume was a pelisse of black *gros de Naples,* and this still continues. Many ladies, when the weather is sufficiently mild, now wear only a high gown of black bombasine, poplin, or silk, with the sole out-door addition of a pelerine. The newest pelisses button down the front with a row of black velvet buttons, not very close together.

Large black velvet bonnets are yet in high favour for walking. Large bows of black love-riband are the sole ornaments on these head-dresses. In carriages, hats are often seen adorned with cypress plumes. According to established etiquette, no other feathers ought to be worn in mourning. Bonnets of light grey satin, lined with black, are now also to be seen in carriages; they are ornamented with two small black osprey feathers. A transparent hat of white crape was seen, with long strings of black gauze riband floating loose, and the crown of the hat handsomely ornamented with black flowers. Grey and lilac ribands striped with black are now beginning to appear on black satin bonnets; and white feathers tipped with black, on black velvet and on grey satin carriage hats. However, many ladies belonging to and living near the verge of the court, still retain their black attire, with love-ribands.

At evening parties and private balls, the gowns of the young ladies are seldom black, unless of lace or figured gauze, which actually is not mourning; but any thing is better than wearing colours when we feel a national loss. However, all the new ball gowns are of white or grey crape. The former is quite as deep mourning as black. The latter, when ornamented with black, is mournful enough on such occasions, especially as the mourning will so speedily change and finish. The trimming on grey gowns is often composed of black satin rouleaux; on white gowns it is a wide bouillon of the same, with either grey or white rosettes sprinkled over it. Black Norwich crapes trimmed with satin rouleaux are much worn for home costume. Poplins of grey spotted with black will be much in request for dinner and evening parties. Black velvet gowns are also much worn at evening parties; the ornaments worn with them are often white.

Rows of large jet beads are often seen decorating the heads of young ladies who have light hair, and produce a good effect. Beret turbans, both in white and black, with a cypress feather, prevail much.

Small caps of plain bias gauze, with black flowers, have been worn in home dress since the commencement of the mourning. Some few ladies have replaced these with trimmings of white love-riband and white crape flowers; the flowers are immensely large. Dress hats of white crape, and of grey satin, with white, or white and black flowers, have appeared at some evening parties.

——*Ladies' Pocket Magazine.*

Diversion 11.

Some text on mourning etiquette has been omitted as being identical to that in Chapter XXX. On the other hand, the information on mourning clothing in the two chapters is somewhat different, so has been retained.

——Frances Grimble.

Chapter XII.
The Conventions of Costumes.

Age, size, the shape of the figure, and the colour of the hair make such a difference amongst women, that it is impossible that they should all wear exactly the same fashion. And if we see so little that is pleasing, it is because very often young or old, large or small, brunette or blond, with Roman features or an irregular little face, they all equally adopt the same styles of gowns and hats, and the same colours and ornaments when the mode demands it. Fashion is as powerful as want, I know; it must be obeyed. But good sense and good taste may always modify the oracles a little.

If you are of a certain age, not only should you abandon the coiffure *en cheveux* and flowers, but also scarfs, *fichu-pelerines,* and every thing which clutters your waist and other beautiful aspects of your shape. To avoid being overly warm, wear a great shawl of barège, tulle, or blond. As every thing becomes youth, I shall dispense with specifying any thing for it (but see Chapter XI).

If your features are noble, grave, or even a little severe, wear toques and berets decorated with feathers, especially weeping willow plumes; have rather long and very brilliant ear-rings; expose your forehead as much as possible; and wear steel, gold, or silver ornaments amongst the curls in your hair, as the fashion indicates. Ornament your neck, especially if it is rather long, with ruches and high, rather open collars of very beautiful blond. This will suit you best; your charm is dignity. If your shape accords with your face, that is, if it is full and imposing, choose long gowns of beautiful materials, with high trimmings; very ample shawls which drape over your shoulders; a very large mantle; and extremely luxurious and large *somnambules.*

On the contrary, if you are small and pretty, the beauty of your features consists of gentleness, and that of your shape of grace. Rather short, transparent, light gowns with very low trimmings; scarfs; small *fichu-pelerines;* falling collars which are not overly large; and above all pretty embroidered triangular shawls, are most appropriate for you. Your shawls should never be larger than four quarters. Wear a cloak as seldom as possible, substituting a fur scarf. Decorate your hats and coiffures with flowers, and delicate flowers too, even when fashion opposes it. The sweetness of your face will be brought out by garlands of jasmine, rose-buds, or lily of the valley, but you would appear crushed under great bouquets of daisies, lilies, or poppies.

If you are inclined to embonpoint, choose dark-coloured gowns, rather tight bodies with the fewest possible plaits, lightly trimmed *fichus,* and wide hats, because all these make you appear thinner. For the same reason, meagre persons prefer white and light colours, gowns with drapery, collars with double or triple ruches, &c.

The colour of your hair and the shade of your complexion also make a great difference in the choice of colours. (See Div. 1.) A deep yellow hat, an *écru* batiste gown, in short all conceivable kinds of yellow, from golden yellow to straw-colour, suit brunettes perfectly. Yellow flowers in their dark hair render them charming, whereas with all this a blond appears nearly livid. On the contrary, tender greens, lilacs, roses, and at the same time black, brown, violet, and deep blue, which bring out the brightness of a blond, would give a brunette a wild and hard air. Some say that light blues are better for blonds than brunettes; according to others, they are as becoming to brunettes as to blonds. I am of the first opinion. Scotch colours, where dominated by red and green, are enemies to brunettes and stout friends to blonds.

Red shades, from ponceau to pink, and white, agree with most women. However, persons whose skin is slightly brown, which is common in those with jet-black hair, look very ill in white or red, and greatly resemble mulattos. For those with light brown hair it is different; nearly all colours look pleasing on them. They look especially well in celestial blue.

Here are the choices which ladies should make in precious gems: brunettes should choose topazes, turquoises, and rubies; blonds should wear chrysolites, amethysts, coral, pearls, and emeralds. Turquoises also suit them. For fancy ornaments, they should abstain from amber necklaces, leaving them to brunettes; pink paste, black or white jet, and garnets become them better. It is needless to speak of brilliants, which embellish all women. Blonds will also retain ornaments of gold, whether matte or *soufflé.*

To choose Fashions which are neither *Recherché* nor *Passé.*

When gigot sleeves began to appear, every one was diverted by the oddness of such a fashion, which not only concealed the shape of the arms, but made them appear much larger than the bust. Ladies who were the first to line their sleeves with buckram to inflate them, seemed to have encased each shoulder in a balloon. However, when this ludicrous style of sleeves had become general, the ridicule disappeared. Their elegance was agreed upon even by those who mocked at first. This is, by the way, an occurrence which supports the philosophy of M. de Lamennais, "The individual yields to the authority of the majority." Now women would be ridiculed for not following this exaggerated fashion.

That is the history of almost all fashions, save that some are not accepted, and no one knows why. The mantua-maker's empire has its mysteries; oddity and ugliness are not reasons for failure. All is not suitable and beautiful, thanks to the saying, "It is the fashion." But if a fashion does not catch on, you will be forced to throw away articles which cost double their value when it first came in.

My readers have already seen, in this brief discussion, what advice I shall give them. They will guess that I recommend that they wait to adopt new fashions until these are somewhat established, and until the preceding fashion has been altogether abandoned. This precaution is indispensable if you do not wish to spend prodigious amounts of time and money to nearly always appear ridiculously got up. (See Div. 2.) They will also think that I shall ask them to choose amongst fashions, not blindly adopt such exaggerated or odd styles and designs, that the materials and trinkets which they spoil will be good for nothing as soon as the style is *passé*. For example, the gowns *à la Robin des Bois*, the scarfs *à la Dame du Lac,* and ear-rings with pendants over two inches long. The blood-red gowns with wide stripes, leaves, and black zig-zags, which were worn last October, were enormously expensive. At the end of five or six weeks they cluttered the used clothing shops; the means of obtaining such a costume when fashion no longer excuses it! (See Div. 3.) Then these exaggerations, these strange styles are extremely unbecoming. The great charm of a toilet is elegant simplicity, the art of subtly putting your charms forward, of regulating your clothing entirely by its grace, and the kind of grace allotted to you.

Bend the fashion to your means of pleasing, and not those means of pleasing to the fashion. If your hands are dry and long, do not wear sleeves with cuffs, but neither should you keep them as they were formerly. Usage affords you a palliative, a middle way; this is a narrow bias band fitted to the bottom of the wrist, which adorns your hand without returning to the old style. Here is an excellent means of modifying the fashion, and at the same time being neither too close to it nor too far away.

Act in the same way with the ugly styles of gown body. Whatever the fashion demands, do not render your body so short as to compress your bosom, or put your belt at the level of your shoulder-blades, as was done formerly. Do not make it too long, in such sort that it approaches your hips, especially if you have a slender shape; because you will excite a mocking smile even from those least disposed to mock.

Be careful also not to make your gown too low-necked, or so that the shoulder-pieces fall to reveal the round of your shoulder: that is the work of coquetry in bad taste. Broaden your shoulders properly by placing the shoulder-pieces on the edge, but never wear sleeves which have the air of falling over your arms. When the gown is of transparent material, low-necked or without a *fichu,* this practice is opposed by not only good taste but decency—the vigilant and sensitive guide for all a woman's actions.

Gowns which are too low-necked have the additional drawbacks of discovering the angles of your shoulder-blades, spoiling the grace of your bosom, and making your waist appear less slender. Half-high bodies which are worn on the edge of the collar-bones are not at all pleasing; they are too low or too high. Your shoulders appear narrow; your bosom seems compressed; your neck revealed just at its base has no longer the seductive curve which is remarked when the gown is cut a little higher on the bosom, or even better, still lower. But then it is necessary to trim the neck of the body, even though you wear a *fichu.*

Can you not follow the practices indicated by good taste, in spite of the precepts of fashion? Some modifications of this kind would lose you little in elegance, and gain you much in beauty. The heap of ornaments, the enormous abundance of trimmings, the confusion of colours, the oddity of styles, things unbecoming to your shape and features, must all be modified in some way, because otherwise your toilet will act directly counter to its purpose.

Suppose fashion wishes, for a certain time, that skirts drag on the ground. Immediately afterwards, it declares that they must be above the ancle. In the first case, a woman has the air of being entangled, her gown is soiled, and it becomes horribly shabby, likewise cumbersome. In the second case, she loses all the charms of her shape, looks smaller, and has the aspect of a rope-dancer. Is it sensible to conform to either of these two excesses?

The Style of Gowns and the Choice of Trimmings.

I shall take a moment to discuss the means of matching the style of the body and the trimmings, to the quality of the material and its purpose.

A common gown should be made to be put on and taken off quickly. It should require the least possible paraphernalia; therefore it should be made redingote style and go all the way up to your neck (see Chapter XV). When you tire of hooking or buttoning the two front breadths over each other from top to bottom, you may sew them together for two-thirds of their length. Beginning at the bottom, make a flat seam from the outside of the gown, and precisely on the line of the stitches of the front hem, so that the seam is unnoticed. Leave the last third unsewed, to facilitate putting on the redingote, and continue to fasten or button that as before.

This mode may besides be advantageously applied to every kind of redingote gown, whether of thick or thin material. It prevents the fronts from coming open at the bottom, which they never fail to do when they are joined by any other mode. It keeps the fronts neater, because they touch less and consequently crease less. This is important for *douillettes*, and others fastened with riband bows. When you wish to trim each side of the front, or rather to show a double trimming, you must necessarily have recourse to this mode, because if fronts crossed over each other often spread apart, what would happen if they were merely brought together? You would have to secure them with a vast number of hooks or buttons, and this would be a never-ending task every time you dressed. Instead, sew the fronts together. Place the two trimmings facing each other, at a distance relative to their shape, their size, and the character of the bows or buttons, which you must then place between the trimmings to appear to fasten the fronts.

The trimming of a redingote is always simple, though elegant. Sometimes the front of a round gown is embroidered to resemble a redingote.

Gowns for demi-toilet, such as those of gingham, printed muslin, or merino, are ordinarily made as round gowns (this style is the opposite of the redingote). The body is quite high, and necessarily fastened at the back. There is, however, a means of having at the same time a moderately low body fastened at the back, and a high body entirely fastened in the front. Nothing could be simpler or more convenient. The gown is ordinarily made with the low body; then you make a redingote body in similar material. It is made like any other body, only you do not sew on sleeves or mancherons, and you trim the arm-hole with piping.

When you wish to dress lightly, put on only the gown. When you require more warmth, or wish for variety, place the second body over the first. The piped arm-holes go round those of the sleeves, which appear to have been sewed to them. The waist-band on which the second body is mounted fits well over the first, and no one perceives that the body is not sewed to the gown.

Many ladies customarily separate the body from the skirt, which is supported by straps. This is convenient only for bodies which fasten at the back.

This kind of gown does not demand too much elegance or height in the trimmings. Biases, folds, or flounces are suitable, but they should be simple and not varied in their placement. (See Chapter XV for directions.) The present styles seem to tax this advice with futility, but I should very much like a report in two years. The biases which form points with their close zig-zags, the flounces *en fille d'honneur, en if,* or triple or quadruple, arranged in a thousand divers fashions, do they not justify my advice?

Besides, since I have the occasion, I must say there is nothing more unbecoming than those exaggerated trimmings which reach to the knee, and very often past it. (See Div. 4.) The gown loses its grace and suppleness: it appears heavy and stiff, and ceases to drape becomingly. This silly and pretentious decoration spoils all shapes, but it especially renders small women grotesque. The height of the trimmings is about eight to ten inches, therefore it is necessary that you be at least of middle height. The grand toilet, it is true, requires the trimmings to be tolerably high, but not ridiculously so; and trimmings which reach the base of the hips (I have often seen this, especially on gowns with *entre-deux* and embroidery) entirely merit this term. This great mass of trimmings is still more insupportable when the rows which compose it are narrow and widely spaced. This appears to be entirely the work of indigence combined with vanity. Nothing which is luxurious should be connected with penury.

Very low bodies with drapery of material similar to the gown or the trimming; flounces with coloured embroidery; real or false blond; ruches; riband *torsades;* rouleaux forming designs; and mixed trimmings of tulle and satin, are suitable for full dress.

All the world cannot have trimmings of real blond, the price of which is very high. Therefore, people try to imitate it with bands of silk tulle embroidered in silk or cotton; but this trimming, always mean, is pretty for only a few days. Edgings of simply cut pointed bands draw, tighten, and pucker dreadfully. It is better, when through necessity or sense you cannot allot a considerable price to the trimming of a gown, to replace blond flounces with double ruches of pointed *crêpe lissé,* white or coloured according to the gown. These ruches are much more elegant and light than ruches of the material. You may put them on all sorts of silk materials; three rows is sufficient.

Never wear a belt of moiré riband, plaid riband, or riband with divers designs, with a grand toilet. Only satin or gauze ribands are permissible (see Chapter XX for directions).

——*Manuel des dames.*

Diversion 1.

Taste in the Colours of Dress. As there is a fashion in the colours, as well as in the forms of dress, and as every colour does not suit every complexion, it becomes a most important point to determine how far a fashionable colour is to be adopted, when it tends to injure rather than improve the beauty of the complexion. Nothing connected with dress, indeed, will more unequivocally display a lady's taste than proper choice of colours.

Fashion, it must be confessed, gives a character to the reigning colours considerably different from that which they naturally possess. You may have observed that fashionable colours, when they first come in, are all often disliked until people become familiar with them, or have seen them worn by high rank, and consequently associate them with the character of the wearers for fashion and magnificence. We feel, says an elegant author, a kind of disappointment when we see such a colour for the first time on those who regulate the fashions, instead of that which used to distinguish them; and this will even occur, though the colour may be such as in other subjects we consider beautiful, our disappointment still overbalances the pleasure it might give. A few weeks, however, or a few days alters our opinion. As soon as it is generally adopted by those who lead the public taste, and has become in consequence the mark of rank and elegance, it immediately becomes beautiful.

Now this, it may be remarked, is not confined to colours which in themselves may be agreeable. It often happens that the caprice of fashion leads people to admire colours which are disagreeable, and that not only in themselves, but also from associations with which they are connected. You might scarcely believe, on first thinking of it, that the colours of a glass bottle, of a dead leaf, of clay-stone, and the like, would ever be beautiful. Yet within a few years, not only these, but some much more unpleasant colours which might be mentioned, became fashionable and were admired. As soon, however, as the fashion changes—as soon as those whose rank or accomplishments give this fictitious value to the colours they wear, think proper to desert them—so soon the colour which has been so admired, is declared vulgar and intolerable.

The Carnation Complexion.

All this, however, does not prove that there is no real beauty or elegance in particular colours, or that one colour is not more suitable than another to different complexions.

The Carnation Complexion. For complexions in which neither the rose nor the lily predominates, you may choose as a harmonizing colour a pale rose, or a fine white; but do not let the latter be in such profusion as to throw the tint of the complexion into the shade. Its contrasting colours are pink, pale green, and lilac. It will have more effect, however, if the latter are introduced as ornaments or in the trimmings, while the principal dress is of the harmonizing colour. Whatever is glaring or gaudy, will have a bad effect on complexions of a fine carnation. If black or any other dark colour is worn, let it be trimmed with some of the contrasting colours; or its dull effect set off by white, and by brilliants, or other jewels.

The Florid Complexion. As in this kind of complexion, the carnation is too high and obtrusive, it must be your care to select such colours as will tend to diminish it by contrast or comparison. If you compare a white piece of paper or linen with snow, it appears that the purity of the white in the former is much diminished. In the same manner, suppose a lady of florid complexion wears a bright pink, crimson, violet, or purple, or whatever may be the colour in fashion. If she is determined to follow fashion at all hazards, at least let her ribands be chosen from some of the shades of bright red or violet. The colours advised above for a fine carnation, would make her florid colour appear much greater than natural, and therefore she must by all means avoid pale pink, rose, and lilac, as well as too much white. A coral or garnet necklace will be of great advantage, and also such ornaments and trimmings as may be of a brighter or more attractive hue than the high colour of the complexion, which it is by all means requisite to outshine.

The Fair Complexion. By this term, which has by courtesy been long applied to the female sex, I mean the complexion which is distinguished by the delicacy and transparency of the skin, rather than by its fine carnation or its bright colour. The complexion, in a word, which usually accompanies light-coloured or red hair, but is seldom met with in those who have auburn or black hair, or who have dark eyes. The French use the term "blond" for a complexion of this species.

The greatest care ought to be taken in fair complexions, to set off the tinge of carnation which may be present, and prevent its appearing too white and lifeless, as if it were formed of marble or ivory. For this purpose it will be necessary to choose either very pale colours, or such as are dark, as the one will improve the complexion by comparison, and the other by contrast. It will require attention, however, not to make the contrasts with dark colours too harsh, for in that case the complexion, instead of being improved, will be injured. Delicate greens and lilacs, and in some cases, such as when freckles are abundant on the face, light yellow, may be worn with advantage. A pearl necklace will suit well.

The Pale Complexion. The difference between a fair and a pale complexion, is much the same as that between the linen and the snow in the experiment above. In the fair, there is a brilliance and a transparency, and at the same time a slight tinge of carnation, which is denied to the complexion which is properly denominated pale. In this complexion, experience dictates that the more pure and bright colours cannot be properly used for dress. All the different shades of grey will be proper, and pale yellows for contrast, with puce and lilac. Black, trimmed with pale rose or pink, will also be proper.

The Sallow Complexion. For contrast, all the shades of green and blue will suit this kind of complexion. Several shades of red and purple will also be proper. But if grey, black, or dusty colours are worn, they will cause the complexion to appear more sallow, or dark and tanned. Lace or linen of too brilliant a white ought to be avoided, and also white gowns, and rose-coloured or light ribands, as these will harmonize ill with the complexion.

The Brunette Complexion. This complexion, which is much admired when accompanied, as it usually is, by dark sparkling eyes and jet-black hair, may be suited with bright colours rather than dark, which do not contrast sufficiently with the dark of the skin. Yellow, in particular, and orange in all their shades will set off a brunette; and necklaces, bracelets, and other jewels of brilliants, and the more showy species of stones. Pearls, however, are improper except as hair ornaments.

Additional Remarks. You may observe also that colours, though contrasted or harmonized according to rule, may be overdone with respect to profusion, and may obtrude themselves too glaringly on the eye. The fewer that are used, the more simple and graceful will be the effect; whereas many colours, however well assorted, give a tawdry and patched air to the whole costume. Never forget that it is the countenance and the shape which ought to attract, and not this or the other article of dress. When the latter is the effect produced, your art may be said to have completely failed.

——*The Duties of a Lady's Maid.*

The Theory of Colours. It is almost impossible to form a theory of the proper combination of colours applicable to dress. They are subject to a thousand contingencies. We daily discover agreeable harmonies of tint where we least expected them, and excruciating discords produced by the juxtaposition of hues, which from our previous experience, we were induced to imagine would prove pleasing rather than offensive. The influence of some neighbouring tint, the position of the colours combined, their relative stations, and the materials adopted for each, frequently tend to produce these effects.

The colour of a single rosette often destroys the general tone and appearance of the dress. Occasionally it may be managed with such skill as to blend the tints of two or more principal parts of the costume, which without some such mediator, would render each other obnoxious to the eye of taste. It is quite certain that the same colour which imparts a liveliness and brilliancy when used for light embellishments, and in a small quantity, becomes vulgar, showy, and disagreeable if adopted for the most extensive portion and leading tint of the attire. On the other hand, the delicate or neutral colours, which look well when displayed over a considerable surface, dwindle into insignificance if used in small detached portions for minor ornaments. Generally speaking, trimmings will bear a greater richness of colours than the principal material of the gown, the breadth of which is apt entirely to subdue its decorations if they are not a little more powerful in tint.

But it is a grave error to endow the minor parts of the costume with undue superiority over the rest. It should never be forgotten that the trimming is intended to embellish the gown, rather than that the gown should sink into a mere field for the display of the trimming. Sufficient importance should always be given to the latter, so that it may enhance the beauty, add to the richness, or harmonize with the purity and neatness of the former. But if its colours are too strong, or even when of the proper shade, if the material is too profuse, or not of a quality sufficiently delicate, it gives to the wearer either a frittered, gaudy, or coarse appearance, according to the nature of the fault. The same tint which looks well in a delicate material, will not become an article which is made of "sterner stuff."

The occurrence of glaring offences against good taste in the trimmings or fixed embellishments of any principal part of the attire is rare, compared with those which are perpetrated in the minor articles of gloves, shoes, ribands, &c.; which are the more important of the two, because they are not the trimmings or finishing decorations of a part, but to the whole of the costume. The former are usually left to the experience of the milliner, or copied from the production of some tasteful mantua-maker; the latter depend solely upon the judgement of the private individual. How often have we seen a gown, exquisite in all its parts, utterly ruined by the wearer, as a finishing touch, drawing on a vulgar glove! Much mischief of a similar nature is frequently done by feathers, flowers, ribands, shoes, and articles of jewellery.

It is not enough that a flower is pretty. It must harmonize with, or form a pleasing contrast to the other parts of the costume. Otherwise its use must be rigorously forbidden. It is the same with jewellery; pearls, for instance, will suit those kinds of gowns which rubies would spoil; and the latter are appropriate in cases where the former would look faint and ineffective. Coloured shoes, I need scarcely say, are exceedingly vulgar. Delicate pink and faint blue silk for these articles have numerous advocates; but white satin, black satin or kid, and bronze kid, are neater and more elegant than any other colour or material. Gloves should be in the most delicate colour which may be procured; their colour has always an effect upon the general appearance. One kind of hue must not therefore be indiscriminately worn; or however beautiful it may be in itself, obstinately persisted in, when every other part of the attire is constantly subject to change.

——*The Young Lady's Book.*

The Change of Colours by Light. I must not omit a very important observation respecting the change of colours by light. Thus crimson is extremely handsome at night, when it may be substituted for rose-colour, which loses its charms by candle-light. But this crimson, seen by day, spoils the most beautiful complexion; no colour soever strips it so completely of all its attractions. Pale yellow, on the contrary, is often very handsome by day, and is perfectly suited to persons who have a fine carnation; but at night it appears dirty, and tarnishes the lustre of the complexion, to which it is designed to add brilliancy. It would be difficult to specify all the particular cases, for all these effects depend upon different circumstances. For instance, on the complexion of a woman, on the greater or lesser vivacity of her carnation, on her stature, on the other colours employed in her dress, &c.

——*The Art of Beauty.*

Diversion 2.

Rivalry in Dress. It is not very unusual to see neighbouring young women engaged in a constant state of petty warfare with each other. To vie in ostentatiousness, in costliness, or in elegance of apparel; to be distinguished by novel inventions in the science of decoration; to gain the earliest intelligence respecting changes of fashion in the metropolis; to detect in the attire of a luckless competitor, traces of a mode which for six weeks has been obsolete in high life: these frequently are the points of excellence to which the force of female genius is directed.

Good Housewifery. Needle-work is generally considered as a part of good housewifery. Many young women make almost every thing they wear, by which they can make a respectable appearance at a small expense. Absolute idleness is inexcusable in a woman, and renders her contemptible. The needle is, or ought to be, always at hand for those intervals in which she cannot be otherwise employed.

——*The Female Instructor.*

Propriety in Dress. Mrs. L.—But surely a woman would not be justified in paying much attention to dress, when she has a family to regulate and control?

Mrs. B.—Too great an attention to the cares of the toilet is not only an error in itself, but in many instances its attendant experiences are truly vexatious. Dress, it is true, may be considered as the criterion of a woman's taste. One moment's survey decides the question, "Is it good or bad?" And even in this glance, the spectator does not neglect to take into the account, whether the dress in question is suitable to the station in life, the shape, and the complexion of its wearer. If he perceives that fashion has not been servilely or implicitly followed; that peculiarity has been avoided, and simplicity preferred to splendour, the opinion he forms must be in favour of her taste. The supposition follows, of course, that the good sense which directs her choice of attire, will have its influence upon every thing of which she has the direction and control.

On the contrary, the want of propriety in dress, whether shown in the neglect of the person, or by a too studied and extravagant pursuit of fashion, makes a more unfavourable impression on an observing mind, than mere absence of taste would produce. In the one case indolence, self-indulgence, and many other symptoms of an ill-regulated mind are betrayed; and in the other, the suspicion cannot fail to arise, that the mind is frivolous and vain, which has evidently bestowed so much time on exterior decoration.

I am inclined also to suspect that those women whose dress, when in public or in company, appears so minutely studied, are frequently negligent and slovenly in their hours of domestic retirement. Thus, for the vain-glory of a few hours, are money, time, and thought squandered, which would have been amply sufficient to have adorned, cheered, and refined whole seasons of domestic life.

Another error, or rather folly, is not uncommon; I mean that of attempting to vie in dress with those whom superior station and fortune entitle to exterior distinction. To do this is to abandon propriety and good taste, and to render ourselves liable to, and deserving of ridicule and contempt; besides incurring the more serious inconveniences arising from any expense which is incompatible with our fortunes.

Mrs. L.—I have now an ample, well-stocked wardrobe; but how shall I keep it in its present state, with my moderate means?

Mrs. B.—A woman's wardrobe may be divided into two parts—the ornamental and the useful. In the first I include all the various articles which are affected by fashion; every thing, in fact, of external dress. In these a good economist will avoid a superabundance. She will endeavour to check that feminine weakness—the love of variety—which so frequently displays itself by an ever-varying costume. She will confine the ornamental part of her wardrobe into as narrow bounds as the extent of her general style of living and visiting will permit. Every one who lives much in society must follow fashion to a certain extent, or be prepared to encounter the laugh, and perhaps the scorn, of those who pronounce judgement on appearances. But it is extremes on either side, which are to be shunned by all who wisely prefer propriety and consistency, to notoriety and peculiarity.

Another disadvantage of having too many of the ornamental parts of female attire, by one who has a moderate allowance only, is the fickleness of fashion, and the constant necessity which this must produce of altering the forms of gowns, which the means of the possessor do not allow to be thrown aside. For these alterations of dress much valuable time must be wasted, or much money squandered. In either case, the very attention which is requisite for so unworthy an object, takes the mind from more important and rational pursuits. Some women seem to think that life is of no use but to make or re-model gowns, and act as if they were born to be walking blocks for showing off to advantage the workmanship of the riband and lace manufacturer, the mantua-maker, and the milliner.

The second part of a woman's wardrobe, comprehending every article not subject to the laws of fashion, deserves also much management and care. For your management of this branch I recommend a good rule: do not neglect to make each year a small addition to most of the articles of which it is composed. By doing this you will scarcely perceive the effects of time, because the yearly supply will bear some proportion to the deficiencies which that ruthless power causes. But if you neglect this rule, the consequence may be that all at once you will find your wardrobe to require a complete renewal, and your annual allowance will then scarcely suffice to provide it. Most of the things to which I allude are of an expensive nature, and sweep away no inconsiderable sum, when whole sets are to be purchased at once.

Dress for the Lower Orders. Mrs. L.—What do you consider an appropriate dress for female servants?

Mrs. B.—This enquiry embraces two considerations; the first concerning the material, the second the form or style of dress appropriate for female servants. With regard to the first, I should say that silk and muslin gowns, lace trimmings, worked muslin, silk stockings, and silk aprons are all imitations of those above their own rank, which should be discouraged, if not positively forbidden in our humble attendants. Equally unsuitable are feathers, flowers, lace caps, ear-rings, and necklaces. With respect to the second, I am of the opinion that all ornamental appendages to that attire which is intended for utility chiefly, are improper in a female servant.

Yet I would by no means infer that it is not desirable to women, in every scale of society, to cherish some pride of appearance. The desire of being neatly, and even tastefully attired, is as natural and commendable in the humble servant, as in the more distinguished members of society. The notion that it does not signify how negligent or unbecoming their garments may be, would introduce slovenliness and uncleanliness all around us. But to this the domestics of the present day are less inclined than to expenditure more profuse than their means, on the luxuries instead of the necessaries of dress.

It becomes, then, the duty of every mistress to point out to her female servants the propriety of plainness in their habiliments. A few hints, delivered in a kind and not peremptory manner, might suggest to a female servant that the following materials of dress are the most suitable in her situation, and only can be permitted. Muslin, not lace caps; cotton and stuff gowns, and petticoats of the same texture; shawls of a durable, but not of a brilliant colour; and bonnets of straw, which may be cleaned and turned.

Mrs. L.—Political economists censure the charity of English women as having tended, with many other circumstances, to destroy a laudable spirit of independence amongst the lower orders of the community, who now claim relief and assistance from the benevolent, rather as a right than as a gratuity.

Mrs. B.—I am not a great admirer of those societies which are formed for clothing the poor. I believe much greater benefits would be conferred by teaching them, or at least their children, how to cut out and make their own clothes. These arts are becoming almost unknown amongst the lower orders; and this, though it may chiefly be caused by the females working in manufactories, has been increased by the ease with which they have procured from the charitable, ready supplies of every article of clothing. A woman who is compelled to make and repair the clothes of her family will be much more careful of them, than one who imagines she can draw upon the treasury of benevolence for all her wants.

——*Domestic Duties.*

The Thrifty Cottager. Something weekly should regularly be laid by, according to the size of the family, for shoes and under garments; for those of necessity will always be wearing out. I say nothing about outer garments; they are not things of every-day purchase. The good man, most likely, had a best suit at the time of his marriage, or not long before, intending that it should serve him for years and years to come. His wife did not live so long in respectable service to come and burden her husband with the cost of her wardrobe. No, she was well furnished with every thing good and suitable of its kind. She was never given to finery in her young days, and now she cares less about it than ever. It is the least of her concerns who has got a new bonnet or gown, or what the shape or colour of it is. She is not likely to want a new one, for she has plenty by her; and what she has is so truly neat and respectable, that it is never out of fashion.

If you are a thoroughly handy needle-woman, you might often make a shilling without much hazard, by buying a cheap little remnant of calico, print, or stuff, making it up into a frock, petticoat, pin-before, or bonnet, and exhibiting it in your window. Some neighbour who is not so handy will soon be glad to buy it. I have known this to answer particularly well in country places, where a handy notable woman gets as much as she can do, and prefers it to going out and leaving her family.

The cottager no more degrades himself, or injures his independence, by accepting aid from benevolent associations, than he would if, toiling homewards with a heavy burden, he accepted the friendly offer of placing it in a neighbour's cart, which would pass his door otherwise empty. The same idea holds good with respect to women accepting the use of linen, furnished by societies for the purpose of assisting them during their confinement. It is no degradation to themselves, nor any imposition upon such societies, nor alienation of their funds, if women several degrees above the absolutely destitute and wretched receive such accommodations.

——*Cottage Comforts.*

Negro Women's Clothes, for Plantations in the West Indes, or in America. The bedgowns are generally cut of blue nap, commonly called pennystone, twenty-seven inches wide. They will require two yards each. The nearest way to cut them is to make the length of the gown the width of the piece, that is, twenty-seven inches. (See Fig. 1.) Make them twenty-two inches wide at the top and thirty inches wide at the bottom. Make the shoulder seven inches, and that will leave eight inches for the neck. Slope out the neck four inches deep before, and two inches behind. Make a string-case round the neck to draw it close. The body will take nearly a yard and a half. The sleeve is half a yard long; make it five inches wide at the bottom, and eight and a half at the top in the double. They will cut one out of the other (both bodies and sleeves), and the piece sloped out of the neck will make a small gusset.

The petticoats will take two and a half yards each. If two are wanted at the same time, cut off five breadths, each a yard long. Divide one breadth in half, and that will allow two and a half breadths for each petticoat. Plait them in at the top to a proper size—say thirty-six inches.

——*Sectum.*

Diversion 3.

"Cachemiremania." There are at Paris brokers in cachemires whom young women should beware and avoid. These people enrich themselves more than any other class of charlatans, owing to the number of customers they dupe. They have a marvellous talent for getting you to exchange a cachemire which is new, beautiful, and in the best taste, for one worth half as much. They have the art of making it seem infinitely preferable, by a thousand of the most adroit and beguiling speeches ever heard. Not only do they dupe *Parisiennes,* even provincial *merveilleuses* pay them tribute, because these exchanges are the fashion, and bartering cachemires forms the most considerable part of the commissions provincials give to their friends at Paris.

Therefore, guard against this seduction. If you purchase cachemire shawls, choose the best, take care of them, preserve them, and do not exchange them.

——*Manuel de la maîtresse de maison.*

One-eighth Scale

← 36 →

7   7   8   7   7

Fold

18

B   B

A   A

27

Centre Front

D   D

9

C C   C C

Selvages

3   30   3

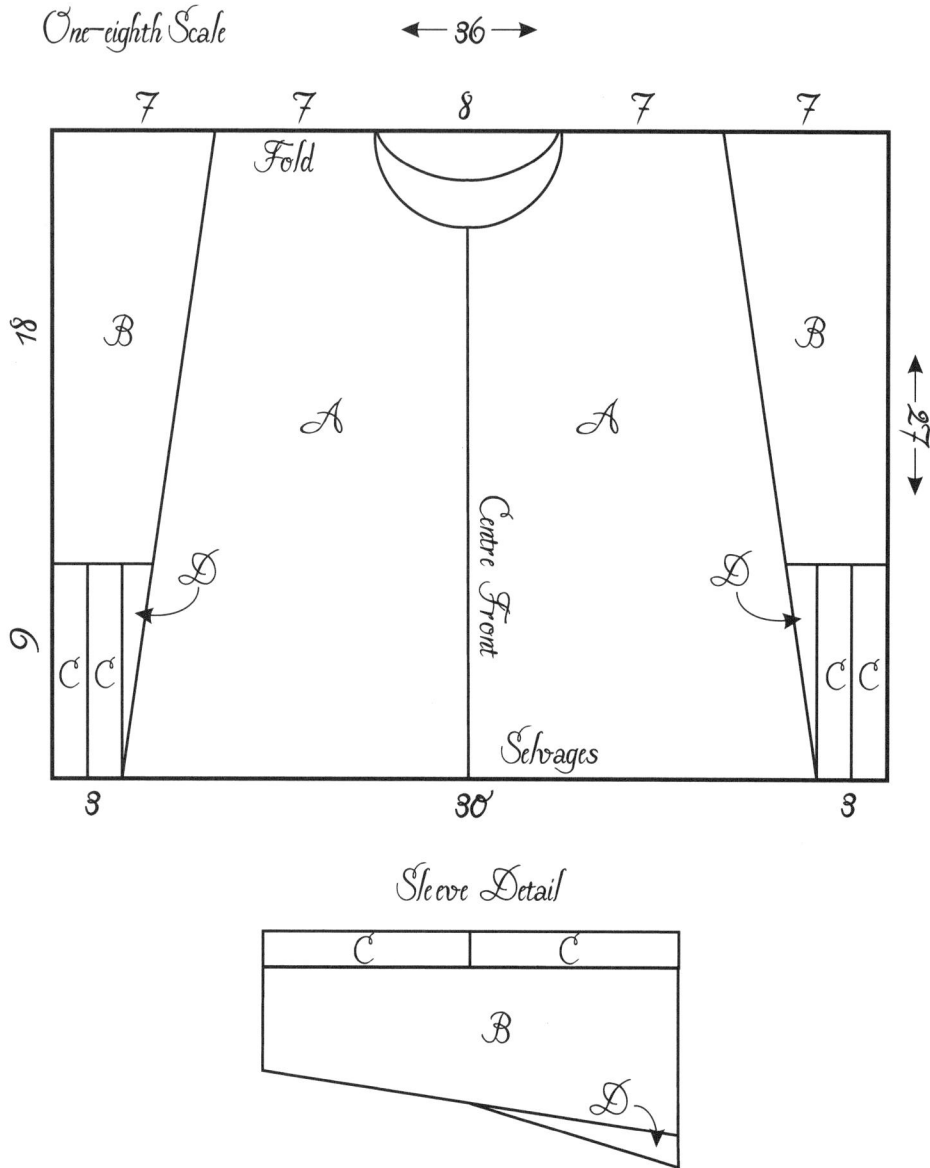

Figure 1. A tentative pattern for the bedgown.

Sleeve Detail

C | C

B

D

Diversion 4.

The Lady's Maid as Mantua-maker. As a considerable portion of your time will be occupied in making and altering your lady's gowns, you ought to study all the branches of needle-work with great care; for upon your taste and skill in this department, much will depend. The daily change of fashions will claim your constant attention; though you must study your lady's shape, and all the other circumstances connected with her person, in order to suit the fashions to these, according to the established principles of good taste. A gown, indeed, may be made in the first style of fashion, and yet may infringe on every rule of good taste, and altogether disfigure the lady for whom it has been made.

For example, when a lady is of a shape disproportionately broad in the bust, the more plainly the shoulders of a gown are trimmed, the better; as in that case a diminished effect is required. On the other hand, if the bust is disproportionately narrow, the epaulette ought to be very full, the sleeve falling rather off the shoulder, and the trimmings to correspond in producing an increase of breadth, to make up for the natural deficiency. This plan will be frequently more successful than any attempt at padding and stuffing, which unless very well done, are apt to give a stiff unnatural appearance to the whole shape.

According to similar principles, all trimmings ought to be suited to the shape of the lady for whom a gown is intended. That is, if the shape is slender, the trimmings will not require to be so very full as when there is much embonpoint.

——*The Duties of a Lady's Maid.*

Chapter XIII.
The Art of a Fine Carriage and Proper Gestures.

A respectable appearance is not only the complement to beauty: it bespeaks good-breeding, and proves it with a habitual sense of order, modesty, and dignity. Equally removed from coarseness and affectation, an easy assurance and a graceful carriage appear so simple and natural, that at first it seems ridiculous to try to establish precepts. There are however, so to speak, some practical requirements. I am going to describe them in imitation of the carriage of persons with habitual good-breeding, moral dispositions, and lastly charm; which carriage paints them (if it may be so expressed) in their true colours.

Good comportment of the feet considerably affects the charm of your figure. When seated, cross your right foot over the left, posed on the toe and the side, in order to make it appear smaller and more graceful. When thus holding your feet, avoid resting the stocking of one foot on the shoe of the other, especially if the shoe is black, because the stocking will be soiled in a few moments. Efface the heel well, and lower your gown over your foot so that only the toe is seen, or at most only the half.

If your knees must not be turned inwards, neither must they be turned outwards in too marked a manner; that is too masculine. To cross one over the other is in the worst taste. This may also be said of the habit of clasping your knees with joined hands. Simply let them rest near each other, very slightly apart.

Occupy your chair entirely, and appear neither too restless, nor too immovable. It is altogether out of place to throw your drapery around you in sitting down, or to spread out your gown for display, as upstarts do to avoid the least rumple.

The position of your arms requires a little attention. Several modes of carrying them are quite incorrect, amongst others that of resting them on your thighs while bending forward, and especially that of crossing them so that an elbow is grasped in each hand. That of spreading your hands over your knees is nearly as displeasing, but the worst of all is to hold your arms too far back and press them against your waist. A witty lady mockingly called this "the grasshopper pose," and indeed, the arms thus bent do bear no small resemblance to the wings of a big green grasshopper at rest. This has besides the distinguishing characteristic of affectation; and if I were a caricaturist, I would constantly lend it to prudery and squeamishness. Never hold your arms quite stiff, but round them elegantly and lift your neck a little. Your fingers also should not be stiff, but slightly curved, and no less slightly spread apart. The best way to carry your arms is to hold them at the level of your belt, your hands half crossed over each other, or placed one upon the other. It is well to vary this attitude from time to time; but not by repeatedly rubbing your fingers, because that habit is a veritable tic of pretentiousness.

Your shoulders and bust ought to be effaced at the same time, and not one at the expense of the other. You may attain this by straightening your back unaffectedly and holding your neck upright. The carriage of your neck is of the greatest importance: it affects at the same time your shape and your face. A neck inclined forwards rounds your back, makes your chin pointed, and imparts an air of awkwardness and stupidity to your whole person. Bent backwards, your neck swells as if with a goitre, reverses your head ridiculously, and fatigues the eye with its forced attitude. Completely straight, it lacks grace. Instead of all this, incline your neck a little to the right. This imperceptible movement gives your neck a kind of softness, a timid expression, caressing, full of charm—but beware affectation!

Let me now speak of the accessory so important to carriage, that is, gestures. (See also Chapter XXXI.) I can give you the rules only in describing their abuse. Therefore, bear in mind persons who believe they have spirited, energetic gestures, and fatigue their unfortunate auditors by the eternal repetition of vehement and strange tics which they are pleased to consider thus. For example: to stretch out their arms frequently, strike the air as if they were rowing, give great blows of their fist to the furniture, clap their hands, shake their head rapidly, shrug their shoulders, turn their back, bob their knees, pull on their fingers, raise their eyebrows, or pinch the skin of their neck, face, hands, &c.

Other faults in the carriage include to look steadily at any one, especially if you are speaking to a gentleman; to turn your head frequently to one side and the other during conversation; to roll your eyes, or raise them affectedly; to admire yourself complacently in a glass; to adjust in an affected manner your hair, gown, or *fichu;* to play continually with a chain or a fan; to smile simperingly; or to carefully fold your shawl, instead of throwing it with graceful negligence upon a table.

The Art of a Fine Carriage.

All this is at the least very annoying and disagreeable. However, energetic gestures are often encountered in lively persons, and they should pay *some* attention to their manners. I emphasize *some*, because too much attention would make them appear stilted, and make the remedy as bad as the ill. Some rare gestures, unforced, graceful, determined by inspiration and not exaggerated by habit, are at the same time the complement and the ornament of discourse. They make your face more pleasing, and give, so to speak, an expressive physiognomy to your carriage.

In walking, always step on the toe of your foot, but not quite the extremity, because that is fatiguing, affected, and often forces your body to stoop. (See also Div. 1 and Chapter XXV.) Your gait ought to be neither too quick nor too slow; the most easy and most convenient pace is that which fatigues the least and pleases most. Your body and head should be erect without affectation or haughtiness; your movements, especially those of your arms, easy and natural. Your countenance should be pleasant and modest. At a ball or an assembly, people who cannot converse with you judge your merit and education by your carriage. How many dancers move off, and how many persons sigh with pity, at the sight of a beautiful woman who has a mincing way, affects grace, inclines her head affectedly, and who seems to admire herself incessantly, and to invite others to admire her also?

Young ladies ought to be on their guard against excessive timidity. It not only paralyses their powers, renders them awkward, and gives them an almost silly air, but it may even cause them to be accused of pride, amongst people who do not know that embarrassment frequently has the appearance of superciliousness. How often does it happen that timid persons do not salute you at all, answer in a low voice, or very ill, omit a thousand little duties of society, and fail in numberless agreeable attentions, for want of courage? (See Div. 2.) These attentions, and these duties, they discharge in *petto*, but who will thank them for it? A proper degree of confidence, but not degenerating into assurance, still less into boldness or familiarity, is therefore one of the most desirable qualities in society. To obtain this you must observe the *ton*, and the manners of polite and obliging persons. Take them for your guides, and under their direction make continual efforts to conquer your timidity.

It is not good *ton* for a lady to speak too quick or too loud. But what is especially insupportable in our sex is an inquiet, bold, and imperious air; for it is unnatural, and not allowable in any case. If a lady has cares, let her conceal them from society, or not go into it. Whatsoever her merit, let her not forget that she may be a man in the superiority of her mind and decision of character, but that externally she should be a woman! You ought to present yourself as a being made to please, to love, and to seek a support; a being inferior to men, but near to angels. An affectionate, complying, and almost timid aspect, and a tender solicitude for those who are about you, should be shown in your whole person. Your face should breathe hope, gentleness, and satisfaction; dejection, anxiety, and ill-humour should be constantly banished.

> ——*The Gentleman and Lady's Book of Deportment,*
> *Manuel complet de la bonne compagnie, Manuel des dames.*

Diversion 1.

To walk well. The manner of walking well is an object which all young ladies should be anxious to acquire; but unfortunately, it is a point too much neglected. In the drawing-room, the ball-room, or during the promenade, an elegant deportment—a "poetry of motion"—is, and ever will be, appreciated. Your step ought not to exceed the length of your foot; your leg should be put forwards, without stiffness, in about the fourth position; but without any effort to turn your foot out. The latter will tend to throw your body awry, and give you an appearance of being a professional dancer, as exemplified in Fig. 1, *a,* which is tolerably correct in other respects, except in the position of the feet.

Your head should be kept up and your chest open; your body will then attain an advantageous position, and that steadiness so much required in good walking. Your arms should fall in their natural position, and all their movements and oppositions to your feet should be easy and unconstrained. The employment of soldiers to teach young ladies how to walk, which I am sorry to say is a practice adopted by many parents and heads of seminaries, is much to be deprecated. The stiffness acquired under regimental tuition, is adverse to all the principles of grace, and annihilates that buoyant lightness which is so conducive to ease and elegance in the young.

> ——*The Young Lady's Book.*

Diversion 2.

The Courtesy. The following is the usual mode of performing the courtesy. First bring your front foot into the second position. (In Fig. 1, *B, C, D, E,* and *F* respectively denote the first, second, third, fourth, and fifth positions of the feet.) Then draw the other into the third behind, and pass

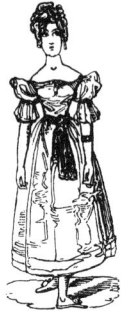
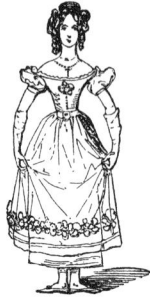
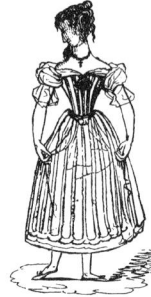

A   *B*   *C*

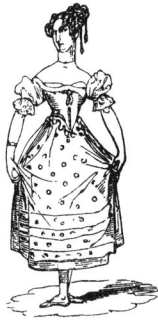
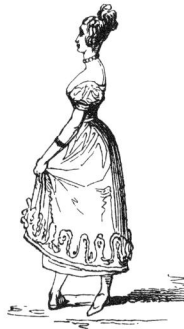

D   *E*

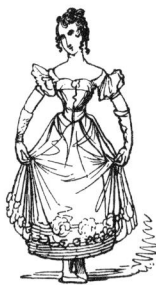
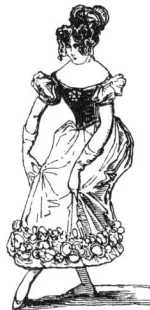

F   *G*

Figure 1. The five positions of the feet, and the courtesy.

it immediately into the fourth behind; the whole weight of your body being thrown on the front foot. Then bend your front knee, your body gently sinks, transfer your whole weight to the foot behind while rising, and gradually bring your front foot into the fourth position. Your arms should be gracefully bent, and your hands occupied in lightly holding out your gown. Your first step in walking, after the courtesy, is made with the foot which happens to be forwards at its completion. The perfect courtesy is rarely performed in society, as the general salutation is between a courtesy and a bow (see Fig. 1 *G*).

——*The Young Lady's Book.*

Part II.
Needle-work.

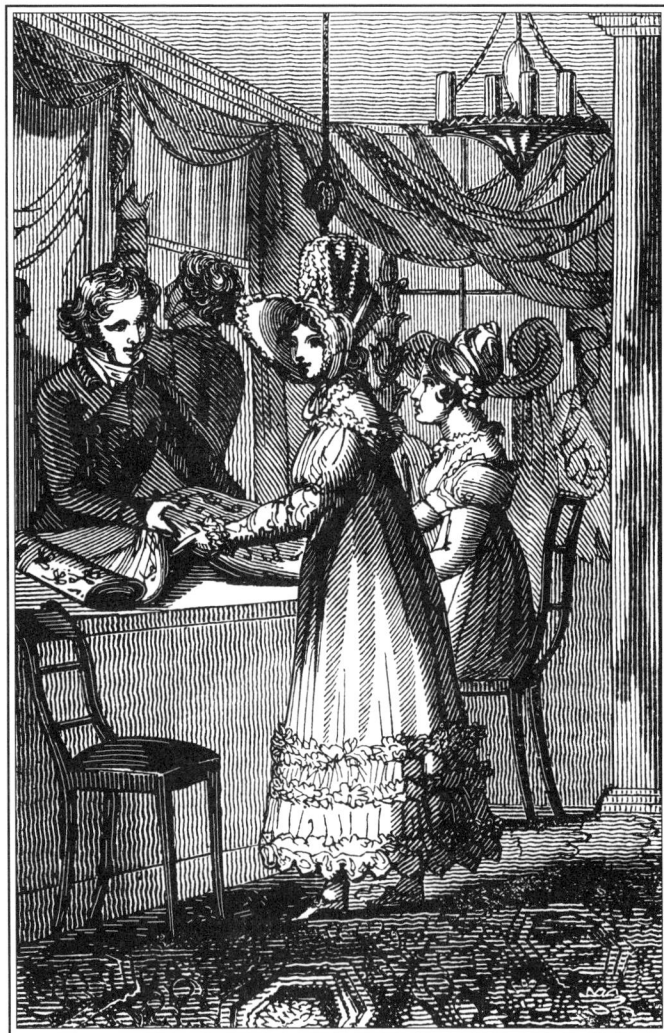

Chapter XIV.
The Art of the Stay-maker.

Those ridiculous and painful prisons called boned bodies, in which women formerly confined themselves, were as difficult to make as they were cruel to wear, forming a special art on which I would not have dared to instruct ladies. But now that simple and easily-made stays have replaced those dismal machines, I hope, by my directions, to be able to put my readers in the way of making all their stays. (Also see Div. 1.) You will reap several benefits: economy; a good choice of materials, for stay-makers always employ the mediocre; the sturdiness of the binding, for which they use cotton tape, whereas it is indispensable that the tape be of linen, since this part wears out quickly; finally, you will avoid the difficulty of having stays made, of being turned and examined by a stranger.

The Materials for Stays.

Stays are made principally of linen dimity with very narrow cords, called *basin de Troyes.* Cotton dimity looks handsomer, but does not last nearly so long. You may also use fine white linen *coutil,* India nankeen, and unbleached toile. These last two materials are ordinarily lined, because they lack firmness. The first has the same disadvantage when it is no longer altogether new. Sometimes, but very rarely, coloured taffety is used for stays.

The Furnishings for Stays.

These furnishings are, 1st., the busk of whale-bone or steel, a thin strip about two inches wide and fifteen to eighteen inches long. (I explained in Chapter VII how it should be chosen and furnished.) 2nd., the whale-bones: first two pieces half an inch wide and nearly the length of the busk, to put in the back; then the other pieces of whale-bone, to the number of six or eight of different lengths, to put in the upper part of the front of the stays, to the right and left of the busk. 3rd., a linen tape the width of the busk to serve as a pocket, and at the same time to support the eyelet-holes and contain the whale-bones at the back. 4th., a narrow linen tape to bind the stays all round. 5th., elastics for when the stays have no busk.

Divers Kinds of Stays.

There are ten kinds of stays: stays with only one gore; stays with two gores; pieced stays; lined stays; half-stays, or morning belts; stays with straps; stays *à la paresseuse;* stays for pregnant women; and elastic and half-elastic stays.

The Parts of Stays.

Whatever the kind of stays, they are always composed of two backs cut lengthways (see Fig. 1 *A*); two fronts the same length but three or four times wider (see Fig. 1 *B*); two bands hollowed out on one side, which are the shoulder-straps (see Fig. 1 *C*); two wide gores for the bottom, cut like the little gores of a gown (see Fig. 1 *D*); smaller bosom gores for the top (see Fig. 1 *E*); and a piece of lining to hold the front whale-bones on each side of the busk (see Fig. 1 *F*). I have already said that the number of gores varies; their shape varies no less.

Stays with One Bosom Gore.

This kind of stays is the easiest to cut out and to sew. I shall commence with its description, which once thoroughly understood will aid you to understand the directions for the others. Hence I shall give it in minute detail. (The stitches used are described in Chapter XV.)

To take the Pattern. Take about half an ell of strong linen dimity; have also the pattern of the stays which you wish to make. (See Div. 2.) It is easy enough to procure one, either by copying the stays you usually wear, or by resorting to persons of your acquaintance; even if you will cut out the principal parts of the stays a little differently, such as stays with two bosom gores, lined stays, &c. To take this pattern (or any other) you must fold up the gores on themselves, bringing one seam over the other, and fix them firmly with a pin, so that the enlargement produced by the gore is not visible. This part of the stays then appears as though the gores were not there; consequently you may cut out the rest of the pattern.

If your model stays have a gore which you wish to omit entirely, you must add the width of the gore which you have omitted to that part, or to

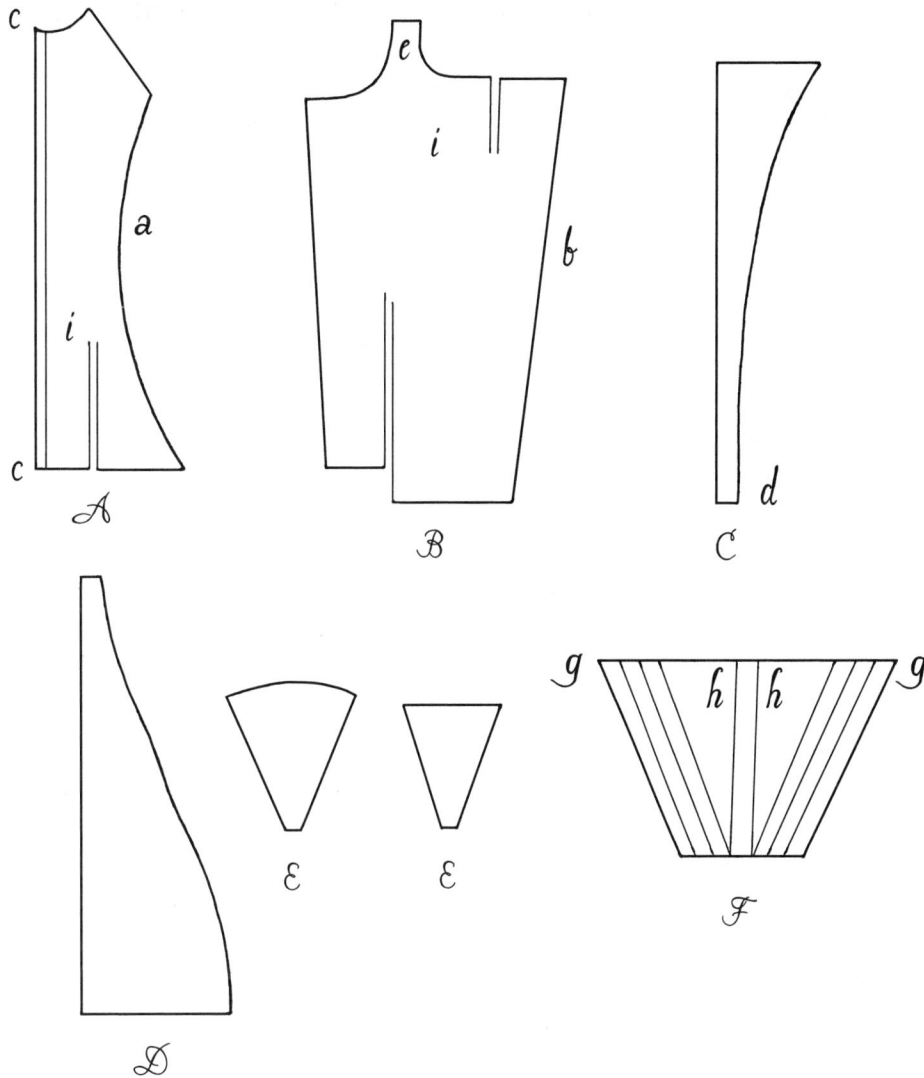

Figure 1. The principal parts of stays.

one near it. For example, if you leave out a gore at the back of the model stays, add to the width of the bias seam (see Fig. 1 A, a) at the bottom of the back, and if you leave out one gore in the upper part of the front, add half its width to the single remaining gore. Put the rest of the width on the bias busk seam, or on the bias under the arms if you have a seam in that part.

These preliminary operations achieved, pin a piece of paper all round the part of the stays from which you are taking, or lifting, the pattern. Be careful to attach this paper along the direction of the material, making sure that neither one nor the other puckers. Cut all round this part, leaving several lines of extra paper for the seam folds. If the model stays have the gores folded up (whether to be removed or not), upon comparison, one of the seams will be found shorter than the other. Be careful not to copy this difference, but on the contrary cut as the longest seam indicates, save for clipping a few threads later, if there are any.

If the folded gore is to remain, slit the paper lengthways the length of the seam to the narrowest part of the gore, whether it is a bosom or a hip gore. This slit is always begun at the widest part of this piece. Since the top of the seam of the model gore is covered by the pattern, you would not know where to begin; but you may see this very well at the bottom, and you are guided by the seam as you slit.

The pattern of this piece thus cut out, remove the pins, fold it, and lay it aside, because the slits prepared to admit of the gores produce little strips, which tear very easily. Continue as I have just described until you have the patterns of all the pieces which compose the stays. As all these parts are double, it will suffice to take the pattern of half the stays. It is needless to say that you must unfold the gores to copy their pattern.

To cut out the Stays. It would undoubtedly be quicker to place your material on the model stays, and to cut it at once, just as I have explained for paper; but if you make any errors, they will be irreparable. The size and firmness of the dimity would be a great hindrance. Finally, you will have deprived yourself of the advantage of cutting between, that is, of placing the projecting angle of one piece in the hollow of another. This saves a great deal of material, and you may easily accomplish it by spreading the dimity on a table, with the different parts of the pattern on the dimity. It is still necessary to fix these with pins, so that they do not slip or become disarranged, and lead you to make a false cut.

The dimity must be placed crossways; that is, so that the selvage is found at the top or the bottom of the stays. Ordinarily material is placed in the contrary direction, but a skilful stay-maker maintains that crossways is far better; I cannot speak from experience. First cut out the fronts of the stays, next the backs, then the shoulder-straps and the gores, cutting the material all round the paper pattern. Next make a seam fold—a trifle wide—in one front, one back, and all the places destined for the seams. Lay each piece on its duplicate, fasten them with several pins, and turn down the excess edges of these second pieces. This is at the same time a means of having the seam fold quite equal on corresponding pieces, and of remedying any errors which may have crept into the cutting.

Proceed in the same way with regard to the gores. Moreover, it is well to trace with a pencil the amount which you wish to put in the flat seam of the gore, or, to say it better, at the distance from the seam fold where you wish to sew. As the gores are placed, basted, and sewed from above, this step is necessary.

Each side of the bias seam which joins the fronts (see Fig. 1 B, b) must have a fold about an inch wide, because this seam fold serves to support and line the lengthways busk pocket. To this end, it is fastened on the right and left by the wide linen tape which will later be placed to make this pocket.

The seam fold of the part on the straight-way of the backs (see Fig. 1 A, cc) must be still stronger, because it must support at the same time the whale-bone and the lengthways row of eyelet-holes (little rings through which the lace is passed). This seam fold must be no less than two inches wide. I shall explain how it is covered by a wide linen tape.

To baste the Stays. Once all the seam folds are prepared, baste the wider ones of the fronts and backs. Be content to mark the others by pressing them and folding them firmly between the thumb and forefinger of your right hand. Then join the bias seam of the two fronts by basting with small stitches on the wrong side. Place the straight edge of the fronts on the curved edge of the backs, on the right side, where they will be prick-stitched. Place the gores in the same way, that is, on the right side. The gores which are put at the bottom of the front, and which are called stomach gores, have their straight-way on the bias side of this piece, and their bias on its straight-way. The gores at the top, called the bosom gores, sometimes have the bias to the left, sometimes to the right of the busk; sometimes they have a bias only on their lower part, sometimes they have none. I shall describe their different shapes when I treat of stays with two gores.

It now remains only to put on the shoulder-straps. Lay them on the right side of the stays, the part marked d on the strap, on the part marked e on the front, shaped for this purpose (see Fig. 1 B and C). They are finished by joining on the back. Baste the shoulder-strap only on the wide end; the narrow end remains free. You only sew it on the front part which comes immediately next to the curve under the arms, after you have tried on your stays to determine its length. It is always cut out at least an inch too long, in order to lengthen or shorten it at will in putting it underneath. Stay-makers baste it temporarily for trying on, and sew it permanently only when they deliver the stays to the purchaser.

To try on the Stays. When the stays are thus basted with very small stitches, work the eyelet-holes (I shall describe them when I come to sewing the stays), so that the stays may be held on you, and ask a skilful person to fit them to you. It is quite important that she know how to fit them, because otherwise, in order to rectify a few little faults, she will advise you to make great ones which it will be impossible for you to remedy, because your guide will mislead you farther and farther, and you will not be able to judge for yourself. If you are making the stays for a person other than yourself, or if by chance you have a sister, mother, friend, or even a maid of exactly your shape (which would be great good luck) try your work on her. Rectify the faults by folding up the parts which are too large with pins, and releasing the basting a little for the parts which are too tight. If the width (especially of the bosom gores) is insufficient to allow a fold, pencil a mark at the place where you must re-position the seam. It is well to also mark with the pencil the places folded up with pins, when you have finished fitting or have taken off the stays. Otherwise, in removing the basting to bring in the seam, you might lose the measure of the fold. It is true that you may place a pin lengthways on this fold ahead of time; but the pencil mark seems to me preferable for all wash materials, because it is more convenient and lasting.

If there are many errors to correct in the stays, you must try the stays on again when you have put them right. In the contrary case you may sew them immediately, after having, by measuring, corrected any little faults. Here is the way to sew your stays: these principles are applicable to every other kind of stays.

To make up the Stays. The manner in which you basted should have told you which kinds of seams to use, according to the nature of the pieces. The bias of the two fronts basted to the wrong side of the stays, is sewed by a seam of very close back-stitches; the gores basted on the right side, are prick-stitched from the right side with back-stitches. At the end of the vertical slit, which is cut across a little to the right and left for the gore, work a succession of ten to twenty button-hole stitches, according to the width which you have given this part; because, when the gore is large, this slit is sometimes nearly two inches; this never happens except with lower gores. The upper gores preserve the slit made, without any necessity of enlarging it and making it square. But these gores likewise require a few button-hole stitches, because the starting point of the slit cannot furnish the material for the seam fold, and the crossways threads of the material there would fray. The gores must have a flat seam all round the wrong side. There are stay-makers who use herring-bone stitches instead of side-stitches at the part of the gore near the back seam, which thus brings the two flat seams closer together. This practice is very sound in this case, and in all others where there is a matter of flattening the seams. The seam which joins the back to the front is prick-stitched, and folded down like the gores. It is the same for the seam which joins the shoulder-strap to the united back and front.

Let us now concern ourselves with the manner of placing and sewing the piece of lining which holds the whale-bones at each side of the busk. This piece, which has the shape of a capital A, is divided in half lengthways. The middle is applied to the wrong side on the bias seam of the fronts, at the upper part of the stays. Begin by turning down the wide fold on each side of this seam. The widest part of the piece of lining is placed at the top of the stays, in such a manner that the A looks like a V (see Fig. 1 *F*). On its upper part, this piece must show about two inches on each side of the busk pocket. On its lower part, it must be concealed by the tape which forms the pocket. Baste it carefully so that it does not make any creases on the stays, then sew the side parts with side-stitches. Slit the lining in half lengthways and up to its crossways half, which permits you to make the lining in two pieces when you wish to economize on material, and that is a better arrangement. As the tape of the busk pocket crosses the lining, it conceals the join of these pieces. For this reason, and especially so that they do not form any lumps on the busk pocket, be satisfied with basting them on each other flat, without any seam folds.

The slit you have just made in the middle of the lining is to admit of the small whale-bones which will be held there. You must make them small cases. To this end, take one whale-bone and push it in between the lining and the outer material. Bring it as close as possible to the side seam of the lining, then baste all along the whale-bone, joining at the same time the lining and the outer material. The case being formed, pull out the whale-bone. For the next case, enter it in the same way, bringing it close to the basting you have just made. Repeat this operation once, and even two or three times, according to the number of whale-bones which will accompany the busk. This operation is performed in the same way, and at a similar distance, to the right and the left of the front seam. When the cases have been basted on the wrong side of the stays, turn the stays over and sew with very small back-stitches over the bastings which are on the cases marked *g* in Fig. 1 *F*. Because the cases are sewed on the bias, there is always an empty part, marked *h* in Fig. 1 *F,* near the upper end of the busk. Do not put the whale-bones in permanently until the stays are finished, because their stiffness renders sewing quite difficult.

Regarding the linen tapes of which I have already spoken in the article on furnishings for stays, the tape destined for the busk is divided in half lengthways. Make a fold lengthways in the middle and lay it over the bias front seam, to the left and right of which you turned down the wide seam reserved for the busk pocket. Apply it also on the piece of lining holding the whale-bones, which it seems to divide in two parts. Fix the tape in place with pins, then baste it a few lines from its selvages. Finish by sewing with side-stitches on each selvage, prick-stitching at the same time the material of the seam fold, and that of the stays. It is necessary to observe that the raw edges of the seam fold under the linen tape must not extend beyond it.

Do not sew either side of the tape at the part next the lower end of the bone-cases; this omission allows the bones to be entered. Later, when you have put them in their proper places, sew this place on the tape to fasten them.

The linen tape which forms the busk pocket must be at least three inches longer than the stays, because it is folded upon itself at both ends, so that it is strong enough to withstand the pressure at both ends of the busk. At the lower end, side-stitch this folded part on the inside with a seam fold. Then work at the end, in the middle of the tape, two eyelet-holes separated from each other by several lines. Do the same on each side of the front seam which is under the linen tape. These four eyelet-holes, thus placed one over the other, admit of the cord which will hold the busk when you have placed it in the pocket.

The upper end of the tape is sewed firmly with back-stitches at the same time as the lining for the whale-bones. Fold down a little of the tape at this end, but without sewing it onto itself, as is done at the bottom. The reason for this is that to fit well, the stays must be longer than the busk. Then resew the folded part of the tape securely with back-stitches, crossways to the exact measure of the busk. This back-stitching is always done from the right side of the stays. It is brought closer to or farther from the edge according to the length of the busk, the taste of the wearer, or the style of the stays. But always guard against letting the busk work up; that is not only very ugly, but very dangerous.

The linen tapes which form the cases for the whale-bones at the back also require some directions. First, they must not be longer than the stays, because excess length would be less a support than a nuisance. You have seen that each back piece has a very wide seam fold. It is over this fold, turned to the wrong side of the stays, that you affix the linen tape, and baste it by the selvage as you baste an over-cast seam, to the place where the seam fold begins. Then sew it with very close over-cast stitches. The over-casting finished, lay the tape over the seam fold and sew it with side-stitches to the other selvage, avoiding any exposure of the raw edge of the seam fold. These two operations finished, take the whale-bone for the back, and enter and baste it as described for the small bone-cases. Remove it and sew, on the right side of the stays, small back-stitches over the basting, as I have explained. If you intend to use two whale-bones, make another case; but I do not advise this unless you are extremely fat. At all events, immediately after making the case for the bone, it is necessary to pierce the eyelet-holes. It is well to leave several lines after the row of back-stitches, because the lace enlarges the eyelet-holes and gradually brings them closer to the edge.

There must be as many eyelet-holes on one side as on the other; but the lower end of the left side (the wrong side of the stays facing you) has no eyelet-hole which corresponds to the one in the same place on the right side. Instead, this eyelet-hole is found at the upper end, because it is on the left side that you fasten the lace after lacing. The right side has the eyelet-hole at the bottom because it is there that lacing begins.

I shall not discuss the manner of making the eyelet-holes at much length, since every one knows it; but I shall indicate several modes for making them sturdy, which are less generally used. Suppose that you have measured the distances between eyelet-holes, you have marked these with pins, and you have entered a punch twice in each hole, circling it as you withdraw it so that your eyelet-hole is well rounded. When the eyelet-holes are thus prepared, some stay-makers add the little metal loops known as eyes, which are used to hook gowns. They sew them by their double looped link round the eyelet-hole, on the side opposite to the bone-case, so that the rounded part of the eye circles the hole previously formed by the punch. They work the eyelet-hole over this loop, and then it becomes impossible for the lace to tear the eyelet-holes. This practice is therefore very sound; but to make it so, you must take care to enter the brass wire loop well into the inner wall of the eyelet-hole. Otherwise the lace breaks the thread which holds it, the brass loop detaches, wears out the lace, and finishes by completely detaching itself from the eyelet-hole, causing an insupportable nuisance.

That is the sole result of the little metal rings which some stay-makers instead put in eyelet-holes. As those are perfectly circular, and consequently do not afford the same support as the eyes, they are immediately detached from the eyelet-holes; or rather, their joining point not being solid, one edge of the ring rises up, pierces the edge of the eyelet-hole, impedes the lace, and tears every thing it catches.

Other persons put a flat braid or a narrow linen tape over the line through which the eyelet-holes are pierced. This braid or tape must be firmly fixed with pins, or instead basted, so that the row of eyelet-holes is quite straight. The punch goes through the support on which the eyelet-hole is then made. It is easily seen that nothing is more simple; also nothing is more sturdy, more convenient, and subject to fewer disadvantages. Put this tape on the wrong side or on the right side, as you prefer; in my opinion the wrong side is better.

When the whale-bones are very thin, you may enter one in a case made by back-stitching immediately after the eyelet-holes. Also, when the stays are made carefully, you prick-stitch the second selvage of the linen tape from the right side, instead of side-stitching it on the wrong side. In this way, the eyelet-holes are between two lines of back-stitches, which produces an agreeable effect.

The stays must be a little longer than the whale-bones, so that they do not make a disagreeable point at the back. But it is necessary that the whale-bones be held firmly in place by some sturdy back-stitches, because otherwise they would cause crossways creases on the stays, which would be annoying and painful.

To finish the Stays. Almost the only thing which remains to be done is binding the stays; it is quite easy. It is merely a matter of placing a linen tape about half an inch wide at the bottom, the top, and around the hollows of the shoulder-straps. The tape is placed *à cheval*, which quite simply is to fold it double lengthways, put the edge of the stays within it, and sew the right side of the stays, and both sides of the tape, at the same time. You must be careful to hold the tape firmly, lest it stretch too much and pucker disagreeably.

Leave the linen tape unsewed, or sewed only on one side, when you come to the cases for the back whale-bones, to avoid closing off the openings. This precaution need be taken only for the bottom edge of the stays. You must also take care not to close off the busk pocket, so that you may enter the busk. The top binding is not interrupted by any thing. First bind the shoulder-strap of the left side (the wrong side of the stays being in front of you), turn round at the end of the shoulder-strap, bind the hollow, and so follow all the front. It is well to remark that where the seams meet, you must pass the needle alternately over and under, in order to be sure to catch every thing. You may also crease them with the thimble while pressing them with your finger-tips.

The stays being at this point, slide in the whale-bones on each side of the busk, then secure them by sewing the part of the pocket adjacent to them. Put in the back whale-bones and secure them firmly. Finish the two little ends of binding previously left undone. Sew the shoulder-straps permanently. Enter the busk into its pocket, and pass a cord through the eyelet-holes of the pocket, making it into a loop.

Stays with Two Bosom Gores.

As I promised at the beginning, the pains I have taken to describe the preceding stays will largely serve for these. Indeed, stays with two gores are soon explained. Slit the back (see Fig. 2 A), which you have cut a little narrower at the bottom, and introduce into this slit *i*, a long hip gore on the straight-way and a little sloped (see Fig. 2 B). This operation should also render the front gore narrower.

It remains to place the second bosom gore. You already know that you cut a slit in the top of the stays, two or two and a half inches from the busk, to admit of the bosom gore (see Fig. 1 B). Well then, you have only to cut another slit half an inch away. This gives a little strip which separates the two gores, which you place as described previously. You may also make the interval two, three, or four times larger, but I believe it is

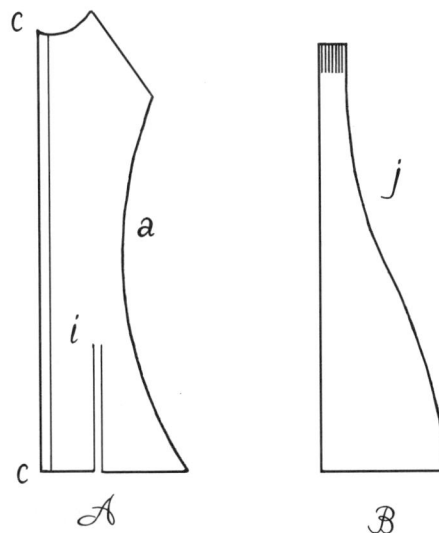

Figure 2. The back and bottom gore of stays with two bosom gores.

better that it be small. For very fat persons, put three gores on each side of the busk.

It is always necessary to make the bosom gores at least five inches long. When they are shorter, they compress the bosom, and their least disadvantage is to deform and wither it. When the ridiculous fashion of extremely short-waisted gowns compelled women to raise their bosom, the gores were made very short, and many problems resulted. In order that your bosom may be properly supported, you may narrow the gores at the bottom, but not too much.

Some stay-makers enter small, and more or less flexible, whale-bones into the flat seams of the gores. This practice is worthless. The whale-bones make a point at the top of the gore, often prick you at the bottom, and curve themselves in a disagreeable and vexing manner. You ought not to put any bones in the front of your stays except those which accompany the busk.

The whale-bones which stay-makers place along the stays, from below the shoulder-straps to the beginning of the hips, to show them off, should be left to coquettes, or persons whose excessive embonpoint burdens their waist with rolls of fat. When the gores are at a little distance from each other, some persons place one more bone in the interval. They are wrong to place it there unless the bosom is very flabby. Furthermore, all the whale-bones are entered under linen tape of their exact width, which is sewed to the wrong side of the stays at both selvages.

Kinds of Shoulder-straps which include Gores.

There are some stay-makers who place a little gore in the middle of the space under the arms. That is well for persons who require large arm-holes, but shoulder-straps which include gores are twenty times better. These require a little attention.

I have said that the shoulder-strap is a band hollowed out on one side, which is fitted to the stays; but in this case it is part of the stays themselves, because it forms the complete arm-hole by itself. Thus it is a hollowed square and a bias (see Fig. 3 *A, m*) where the shoulder-strap begins, and there is no seam other than the one which unites it to the back and the front previously joined. You will perceive that it is necessary that it be measured quite precisely.

Many persons leave it longer, cut it crossways, and cross it about four inches from the front to avoid the necessity of exact measurement, which may only be taken over the arms. This kind of shoulder-strap answers very

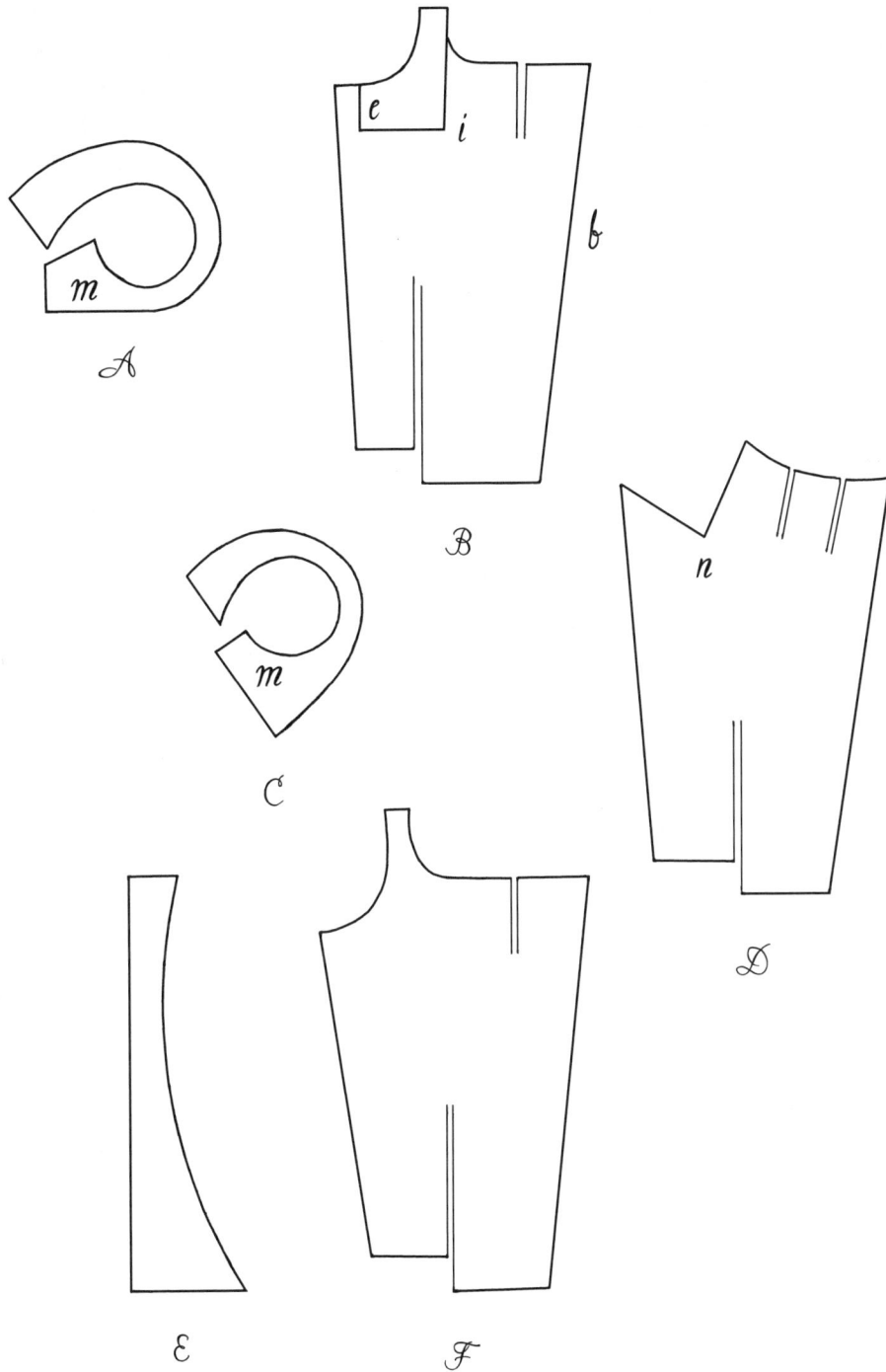

Figure 3. Shoulder-straps which include gores,
and stays with a side-piece.

well and is not uncomfortable. Cut the stays accordingly: because the arm-hole is part of the shoulder-strap, the front of the stays shows a square at this point (see Fig. 3 *B, e*). This part of the shoulder-strap is basted, so as to be prick-stitched on top of the stays, and the seam is turned down with the piece. Furnish this shoulder-strap with linen tape *à cheval,* like any other.

This shoulder-strap is called a square piece; the following shoulder-strap is called a shoulder-strap with a gore (see Fig. 3 *C*). It entirely merits that name, because instead of beginning with a square piece, it begins with a gore similar to a bosom gore. It is all in one piece (see Fig. 3 *C, m*), unless you do not wish to cut it crossways, as I have just explained. It is needless to say that the front of the stays must be cut out to correspond; however, a diagram is given for greater clarity (see Fig. 3 *D, n*).

Sometimes a band is placed between the back and the front of the stays; it is in some sort the back of the front. You then make the front much narrower, as shown by Fig. 3; the band is *E*, the front is *F*. This varia-tion serves to use pieces of material cut between, and to give a bias to the under-arms to replace the shoulder-straps cut with gores.

When you have in the stays other seams than those of the gores and the joining of the pieces, they should be made by over-casting on the wrong side, or better still with back-stitches. Crease the seam well, turn down the seam folds, and cover it with a narrow linen tape, sewed with side-stitches on both selvages. You may feel that the tension of the material on your body will render the thickness of the seams painful, consequently that it might be proper to finish all seams in this manner, if that does not demand far too much time.

Elegant ladies have a band of embroidered percale sewed to the front of their stays from one shoulder-strap to the other. This practice should be followed; it is both modest and pretty. The percale takes the place of a chemisette, which you will not always have the leisure to put on. But as it must be sewed with small stitches, and becomes soiled ten times quicker than the stays, it is disagreeable to unpick it in order to renew it; therefore it may be better to lightly baste a half-chemisette over the gores.

Pieced Stays.

This third fashion has the purpose of preventing the stays from working up; but if it is not carried out properly, it will produce the contrary result. You know that stay fronts are cut on the bias, and the property of the bias being to stretch, the stays must necessarily work up. To obviate this inconvenience, cut out the fronts in three pieces. One extends most of the way across the upper part of the front, with no middle seam, as shown in Fig. 4 *A;* it is cut on the straight-way. The bottom fronts are in two pieces and on the bias as usual, but are cut out to receive the upper piece, as shown in Fig. 4 *B.*

The division is made a little below the bottoms of the bosom gores and across to the middle of the region under the arms, as shown in Fig. 4 *B, q.* The upper piece includes the end of the shoulder-straps, as shown in Fig. 4 *A, r,* and half the hollow of the arm-hole. The two side edges of the half arm-hole must be a little on the bias, in order to replace the widening of the shoulder-strap incorporating a gore. Cut slits for one or two bosom gores on each side. In short, this piece exactly resembles the portion of the front which it replaces.

Sew the two bottom fronts together as usual. Hollow out a little from the replacement piece in the middle, where it corresponds to the seam joining the fronts. Make a seam fold at each of the two side edges, and at the lower edge; then place this piece across over the edge of the united fronts. Prick-stitch it as you do for gores, and turn it down on the wrong side with small herring-bone stitches. Then place the gores, the lining to hold the whale-bone, and the busk pocket.

Especially for this kind of stays, it is important that the bosom gores be the proper length, because otherwise the upper piece would work up over the bosom and hurt horribly. The hollowing which I recommended for the middle of the region which is joined to the front seam must be accentuated more or less, according to the embonpoint of the person and the size of the stays. Sometimes this hollowing is repeated at the upper part of the piece, and then the line of the gores exceeds it a little. This mode may be used, when you wish, for every other kind of stays. But I prefer to place the busk a little lower and leave about an inch at the top, as I described previously.

Lined Stays.

You must recollect that lined stays are most commonly made of nankeen or unbleached toile. However, many stays of fine linen dimity are lined with toile so that they last longer; taffety stays are lined as well. Here is how to proceed:

Commence by cutting out four of each piece, two of the outer material and two of the lining, excepting the shoulder-straps. For each of these, fold a band of material double, and hollow out a curve on one side, the

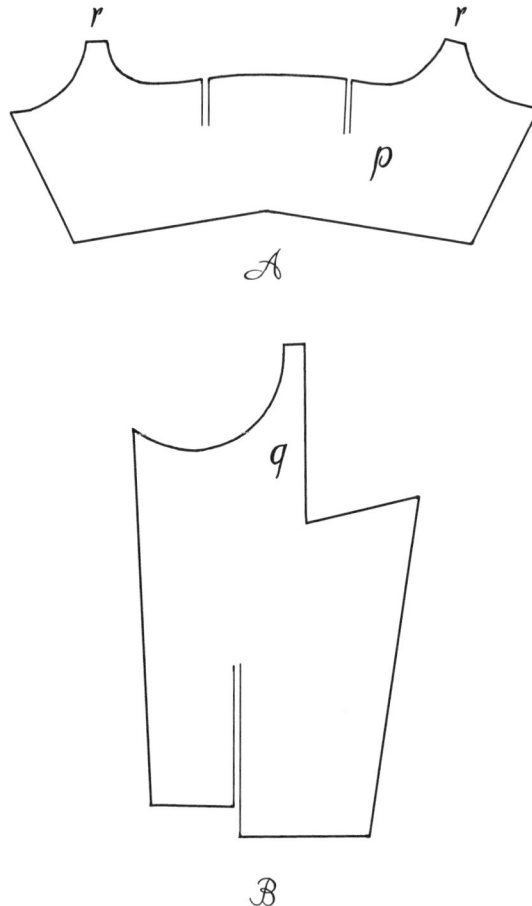

Figure 4. The top and bottom of the fronts of pieced stays.

straight-way of the upper portion of the shoulder-straps permitting this operation, to get the shape shown in Fig. 1 C.

Sew together the two fronts of the outer material, and those of the lining, as if you were making two pair of stays. Turn the seam folds down well. Then lay the joined outer front over the joined lining, in such a manner that the seams touch and conceal each other. Spread the fronts on a table, and baste all round the edges, and along the length of the slits made to admit of the gores. Lay the outer gores over those of the lining, baste them together, then sew them by prick-stitching them to the lining, taking back-stitches on the right side. Instead of making a flat seam with their seam folds, sew them to the wrong side with side-stitches, since you have made back-stitches on the right side.

As for the side portion of the backs, place a linen tape between the outer material and the lining (many persons omit it, but that is at the expense of sturdiness). Make a wide seam fold on each piece, and over-cast them together. The back whale-bone is also entered between the lining and the outer material. The seam which joins the front to the back is made as follows: prick-stitch the outer material of the front onto the outer material of the back, catching the back lining at the same time. Then turn down the front lining and sew it with side-stitches, in such a manner that it conceals the seam folds of the pieces.

The busk pocket is commonly made without linen tape. Measure the lengthways half of the busk, and lay it over the front seam of the stays. Then pencil a mark at the right of the busk. This mark serves to guide a basting, which in its turn guides a line of very small back-stitches, which form one side of the busk pocket. Enter the busk between the outer material and lining, baste to the left of it along its length, then withdraw the busk. Take a new line of back-stitches along this basting to complete the busk pocket. You will perceive that it is unnecessary to add a separate piece of lining to hold the small whale-bones which accompany the busk; their place is found there quite naturally. (When stays are lined because the material is very fine, it is proper to put a linen tape under the part of the front which forms the busk pocket.)

Lined stays are not commonly bound with a linen tape *à cheval*. Instead, make a seam fold all round the outer material, and all round the lining. Then sew with side-stitches, which you tighten a little. Three or four lines below this kind of hem, take a line of small running stitches, or back-stitches if you wish your stays to be beautifully made. However, it would be quicker and more secure to apply a linen tape *à cheval*, after trimming the inner and outer material evenly, so that they do not form a lump under the tape.

Half-stays, or Morning Belts.

Cut out the top as for an ordinary pair of stays (of whatever kind you prefer). Allow only about an inch and a half below the beginning of the gores. Then cut two strips about half an ell long, at least half a foot wide at one end, and sloping off to no wider than an inch at the other end. These strips, or straps, are intended to replace the eyelet-holes and the lace. They are sewed to the back, and are often cut out as part of the back, if the extent of the material permits. The straps cross over each other, join the stays at the back, then come round to be attached in the front with a linen tape sewed to their ends. When the stays are lined, and the straps are lined likewise, bind them as I have explained for the preceding stays. Otherwise, it is well to fasten the seam fold which each must have all round, with very close herring-bone stitches, because the fulness of a hem would hurt you.

Do not put any busk on these stays, but only two, three, or four slightly stiff whale-bones, and only in the front. Do not bone the straps, because they bend in crossing and press any bones into your back. Otherwise, half-stays are made altogether like the upper portions of whole stays.

Stays with Straps.

The name of these stays indicates their relationship to those which I have just described. However, stays with straps are always complete, and no different from ordinary stays excepting the straps which re-place the eyelet-holes, so that you may dress yourself. To this end, make six or eight straps, according to the size of the stays and the width you desire for the straps. Position the straps alternately; that is, when you sew one of the straps to the upper part of the right back piece, the corresponding position on the left back piece does not have one, and so on to the end.

Because these alternating straps meet up very ill in the front, it has been thought to make the straps pass under each other at the back, by means of an opening which is placed between the stays and the strap, and furnished with whale-bones. It is then the openings which alternate, because all parts of the back are equally furnished with straps. The straps cross well, but the whale-bones which impart the necessary stiffness to the openings twist, and soon become painful. On the whole, I have taught the manner of making this kind of stays only so as to omit nothing.

Stays *à la Paresseuse*.

Here is another kind of stays which allows you to lace yourself. If it is out of fashion it may return, and moreover it is well to have such a pair of stays for hurried moments. These stays are made like any others; or to say it better, you may put this kind of lacing on any kind of stays. It is necessary that they be furnished at the back with whale-bones and eyelet-holes.

Commence by counting the number of eyelet-holes on the stays. Then cut as many pieces of tightly-woven flat braid; make each piece about half an ell long. Sew a piece of braid at each eyelet-hole, always from the side towards the middle of the stays. That done, thread all the braids sewed to the left back through the corresponding eyelet-holes of the right back, and thread those sewed to the right back through the eyelet-holes of the left. Then pass all the braids back to their original sides, without threading them through any eyelet-holes.

Collect all the ends of braid on the left into an even bundle. Sew the ends together firmly. Then fit the ends into a wide linen tape about two inches long, which folded crossways in the middle, and over-cast on each side along its selvages, encloses the bundle of braids. Sew the braids to one end of this tape with back-stitches, turn it over, and sew the other ends of the braids to it with side-stitches. Repeat this entire operation for the braids on the right side.

Finish the work by sewing another piece of braid, about a quarter of an ell long, to the middle of the folded part of the left tape. Sew a second braid to the tape on the right. You will tie the braids at the front of the stays when you put them on.

All the eyelet-holes are laced in the following manner: when you want to put on your stays, separate the backs as much as possible and put your head through. After having passed your arms through the shoulder-straps and arranged the front, tighten the two final braids at the left and right, and you are instantly laced. That is the advantage; here are the disadvantages: the numerous braids get mixed up and tangled in a way which requires much patience and time to untangle them. They frequently break, and get in the way at the side.

Stays for Pregnant Women.

Belts, or half-stays, are the most suitable stays for women in this condition; they should not wear any other kind, above all during the last months. But at the beginning of pregnancy they may have a pair of stays prepared as follows. Belts, much widened at the bottom, have stomach and bosom gores slit lengthways in the middle. Both edges of each slit are bound with a narrow linen tape *à cheval,* and furnished with closely-spaced eyelet-holes. (Persons who fear being too tightly laced have stays which lace both back and front. The front is arranged in this manner.) You lace these eyelet-holes, and as your size increases, you loosen the lace. These stays are also cut out in a circle in the middle of the front to accommodate the shape of the stomach. It is proper not to put a busk there, but to replace that article with elastics, as I shall describe.

Elastic Stays.

Elastics are made of copper wires, extremely slender and arranged in a very tight spiral which, confined to a space more or less long, stretches and tightens exactly according to the form of the object which it encompasses. It is the gentlest manner of supporting the shape. Consequently it is used for children, pregnant women, and persons in frail health. Stays may be elastic in whole or in part.

In the first case the stays are lined, and you furnish them all over with small cases which contain the elastic and which you make like bone-cases; with this difference, that you never withdraw the elastic after having measured the case, because the suppleness of the elastic readily permits sewing, even though it is between two materials. It is necessary to fasten the elastic at both ends, at the top and bottom of the stays. Pull it a little, so that the material which it shapes forms little folds when the elastic tightens. Without this step, the material would prevent the elastic from stretching, and it would remain rigid. But take good care not to pull it too much, because then the spiral would not stretch any more, and the elasticity would equally be lost by the contrary excess.

Elastic is sewed with running stitches. Do not put elastics into gores, nor into shoulder-straps. Entire elastic stays are ordinarily made of brown taffety.

Partial elastics are employed in every kind of stays. For example, you may sew five or six rows of elastics between two bands of percale or fine toile, and fit this elastic band to the bottom and all round the stays. The purpose of this practice is to prevent the gores from working up over the hips; it serves very well, but it is for stays *de toilette*.

Other elastics replace the busk. Mark a band of dimity four, six, or eight inches wide, or even more, according to the width you desire. Double it with a single fold, then measure it at least a third longer than the stays, because the contour of the elastics requires much material. After that cut pieces of elastic of equal length, and put them three by three, or four by four, crossways inside the doubled band, allowing a space of about an inch or two between each group of three or four. Always begin by fastening the elastic at both ends to control it. Continue thus to the end of the band, which you then place between the two fronts instead of the busk pocket. Ordinarily two small whale-bones are placed lengthways, to the right and left of the elastic band.

This band is not always simply straight. Most commonly it is given the shape of an A, but very long at the bottom. The part widening from the V is applied to the top of the stays: this is done to replace the small whale-bones which ordinarily accompany the busk.

Stays made to conceal Defects of the Shape.

Without being accused of that ridiculous and deplorable coquetry which asks of art the shape denied by Nature, you may, when you have the misfortune to be more or less misshapen, seek to conceal this unfortunate state. A woman who wears a false bosom is a fool, or a contemptible coquette. But one who pads her stays a little to hide a disparity in her shape is not, in my opinion, any more reprehensible than a sick person who summons a physician. Are not all degrees of deformity infirmities?

Take a little cotton wadding and apply it to the place on your stays which corresponds to the fault in your shape. Make the first and largest layer, and sew it with small stitches. Place and sew other layers there in the same way until the necessary thickness is attained, gradually reducing their thickness towards the edges. Find a skilful and discreet person, and ask her to fit the padded stays to you. Finish by placing a piece of toile or dimity over this kind of pad. It is better if the stays are lined: you may more easily enter the cotton between the two pieces before making up the stays.

If instead of a hollow, the fault of your shape is an enlargement, pad the parts of the stays near it, first at the top of it, then thinning imperceptibly as you move far enough away that it may be interrupted without difficulty. If the enlargement is very pronounced, you must resign yourself to padding the entire pair of stays, because otherwise one side of your shape would be very much higher. Thus the enlargement will find itself, as it were, in a case, and will be as one with the padding. You will be a little warm, it is true; but you may partly remedy this by replacing the cotton with hemp or flax tow.

The habit of sewing, and especially embroidering, as an occupation makes many women have a right shoulder-blade more prominent than the left. If you are subject to this little inconvenience, your stays may be made a little high in the neck, and a little cotton put at the level of the first eyelet-holes. You may cover it with a little white leather, then put a similar piece of leather on the other side. This measure will appear to have the purpose of preventing the whale-bones from injuring you; and you will be able, if necessary, to permit your stays to be seen without fear.

———*Manuel des dames.*

Diversion 1.

The Art of making Stays. I sincerely agree with my young readers that is it not as amusing to make a pair of stays, of whatever kind, as to make a ball gown, a hat, or any other part of your attire. But that does not matter; it is necessary for a young lady to understand and be able to make every thing which she needs. Perhaps some one will argue that a young lady who is receiving even the slightest education cannot engage in such occupations: I shall respond that there is time for every thing.

Economy is the foundation of a good education: it is for mothers to instruct their daughters by example, and to make them prefer what is useful to what is of only passing merit. By accustoming them early to being present at the summary of the daily accounts, mothers will find that young girls are carried along by a kind of curiosity natural to their time of life. Sensible and far-sighted mothers hasten to profit by this sentiment. They rely on their children for the care and the honourable task of keeping the accounts of the household expenses, which up until then they took upon themselves. Arithmetic is not a purely speculative science for young persons: they ought to know the price of all things, from necessities to luxurious articles. They should learn to judge the annual sum indispensable for maintaining their wardrobe, and the increase of expense which inevitably results from abandoning these tasks to the hands of strangers.

Unhappily, such young ladies will find that there are still people enough to whom this wisdom is unknown. They may then establish comparisons entirely in their favour, and render tender thanks to their far-sighted mothers, bringing many converts to their circle. By this means they will propagate the invaluable order and economy upon which the happiness of an entire life depends.

What man, indeed, could be so unreasonable as to prefer to a young lady brought up by these principles, one whose frivolous education has left her a stranger to all this work and knowledge, true treasures in a mother of a family?

Suitable Materials for making Stays. Stays are ordinarily made of finely-corded dimity called *basin de Troyes;* sometimes also of *coutil,* India nankeen, white moiré, or satin. The last are worn for grand toilets. For ordinary stays, I recommend *basin de Troyes;* the best is four-ply.

It is well to warn my readers that the heavier dimities are not those which wear best; a tolerably fine dimity is preferable to thick. The fine has two advantages over the thick; it lasts longer, and it becomes less soiled.

Since *coutil*, as well as nankeen, must be lined because it has little firmness, I advise my readers not to use it, for lined stays never assume the shape of the figure as well as unlined ones. Lined stays are useful only to misshapen persons, for the lining prevents the little pads which are added from being as apparent.

The Measures for Stays. The order which I propose to follow in the course of this little treatise requires that I describe the way of taking the measures for this essential part of dress. However, if you at the very least possess a pair of stays, it will be much easier to work from that model, however bad it may be. I shall return to this below.

Commence by taking a strip of paper, which will serve to take the proportions of the body which must be enclosed by the stays (see Fig. 5). This is called the measure; it is about an ell long and two inches wide. Fold the measure double lengthways. Press the fold between the thumb and forefinger of your right hand. The two extremities of the measure must be marked with different labels. Let us call them a and b in order to recognize end a, which will be used during the whole operation.

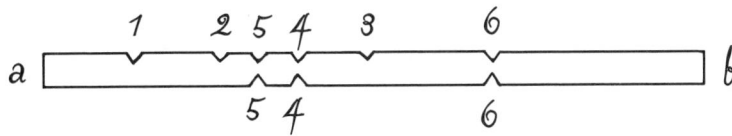

Figure 5. The measure.

It is always more decent to take the measures while the person is wearing stays, howsoever faulty, than to take them bare. First take end a of the measure between the thumb and forefinger of your right hand, then lay it over the shoulder-blade below the base of the arm. Extend the measure in a straight line to the other side of the back, after which take half the length measured and cut a notch there (see Fig. 5, *1*). Place the notch on the same point on the left back where it previously rested. Beginning from that point, lay the measure to the base of the bosom. Cut a second notch there (see Fig. 5, *2*) and continue to measure from the base of the bosom to the middle of the busk. Cut a third notch at that point (see Fig. 5, *3*). This third notch marked, take the measure at end a, and encircle the waist under the bosom, leaving the measure two fingers narrower than the curve of the waist. Proceed the same as before; that is, take half the distance measured and cut a double notch on the fold (see Fig. 5, *4*). Take end a again, replace it on the lower end of the busk, and bring it round over the hip to the middle of the back, that is, between the two bones which terminate it; this notch is made double (see Fig. 5, 5). Take end *a* again, and go round the arched part. Fold the measure double along the entire length, and cut the two notches marked by two 6's. It is essential to take this measure while the person is wearing stays. The fleshy parts being in place, it will be easy to judge the proper proportions to keep.

To cut out a Pattern. Since it is very difficult to cut out a pattern for stays which fits well straight away, cut one by the model stays in Chambery gauze, a kind of cheap gauze. First fold all the gores of the model on themselves and bring all the seams together, one over another, and fix them firmly with pins, so that the enlargement produced by the gores is no longer seen. This part of the stays then appears as if it did not have a slit at that place.

Next lay the gauze over the stays. Take care to place the gauze in precisely the same direction as the stays; that is, the straight-way part of the stays is straight-way on the gauze. The part with the straight-way must be under the arms, and the part in the front must be on the bias. Take great care in attaching the Chambery gauze along the stays. Then cut to the right and left of the seams, without leaving any seam folds.

When the pattern is cut out, remove all the pins which fasten it to the model. However, after cutting the slits which must admit of the top and bottom gores, lay a piece of the gauze over the gores.

I warn you that it is always necessary to cut out the gores at the bottom of the stays along the straight-way on one side, and on the bias on the other (see Fig. 6 *A* and *B*); the bias side is placed over the hip and the straight-way over the stomach. The bias at the hips provides more ease of movement and prevents the stays from pulling up, the material being much more elastic in that direction than on the straight-way. If the stays have two gores at the bottom (so that there are four for the two sides), the bias of the second is also placed on the hip. Consequently, the straight-way of the second gore is near to the eyelet-holes.

The bosom gores must be cut out on the bias on both sides. The straight-way in the front is in the middle to give more support to the bosom (see Fig. 6 *C*, *wyx*). If the person who will wear the stays is fat, or if she has an occupation which obliges her to move her arms frequently, slit the middle of the under-arms, in order to place there a little gore about three fingers high by only two fingers wide.

When the first pattern is cut out, put it over a sheet of stout paper, and fix it to the latter with pins. Then take the measure and place it on the gauze pattern, in the same way you would place it on the person, to

Figure 6. The parts of a pair of stays.

determine whether the pattern requires some corrections. When at last it has all the proportions which are indicated by the measure, when you measure the top or the bottom of the stays, you will see how wide to make the gores by the length of the paper which remains to go up to the place measured, that is the notch indicated for this part of the size. If this measure shows that the pattern must be enlarged, mark it with a pencil on the paper destined to become the pattern. If, on the contrary, the pattern is found too wide, fold it over itself to alter the size, then cut out the paper pattern.

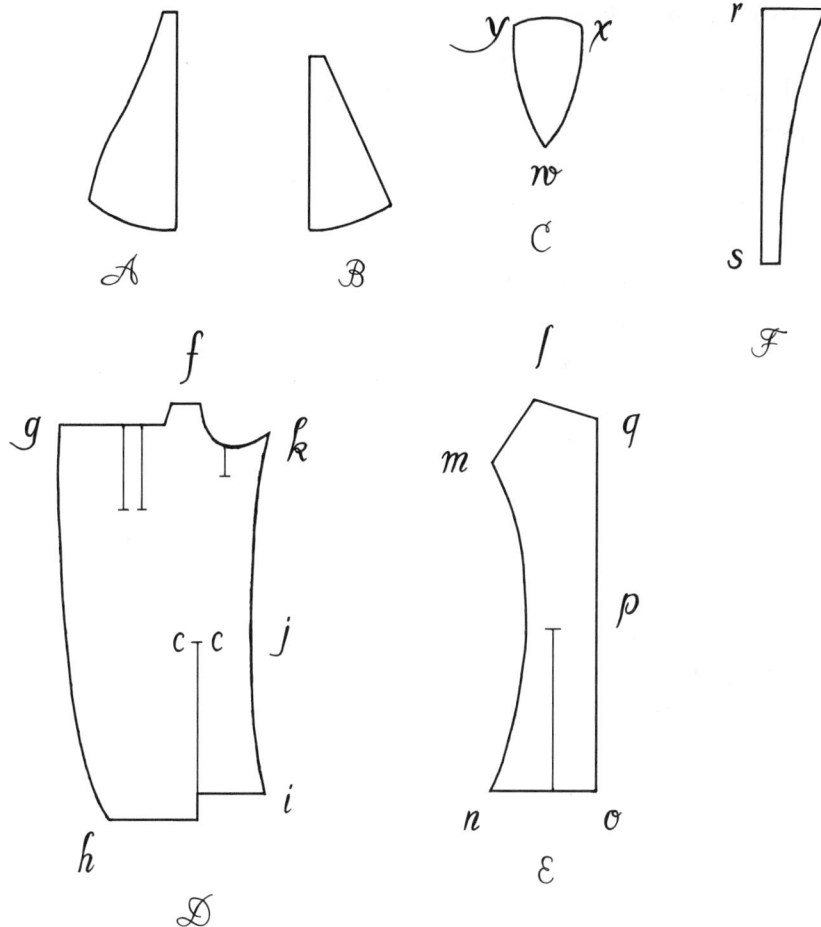

In observing all the marks which have been made, this second pattern will be sufficiently correct that you may venture to use the dimity, or any other material listed above.

The Art of the Stay-maker.

Different Kinds of Stays. I am going to list all the kinds of stays which may be used. The stays I have just spoken about, and of which the pattern has been taken, are called stays with double gores. Then come the stays with single gores, lined stays, stays *à la paresseuse*, stays with straps, stays for pregnant women called *brassières de Venus*, elastic stays, half-stays or morning belts, and night stays or *brassières*. I shall return to these later.

The Different Parts of Stays in general. The pattern of the stays I spoke of above is composed of a front (see Fig. 6 *D*), a back (see Fig. 6 *E*), and a gore at the bottom of each piece, near the side. The wider gore is placed on the bottom of the front of the stays, and the narrower on the back. The bosom gores must be equal. One side of the shoulder-strap must be on the straight-way.

If you must use this pattern often, I advise you to line it with toile or calico, it matters not which, for the little strips formed by the slits for the gores are very much subject to tearing. Fasten the toile to the paper with short running stitches, taking care to take one at a time. This lined pattern will last a very long time. Take care also to write a label on each piece indicating its respective place; expert stay-makers never neglect this precaution. Nothing in a woman's toilet is more meticulous to make than this garment. It is well to have a table on which to put the material intended for the stays, a pincushion, and scissors with blades about five inches long. One blade must be rounded, and this blade must touch the table all during the work of cutting.

If the material which you prepare to cut is only two-thirds of an ell wide, you will need three-quarters of an ell for the stays of a person with a rather stout figure. The width mentioned can guide you for every other. Fold this material double, and place the front of the stays pattern on it, with the top of the stays touching one selvage, so that the stays will be cut crossways. Stays require to be very sturdy; when the material is placed in this direction, they acquire more strength than in the other. The pattern must be fixed firmly with pins. It is necessary, as I have already said, not to lift the material from the top of the table, which may occasion errors in cutting. In addition, this mode is used by all good stay-makers: I have no doubt that my readers will adopt it.

Do not neglect to pin the little strips already mentioned; the cut of the scissors in that part must separate them. This is the only part of the stays which is cut out at the edge of the paper. Allow a margin of one finger from the paper every where else. Fold the surplus material down even with the pattern, and press it firmly between your thumb and forefinger, making it equal every where. But as a precaution, also mark these folds with a pencil. Then detach the pattern from the top of the material. Now you have cut out the front of the stays.

Then comes the back to cut out. Place the material in the same direction for the back and its gores as for the front. Only the shoulder-straps should have the selvage along their length (see Fig. 6 *F, rs*). Detach the backs after leaving one finger all round, as for the fronts. If the backs are found to be very curved, make several cuts along the marked fold in order to prevent puckers. Fasten the fold by basting; also baste the part for the eyelet-holes. Pin together all the parts of the pattern which you have already used.

Place the back on the front of the stays, precisely following the pencil mark (see Fig. 7, *ox*). The thread which you use for this basting must be extremely strong, and the needle must be very short and reinforced. I advise, above all things, that you not take two stitches at a time; that mode distorts the work. Put one front on the other so that the right side of the stays is inside, then baste them together with running stitches.

The folds along the edges of the little strips, between which the gores will be placed, are made very narrow. At the top of each vertical slit, cut two horizontal ones, which serve to prevent the creases which would be caused by the folds; and without which the gores would have no grace, neatness, nor even durability. To cut the slits, see Fig. 6 *D, cc*. Pin the

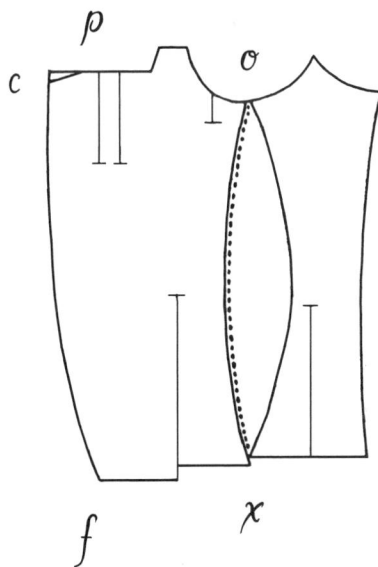

Figure 7. The front and back of a pair of stays.

gores before basting them; this is essential for working methodically. The bosom gores must be placed in the same manner as the hip gores. Baste the shoulder-straps firmly to the back, taking care to make a fold for each strap, after which sew it by prick-stitching.

Divers Furnishings, their Choice and Use. Before making the eyelet-holes for a pair of stays, place a tape of well-twisted thread, three fingers wide, flat on the back. The tape must be loose; that is, it must undulate slightly over the back to prevent any puckers in making the eyelet-holes. Then baste on a strip of any kind, but sturdy and an inch wide: put this strip on the back so that it does not exceed the edge. This false strip serves for piercing the eyelet-holes, so that you may try on the stays. You see, therefore, that this strip must not be pierced all the way through the backs, for fear that they may be left too narrow. If indeed they are, it will suffice to alter them; it is true this will cause a waste of material, but not of time.

Eyelet-holes for stays must be pierced like those for gowns; that is, there must be as many on one side as on the other. (See the mode of working eyelet-holes in the following article.) Baste a case for the bones on each side. These bones must be half an inch wide and very thin; I shall describe the manner of preparing them later. Secure them at the top and bottom with running stitches across the back. Attach the whole on the right-hand side, and at the top of the stays.

Nothing remains but to baste the linen tape which will serve as a case for the busk. The width of this tape must exceed that of the busk by about three or four lines. The tape must be of well-twisted thread just like that placed on the back. Fold the tape double lengthways, press the fold between your thumb and forefinger, and place it over the seam which joins the fronts. Fix it there with several pins. Then baste it to each side very close to its selvages, in order to be able, after basting, to enter the busk.

There are two kinds of busks, those of steel and those of whale-bone. The latter flake off and give way easily, but do not require to be furnished like those of steel. If you do not take care to furnish a steel busk with un-sized paper, and then with white leather, or better still oiled taffety, it will cause a great stomach-ache. It is therefore urgent to cover it with oiled taffety, for this covering is known to guarantee against rust, a thing the leather does not do; it only prevents the rust from penetrating immediately.

To lace the Stays correctly. Put on the stays by passing your arms through the arm-holes, then evenly disperse the folds formed on your shift so they will not be troublesome when the stays are laced. To lace the stays with ease, bring the shoulder-straps over your shoulders, while taking care that the shift does not make any folds at that place. Commence lacing at the top, from right to left. This manner of lacing is the most suitable, not having the disadvantage of the contrary way, of pushing the flesh up and carrying the blood to your head.

The lace which you use must be at least three ells long. Some persons employ two laces of an ell and a half each, and begin by lacing the hollow of the waist, going upwards, and then go back down to the waist to take up the second lace, which serves to fit the hips. In whatever manner you are laced, begin by using the length of the lace, seeking only to hold the stays on your body without tightening them. Then pull your shift up or down as needed. Take care to pull down the stays by the bottom gores, and put your forefinger underneath along the shoulder-strap, at the same time giving to the last a small movement which will make it descend over your arms. Then pass your hands over the front between the stays and the shift, to spread the folds; leave that part very little tightened. This advice is given for health rather than for appearance.

Move your hand to the top of the busk, pressing hard from top to bottom. This adjustment is necessary, and those of my readers who may lace themselves will do well to continue this pressure until the moment when the stays are half tight. Quit this position when it is necessary to hold your shoulders in front. Then with your left hand, take the two bones at the hollow of the waist and bring the backs together. (See the position of the maid's hands in Fig. 8.) Pull the lace by degrees with your right hand. To be well laced without the slightest discomfort, recommence this last operation five or six times, in order to avoid all jerks. When the stays are finally laced and properly tightened to the hollow of your waist, pick up the lace to continue lacing the hip portion. Above all, do not squeeze your hips too close together. That is very ugly, and removes all the grace a woman may have in her shape. The stays when properly tightened, must leave the space of a hand between the backs, because the materials of which they are made stretch immediately.

To fit on the Stays. If the gores are too wide, but there is not quite enough material at that place to make a fold, use a pencil to indicate it.

The front of the shoulder-strap is held by only one pin, and is always longer than it need be. Alter the shoulder-strap on this end if necessary.

If you wish to be well dressed, the back of the stays must be very high. This style is also proper for fat persons, who cannot, because of the roundness of their shoulders, keep any clothing over the latter, rather than meagre persons who wish to hide their bones.

If the stays are too long, put pins at the place where you must cut them.

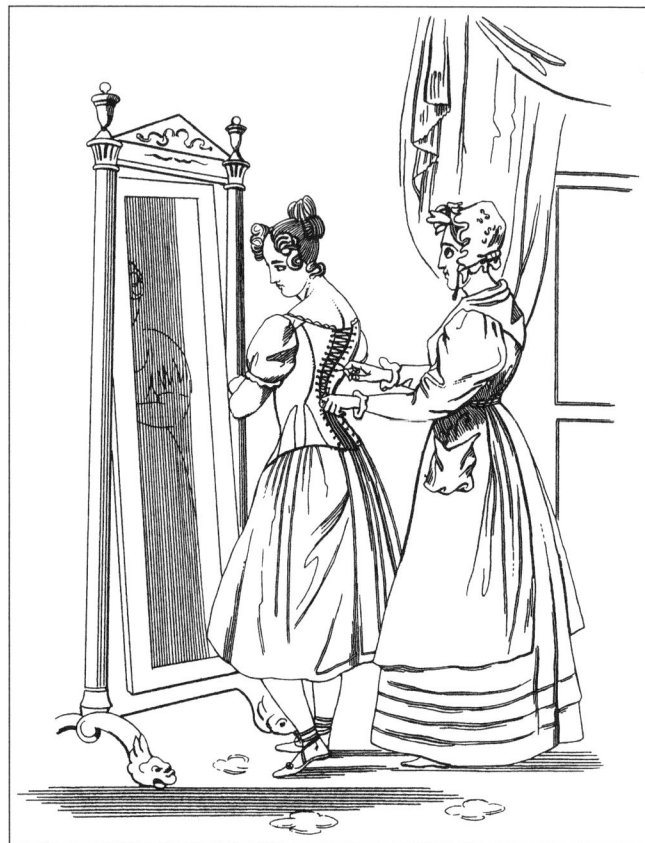

Figure 8. The manner of lacing the stays.

You must hollow out, that is to say cut out, the middle of the top of the stays just over the busk. This will prevent them from coming up and hurting your bosom. Indicate the hollowing with the aid of a pencil or a pin, which you place just over the busk. (See above Fig. 7, *cp*.)

I also advise attaching a linen tape, folded double along its length, on the hips. One end of the tape is passed through a bar which has been put on the stockings, and tied; this replaces garters. The place on the stockings where the bar is located must be sturdily finished; this prevents the stockings from tearing. Another precaution is to put a bar on each side of the stockings, for fear of mistaking which leg each is put on.

I hope that my readers will adopt this manner of gartering as the most healthful and least awkward. Persons whose blood circulates with difficulty find it well to do so. It has the added advantage of preventing the stays from working up. However, this kind of garter must not be attached to the stays until they are finished. You need only mark the place with a pin when trying them on.

If the alterations are too great, or if the stays are sized too wide, it will be necessary to correct the largest faults and try on a second time.

To take the stays off quicker, cut the first stitch which holds the false band through which the eyelet-holes are pierced. The stitches will give way without difficulty, and the stays may readily be taken off.

Once the stays are removed, determine at once whether the pins are well fixed. Enter them more securely than you were able to do with the stays on you (or another person), for a single omission could cause you much difficulty. For greater security, pass coloured thread at the places where you put the pins.

Un-baste the stays, lay the pattern on top of each piece, and see if it accords with all of them. Then prepare to sew the stays permanently.

Seams to work on Stays. The seams for stays of any kind must be made very sturdy. Use only back-stitches, prick-stitches, side-stitches, and button-hole stitches.

Sew all the gores by prick-stitching; and work very close button-hole stitches at the end of each, that is to say, over each little crossways slit. Apply a tape of well-twisted thread, half a finger wide, on the reverse of each seam made. Sew this tape with side-stitches, making the first on the gore at the prick-stitches, and the second on the stays. This manner of finishing the gores with linen tape takes much longer than turning down the surplus of the gore, but you are repaid for the time to put it there by the sturdiness you impart to the entire pair of stays. The seams for the bosom gores are the only ones not covered by a tape; that would hurt the bosom.

The linen tape which is basted onto the back is held by a row of prick-stitches made on the edge. Work a second row at the distance of half an inch; the space between the two will serve as the bone-case. Proceed thus: when the first row has been made, pass the bone between the dimity and the tape, pushing it firmly towards the seam side. Leave it there until you have basted for the other row of prick-stitches, with running stitches, then withdraw it. This second row must be made outside the case; otherwise the bone will not go in. That done, sew the surplus tape with side-stitches.

On the wrong side of the stays, back-stitch the seam which joins the two fronts. Take advantage of this position to pin all the parts together. Pay attention that all similar seams face each other; trim them even all round the stays. This operation done, detach the stays. Take some tape similar to that which you used to cover the seams. Bind the stays by folding it double and placing it *à cheval,* and make it fast with side-stitches. When you bind the bottom of the stays, stretch that part in order to allow the hips more freedom. To do this, attach the part to bind, to a ball full of lead, which is called a weight.

The top of the back and the shoulder-straps must be neither loose nor tight. Because the shoulder-strap is not attached to the front of the stays (except by lacing), you therefore will be able to bind the entire top without cutting the tape to bind the arm-hole. Since the bosom binding requires much more care, it will be easier to do it well by basting, because you must leave the material a little loose, and consequently pull the linen tape with your left hand while your right is occupied with basting. Then sew this part with side-stitches like the others.

The binding being finished, bring the left shoulder-strap over the right, and pierce their edges at the same time in the front, for each of their two eyelet-holes. Two eyelet-holes separated by a similar distance are also pierced from the right side of the stays, where the front of the shoulder-strap must fit. These eyelet-holes will serve to hold a linen lace, or better still a silk one for durability. By this means you may increase or decrease the length of the shoulder-strap at will, by bringing it closer to or farther from the stays. This manner of attaching the shoulder-strap is very useful, above all to persons whose occupation is to handle some instrument. They may enlarge their arm-holes as much as they want, and after the hours devoted to study, tighten them at will. This mode may appear taxing, but you will be well repaid. Musicians, &c., will recognize all its advantages by the results. I could name many persons who have adopted this practice, and none have abandoned it.

The busk tape which you used while trying on the stays is placed as before, and with a good margin at the top as well as the bottom. When the basting in the middle has been done, take over-cast stitches at the top, and side-stitches along the selvages, if they are strong. Or else, baste these two sides and take prick-stitches on the right side of the material. That is even prettier, but it is true, takes much longer to execute.

This tape must be folded over at the bottom by about a hand. Fasten the tape over itself by side-stitching; only the width of the tape at the end remains unsewed. Pierce two double eyelet-holes at that place; that is, the punch should pierce the material of the stays as well as the tape; but four separate eyelet-holes will be made. Take care, before piercing the eyelet-holes, to take the exact measure of the busk, in order to prevent the stays from forming creases across the stomach because of excess length.

To make the Eyelet-holes. There is little left to do except the eyelet-holes at the back. For these, turn the stays to the right side, and lay

To make the Eyelet-holes.

their backs together quite evenly. Pin them at the top to your weight, if you have no one to aid you with this operation. With your left hand, grasp the backs towards the middle and near the prick-stitches. Take a bodkin whose point has been carefully protected with a piece of cork. Despite this precaution, first try it on a piece of material which you are not going to use; for if the point is blunted you risk ruining the backs.

Let us suppose that the tool is in good condition. Take it in your right hand; rest your palm on the end of the handle; your little finger and ring finger serve to hold it in this position. Your thumb, forefinger, and middle finger encircle the point where the handle is joined to the rounded piece of steel called a punch. Pierce the first eyelet-hole at a distance of a little finger from the top of the backs; pierce another eyelet-hole, the same way, at the bottom. When these two eyelet-holes have been made, you will see that they are symmetrical on the left and right back. The rest of the eyelet-holes are staggered, so that each faces an empty space directly opposite.

Detach the backs from the top of the weight, or from the hands of the person assisting you. Pull the back which is behind to the left; then attach the backs to the weight again. Pierce the second eyelet-hole at the top of the right back, at a distance of an inch from the previous one, and so on, progressing to the next-to-last, which must be very near to the last eyelet-hole.

The left back will have the same two closely-spaced eyelet-holes, but even closer together, and these will not be at the bottom but at the top; and it is at the top of the back that you attach the lace. Detach the backs from the top of the weight; re-enter the punch from the wrong side while rotating it. In a word, pierce your eyelet-holes exactly like those for a gown body.

You should have besides a short needle, called a between needle. Thread it with well-twisted linen thread; this thread lasts a very long time and does not have the disadvantage of silk, of yellowing during washing. Be careful to take only a very little material on your needle, as much of it on top as on the bottom; tighten the stitches equally.

I think my readers must know the button-hole stitch, which is nothing but a very regular *cordonnet*. Above all, do not knot the thread which you use; that would not be neat work; and if you cut the knot after the eyelet-hole is finished, that could injure the solidity. Re-enter the punch once or twice during the operation in order to make the eyelet-hole sufficiently large for the lace to pass through easily.

Do not neglect to have near by a small ball filled with emery, the diameter of a five-franc coin. Pass the needle through the bag from time to time, which will renew the needle's original brilliance: by this means it enters the material with great ease.

It is not necessary, for making an eyelet-hole well, to grasp both sides of the material surrounding it; that would make the backs pucker. You need only take the part of the back where you wish to work the eyelet-hole, between the thumb and forefinger of your left hand, and leave free the other side of the back, which is on the right. When the eyelet-hole is finished, securely fasten the thread by passing it under a few button-hole stitches on the wrong side.

Make a small slit across the bone from behind the back, lengthened to two fingers from the edge of the stays. Make a case for an extremely thin bone at both sides of the bosom, below the shoulder-strap. I do not advise bones on each side of the busk; that compresses the bosom too much.

A small task still remains before you enter the bones, as well as the busk. To cleanse a new pair of stays thoroughly, rub them with a piece of stale bread. Cut it square and leave the crust on it, in order to hold it in your hand more easily. Rub the stays for a long time and very gently, then shake them out. Iron all the seams, pressing forcefully to flatten them as much as possible.

To completely prepare the Bones and secure them. Prepared bones are found at all haberdashers, but they are very dear. Here is an easy way to prepare them yourself.

Purchase barbs of whale-bone, and cut them to the length of the stays, after which put them in boiling water to soak. The vessel which contains the water must be long enough to hold the bones lying flat. Do not remove them until the water has become lukewarm. It is still better to cover the vessel, and to leave them there about half an hour.

When taken out of the water, the bones are extremely easy to cut. You must have a knife which is used exclusively for this purpose. When you have split them, round the ends before they cool, and make a hole in each bone near one end. The holes are made by means of a punch.

Then take a piece of glass to polish them, pressing more forcefully at the edges than in the middle. Make them very thin and smooth; otherwise you will risk piercing their cases when entering them.

Now give them the shape needed to follow the curve of the waist, which must be done while the bone is still soft. Make the curves more or less pronounced according to how the person is shaped, or else they may hurt her. If, after being polished, the bones are still not soft enough to assume the desired curves, put them back to soak in the boiling water.

If you add a bone under the arm, make this last one still thinner than those of the back, and round the ends like the others, without forgetting to make a hole. When the bones have regained all their flexibility, bone the stays; that is, enter the bones into their cases.

The bones must be cut shorter than the stays. Enter them by the button-hole which you made on the wrong side, near to the eyelet-holes. Push them up to the edge of the top of the back, in order to make the other end go in. Then push the bones back towards the bottom edge, to prevent them from coming out. Do not neglect to forcefully pull the bone-case to prevent the back from puckering, that is to say, from forming crossways folds.

While you firmly hold the bone between the thumb and forefinger of your left hand, search out with your right hand, and the aid of your needle, the hole which was made in the bone. Make the needle come out on top; re-enter it in a way which encompasses the bone on both sides and over its thickness, so that it forms an eyelet-hole. By employing this procedure, you may be certain that the bone will not come out of its place.

The steel busks which are found at the ironmonger's are rounded at the ends. Such a busk, as I already said, must be covered with oiled taffety, in order to prevent rust from forming. Leave it well wrapped in this covering, and fasten it with several long running stitches. Than pass the busk between the stays and the tape meant to hold it. Pass a lace through the four eyelet-holes made in the bottom of the stays; tie the lace at that place. Also take care to make two little pads of white leather, stuffed with wadding. Each must be only the width of the busk, square, and exceed the busk by several lines. Place one pad at the top and the other at the bottom, in order to avoid direct pressure of the latter on the thighs.

The Modesty-piece. There is nothing left to do but to attach a modesty-piece to the stays. Take a sixth of an ell of percale or batiste. Fold it double, so that its selvages are together, to mark the middle. Place the middle fold over the busk; pin it at that place; work downwards, fixing it to the busk to the level just below the bosom. Beginning again at the middle fold, fix the top up to where the shoulder-strap begins. Fix the part on the edge a little on the bias. Only the part below the bosom must not be pinned. There will remain a certain fulness, for which you must form two or three plaits around where the narrow strip separates the two gores of the stays. Mark them clearly by pressing them between your thumb and your knee; this last imparts roundness.

Before removing the pins, mark by a fold the material which you must cut below the pins. First baste the folds; sew them by prick-stitching; then work a hem at each side of the modesty-piece. Finish the bottom part by binding it flat with very fine linen tape. Make a hem-case at the top. Work two eyelet-holes at each edge and in the middle of the case. Before passing the strings through, sew an embroidered edging flat onto the edge of the case; it must not be at all gathered (see Fig. 9, *ef*).

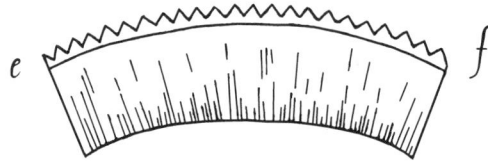

Figure 9. The modesty-piece.

Sometimes a narrow strip of batiste, an inch high, is substituted for the embroidery. This strip must be gathered to be pressed into very small folds when ironed. The strip is attached to a linen tape as narrow as a lace; the strip must be extended to the back bone.

This extra care for things which are never seen denotes an extreme neatness, a quality without which a woman cannot be really respectable.

Stays with Single Gores. This kind of stays is no easier to make than stays with double gores, except that they take less time to sew; and they suffice for persons whose bosoms are not large and whose hips are not very pronounced. The gores must be put in like those for stays with double gores.

Lined Stays. Lined stays are absolutely no different from the others, excepting their lining. I do not advise my readers to wear them—if however they are not constrained by reasons of which I shall speak later. If some of these reasons compel you to line your stays, line them with toile in preference to every other material. You will need about the same quantity of toile, as the material used to make the outer part of the stays. The toile must be of very smooth thread. After you have cut out the outer material, lay it over the toile. Above all, place the toile in the same direction as the outer material, else one of the two will soon tear. Baste them together about two fingers from the edges, in order not to interfere with the seam folds which you will make.

The basting for the gores will not require this step, for the latter are sewed with their linings, and the lining of the stays is turned down on the gores. Despite this lining, you must not omit the wide tapes on which the eyelet-holes are made; the lining is not sufficiently strong to replace them.

The back-stitched seam which joins the fronts must be made without the lining. It is only necessary to sew the latter with slightly-crossed running stitches, but without turning down. Be careful to first spread the margin of the seam of the stays to the right and left, to avoid lumps.

Place the tape which will contain the busk as for other stays. The binding of these stays does not differ in the least from that of the others.

Stays *à la Paresseuse*. This kind of stays is useful when you are travelling, when there is little time to devote to the toilet; and if you are obliged to pass the night in a carriage, you need only tie and untie to make yourself comfortable, and by this means rest more tranquilly. I am supposing that to do this, my travellers have their gowns made to open in the front, because other gowns would much be too awkward.

These stays are likewise well to put on in the morning, before dressing. If only for an hour, a woman must not appear without this garment; she would have an air of untidiness which does not at all suit her sex. In England they are even more strict on this point than in France, because decorum does not permit a woman to appear without stays or with undressed hair, even in front of her brothers.

Stays *à la paresseuse* can be made long, short, lined or not lined, with double gores or with single gores. The difference between these and the others is that the eyelet-holes are laced in a different manner.

Commence by putting the backs of these stays over each other with the wrong sides on the inside. Pierce the eyelet-holes at two fingers' distance from each other. Work them the same as for other stays.

Take some very strong lacing of well-twisted thread; cotton is handsomer, but it is not nearly sturdy enough. Cut as many pieces, half an ell long, as you have eyelet-holes. Sew the ends to the wrong side, directly between each eyelet-hole, in such a manner that the bone-case remains free. When that is done, pass all the cords sewed onto the left back into each eyelet-hole of the right back, and all the cords on the right back into the eyelet-holes of the left. Then re-pass all the cords to their original places, without putting them through the eyelet-holes; this will serve to hold the bone by flattening it on the back.

Collect half the cords on the right into a bundle; bind them together with a linen tape two fingers wide and equally long. Once the cords are sewed, over-cast the tape at its selvages, and fasten it permanently at the top. Make another bundle with the remaining cords on the same side. Then begin the like operation for the other side.

When the four bundles are finished, sew to each a cord similar to those which were passed through the eyelet-holes; fasten it with back-stitches.

The four bundles are that much more convenient, in that if one is too tight at the top without being too tight at the bottom, you may, by this means, relieve only the place which hurts.

In order to follow the curve of the waist, the cords at the top of the stays, and those at the bottom, must be the longest. Those which follow diminish gradually, the middle cords being shortest, to leave more room at the shoulder-straps as well as at the hips.

To prevent the cords from becoming tangled, which is most disagreeable and takes too long to remedy, make a species of bar of linen tape on each side of the stays near the base of the hip. This bar serves for passing the two laces which are attached to the end of each bundle. Take care to put them there as soon as you have untied the stays; this little fastening spares much trouble.

Begin by tightening the bundles at the top; otherwise, as I have already said, the flesh will push up and become red. This pernicious habit can occasion violent megrims. Although this kind of stays may be convenient, I do not advise my readers to wear them all day, because eventually they become annoying on the side, where the laces form bands.

I shall finish by encouraging my readers to put a piece with elastics about four fingers long on the end of the shoulder-strap at the back. This piece greatly aids the easy movement of the arms.

Stays with Straps. These stays are made the same as those which I described previously. They are no different but for their straps, which replace the eyelet-holes. Seven or eight are made for each side, according to the size of the stays and the width of the straps.

The straps are placed alternately; that is, when one is sewed to the upper part of the right back, the corresponding place on the left does not have one, and so on to the bottom (see Fig. 10). But these straps meet up poorly in the front. A kind has been invented where the straps pass over each other at the back, by means of openings furnished with bones, between the stays and the straps. But then the openings themselves are found to alternate; they enlarge and injure the shape. I hope my readers will not take the trouble to make them. It is rather to describe every kind of stays that I have not omitted these, than to advise my readers to wear them.

Stays for Pregnant Women, called *Brassières de Venus*.
These stays are also made like the first ones, except that the bosom gores are slit lengthways in the middle. This slit is bound with a linen tape placed *à cheval,* and sewed with side-stitches or prick-stitches; the latter is preferable for this part. The slit is then furnished with eyelet-holes; and with the bosom enlarging every day, every day you may lace the opening

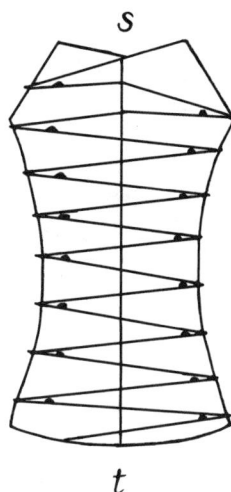

Figure 10. The back of a pair of stays with straps.

larger. But if the person for whom the stays are made intends to fulfil the most sweet and sacred of duties, that of nursing her infant, she will for that time substitute a row of buttons and button-holes for the eyelet-holes. Nothing is more convenient.

The shoulder-straps must be made, in large part, of elastics. The bottom gores of the stays must be very short and cut very high (the stomach being higher during this time), for example at three fingers near the base of the bosom. These are also made of elastics, though the front ones are laced just like the bosom gores. These stays have for a busk a length of elastic about three fingers wide, and at each side of the strip a bone about half an inch wide, and very flexible.

Half-stays or Morning Belts. To make these stays, cut out the top of an ordinary pair of stays; it makes little difference whether it has one gore or two. Allow only an inch or two of material below the base of the bosom. Then cut out bands half an ell long and a sixth of an ell high, which slope off to only an inch at the opposite end (see Fig. 11 *A*, *ab*). These straps are intended to replace the eyelet-holes; they are sewed to the back, and are often made part of it, if the material is sufficiently wide (see Fig. 11 *B*). The straps, crossed one over the other by means of a vertical slit made in one of them (see Fig. 11 *B*, *pq*) join the stays over the back, and come round to be attached in the front by a linen tape a finger wide. Do not put a busk on this kind of stays. Substitute in the front several bones about half an inch wide, and one of the same width on each side at the back. The bones support the straps and prevent them from getting into a string at the back.

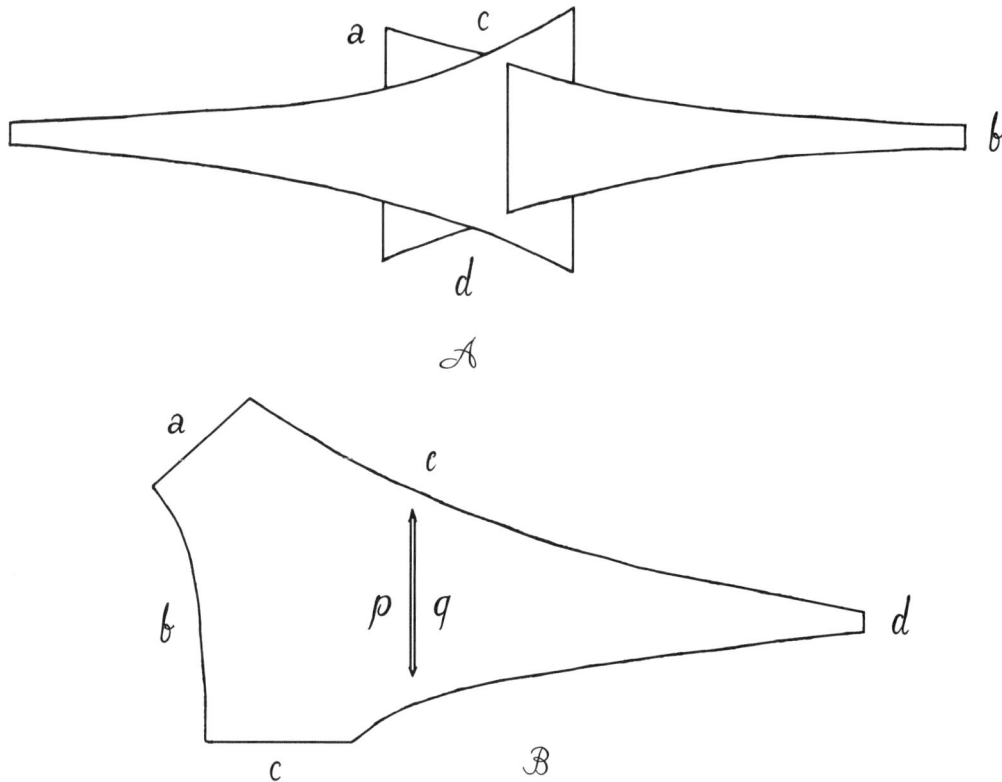

Figure 11. The straps for half-stays.

Elastic Stays. These stays are ordinarily made of dark-coloured taffety, and are worn by persons who are pregnant or in ill-health. They are beneficial and healthy, especially for children, whose size grows every day. It is quite difficult to make this kind of stays. I do not believe my readers to be endowed with the great patience required to themselves make a pair of stays entirely of elastic. Besides, that is done so rarely that I shall not give the mode. And then the work requires so much time and care, that it would be better to entrust it to practiced hands, for it takes much time meant for other, no less essential, occupations. Therefore, I shall merely show you the manner of placing pieces of elastic in rows, in order to form parts for adding to all kinds of stays.

Take two pieces of fine toile or calico, which must be cut about twice as long as the elastic, to facilitate the movement which you want to allow for it. Fasten them together at one edge. Pass a piece of elastic between the layers of material near this edge, fasten it with running stitches, and take any kind of stitch at the ends of the elastic to prevent it from coming out. Repeat the same operation for each piece of elastic which you put in the piece of material. When you reach the point of putting in the last piece, make a hem into which you will enter it. The hem must be just wide enough to enclose the elastic, and no wider.

Night Stays or *Brassières.* These are the same as stays with long straps, only when they are finished you add a piece of percale or batiste to the top of the bosom. See Fig. 12, which shows this piece placed properly over the stays. The line *ab* is the selvage of the material, of which point *a* must be placed on point *e* of the seam which joins the fronts; and the part *bc* must be gathered so that it is no wider than a finger. The bias edge *cd* is placed along the shoulder-strap, and descends to the right angle found below. The curved part *ad*, which is found at the top of the front, must be sewed to the front by over-casting. This curve is made to accommodate the bosom.

Some persons make the top of the stays separately. That is, the top is fastened to the stays only by the slanted part *bc,* which is gathered onto a linen tape wide enough to work a lengthways button-hole; the button is placed on the shoulder-strap. These stays may be made closed at the back, and fastened in the front by alternating straps, like the stays with straps described above.

The Mode of concealing Faults in the Shape. It is easy to accommodate such disadvantages, especially when it is only a matter of one side of the bosom or one shoulder being smaller than the other. Unhappily

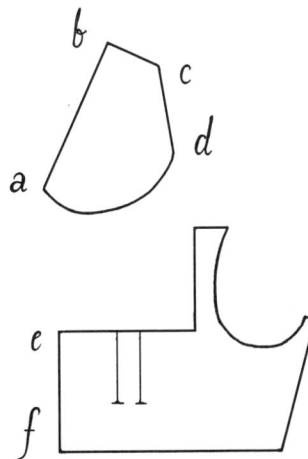

Figure 12. The front of a pair of night stays.

that is often seen, and results only from bad carriage during early youth. I also recommend the use of a weight covered by a pincushion when sewing. The work is attached to this, and not over the knee: that practice is pernicious and injurious to the health, so much so, that it injures the development of the shape.

However, if one of your sides is smaller than the other, when you try on your stays, mark the place to fill with pins, then cut out in toile the shape outlined by the pins. Place a layer of tow over the toile; then place over it a second smaller than the first; then a third smaller than the second. If the side to fill in is not very hollow, these three layers will suffice. If that is not found to be enough, add as many layers as that place requires, but take care to always make them diminish in size. When this pad is finished, fit it to the prescribed place on the wrong side so that the larger layers of tow are closest to the body. Here is the situation for wearing lined stays: the alterations will be much less visible between two layers of material.

As these pads are always placed near the edge of the stays, if you have put one on the back, bind the two pieces symmetrically, that is to say, the similar place on the other side. If the pad is on the front or the hips, do the same as for the back. Bind the stays in white satin. In every case this binding, far from injuring the stays, will only increase their sturdiness by preventing the bones from pressing directly against your flesh, and no one will perceive its purpose. This attention to appearance is quite excusable; besides, its end is to make gowns fit well.

To wash Stays. It is more important than is thought to take care in washing stays; it makes them last much longer. I am sure most of my readers will not do this work themselves; but at least they will know how to order it to be done, whether by their maid or any other person. (See also Chapter X.)

First soap the stays in cold water, then rinse them well. Take the soap again, plunging it into the water now and then, after which rub the stays several times.

Put the stays into an earthen or copper vessel. Add blue to the water which you pour into the vessel, and several shavings of soap and pieces of suet. Put the whole over a very low fire, and leave it an hour or two. Soap the stays again; that is, take a part in each hand, and rub them together. After ten or fifteen minutes of continuous rubbing, wring them out and rinse them again in clear water.

For this last operation, take rice-water into which you have put a little blue, and plunge the stays into it, taking care to soak them throughout.

Rice-water will impart a stiffness much less brittle than starch, and as if the stays were passed through a calender.

Do not wait to iron the stays until they are completely dry. Take care that the irons which you use are very clean and smooth. To achieve these two things, first, their usual place of storage must not be at all damp; second, when they are warm you must wipe them with a soft linen, then rub their surfaces and sides with white wax. That done, press them on the linen, and move them to the right and left; the sides the same way. After all that the iron will glide extremely well. It will do nothing but move easily over the stays, a thing difficult enough if you do not follow the preceding advice.

To keep your Work clean. I believe my readers will thank me for a little piece of advice which I shall give to those amongst them who may have the inconvenience of perspiring hands. The first thing is to entirely leave off washing them in cold water. Boil some bran in the water intended for this use, and do not wash them too often; for, far from decreasing perspiration, that operation increases it.

When you have washed your hands with the bran-water, dry them with a very soft linen. Obtain a small pad made of swan-skin, which is covered with corn-starch, and use it to powder your hands. This last operation has the object of drying your hands without hardening them.

Keep just a little clear water into which you put a few drops of brandy or Cologne water. This little bit of water serves for dipping your fingers up to the base of your finger-nails, in order to strengthen them, and to remove the powder attached to them.

If you are careful to do all that I have just recommended, and if in addition you do not forget the little emery ball, your work will emerge fresh from your hands.

——*Art de faire les corsets, les guêtres, et les gants.*

Diversion 2.

Ladies' Stays. The twenty-eight-inch stays are about the middle size, and these are cut according to the following dimensions: sixteen inches long in the front, seventeen inches long at the back, and thirty-eight inches round the bottom. (See Fig. 13.) Seven and a half inches will be the half width of the front piece at the bottom, and two gores let in four inches, two and a half inches wide at the top of each gore, which will make half the width of the front two and a half inches. There is another kind, of a different make, called a jubilee front. This requires a seam up the front

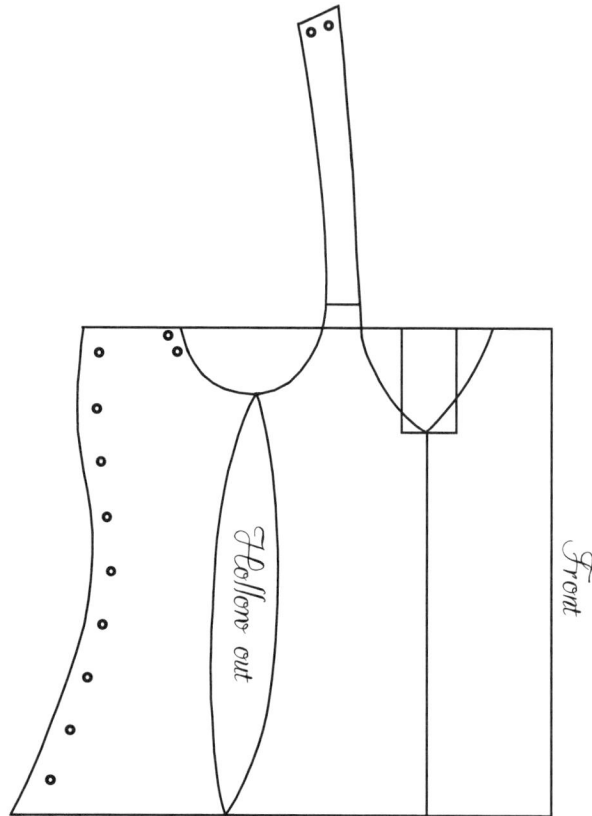

Figure 13. A pattern for a pair of stays.

piece, and two and a half inches allowed on each side, to make them the proper width at the top of the front piece. The back is four and three-quarters inches wide between the shoulders. The arm-hole is six inches wide, and four and three-quarters inches deep. The size is taken in the small of the waist.

These stays will take a yard of eighteen-inch sateen. The sizes are from twenty-four to thirty-two inches, and they vary an inch each in width, and a quarter of an inch in length.

——*Sectum*.

Chapter XV.
The Art of the Mantua-maker
or Cutter of Gowns.

The art of the mantua-maker encompasses the manner of cutting out gowns, of sewing them, and of trimming them. (See Divs. 1, 2, and 3.) I shall treat of each in turn, commencing with how to sew. However, I shall not speak of the tools required by the mantua-maker and the *lingère*, such as the scissors, thimble, &c; they are too well known. I shall say only that when you sew firm material, you should protect the right portion of your left forefinger, below the nail, from needle pricks by putting a finger-stall there—a little device of horn or bone similar to a ring, widened to almost an inch in the middle; the old *bagues à bateau* give the idea of the shape.

Common Stitches and Seams.

There are several kinds of stitches: the running stitch, the over-cast stitch, the side-stitch or hem-stitch, the back-stitch, the herring-bone stitch, the button-hole stitch, and the chain-stitch, which is very seldom used. There are also divers kinds of seams, including the flat seam, the seam *à la reine*, the lace seam, and the seam called the mantua-maker's hem; as well as hems properly speaking.

The Running Stitch. This stitch is very simple. When the needle is threaded, and the thread is terminated by a knot, pass the needle through the material, taking more or fewer threads according to its thickness. Bring out the needle and re-enter it a distance equal to the number of threads which you took previously; and so on. (See Fig. 1 *A*.) A very long running stitch is used for tacking or basting; that is, passing the thread through the pieces of material to fasten them together temporarily. You remove these threads when the sewing is done. The running stitch is combined in a seam with other stitches. To work it more comfortably, attach the material over your knee with a pin.

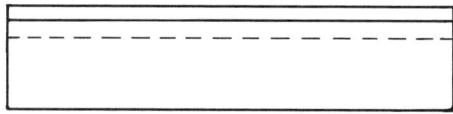

A

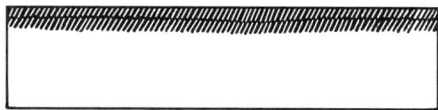

B

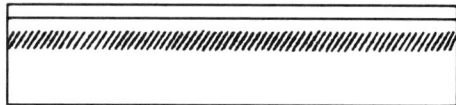

C

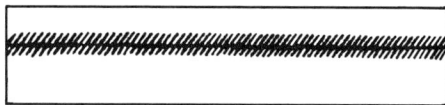

D

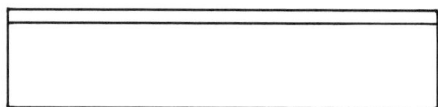

E

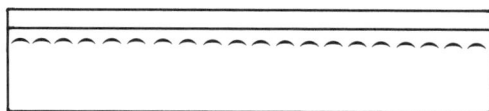

F

Figure 1. Stitches, seams, and hems.

The Over-cast Stitch. This stitch is no less easy. Take two pieces of material, each of which you fold over several lines the entire length of the material, to prevent it from fraying; this is called the seam fold. Then place one piece over the other, fold against fold, basting them together if you are not at all accustomed to sewing. Take them between the thumb and forefinger of your left hand; then sew the two pieces of material with a threaded needle, sticking it quite straight into the side of the material which presses your forefinger.

For this stitch, unlike all the others, it is needless to knot the end of the thread in order to fasten it when you begin. That would produce a disagreeable thickness in the over-casting which, when well executed, resembles a kind of *cordonnet* (see Chapter XIX). Before pulling all the thread in bringing the needle out from the pieces, leave a short end of thread, and fold it across between the two materials; it will be concealed and secured by the subsequent stitches. This mode also serves to join on a fresh thread when one chances to break, or when the thread in the needle runs out.

To continue over-casting, when the needle has gone through both materials, pull it out quite straight, and re-enter it very near, in the same manner, always from the side of your forefinger. Continue taking stitches close together, always entering the needle as close as possible to the edge of the two pieces of material, and bringing it out so that no stitch exceeds another (see Fig. 1 *B*). Over-casting ought to be a close and unbroken line of stitches. Take good care that your stitches are equal as to spacing and width. When over-casting is seen from the wrong side, the stitches should be seen to penetrate along the same thread of the material. Attach the material vertically to your belt when you do over-casting.

When you over-cast two bands of material with selvages, do not make a seam fold, and bite still less with the stitches than when you have made a fold. Biting is the action of taking up more or less material with the stitches. When the material has no selvages, and therefore must have seam folds, you ordinarily sew a flat seam on the wrong side of the over-casting, taking care to fold down one side of the material a little more than the other, so that the wider fold will cover the narrower one. When one of the two pieces has a selvage, it is the selvage which will cover. Do not turn down the selvage unless you wish. The other edge is the only one at risk of fraying, and you will find it a proper width to be covered. It is better, however, to turn it down by two or three threads, because it often happens that you are obliged to trim the one which exceeds it, which wastes time and injures sturdiness.

Proceed thus to work the flat seam: first flatten the over-casting a little; then turn the two pieces of material it has joined to the wrong side. Spread them over your knee, then turn down the wider seam fold over the narrower one. Go in several threads along this flattened fold; then you may sew it like a hem, one side of the material placed before you (see the article on hems).

When the flat seam is too wide it is more easily made, but coarse. When it is too narrow it makes the over-casting pucker, and gives considerable difficulty. If the seam fold (above all that of a flat seam, and principally when it is on the selvage) has not been made evenly, the flat seam is disagreeably scolloped.

When the over-casting joins two pieces of satin, taffety, or in general any silk material, do not work a flat seam. Content yourself with flattening the over-casting with your thimble, spread the two folds which you have turned down, and pass a thread over each seam fold to prevent it from fraying. For this use over-cast stitches, but less slanted, and twenty times more separated; in this case the over-casting is always on the wrong side; mantua-makers constantly do it this way. Only *lingères* put it on the right side, the over-casting of two selvages excepted; because such over-casting, not having a seam fold, appears on the wrong side as a crease in the material. The flat seam is attached over your knee for working.

The Seam *à la Reine*. This is an over-casting without any seam folds, which all the same must not fray. To achieve this, it suffices to space the stitches very closely, slanting them in an imperceptible manner. It is necessary to bite in a little more, so that the material will support the seam, and to aid in forming the *cordonnet*. This kind of seam, much used for fastening together bands of gauze, muslin, or light taffety trimming, must be used only in that way. Its want of sturdiness prohibits its use on materials of a certain strength and a certain length.

The Lace Seam. This seam is intended to increase the width of laces or pointed tulles. It therefore joins the selvage of a lace to the selvage of a tulle (the term selvage is especially applied to a band of lace without borders or points, having selvages on both edges). The selvage of a lace is composed of little crossways threads and round holes, which alternately succeed each other. Therefore you sew, with very fine thread, the bars of one selvage to the bars of the other, and the holes to the corresponding holes.

The seam which unites laces lengthways is no less simple. When you have to work it, take the two ends of your lace, and lay them over each other flat, overlapping them more or less according to the width of the lace; because this seam must be worked on the bias, that is, the slanting line which crosses the lace. It is proper to lightly baste this seam, so as not to risk distorting the slanting net-work of the lace underneath. When you have accurately positioned both ends of the lace, so that their respective slanting lines are precisely aligned, thread a needle with lace thread. Fasten it at the join of the selvages; and holding the laces folded over your left forefinger, between your thumb and third finger, catch at the same time the little bar on top and the little bar underneath, at the right of each mesh which forms the slanting line. Only pass the needle under these two united bars, though the thread does not seem to encompass them, because the next stitch fastens the thread over them in finishing the previous stitch, and so on. This prevents it from being seen; but if you wish for a rather more visible but sturdier seam, pass the needle twice at each mesh. The designs which you encounter are sewed in the same manner, only your stitch must catch the whole flat thread of which designs are ordinarily formed.

Finish by passing the thread several times at the middle of the edge of the lace, on top of the *picot*, and fasten it by winding and re-winding it over itself. The thickness of the edge will prevent it from being seen. It remains only to cut off the excess pieces of lace on top and underneath, with sharp scissors. If the seam is well made, it cannot be distinguished from the slanting continuation of the net-work.

The Side-stitch. For side-stitches (see Fig. 1 C) first knot the end of the thread. Then stick the needle into the bias of the material, taking care to turn the point towards your left shoulder when you bring it out, after having taken several threads. Re-enter it in the same way, and at a distance equal to the number of threads which you have already taken. Side-stitches serve for flat seams, replacing over-cast stitches, and are turned down like over-cast seams. They are used principally to make hems, and they also bear the name of hem-stitches for that reason.

For flat seams, lay one of the pieces of material you wish to sew over the other, taking care that the one on your side is over the one which you sew. This side must be a little lower than the other, in order that the other may be turned down over it, as I explained for over-casting. It is important to baste a flat seam if you have not made them often, for it is difficult to make the stitches follow a perfectly straight line owing to their slanting position; otherwise the seam will form very disagreeable undulations. Moreover, you will often do well to baste your seams, of whatsoever kind, to prevent gradually taking up more material on the side where you sew, than on the other. Without this precaution, you will unwittingly do so, especially when the pieces of material are cut on the bias.

When you wish to join the edges of two pieces of material, such as the bottom of a lined sleeve, or the top of the collar of a night jacket, make a seam fold on each piece, as when you prepare to over-cast. Then place the piece closest to yourself several threads lower than the other, and sew them with side-stitches. It is fairly common to sew a row of running stitches several lines farther from the edge than the first seam, in order to prevent the seam from stretching too much, especially when the pieces are cut on the bias.

The Mantua-maker's Hem or Seam. This seam is worked as follows: lay two pieces of material one over the other as for a flat seam; then turn down the piece which you have left a little higher over the lower piece, placed before you; make a narrow seam fold on the first piece. Then re-fold the portion of the two pieces over the first fold, like a hem; sew this seam fold along the two pieces with side-stitches (see Fig. 1 D). The roll which forms the mantua-maker's hem is narrow and rounded, and pleasing besides. You must take great care to enter the needle forcefully for this kind of seam, especially if the material is firm, because it must pass through both pieces of material, and the portions turned down for the seam, all at once. Do not knot the thread to join on a fresh one for this seam, nor for a hem. At the first stitch with the newly-threaded needle, leave a short end of thread, which you re-enter in the hem. The mantua-maker's hem is made over the finger; that is, in sewing you fold the material over the forefinger of your left hand and hold it there with the neighbouring finger and your thumb: this process is very convenient and saves considerable time. Few seams permit it because of the risk of unintentionally taking up too much material.

Hemming. Hems which are attached by side-stitches are an essential part of sewing; there are scarcely any articles of clothing, large or small, where they are not used. To work one well, begin by making a narrow fold, of several threads of material. With your right hand, pick up as much material as it can hold, in large folds; turn down and crease the narrow fold with your thumb (see Fig. 1 E). When your right hand is full, let go of the material and start over as before. This first part of the fold finished, continue in this way to the distance required by the length of your hem. Your first fold thus completed, make a second one.

Place the material which you have folded over your left forefinger, and hold it with your thumb and left middle finger. Stick the needle crossways into the material, then into the edge of the seam fold; continue the side-stitch. When the hem is large and a cord is passed through it, it is called a string-case.

When you hem gauze, bands of trimming, in short every thing which requires little care or sturdiness, use running stitches. Since in this case you pass the needle through the material five or six times without the necessity of withdrawing it, you take six stitches at a time; this greatly hastens the work. Attach the hem over your knee when it is sufficiently long that you can conveniently do so.

The Back-stitch. Back-stitches require more attention than the preceding ones. The pieces sewed with this stitch are placed over each other evenly, because back-stitches are never used to make a flat seam. After having knotted the thread, pass your needle flat into the material, and bring it out at a distance of several threads. Re-enter it at the same place where you brought it out, and bring it out ahead the same number of threads as for your first stitch. Return backwards, always covering your stitch in this way. Back-stitches all appear taken one into another (see Fig. 1 *F*), and are at the same time very sturdy and very pretty; but they call for great care. It is necessary to count the threads often when positioning the needle. *Lingères* employ back-stitches extremely rarely in sewing, but great use is made of them in prick-stitching.

Prick-stitching is always done from the right side of the material. Make a seam fold on the piece you wish to prick-stitch, then tack or baste with stitches of moderate size, because it is essential and very difficult to work a perfectly straight line with back-stitches. Place the piece due to be prick-stitched, horizontally flat upon the one to which it is to be joined. Begin a row of back-stitches several lines from the edge which forms the seam fold. Quite commonly a second row of back-stitches is made at an interval of several threads from the first row (see Fig. 2 *A*). This is the manner of making up all the pieces which compose the body of a gown; it is also much used for gentlemen's shirts. Fasten the piece which you wish to prick-stitch over your knee.

The other use for the back-stitch requires less care. It serves to make seams which, since they are always placed on the wrong side of the material, do not require the perfect regularity of the prick-stitch. Place two pieces of material evenly one over the other, but without making a seam fold, and without one side exceeding the other. The seam must be made a little below. Sometimes it is composed entirely of back-stitches, sometimes of alternating back-stitches and running stitches (see Fig. 2 *B* and *C*).

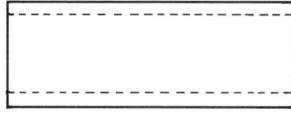

A

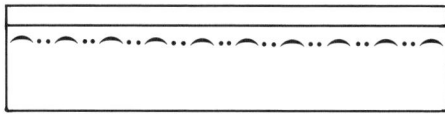

B

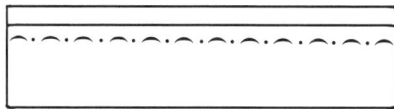

C

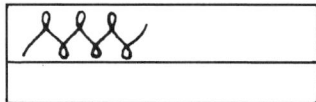

D

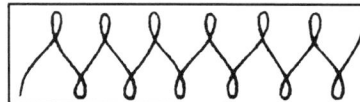

E

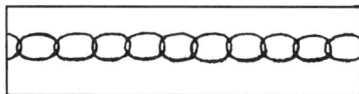

F

G

Figure 2. Stitches and a button-hole.

I have said that these seams must bite more material than the others, because you then make a fold on each side of the seam to prevent fraying. After that sew the two pieces together by a long, slightly slanted over-cast stitch; this is a kind of permanent basting. You ordinarily re-use the thread passed in tacking or basting a back-stitched seam. Pull by the knot which begins the basting stitches, and they will all come out at once.

The Herring-bone Stitch. For this the material is ordinarily a piece more or less wide, either furnished with a wide seam fold to be fastened by the herring-bone stitches, or one meant to be attached to a larger piece by these stitches. I shall describe the first situation.

Take the material you wish to work on between the thumb and middle finger of your left hand, so that it folds over your forefinger. The side of the seam fold is placed to the left of your forefinger. Put the end of the thread, under the end of the seam fold on the right, and turning the eye of the needle to the side opposite to you, stick it into the turned-down edge of the seam fold, as if to take an ordinary running stitch. Then re-enter it on the left, at the back, slantways above the first stitch, at the top of the fold. Again take a running stitch there, so that you make a stitch extended slantways from the first stitch. Then, always holding the point of the needle towards you, take another running stitch on the turned-down edge of the seam fold on the right, at the level of the first stitch, so that a new stitch extended slantways, beginning from the upper-left stitch, is parallel to the other slantways stitch. Putting this upper stitch between the two lower stitches gives the shape of an A to the three stitches which form the herring-bone stitch. Since you always bring the needle back behind, the running stitches are found to be covered and the threads crossed (see Fig. 2 *D*).

To begin another herring-bone stitch, enter the needle to the left at the level of the previous upper stitch, then lower it to the right, slantways and parallel to the level of the lower stitch, and so on. This operation will give you a series of slanting stitches, crossed in a parallel way (see Fig. 2 *E*).

Herring-boning is always worked from left to right. It is used to sew down seams with only a single fold, to avoid excessive thickness, and not for seams which have a second, narrow fold to prevent fraying. The seams of stockings, stays, and toile slippers are almost always furnished with herring-bone stitches, because these articles are tight fitting, and it is necessary to avoid projecting seams as much as possible.

The Button-hole Stitch. It is thus named because it necessarily reinforces the short slits through which you pass the buttons sometimes used to fasten clothing over the body. To work this stitch easily, commence by very firmly holding your material over the forefinger of your left hand, with the aid of the thumb and third finger of the same hand. Then take an over-cast stitch well in; but when passing the needle through the material, before pulling the thread all the way, pass it through the little loop of thread before it is drawn close; then pull the needle backwards so that the eye faces you. Continue the same operation, taking your stitches from left to right, contrary to what you have done until now; all the stitches previously discussed are taken from right to left.

Button-hole stitches must be perfectly regular, taken neither more nor less deep into the material, and with none closer together than the others. When you have continued in this manner completely round the little slit, take a little upright over-cast stitch at each extremity, into the stitches closest to the ends of the slit; this is called the bar. (See Fig. 2 *F.*)

The Chain-stitch. This stitch is scarcely ever used except to form a kind of embroidery on the edges of the cuffs of a gentleman's shirt-sleeves, and on the upper sides of gloves (see Chapter XIX). It is done in this fashion: begin by entering the needle from below the material which you wish to decorate with this stitch. Pull through the entire length of thread (which must be fastened). Then bring the thread under your left thumb, and enter the needle as close as possible to the place where you pulled it out. Bring it out again several threads farther, in the middle of the loop formed by the thread held under your thumb; always holding the thread under your left thumb, pull it towards you, and the first chain-stitch is formed. Then stick the needle again into that stitch, very near the place where you brought it out; *voilà,* another stitch; and so on (see Fig. 2 G).

These are all the kinds of stitches which mantua-makers use to sew gowns. (See Div. 4.) Let us now see how to cut gowns out and make them up.

General Rules for Gowns.

A gown is composed of a skirt, body, and sleeves. I shall describe only the way to cut out the skirt, because the other parts change their shapes continually. To try to describe them all would be an impossible task, and useless besides, because fashions which I would try to represent would soon be outmoded for ever. (Chapter XVI gives some ways to make up gowns so that you may easily alter them.) I shall not discuss them excepting articles which are always cut the same, whatever ornaments may be put there besides. (See Div. 5.)

To cut out the Skirt. The skirt is prepared by first cutting out the breadths (a breadth is a piece of material between its two selvages, and of indeterminate length). The breadths must extend from the belt to the feet. If the material is three-quarters of an ell wide, cut four breadths, one to make the back, one for the front, and the two last for the side gores: a gore is a breadth cut sloped.

Fold your front breadth in half lengthways. Next re-fold it, from the top to the sides, to mark a sloping or bias line more or less long according to what you propose to add to the front gores to extend this line. The fold will serve to guide your scissors. Take care to bring the line closer in as you advance towards the top of the breadth, in order to fit the shape of your hips well. In Fig. 3 *A*, *a* shows the front of a gown with the sloping line completed; *b* shows how it is cut. The gore added at the bottom is the same one subtracted from the top.

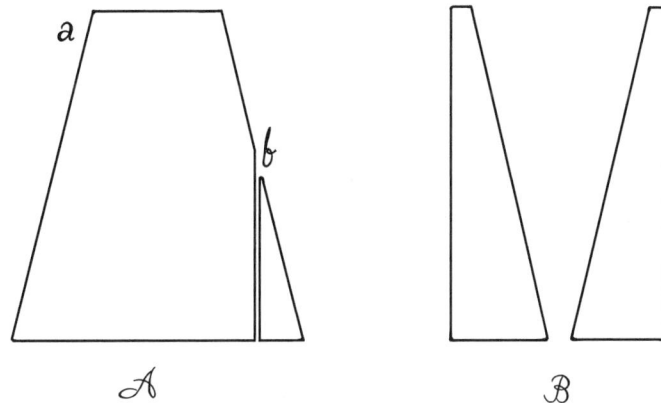

Figure 3. The front breadth and the side gores.

Leave the back breadth between the two selvages without subtracting any thing from it. Then mark a sloping line on each of the two remaining breadths for the side gores. This line must be marked quite narrow, and on only one side of the breadths (see Fig. 3 *B*). If the material has a wrong side, place one breadth over the other in such a manner that the right sides touch, in order to be sure that both sloping lines will be cut in the same direction. Take this precaution for all the parts of the gown which you will cut in pairs, in any material which has a wrong side. Failing that, it will come about that one of the two parts cannot be used.

To make up the Skirt. Your side gores being cut out, join them by the straight-way or the selvage (the straight-way is the edge of the material which is not on the bias). Join the straight-way to the back breadth, putting the narrower end of the side gore at the top. The sewing which joins them is ordinarily the back-stitch and the running stitch alternated. Do not overcast the seam, because you have two selvages, which will not fray.

The back breadth thus united to the side gores presents a sloping or bias line. Join this line to that of the front by a seam of continuous back-stitches, or a mantua-maker's hem. The joining of these two bias edges requires great care. This seam cannot be made while pinned over your knee or even held over your left forefinger, as I described earlier. You must take it between your thumb and forefinger; otherwise the biases will stretch and become distorted. Tighten the stitches of this seam imperceptibly, and take good care not to pull the biases when basting it. Failing that, the skirt will drag on the side, and it will be necessary to unpick the seam and start over.

Some mantua-makers first sew together two breadths, which make up the back. Then they cut a third breadth slantways in the middle, from top to bottom, to make a gore for each side (see Fig. 4 A, cc). Because the narrow end of the gore is always at the top of the skirt, one of these pieces must be placed upside down and on the reverse (see Fig. 4 B). But this fashion of cutting out the skirt has two disadvantages: the first is that the bias slopes too much; the second is that, when the wrong side of the material differs from the face, you must take the second gore from a different breadth.

You may also form the sloping line by adding the gores removed from the front breadth, to the two breadths sewed together for the back. These gores are not ordinarily long enough to go from the top to the bottom of the

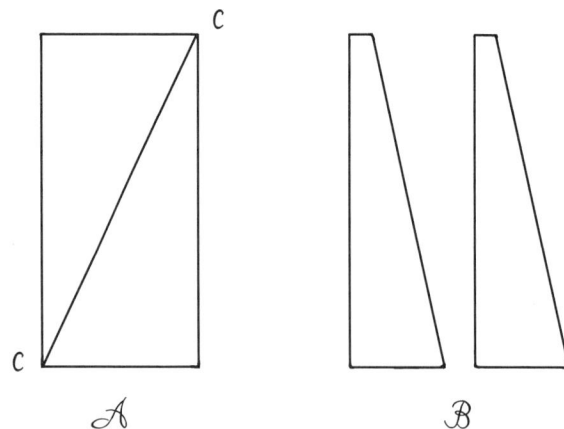

Figure 4. Another mode of cutting the side gores.

back breadths, so you complete the bias by removing a small gore from the top of each back breadth (see Fig. 5). This mode, which requires less time, is disadvantageous for materials with flowers, or designs which are always placed in the same direction. Because the wide end of these gores is taken from the top of the front breadth, but must be placed at the bottom of the back, the flowers will necessarily be in the contrary direction.

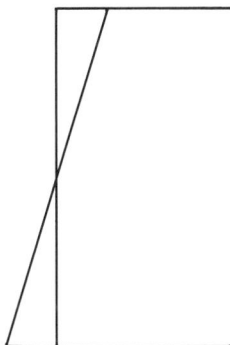

Figure 5. To add a bias to the back breadth.

Pay attention to precisely matching the stripes or designs of the material, if it has any: this precaution applies only to sewing the side gores to the back. You may easily see that the sloping lines of the side gores and the front interrupt the continuity of the design. There is an art to joining them pleasingly, especially stripes, which is to form a chevron (see Fig. 6 *A*). But that is unimportant.

Whatever may be the modes which you adopt amongst these to cut out the skirt, it must always have a width of two and a quarter, to two and a half, ells at the bottom, and an ell and three-quarters, to two ells, at the top; according to the size of the person.

If you wish to cut out a redingote, cut your material as described previously; only make the front breadth a sixth of an ell wider (by cutting the gore narrower) and slit it along the middle from top to bottom. This extra sixth serves to make a hem on each side of the divided front breadth, and for lapping the fronts when fastening the redingote on the body. (Chapter XII explains how to attach the fastenings. Div. 6 gives more details on tailor-made riding habits, pelisses, and spencers.)

When the skirt is not a redingote, make a slit a sixth of an ell long in the top of the back breadth, in the middle, to make the skirt easier to put on. This slit should be furnished with a very narrow hem, but it is best

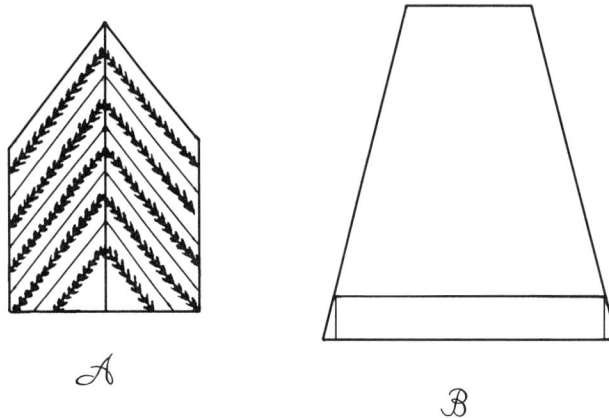

Figure 6. To match stripes and to fold up the hem.

to put a braid there. The addition of a little heart-shaped piece or button-hole stitches at the end of the slit, to prevent it from lengthening, does not always achieve that end.

The skirt being made up, that is to say, all the breadths which compose it being sewed together, work a wide hem all round the bottom. The width which the gores impart to the bottom being somewhat greater than a little above it, you will experience some awkwardness in making your hem meet at the seams. Overcome this by folding the excess width over itself (see Fig. 6 *B*).

To make up the Body. I shall only discuss what is invariably done with the body, whatsoever the shape given it. (See Div. 7.) First, it commonly has a seam which joins the front to a small piece called the side-piece, which forms the part under the arm. The front is laid over the side-piece, and the seam is prick-stitched. The side-piece is in turn laid down and prick-stitched over the piece which forms the back of the body.

The body being made up, baste it over a wide linen tape, so that it will have the strength to resist all the movements of your waist. Just as commonly, a band is used; this is three inches wide, and of a length to precisely encircle your waist. Measure the half of the band, likewise the body, and attach them together at their middles. Place this band over the bottom of the body on the right side, prick-stitch it, then fold it to the wrong side over the linen tape, taking care that it hides the raw edges of the pieces of the body. Baste it, then sew it with very close side-stitches.

I shall not describe the sleeves excepting modes which are always followed despite variations in fashion. Thus when it comes to setting in the sleeves, that is, sewing them round the arm-hole (the circular opening formed by the shoulder-piece and the side-piece), begin by hollowing out the sleeve; that is, by cutting a curved piece from the top (see Fig. 7 A). This hollow, which is always placed on the front side of the body, has the object of easing movement of your arm.

The sleeve is divided in half, as well as the arm-hole. Attach the top of the seam which joins the sleeve, to the top of the prick-stitched seam which joins the side-piece to the front of the body (see Fig. 7 B). The other part of the sleeve is attached to the other part of the arm-hole. Then baste the sleeve, without making any plaits, round the part which goes under the armpit. Next arrange the other part by gathering it (see below), and work a circular seam with very close back-stitches. When the body is not lined, encircle the arm-hole with a flat braid, with the aid of a basting whose stitches pierce the right side very little. Make a seam fold all round the arm-hole before placing the braid there; the basting which attaches it is permanent. (Chapter VII describes how to furnish the arm-holes to prevent stains from perspiration.)

To set on the Skirt. There is nothing more to do but to set the skirt onto the body. First make a seam fold on the skirt, as described above for

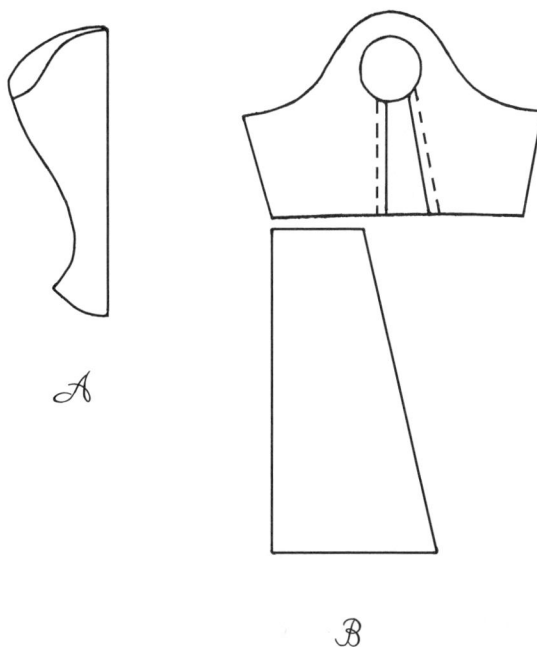

A

B

Figure 7. The sleeve and the manner of assembling the gown.

over-cast or prick-stitched seams, taking care to turn down this fold much more deeply in the front, especially in the middle. Without this precaution, the skirt would crease widthways over your stomach in a most disagreeable manner.

Divide the body and skirt in half, and attach the corresponding divisions to each other. The seam which attaches the side gores to the front of the skirt, must meet the seam which joins the front of the body to the side-piece (see Fig. 7 *B*). If you have set the body onto a belt or band, attach the skirt to the band on the wrong side by over-casting. Otherwise, set the skirt onto the bottom of the body with prick-stitches, and work them up to the place where you must sew the folds of the skirt while gathering them.

To gather, take long running stitches without fastening the thread except by a knot which you may pull at will, which brings together more or less material over the thread, and forms the folds. These must always be even, whatsoever their size. When you have thus gathered each side of the skirt, in the space between the slit at the back, and the place on the waist which you have marked for sewing the folds, fasten them, one by one and very close together, with one or two over-cast stitches. If the skirt is set on by over-casting, continue to sew on the wrong side. If, on the contrary, you are using prick-stitches, turn the gown over to the right side, so that you may sew the folds from that side.

Of lining a Gown. Cut out the breadths for your lining exactly like those of the outer material. Then spread the two corresponding breadths on a table; the back breadth of the outer material, the back breadth of the lining; the side gores of the outer material, the side gores of the lining; and so on. Lay the corresponding pieces one over the other, but not at all carelessly. It is important that the lining be resting on the table. Commence by basting the pieces together, on the side opposite to the side in front of you.

Lift the outer material, folding it over itself several times, lightly passing your hand, fully open, over each fold, so that the creases will serve to guide you later. The folds must be about a sixteenth of an ell apart. When you have thus folded the material until it has no more than a sixteenth interval up to your first basting, freeze it; that is to say, baste it permanently.

To do so, thread a needle with double or triple the quantity of thread which you ordinarily use. Stick the needle into the outer material and the lining, scarcely piercing it. Re-enter the needle at a distance of a little less than a sixteenth, always catching the outer material and the lining at the same time, to take a long stitch concealed between the two materials (see Fig. 8 A). When the thread has run out, knot a new one onto the short end remaining. You do not even need to cut the two ends left above the knot; the thread will not be seen at all, either on the right side, or on the reverse. Your first row of basting finished, turn down the next fold of the outer material, and begin another row along the crease formed by your hand.

Depart from this mode when lining sleeves: do not freeze the lining to the outer material. Fold the sleeve in half lengthways on one side, likewise the lining on the other. Baste them together on the wrong side like two separate sleeves, then sew them with a seam composed entirely of back-stitches (see Fig. 8 B). Put your hand into the lining and turn it right

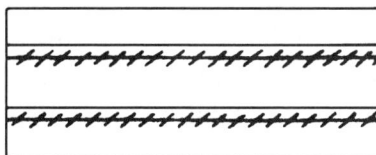

A

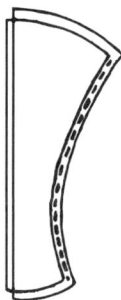

B

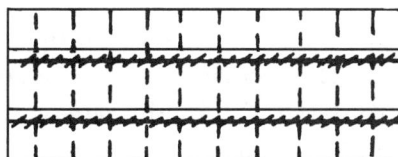

C

Figure 8. To line a gown.

side out. The sleeve will be found to encircle the lining from top to bottom. The seam will have two right sides; one on the side of the sleeve, and one on the side of the lining.

When the gown is wadded, that is, you have placed a tissue of un-spun cotton called wadding between the outer material and its lining, do not follow the mode I have just described for the sleeves; freeze as explained for the manner of lining. (See Fig. 8 C.)

The application of a lining changes a little the manner of making up the skirt. Whether the seam is on the straight-way or on the bias, the two outer pieces of material are sewed together with the lining of the first piece; then the lining of the next piece is turned down and sewed over the raw edges.

For example, suppose you begin to make up the skirt at the back. Lay the outer material of the back and its lining together, wrong side to wrong side. Lay the outer material of the side gore on top, right side to right side with the outer material of the back. Baste all three pieces together on the side where the side gore must fold out. Sew this seam with back-stitches, either alone or mixed with running stitches, as required. Then flatten the three narrow edges of the seam towards the side gore, folding the side gore out to its proper place. Turn down one edge of the side gore lining and lay it over the three raw edges of the previous seam, so that it conceals them. Sew this lining seam fold down with side-stitches.

You now have the side gore and its lining positioned with their wrong sides together. Lay the next piece over the outer material of the side gore, and continue as described above all the way round the skirt. For the last seam, where the last side gore and the back will be joined, fold the lining of one side out of the way when joining the other three pieces, so that it may be side-stitched down over this last seam.

When you are to wad a gown, cut out the breadths of wadding exactly the same as those of the lining and the outer material. The wadding, which is sold by the piece, presents a cohesive surface. It is necessary to divide it in half by splitting the piece from one side and opening it out; it will then present a very soft fleece. This fleece must be placed on the lining so that the warmth may be more readily felt by the person who puts on the gown. Spread the breadth of lining on a table, and the breadth of wadding on top. Fasten them together with rows of long running stitches placed crossways, a thirty-second of an ell apart. Then freeze the layers as I described for a lining. Pay close attention to piercing the wadding and the lining at the same time.

Divers Trimmings.

Divers Trimmings.

The capriciousness of fashion, which is chiefly expressed in the style of the trimmings of a gown, binds me to describe only the manner of placing them at an equal distance from each other, and the steps to take in that regard in order to have less trouble and to make them better. (Chapter XII gives advice on choosing them.) But I also believe that the extreme variety of fashion forces it to return often to trimmings previously abandoned; all the better that its inventions have after all a narrow enough scope in this matter.

Therefore, I shall add sufficiently extensive details of present and past forms of trimmings. Here are their various kinds: flounces; rouleaux; folds; biases; braids; fringe; plain *entre-deux;* embroidered tulle or muslin *entre-deux;* the fancy *entre-deux à dents de loup* or *à poignet, dents de harpie,* and *trou-trou-popoye;* draperies; *agrafes;* divers ruches; and panes. The mixture and variety of these numerous trimmings will, I hope, put young persons in a position to brave all the capricious revivals of fashions.

Flounces. These are the principal and almost the only constant trimming; for though their position and width vary infinitely, bands gathered and sewed onto gowns are almost continuously in use. When flounces are very wide, that is to say a quarter or a third of an ell, or more, they are called *falbalas;* but the cut is always the same.

Sometimes flounces are bands of muslin, embroidered gauze, or percale which are embroidered, scolloped, or hemmed. (See Div. 8.) Sometimes in hemming them a cord is put between the first and second folds of the hem, which covered and concealed by the hem, lends support to the edge of the flounce. Sometimes the bands of flounces are cut into great scolloped points or Vandykes; and in hemming the points, a cord is inserted as I have just explained.

Corded Piping for the Edge of a Flounce, or what you please. Again these points may be hemmed with a corded piping. This fashion of employing cord is much prettier and has lasted much longer than the preceding one. Here is how to proceed: cut a narrow strip of material on the bias, similar or not to the material you wish to border, according to the received style. This narrow strip or piping is about a finger wide, according to the size of the cord to be covered. The piping being cut, take it between the thumb and forefinger of your left hand, folding it double from one end to the other, so that it produces a crease in the middle all along the piping. Place your cord between the two portions of the folded strip. Push it all the way to the crease, holding it quite tight with the nail of your left thumb, so that the piping assumes the shape of the cord there. Then sew the cord inside the piping with tolerably long running stitches; the edges opposite to the cord remain together and in parallel. That achieved, place the covered cord over the right side of the piece to be bordered, in such a manner that the cord is farthest from you, and the raw edges of the piping strip and the piece being bordered are together.

Then back-stitch all along the thread which fastens the cord, catching the three edges together. Take care to hold it very firmly, or attach it over your knee with a pin, so that the cord does not become detached or stretch. If you border points without holding the cord firmly, it is impossible to attach it. The seam of the three edges finished, lift the cord, turning both edges of the piping under the bordered piece. Your cord then appears as if glued to the edge of the piece, for you see no trace of the stitches. Fell down the edges of the piping strip with very small stitches.

Some mantua-makers fasten the corded piping under the piece by basting, or with long herring-bone stitches. When you have thus bordered narrow bands or cuffs, join the two sides together on the right and left, under the edges of the piping, on the wrong side. Then too you may often content yourself with applying them underneath and passing the ball of your thumb flat over the top. You may do this without difficulty, because you place the strip or cuff flat on the material, while sewing the two sides along the length of the cord, in the narrow groove formed by the join of the cuff and the cord. The under side of the cuff is entirely hidden; the back-stitches which must be made in the groove are no longer visible. This succeeds in rendering the border very neat and pretty.

I have given all these details about corded piping because you may now use it to make all the sleeve, collar, and cuff borders which are in some sort the shoulder-straps of gown bodies. Milliners also employ corded piping, and tailors use it to border ladies' mantles. When *douillettes* and redingotes have no trimmings, they are elegantly bordered by a cord in this fashion.

To sew on a Flounce. Flounces have been arranged in a thousand ways. Sometimes there are four, six, eight, or more rows, one above another. Sometimes two or three are grouped together, with greater intervals between the groups. Sometimes they imitate the shape of a cone, which is called trimming *en if,* by successively placing narrow strips of shorter and shorter length, according to the height of the cone. Sometimes they are made to depict waves. Sometimes they are placed slantways close together all round the gown, and called trimmings *à la fille d'honneur,* or at equal intervals. In short, I would never finish if I had to describe all conceivable variations. Though that task is impossible I shall discuss flounces at length, because they are also used to trim night jackets, *fichus,* and caps.

Take care to measure, with a piece of pasteboard of the height determined upon, the distance between the hem and the first row of trimming, that between the first row and the second, and so on. Each time you apply your pasteboard measure upright on the gown, place a pin crossways over the measure, which will give you a row of pins all round the gown. Then replace the pins by passing a thread whose colour contrasts strongly with that of the material, in order to guide you. When the hem is very wide, also take a small pasteboard measure and apply it on top from time to time, to see that every thing is even.

Next divide the skirt into quarters, marking each quarter with a pin or by passing a bit of thread there, which you loop; divide and mark the trimming in the same manner. Attach each division of the trimming to the corresponding division of the skirt. If you are unpracticed, divide each quarter in half, then even out the folds.

If the flounces are of transparent material such as gauze or muslin, make a roll on the side of the band which you wish to sew to the skirt. This roll is made by slightly rolling the band with your left thumb, over the forefinger of the same hand; it must be narrow and quite even. Then gather by passing the needle under the roll.

The seam for the flounce should be made on its wrong side, and by over-casting. First mark a crease on the gown, following the thread tracing all round. Place the band (see Fig. 9, *e*) upside down over the gown. Sew on the trimming by taking a stitch at each fold formed by the gathering. Then turn the flounce down, flattening the over-casting (see Fig. 9, *g*) with your thimble.

When you wish to put a cord at the top of a flounce, take an exact measure round the skirt; the cord must be the same length. Divide and mark both the skirt and the cord into quarters. Fix the flounce to these divisions, and sew it to the cord. Then attach the corded flounce to the gown with long back-stitches. This mode avoids crumpling the gown, an advantage not to be disregarded, especially for silk gowns.

Sometimes very wide flounces (and only these) have a heading. This heading is made instead of gathering the flounce, on the edge opposite to the one which is embroidered, hemmed, or bordered. If both edges are embroidered, hemmed, or bordered, work the band with one border on the wrong side and the other on the right side, so that in falling down, the

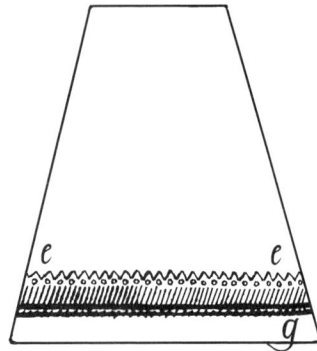

Figure 9. To sew on a flounce.

embroidery of the heading will appear on its right side. Then, under the edge embroidered on the wrong side, make a crease to mark the width which you wish for the heading. This is ordinarily that of the embroidery (when there is any) and generally about two fingers. Gather without a roll on the crease; then place the flounce flat on the gown, because it has no roll to hide. It is unnecessary to turn over the flounce as I explained at first.

Sometimes the flounce is surmounted by a rouleau. For this, gather while rolling the edge of the flounce which is not embroidered. Then below the gathering, at about three or four fingers according to the width you wish to give to the rouleau, gather without rolling. Sew on the flounce, beginning with the rolled gathers, and putting the wrong side over the gown. Then turn it down, and sew the second gathering flat, placing the folds perfectly parallel to those formed by the first sewing of the gathered rouleau. It is needless to say that you puff the portion of the flounce destined to make the rouleau, by leaving half as much material underneath. When you join by over-casting the bands of material which compose the flounce, take care to leave the rolled portion unsewed, other than for some stitches to keep the gathered rouleau uninterrupted. The object of this is to facilitate ironing the rouleau, for it will be necessary to raise it with a goffering-iron, which is passed between the gown and the rouleau.

You will perceive that these modes should be applied to all kinds of trimmings, since whatever their style may be, the order here necessarily presides.

Rouleaux. You have just seen how these are made at the top of a flounce, and so may conceive that it is the same thing when the flounce is not there; only, when gathering you must join the two edges into a roll, then sew one side to the right side of the gown. This is done with side-stitches, and not flat. Take care to begin the seam made inside, near the side which is seen from the top of the gown, because the rouleau naturally falling down will hide a seam made quite on top, if the rouleau is near the hem. You may also put a rouleau over a cord, then sew it flat to the gown, as I explained for flounces.

All the variations I have just described for flounces have been applied to rouleaux; therefore I shall dispense with going over them here. I shall only indicate how you proceed to trim gowns with continuous rouleaux.

These rouleaux are ordinarily made of muslin or gauze, for gowns of percale or transparent material. You will need a little less trimming material, than twice the sum of the height and the width, of the bottom of the gown which you wish to trim. Take into account the direction and the size of the rouleaux, then measure with a small piece of pasteboard as previously explained. But as the rouleaux are continuous, re-position the measure from the place it just quit, and so on all along the trimming, until you have come back to the starting place. Each time you place the measure, make a mark with a pin or a bit of tied thread. If the rouleaux are lengthways, place the measure lengthways; if they are slantways, place it that way; and so on.

When the rouleaux are lengthways or slantways, it is unnecessary to leave small slits for the goffering-iron, because it may be entered very well in the openings at the top and bottom of the rouleau. You may see from this direction that you do not sew the top and bottom ends of lengthways or slantways rouleaux, unlike rouleaux placed widthways. After having measured widthways rouleaux, and gathered at each little mark from the top downwards, join both ends of the trimming with a seam; this must be at a gathering of the rouleau.

The following is done like the wide bottom of a skirt with folds: inside the gown, at the bottom, attach the rouleau a little above the hem, putting a pin at each gathering. The under side of the rouleau, which shapes the gown, is straighter than the upper side, which puffs out. Judge by the eye for the first rouleau; then, on the outside of the gown, measure for the others from the bottom of the first. You must make this measurement a little smaller towards the top of the gown, because of the narrowing resulting from the bias cut of the gores. For the same reason, the rouleaux will puff out a little more towards the top, but that will be scarcely noticeable. Then sew the rouleaux from the bottom to the top of the gown, along the gathering, while evening out the folds.

Boullions or puffs are used on calico, merino, or taffety, and are always of material similar to the gown. In order that they may be pretty, the material must have firmness. The band intended for the puffs must be at least a third more than double the distance round the gown; measure to divide it into quarters. Then sew this band to the gown, or to a cord, in large box-plaits. One side finished, arrange the other likewise in box-plaits, but in the contrary direction; that is a plait on the right side is copied on the left, and a plait on the left side is copied on the right. This operation inflates the middle of the puff considerably, and produces pretty glints on the sides when the material is lustrous. These puffs are nearly always two in number because of their width, about double those of ordinary rouleaux. Some persons put three, but never together; an interval of about an eighth of an ell separates them. Puffs are only put widthways round the skirt.

Another kind of rouleau, very easy to make and very pretty, has trimmed gowns of silk, of merino, and ball gowns; it is still used on these last. This rouleau is made of a riband or a satin bias, which you stuff with cotton wadding. Unite the two edges of the riband with long running stitches, if the riband is wide enough to join; or with crossed or uncrossed herring-bone stitches, if the riband is too narrow to completely encompass the cotton. The rouleau is applied with the join next the gown and so hidden; even so it is better that the riband completely enclose the cotton. This rouleau, similar to a draught stopper for a door, is applied over the gown by sewing firmly under the rouleau in such a manner that the stitches are not apparent. It is placed widthways or slantways; it may also be formed into diamonds, points, or leaves. An indeterminate number of rows may be used, but most commonly three rows are placed widthways. These rouleaux are also made of merino, though that kind may be rather heavy. As they do not have any plaits, you may sew them by the eye, measuring only the distance from one row to another.

Folds, or Tucks. Like biases, folds are still the height of fashion. When you begin to cut out your gown, determine the number and width of the folds with which you desire to trim it, in order to allow enough material for them. Each fold will take about a quarter of an ell. To this end you must consider for a moment the folds placed on the first breadth, fixing them provisionally with a pin, which you then take out. Cut the other breadths by this one. Your gown made up, re-fold it widthways all round at about a sixteenth of an ell from the hem; this will be the interval from one fold to another. Baste or pin each fold as you mark it.

Be very careful when you come to the bias seams of the skirt, because your fold faces the hem, and consequently you put a narrower part over a wider one, since skirts always widen towards the bottom. Necessarily there will be more material on the under side of the fold than on top, and consequently a danger of puckering the fold, which would be extremely ugly. To prevent this, you have only to fold a little of the bias under near each seam, imperceptibly taking in the under part of the fold all round the gown. Sew the fold with very small running stitches from the right side of the gown. The pasteboard measure is indispensable for judging if the fold is equally wide every where, and placed at the proper distance. Often embroidery is put between wide folds.

Formerly the same kind of folds were made on gowns, only extremely narrow. These are still used on caps, handkerchiefs, and other similar articles. They are very easy to make, because their narrowness renders the stitching imperceptible. They do not need any space between them. They must be very numerous to form a row, twenty to thirty for a gown, for example, or an *entre-deux;* this numerous row is repeated three or four times, at an interval of several fingers.

After the wide and narrow folds, it is necessary to speak of middle-sized ones. These are less pleasing, but they have one pretty variation: this is the reversed fold. You know that folds usually face the hem, and their seam faces the top of the skirt. Make your fold in that direction for the space of about a sixteenth of an ell; then straightening it up and turning the fold towards the top of the skirt, sew the seam on the hem side. Sew in that direction as far as you did in the contrary direction; then return to the first direction, and so on all round the gown. Repeat this operation for the second, the third, and all the folds, which makes a very agreeable effect.

These folds are made without any interval, six, eight, or ten in succession, according to their size. Then you leave a suitable space and begin a new row. You may place these rows contrariwise; that is, put folds which face the top of the skirt in the first row, and folds which face the hem in the second. Fashion has revived contrary folds many times, and will continue to do so.

Biases. Nothing is easier to make than a bias trimming. Take a band cut on the bias, of what width you please; at present, the wider biases are, the more beautiful they appear. Fold this band or bias double. Have a cord prepared for piping, as I explained above. Sew the two edges of your bias together round the cord, without any plaits, with back-stitches alone or mixed with running stitches. Raise your cord when the seam is finished; flatten the seam well, pulling the bias between the forefinger and middle finger of your left hand. Then put the bias thus prepared a little above the hem of the skirt. Sew it flat with back-stitches, sticking the needle precisely into the groove formed at the join of the cord and the bias. Measure the distances for placing the other biases, which you sew in the same way.

Ordinarily three are used, and only widthways round the gown: there are no other variations. Fashion, however, has just replaced the hem with a bias of absurd width; in this case it is used alone. When you wish to put a flat, coloured braid on top of the bias, dispense with the piping. Put the bias on the gown, then the braid on the bias, with running stitches.

I shall not linger on the subject of biases except for a single, but important observation. You do not join the bands of material which compose a bias with upright seams, unlike all other bands. The ends of a bias band, which are on the straight-way, necessarily describe a half V, or rather a right angle. The seam must therefore be made in that direction to be inconspicuous.

Braid and Fringe. Trimmings of round or flat braid are of the greatest simplicity. For round braid you wrap the braid in the gown on the wrong side a little above the hem, and sew it there with running stitches. The other rows are made in the same way. Placing flat braid is even easier; you put it over the gown and fasten it there with running stitches: the number of rows and the distance between them depend upon taste. These trimmings have been used for a long time.

Silk ravellings or fringes are sewed flat over the seam of the hem, which is hidden by them. This trimming is still worn, though it is rare.

Entre-deux. I have little to say about the ordinary *entre-deux* used at present; they are indeed so simple. But *entre-deux* of the past, and likely those of the future, will give me a little more work.

An *entre-deux* is a straight band of tulle with selvages on both edges. *Entre-deux* are sewed between bands of percale, or rows of folds, with little over-cast stitches like those used to sew lace; that is, made into the bars and holes which form the *engrêlure,* or footing of the tulle. You have no other precaution to take except to be watchful, so that you neither tighten nor take in too much of the tulle. You may fold it over, or even cut a little at bias seams; but ordinarily you may be content to take in a little more in that region.

An *entre-deux* of embroidered muslin is the same thing, except you must first hem the *entre-deux* band before sewing it by over-casting: it is needless to say that the over-casting is on the wrong side. The interval is measured according to the *entre-deux.*

When the *entre-deux* are very numerous, and of cheap material such as gauze or clear muslin, replace the bottom of the gown (ordinarily of percale), according to the height of the trimming decided upon, by an extension of the material which will form the *entre-deux.* Let us suppose it to be gauze. You add it to each breadth, and make it up, in short make the extension of the skirt, except that you add a false hem of percale. Then make bands of percale bordered on both edges with a corded piping, or showing a fold, bordered (or not) on one side with a cord. These bands are placed on the gauze at equal intervals, and sewed flat in the space between the cords. Trimmings are also made of similar bands (with corded piping) without any necessity of arranging them on a clear foundation.

Before going on to explain other *entre-deux,* I must inform my readers of a little needle-work required by the following *entre-deux: dents de loup, dents de harpie,* and *trou-trou-popoye.* This explanation may be useful even if the fashion for these does not return.

Dents de loup or *à poignet* are executed as follows: cut two narrow strips of percale or other material; but percale is ordinarily chosen. Lay one strip quite evenly over the other. It is not even necessary that the two strips be separate; it suffices to fold a wider one double. Then take a strip of paper which has been cut into triangular points, of what size you please. Lay the strip of paper over the strips of percale. Then fix it there by basting, or by pinning it here and there; or when you are practiced, simply hold it over your left forefinger, between the thumb and the other fingers of the same hand. The paper must be facing you.

These preparations completed, sew your two strips of percale together, with back-stitches mixed with running stitches, following the cuts of the paper. Remove or un-baste the paper, and lay it aside. Then cut along the seam which you have just made, leaving a very narrow margin of material along the points, so that your seam is not spoiled. The cutting complete, take either a bodkin, or scissors which are not too pointed; push the tool between the two strips, into each point. Then turn it to the right side, so that your seam is entirely hidden. Take good care to reach the extremity of each point, pushing the bodkin in quite straight. This operation produces a succession of very pretty points, which are almost a species of scollop.

Dents de harpie are less pretty, but quicker and easier to make. Here is the mode: take a strip, whose length and width depend upon what you have determined for your points. Cut into this strip here and there, nonetheless making the cut or slit no longer than two-thirds of the width of the strip; the last third will support the points. So that your points will be perfectly equal, always measure the interval left between the slits, making it the same as the first interval you marked. Your strip thus entirely arranged, turn it to the wrong side, which you place facing you; and taking the two sides of each interval, turn them down close together, towards you. This forms a little bias line to the right and left, from the lower part of the slit to the upper part of the interval, which thus folded down gives a sharp point. Fasten the two little turned-down pieces together with several stitches, and pass with a long stitch to the next interval. The strip, turned over to the right side, will show a succession of points widened at their base and quite pointed at the tip.

The *trou-trou-popoye* is much more modern than the previous article, and also very easy. Take a strip of gauze or very clear muslin about three fingers wide. Make a seam fold at each edge of the strip, then fold it very neatly in thirds. Then take a piece of paper cut into points, as I advised for *dents de loup,* and follow this model the same way; with the difference that instead of sewing firmly with back-stitches, you use loose running stitches, or rather a kind of gathering; for as you advance you pull the thread of the running stitches, and in this way you tighten your points. This produces, to the right and left, a series of puffed points, without the stitches being apparent. From time to time you must fasten these festooned gathers with several stitches, so that your work does not loosen. When you have a little practice, dispense with putting the cut paper over the strip; gather the points by the eye.

These three fashions of points are used as follows. When you have to make a folded *entre-deux,* take a strip of muslin of a suitable width, about an eighth of an ell; this should be at least double the distance all round the skirt which you will trim. Gather this strip on both edges. Since it has gathers to arrange evenly, divide both it and the skirt into eight equal parts as explained for flounces. If the *entre-deux* is to be placed between *dents de loup,* trim the edge of the gown with a row of these points in place of a hem, then sew one edge of the *entre-deux* to the wrong side. The other edge of the *entre-deux* is sewed to a parallel row of points. If the *entre-deux* are double, do not separate the two strips. Measure them double, gather in the middle, and place a row of *dents de loup* on the gathering. The over-casting with which you sew is always done underneath. The row of points is then turned down: all these points have the extremities turned towards the bottom. They are used on sleeves, *fichus,* and every where they may create the most agreeable effect.

Another fashion of folded *entre-deux* differs from the above only in that the *dents de loup* are replaced by a strip folded triple, and showing a hem.

Great *dents de harpie* are placed flat on coloured gowns. The effect of this trimming is rather mean.

The *trou-trou-popoye* makes novel *entre-deux.* Place it between strips of percale, sewing only at the tip of each little puffed point. This is pretty only from a distance. This kind of trimming, used like ordinary *trou-trou* for trimming caps and collars, bordering strips of gauze or muslin, is excessively common, and gives some difficulty, because it is necessary to make the strip and the points extremely small.

To put *Entre-deux* on Collars. When you have an organdy or gauze falling collar to make with tulle *entre-deux,* you must first hem the collar. This hem must be very wide, and consequently the right side where the hem is to be sewed, is much smaller than the part turned down for the hem. You are forced to make large creases underneath, which pucker, and which are visible through the clear material. The turned-down hem fold shows just as much, which is neither neat nor pretty.

To avoid this disadvantage, first cut your collar to its exact size, without leaving any thing for either side of the hem. Then take a bias strip of similar material; fold it double, which will then be a proper width for the hem. Place it over the extreme edge of the collar, so that all three edges are together, and the right and wrong sides of this false hem are in their final positions. Baste, then sew the under side of the bias strip as if it were a hem. You perceive that the false hem will show no creases. Since the bias strip is in some sort elastic, you will be able to tighten or stretch it imperceptibly, as required by the roundness of the collar. Leaving the three edges in place, seam them all from the right side, first basting at the edge of the new hem, then making a seam *à la reine* along the basting, which seam disappears in the seam of the *entre-deux.* Then trim off all the ravelled threads.

The same mode is used when you must place several *entre-deux.* The bias strip is folded and sewed to the tulle, which is already sewed to the hem on the other side. The two opposite edges are united by a seam *à la reine* as described above, and you gently pull the bias to follow the roundness of the collar accurately. When you arrive at the last strip, which must serve as the hem, put the bias fold at the lower part without sewing, and fasten the edges by the seam *à la reine* to the last tulle.

Draperies. Trimmings in drapery require that, when you cut out the skirt, you add enough length to drape it. This is about a quarter, or even a third of an ell; double this measure is necessary for draperies requiring much gathering. Then measure the distance between the places where the drapery will be raised, and gather them from bottom to top, the same as I explained for rouleaux placed lengthways.

That finished, prepare as many narrow strips as there are gathered places. These strips may be of material similar to the gown, simply folded triple, or trimmed with corded piping, or bordered flat by coloured braid. Be that as it may, place these strips flat over the gatherings, evening out the fulness while securely sewing each side of the strip. It is imperative after that to line this trimming on the wrong side of the gown; for want of this precaution, many ladies have entangled their feet in the folds of the drapery, and have been injured in falling. A loose lining is often put from the top to the bottom of the drapery.

Agrafes. The fashion of trimming *en agrafe* is well for gowns which are not washed, and which are of tolerably stiff material. Here is how you proceed: measure the gown as for positioning flounces. Take a sufficiently wide strip trimmed with cord on both edges (in piping or otherwise), of a length more than double the distance round the gown; measure it in eighths likewise. Place the strip flat on the gown. Between each part of the strip measured in eighths, take new measures, which must be about an eighth of the previous eighth. Mark these measures with a pin, immediately fixing the strip to the gown, folding as much as possible to that place; for as you might expect, the under side of the band formed by the gown is much narrower than the part of the strip, so that the strip will puff out. Repeat the same thing at the next measure. When you come to one of the eighths of the gown, sew the eight places which you have pinned, forming gathers or plaits. The strip thus forms a very elegant large loop or *agrafe,* but it is easily crumpled.

I have said that these *agrafes* are only marked in eighths of eighths, and not all round the gown at the same time, because the pins, holding a quantity of plaits, are easily detached. If you mark too many *agrafes* at the same time, you may have to begin measuring all over again.

A very pretty derivation of this kind of trimming is that called *en coquilles.* It is the same thing, except that you use quadruple the length of the strip; and at each measure for an *agrafe,* instead of spreading them a little over the gown, you place them next each other, without leaving any space underneath. This actually forms a succession of *coquillages,* which pressed against each other, acquire by this position a kind of sturdiness, so much that this trimming, though it may not seem tidy for them, is well suited to muslin gowns, printed or otherwise. In laundering, the goffering-iron is passed into each *coquille.*

Ruches. Box-plaits are used to make all kinds of ruches, to put round *fichus,* caps, pelerines, or gowns. Here is how to make them successfully.

As for every kind of trimming, it is necessary to fold both the article which you will trim, and the strip which you will box-plait, into two equal parts to find the exact middles. Fasten the middle of each together. Place the article (let us suppose it to be a pelerine) flat over your knee, and a little slanted. Put your feet on the rungs of a chair for more convenience. It is also necessary that the pelerine be placed to your left.

These preparations made, take the strip of trimming, and place it flat on the right side of the pelerine over the hem. Lay your right thumb and forefinger over the beginning of the strip, and pass the middle finger of your left hand under the strip between those two fingers. Raise your middle finger to a greater or lesser degree, according to the size of the plaits you wish to obtain. Still holding the plait between your right fingers, bring your left finger out, and lay it across over the middle of the plait, at the same time removing the fingers of your right hand. Replace the tip of your left finger with a fine pin, stuck lightly into the plait to preserve it. Then go right next to it, or a little farther, according to the spacing you intend, to begin a new plait. Continue thus until you reach the end of the pelerine.

Next thread a needle with a long piece of thread. Sew the plaits with running stitches along the pins, which you remove as you advance. Persons who are practiced do not pin the plaits; they mark them, then sew as soon as they remove their fingers.

Double and contrary box-plaits are also made. Double box-plaits consist of two box-plaits, one over the other. To give the idea, it is necessary to say that a box-plait is often made by folding the strip to the right, then to the left, so that the two folds produce the effect which I already described. With the first mode, you are more assured of the regularity of the plaits. However, the second mode is indispensable for double box-plaits, because they must be made by forming two plaits one over the other to the left, and the same to the right. Double box-plaits are used to make large ruches for trimming gowns. You may obtain very high box-plaits by folding the strip four, five, six, or even seven times to the right and left.

As for contrary box-plaits, they are made first on one edge of the strip and not in the middle, unlike all the others. Then you make new box-plaits on the second edge of the strip in the space between the first ones, which produces a very agreeable contrast. But contrary box-plaits may only be made on material which is not washed, because it is impossible to iron them. They are used to trim gowns.

Double ruches are made by putting a second row of box-plaits so close to the first row that they appear to merge.

When you wish to trim a gown of *gros de Naples,* or only of marceline, with ruches, have the strips pinked at a haberdasher's. This costs two sous per ell at Paris. In the provinces you obtain an *arrache pièce à dents* and cut them yourself, laying this instrument over both edges of the strip.

Panes. This trimming was once all the rage. It is now forgotten, but every thing leads me to believe that it will one day be remembered. Here, in the mean time, are the directions: when a gown must be trimmed with several rows of panes, draw on it a succession of diamond shapes, more or less large according to the size suitable for the panes. Then scollop all round the inside of each diamond, and cut out the centre following the scollops. For the other part, or rather the pane, cut out muslin, gauze, or tulle diamonds much larger than the scolloped diamonds, so that the new diamonds may puff out. Gather these diamonds, each in turn. Attach the two most pointed ends of the muslin diamonds, to the corresponding points of the scolloped diamonds. Then sew each muslin diamond to the wrong side, behind the scollops, by this means hiding the seam. Work a narrow flat *cordonnet* round the pane on the right side.

The most elegant panes are those where the muslin or tulle displays a flower embroidered in raised satin-stitch, matching the design of the embroidery on the gown, with which these rich trimmings are mixed. Panes are used not only at the bottom of gowns, but also on sleeves, *fichus,* and caps: this makes a most agreeable effect. They are ironed by passing the goffering-iron inside.

Here is, I believe, a complete treatise on trimmings. It will still be one in the future, despite all the odd and fertile inventions of fashion; for fashion cannot but cause the return, at some point, of some of the trimmings which I have just described so precisely.

——*Manuel des demoiselles.*

Diversion 1.

The Trade of the Mantua-maker. Though in London the trades of mantua-maker and milliner are frequently separate, they are not always so; and in the country they are very commonly united.

In the milliner, taste and fancy are required; with a quickness in discerning, imitating, and improving on various fashions, which are perpetually changing amongst the higher circles.

The mantua-maker's customers are not easily pleased; they frequently expect more from their dress than it is capable of giving. The mantua-maker must be an expert anatomist; and must, if judiciously chosen, have a name of French termination. She must know how to hide all defects in the proportions of the body, and must be able to mould the shape by the stays, that while she corrects the body, she may not interfere with the pleasures of the palate.

The business of the mantua-maker, when conducted upon a large scale and in a fashionable situation, is very profitable; but the mere work-women do not get any thing at all adequate to their labour. They are frequently obliged to sit up very late, and the recompense for extra work is in general a poor remuneration for the time spent.

The frontispiece to the back-matter represents a mantua-maker taking a pattern off from a lady, by means of a piece of paper or cloth. The pattern, if taken in cloth, becomes afterwards the lining of the gown.

——*The Book of English Trades.*

Diversion 2.

The Art of Mantua-making. Economy is a most essential virtue in women, and the want of it is often the origin of too much indulgence in the extravagances of the toilet. The habit of spending a great deal of money on trifles, sometimes becomes so strong that it is a need throughout life.

It is not only in spending money that economy should be exercised: its habitual application is found in the care which a woman takes over the divers parts of her attire. Such care is a very important part of education. A young lady should be charged with looking after her wardrobe herself, and keeping in order all which relates to it.

Lack of order is excusable only in the poor, where all the members of a family find themselves constrained by necessity to use for their subsistence every moment not devoted to sleep. When other classes neglect orderliness, they must suffer for it; it is the natural punishment for their negligence.

As order is the foundation of economy, it is necessary to include in this work all the means of giving young ladies a virtue which is so important, and which will have so much influence on their well-being and that of the persons surrounding them. They should also be given, at a very young age, an adequate and convenient place to take care of the articles used in their toilet. In general, on this point as on all the rest, early habits have a remarkable influence. It is more important than may be believed, to accustom young girls to care for their attire, and not to disdain their old clothing.

To quote a lord who wrote on the door to his kitchen: "Enough, but nothing more." This motto should be that of all wealthy parents who have the kindness to train their children in sensible economy.

Mothers! Never neglect this plan of bringing up your daughters so that they may be happy! Have them use their talents to this end, and they will for ever be grateful to you, as will the society which they will one day ornament.

The Work-room. Before teaching the art of what is, properly speaking, mantua-making, it may be useful to say a few words about the most essential furniture and tools, and the most advantageous way to arrange them.

A room exclusively devoted to this kind of work must contain a table for cutting, raised to elbow height, in the shape of a rectangle about five feet by four. At the best-lighted place in the room, place a second table called the work-table, which has drawers for patterns, measures, threads, &c., &c. A box weighted with four or five pounds of lead, and covered with a pincushion, is placed on this table. You ought to attach your work to the pincushion, not over your knee. By the latter mode, you not only risk tearing your gowns, you form the habit of leaning your body forwards, which is too little known as a pernicious habit against which young people should be warned.

A little book with cashmere, merino, or flannel leaves serves for storing needles. Unlike a needle-case, it will not blunt them. Take care to furnish your scissors with little strips of velvet, or any other soft and flexible material. Your thimble should be pierced with large holes; ivory thimbles are the best; they do not soil your work as others do. I cannot too highly recommend long needles; the skill of using them is soon acquired, and the difficulty their use presents at first is well repaid by the freshness which they leave in your work. Finally, I advise the use of a little bench or stool, on which to place both feet when working.

I shall not speak to my young readers about the manner in which to work the stitches employed in sewing gowns; what young girl is ignorant of them? I shall merely list them: the running stitch, the over-cast stitch, the side-stitch or hem-stitch, the back-stitch, the button-hole stitch, and the herring-bone stitch. It is essential to know what part you must use them on when making a gown.

Of the Measure. Provide yourself with a sheet of strong paper; cut it into strips three fingers wide, then fold them double lengthways. Take one of them which you leave folded, while with your other hand, you take a second half-opened strip, into which you insert the first one. Fix these strips with a stitch or two; repeat this operation until the measure is of a proper length. With the aid of this very simple and cheap tool (see Fig. 10), you may succeed in taking precise measures for all the parts of clothing.

Here is how to take them: hold the strip of paper in your left hand; take a pair of scissors in your right; stand in back of the person whom you want to measure. Take the strip in both hands; bring end a onto the back, beginning from the arms; lay your right hand there and extend your left, holding the measure, to the other shoulder. That done, lift the measure. Fold double the length of the strip included between the shoulders; mark the fold which you just made with a notch (see Fig. 10, *1*). Lay the notch on the left shoulder; extend the measure under the arms to the base of the bosom; cut a notch at that point, similar to the first (see Fig. 10, *2*). Extend the measure anew to the busk; cut another notch similar to the two preceding ones (see Fig. 10, *3*). Remove the measure; take end a again; encircle the base of the waist; fold that distance measured in half; and cut two notches at the fold (see Fig. 10, *4*). Take end a again and bring it onto the arm-hole a little towards the back; pass the measure to the elbow; extend it as far as the wrist, or farther if the sleeve must cover part of the hand; cut two notches at that length (see Fig. 10, *5*). The sleeve measure is taken from all that length. Generally the measure is only folded in half for symmetrical parts, that is, those which are alike on the right and left of the person, and which taken together form the whole. For example, the two parts of the back, the two parts of the body from the pit of the stomach to the backbone, &c.

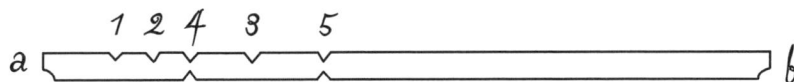

Figure 10. The measure.

Place the end of the measure on the over-cast seam which joins the skirt and the body, and bring it down to the upper of the shoe. That is, to my mind, the length which a gown must have to be graceful or even decent. And I admit, I far from approve today's fashion. These shortened garments, doubtless borrowed from rope-dancers, depart from the grace and austerity of the costumes of the women of ancient Greece, which our mothers were able to see revived briefly during the Revolution.

General Observations. It is needless to say that the longer the material is, the more graceful the folds, and the more varied their undulations. "I have such a pretty instep," think some of my readers, "which it would be a real pity to hide." Very well then; but are you immobile, and do you think it will not be glimpsed during an entire soirée? "That which is rarely seen pleases more and for a much longer time," says Madame Riccoboni; and this truth, which appears trite, is even so not sufficiently well known.

I therefore advise wearing long gowns. If you are statuesque, if you present yourself with a certain assurance, a short gown will only add to your deliberate manners, and all excess is a fault! If on the contrary you are timid and little accustomed to society, how ill a short gown becomes you! Your timidity, so pretty and interesting in a young person, will before long be considered awkwardness, lack of etiquette, &c.

However, I do not pretend to lay down a rule with no exceptions. Every one must choose the attire which best suits her demeanour, her shape, her gait, and her occupations. Fashion, a word which serves as a passport to all extravagances, cannot be a law which governs women of good taste and good sense. I once knew a lady of very high rank, who always wore gowns of a simplicity unprecedented in those times; who, consulting fashion less than what was becoming to her, adopted the use of long waists and gowns well before any one else had ever thought to wear them. She also adopted the body which she knew to be more graceful on her than any other. In a word, she had enough good sense to know she would lose much by changing this fashion. She had the benefit of being admired for her talents, her wit, her charms, and the simplicity of her attire. I observed during the time when blouse gowns, being new, were desirable to wear, that she did not act like most women, who follow a fashion without knowing if it suits them, but only because it is the fashion. This kind of gown looked very ill on her; she never wore it: that is what I mean by good sense in choosing fashions.

It is necessary, in passing, that I tell you why and how fashions succeed each other so rapidly. Do not imagine that the latest is the prettiest. As it is customary amongst people of good *ton* to avoid every thing which has become vulgar, the costume of the day is not preferred because it is prettier or more convenient, but solely because it is chosen by fashionable people. As soon as this costume is no longer distinctive, it changes to another style.

A wealthy woman sees that a gown which she has just had made by the best mantua-maker at Paris (Victorine) is already worn by thousands of people; she has recognized her porter's daughter wearing this costume. She then complains that this fashion has become so common, that a woman of good taste can no longer wear it. The mantua-maker is not at all annoyed at this mishap. Supposing that the gown was trimmed with a flounce a quarter of an ell high; it is therefore replaced with one half an ell high. The body was bare; lengthways or widthways draperies are quickly added to it. The sleeves, which were tight round the arms near the cuff, are changed for sleeves *à la Grecque*, a kind very large at the bottom.

All this is not pretty, but at least no one has worn it before. This fashion soon meets the same fate as the other, that gives place to a third, and so on. And all the mob believes this to be the whim of fashion, when it is only that of two or three rich persons. If every one had simple and moderate taste, all these extravagant fashions would not arise.

Of cutting out the Skirt. If you desire to make a gown, place the material which you have chosen on a chair, which is situated at the right end of the cutting-table. Pull an ell, or an ell and a half, of the material over the table. I shall call the left and right of the table, the left and right of the person who is working there. Fold the material double lengthways, so that the two selvages touch, and the fold is near you. Take care to also have a chair on your left, where you will put the cut breadths.

Approach the chair on which the material is placed. Take the scissors which have one rounded blade; it is this blade which must touch the table. Place it slanting underneath the selvages, taking care that only the small portion of the material which touches the scissors is lifted up from the table. Put your middle finger and ring finger in the handle belonging to the rounded blade; use your forefinger to support this handle, which is on the under side, and pass only your thumb through the handle of the upper blade. Take care that the rounded blade rests on the table during the entire operation. Make two parallel slanting cuts in the selvages, about two inches apart. These cuts are made because the selvages are always tighter than the material; their object is to prevent the material from puckering.

Then take up the measure, and go to the left of the table. Lay the measure over the material, letting it exceed the latter by about two or three fingers. Hold the end of the material, and that of the measure, with your left hand. Beginning from the extremity of the material, drag your right hand to the extremity of the measure, then replace it with your left hand. With your right hand, provided with the scissors, cut, at a very little distance from the measure, the breadth which will serve for the front of the gown (see Fig. 11 A).

Your first breadth being placed there, again pull the material from right to left. Fold it double, just as for your first operation. Then take the breadth already cut, and put it on the material. Proceed just the same with the measure, that is letting the material on top extend three or four fingers beyond it; this last is the back breadth, which is always cut longer (see Fig. 11 C), save for some persons who have a large stomach, or those who are not at all fleshy in back. Those who are fleshy in back, or who have an upper body which leans forwards, require this breadth longer.

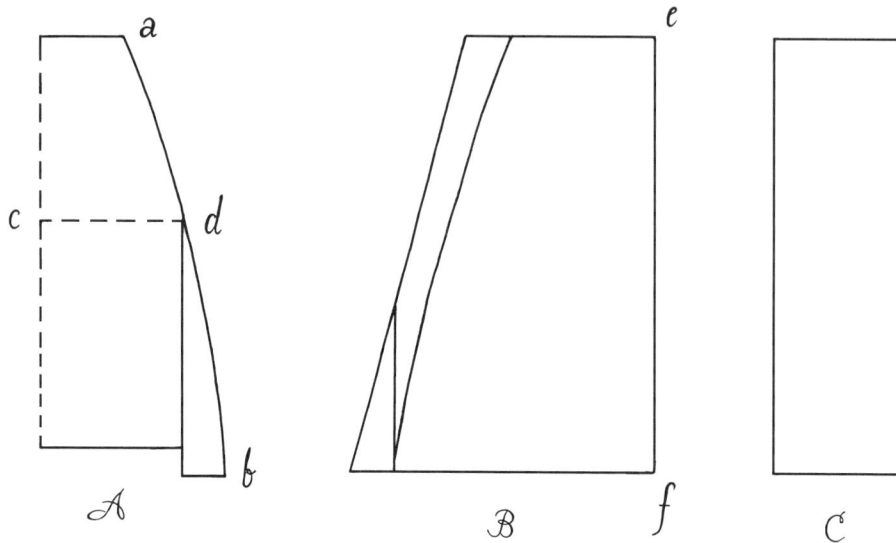

Figure 11. To cut out the skirt.

Remove the two breadths from the top of the table, and again pull the material from the chair to place it on the table. This time do not fold it over itself; leave the whole width there. Take the back breadth, which must always be on top; cut the third, or side breadth equally long (see Fig. 11 *B*); replace the back breadth on the chair. Arrange the material anew across the whole width, and cut the fourth breadth like the third (see Fig. 11 *B* again).

Leave these last two breadths on the table; move them away from you, in order to place there the front breadth, which must be folded length-ways. Lay the two selvages over those of the other breadths and fix them with pins, beginning from right to left. Take care to put the breadths of an equal length on that side. Do not spread the pins too far apart from each other; you cannot be too careful in cutting out this part of the skirt. That done, turn to your measure, on which the distance round the waist, taken from the middle of the busk up to the middle of the under-arms, is indicated by notches. Take this measure, and bring it to the fold in the middle of the front breadth. Drag your hand over the measure up to the notch which you must use; enter a pin in the material, as close to the notch as you are able.

Then take the part of the breadth measured; bring it over the bottom of the same breadth; take twice this measure, and enter a pin as you did at the top. Fold the material over itself exactly where the pins are found.

By this means you form a sloping, or bias, line (see Fig. 11 *A, ab*) which is found over the hip. Pass your hands over the fold several times, after which put your material back flat. The greatest care must be taken for a cut on the bias, because you cannot mark it exactly as you must cut it. (See Fig. 12, in which *gh* represents the fold, and *ijk* the curve according to which you should cut.) It is with your scissors that you give the bias curve shown in Fig. 11 *A, ab,* in order to fit the hips well. The lower the waist of the gown, the more necessary this curve is. Above all, rest the rounded blade of the scissors firmly on the table, so as to lift the material as little as possible.

Having cut the bias, place the selvages of the side breadths in front of you (see Fig. 11 *B, ef*) taking care to put the narrowest part on your right, which will be the top of the skirt. That done, take the front breadth, and likewise put the straight-way in front of you. You may see, by referring to Fig. 11 *B,* that the small gore exceeds the front breadth by three fingers; bring it back up a little closer to the middle, then fold the breadth widthways following *cd.* Put a pin in the middle; place the bias of the front breadth on the middle of the bias of the side breadths; after which place your hand there, not lengthways but across the material, so as not to distort this part. Pin it carefully, without lifting it from the top of the table,

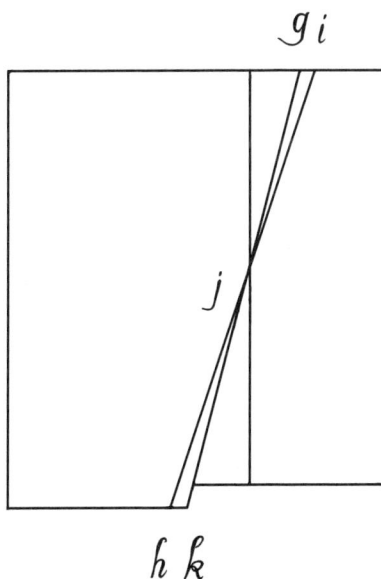

Figure 12. To cut the bias.

and give the same curve to the side breadths as to the front. If the person who will wear the gown is stout, remove a little gore, a quarter of an ell long by a sixteenth wide, from the selvages of the side breadth. *Voilà,* your skirt entirely cut out.

Of making up the Skirt. Commence by unpinning the breadths. Then sew on the small front gores with running stitches, if the material is light, such as florence, marceline, levantine, and even *gros de Naples;* but employ alternating back-stitches and running stitches for thick materials. Velvet requires only back-stitches, little tightened.

When the small gores are sewed, pin the bias of the front gore to the bias of a side gore; do the same for the other side. Take a long needle of the kind used by *marchandes de modes.* Thread it with grey thread (a kind of thread which is used for basting; basting is sewing with running stitches the length of the needle). Never take only one stitch at a time in this kind of sewing; otherwise you risk distorting your work. Begin to baste the bias seam at the bottom; this mode has the recommendation of being easier and better than any other. Dispense as much as possible with taking back-stitches in these kinds of seams, and still less take them in hems, excepting wash-gowns. Then take the side breadth, from which you have cut off a gore if the person is stout. Join it to the back breadth, again by basting it, and taking care to hold the bias side in front of you. That done, cut a short slit, a sixth of an ell long, in the top of the back breadth, to facilitate putting on the skirt. This slit must be furnished with a narrow hem, into which you enter a very narrow braid.

Now there is no more to do but to over-cast the seams without selvages. To do so, use the forefinger of your left hand to spread both edges of the material, which you must fold over itself inside. Then over-cast with very long stitches, or use running stitches, which are sooner done and achieve the same end. Over-cast the top of the skirt without turning it down.

Next proceed to round the top of the skirt. Put a pin at the fold which is formed in the middle of the top of the skirt. Lay the two bias edges together; do the same for the other seams. Fix them with pins; this must be done on the wrong side of the skirt. Take the measure; place it at the top of the skirt, taking care to let it exceed the material by about an inch. This suffices for all persons, excepting pregnant women. For them, cut all the breadths even, because you will be obliged to remove a great deal from the front breadth. Despite all this preparation, do not omit to gather a little over the stomach; by this means the size of the latter is less perceptible.

Put your right hand on the measure and on the skirt. At the same time, beginning from the same point, drag your hand up to the other end of the measure; place a pin there. Reverse the part of the material which exceeds the measure, over the skirt. Fix the fold by means of a pin. Bring the part measured along the bias, and hold it with your longest finger. Do the same to form the fold. Then re-position the front breadth over the middle of the back breadth, and let the latter exceed it by about three fingers, in accordance with the carriage of the person. When all this is done, it still remains for you to draw a curve from the back breadth to the bias.

Place the pins, which must hold the material intended to make the hem in the middle of the latter, so that you may baste round the skirt. Unpin the skirt. Make a little paper measure, which you use to make the hem even. If the skirt is of silk, work the hem with running stitches. You will do well to put a strip of cotton wadding inside it. This does better at keeping the gown more evenly round, than the strip of straw which was put there formerly. The skirt being sewed, must be two ells and a quarter round. I make no distinction between a small woman and one of middle size. That is only done for women of an uncommon size, and for them add a breadth more at the back of the gown so that the slit of the skirt is found between two selvages.

Of cutting out the Body. Different bodies may be set onto this kind of skirt. I shall begin with the plain tight body. This is composed of two lined pieces. One is for the front; Fig. 13 *A* shows the half; and the other, for the back, is shown in Fig. 13 *B*. This body has been worn for centuries, and I do not doubt that our children and grandchildren will see it still. It is adopted for over-gowns as well as slips.

Here is the manner of taking a pattern for it: procure an absolutely plain body, with a neck as high as possible. Perhaps you do not have such a model; it will be easy for you to obtain one from amongst your acquaintances. When you have got it, try it on first, and see if it is too large or small for you. Observe its faults as closely as possible, in order to avoid them when cutting out the first pattern. This pattern will be cut out in Chambery gauze (a kind of cheap, very transparent gauze).

Fold the model body in half, so that no more than one of the fronts and one of the backs is visible. Turn one sleeve to the wrong side and pass it into the other, so that they are as if removed on the side where you must place the Chambery gauze. Then apply the selvage of the gauze following Fig. 13 *A, ab*. Commence pinning at the bottom, letting the gauze exceed it by three fingers; the surplus material is left to accommodate the curve

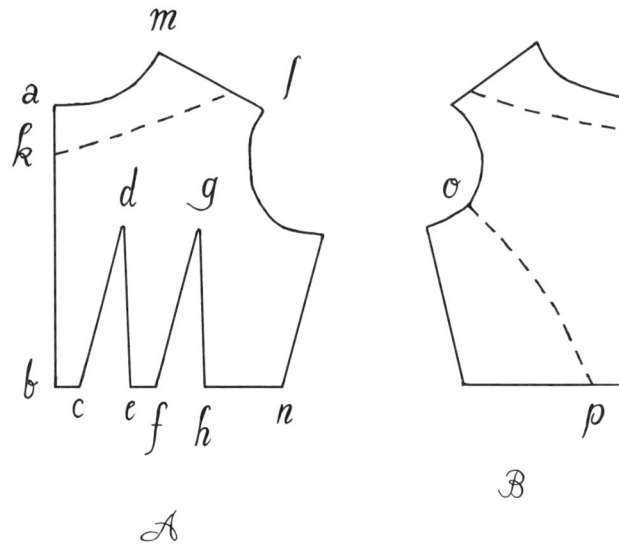

Figure 13. To cut out the body.

below the bosom. Continue to pin along the selvage indicated, that is, following *ab,* up to the top of the model body. Hold the part pinned between the thumb and forefinger of your left hand, while your right is employed in spreading the gauze on the straight-way, to the end of the shoulder.

The gauze being placed smooth on the widest part, a surplus of gauze will be found at the bottom of the body. This surplus is used to form the two plaits which serve to contain the bosom (see Fig. 13 *A, cde* and *fgh*). These plaits must be a finger apart at the base, and at least three at the top. At the bottom they are very wide, and at the top they must gradually disappear. To impart more grace to the plaits, lay them over your knee and form them to its shape. As the material is very clear, you may strongly mark their depth, and then cut the plaited parts.

Finish pinning the gauze precisely on the seams which are made on the body, that is, under the arms and then the part at the arm-hole, from under the arms up to the seam which joins the shoulders. Also pin this last seam, as well as the part at the neck and the bottom of the waist. Cut just at the pins, then unpin the pattern. Do the same for the back.

Take the measure; lay it over the gauze pattern in the same manner in which it was placed on the person. If the pattern is not correct, mark its faults on it. Take some extremely stout toile, and cut out a body using the pattern you took. Baste the four seams and the plaits. At the bottom, put a strong linen tape and a very strong hook and eye.

Try on this imperfect model. Put pins across the front at three-quarters of its height. These pins describe a nearly straight line, because the last pin at the shoulder leaves only three fingers of the width of the latter. Mark the height of the body with notches. You have made, by this means, a pattern for two different bodies: in Fig. 13 *A, amlnb* for a high neck, and *klnb* for a body *en fourreau,* that is a laced tight body. Again pay attention to making it as graceful as possible.

Finally cut out a second pattern in very strong paper; this is the last one. Strengthen it with a lining of toile, and fix the layers together with short running stitches all round. This step is necessary because the pattern will serve you at all times, since it will suffice for cutting out every kind of gown which you want, as will be seen later.

Of making up the Body *en Fourreau.* This style of body requires a strong lining; the stronger it is, the better the gown will fit. Do not neglect the bones: 1st., one in the middle of the front, whose case is between two rows of running stitches spaced apart the width of the bone which will be entered there. 2nd., the seam under the arms. 3rd., one on the edge of each back. You must leave at that place enough material and lining to make a sturdier case than that on the front. When you have folded the material over itself on the wrong side, baste at the width of the bone. Turn the back again and baste on a linen or silk tape adjoining the first basting. Holding the tape, push it from left to right. Turn the back to the right side again, and take back-stitches one into another below the basting; these are called prick-stitches. Then it is a matter of piercing the eyelet-holes, before placing the bones.

To pierce the eyelet-holes, turn to your weight covered with a pin-cushion. Attach it at the top of the back, which is turned to the right side, and consequently the linings touch. Take the bottom of the back between the thumb and forefinger of your left hand. Take a punch whose point has been carefully protected with a piece of cork. Despite this precaution, still take that of making the first hole on a piece of material which you will not use; for if the point is blunted you risk spoiling the backs.

Let us suppose that the tool is in good condition. Take it in your right hand; rest your palm on the end of the handle; your little finger and ring finger serve to hold it in this position. Your thumb, forefinger, and middle finger encircle the point where the handle is joined to the rounded piece of steel called a punch. Pierce the first eyelet-hole at a distance of a little finger from the top of the backs. Repeat this operation at the bottom of the backs. When these two eyelet-holes have been made, you will see that they are symmetrical on the left and right back. The rest of the eyelet-holes are staggered, so that each faces an empty space directly opposite.

Detach the backs from the top of the weight. Pull the back which is behind to the left, then attach the backs to the weight again. Pierce the second eyelet-hole at the top of the right back at a distance of an inch from the previous one, and so on, progressing to the next-to-last, which must be very near to the last eyelet-hole.

The left back will have the same two closely-spaced eyelet-holes, and these will not be at the bottom but at the top; and it is at the top of the back that you attach the lace. Detach the backs from the top of the weight; re-enter the punch into the eyelet-hole which you wish to make first. For this, take a short needle of a size proportionable to the length of thread or silk which you wish to use.

Because I believe that my readers are familiar with all the kinds of stitches listed earlier, I shall content myself with teaching them how to work the eyelet-holes well. Be careful to take only a very little material on your needle, as much underneath as on top. Tighten each stitch equally, and re-enter the punch in each finished eyelet-hole. This is done from the wrong side to the right side, so that the eyelet-hole is rounded, and comes out again right side up. Also, to prevent the back from puckering, take the part to work between your thumb and forefinger, and leave the right-hand side free.

Form the two front plaits, which must be marked by a basting on the material. They are indicated by Fig. 13 A, cde and fgh. Despite the care taken in passing the threads, it is still quite difficult to join the two bastings. You must have recourse to your knee, so as to round them a little in forming them. Always commence at the top, be it in basting, or in sewing them.

Take a strip of double wadding three fingers wide. Apply it along the body between the outer material and the lining; tear it in a few places, so that it assumes the roundness of the gown body. Also put a slight piece under the arms; this prevents perspiration from soaking through the gown. This piece will only improve the appearance of the waist.

How many women have rounded their shapes with a wadded gown, only to appear stouter! Let us try to know better: let us alter our shapes in a way which suits us, and not follow a fashion unless it does. In my opinion, that is the prettier coquetry. With these divers toilets, assemblies would charm the eye no less; quite the contrary, the variety of the whole pleases a man. And ladies, for whom do you take so much trouble?

Let us return to the gown body. When these pieces of wadding are in place, lay the shoulder of the front on that of the back; baste firmly. Likewise baste the seam under the arms. Enter the bones at the places mentioned above.

Take a wide linen tape; take the measure, on which notches indicate the distance from the middle of the front to under the arms, and from under the arms to the back. Mark these same distances on the tape with pins, and baste it to the right side of the body. Over-cast the tape to the skirt. Make gathers spaced by four fingers or less on each side. The longer the waist, the more the gathers must be sloped off, so that the hips may be fitted more gracefully. Attach two large hooks and eyes to the tape. Also add at each under-arm, two ends of tape an inch wide and a quarter of an ell long; attach them at the edge of the linen tape which holds the body. That finished, your gown is ready to try on.

The Best Mode of fitting a Gown. My readers will not fail to find some one who will willingly offer to help fit a gown cut out as I have just described: it is a service gladly rendered between young persons. In general, it is better that the gown be rather too small than too large; the faults (if it has any) will be perceived much better.

While the gown is on the person, have some pins put in it. The first is placed about two fingers from the eyelet-hole at the bottom of the waist. The second gradually approaches the shoulder-blade. The third and fourth must follow the same inclination, and so on (see Fig. 13 *B, op*).

If the body is too long in the waist, and the front plaits do not go up high enough, pass your finger under the shoulder seam. Lift it, so that the body comes up; form a fold at the place where you put your finger. This little correction will suffice to remedy the fault. If the gown has been cut out according to the mode which I have indicated, the fault which I have just pointed out is the sole one to be feared. After a certain time, you will no longer have the trouble of fitting the gown; practice will make you familiar with your size, and to succeed it will suffice to use your pattern.

I shall now speak of the manner of finishing the gown which has just been fitted. The first thing to do, on taking off your gown, is to prepare for sewing it permanently.

To make up the Gown. Begin by taking the skirt off the body. Pay attention to whether the skirt has some pins which indicate corrections to make; pass a thread in their place. Fold the skirt to the wrong side; form as few folds as you can, and if possible, none lengthways. If you have only the body and the sleeves to make up, put the skirt in an armoire. A box would be still better, above all when the skirt has been set onto the body.

Take the body; pass a thread just at the place where you must put your waist-band, which will be of the same material as the gown. When it will be sewed with back-stitches, double it with the linen tape which was used previously. Also pass a thread at the place where you want the body to end. Take some corded piping (see the article on making it below). Turn the body to the wrong side in front of you. Place the piping on the right side of the body; its raw edge must be on top. Take it, as well as the body, between the thumb and forefinger of your left hand, and make it so that the narrow cord is very tight. Sew the piping with short running stitches, being sure to take only one at a time, for two reasons: first, to avoid the risk of biting into the piping, and second, to avoid puckering the body. This stitching finished, neatly cut the part of the body which is meant to be re-covered by the over-casting of the piping, with which you make a hem without piercing the under side of the body. Fold down both ends of the piping; then put a hook at one end and an eye at the other. Place these also at the bottom of the waist-band. Do up the narrow tapes under the arms as before. Take the greatest care when prick-stitching the plaits under the bosom. Do not attach that part of the body to your pincushion; you would spoil it entirely. Set the skirt onto the body.

Now take the sleeves, which we will suppose made, and which I shall teach you to make and to set on gracefully in the articles devoted to long and short sleeves. It is best to have two pair. In this case, you will fasten short sleeves to the body. The long sleeves are fastened at the top with a corded piping, the length of which is measured by the arm-hole (the part formed by the seam of the shoulders and that of the under-arms). These two pair of sleeves are convenient in that you may, while retaining the same gown, change your toilet. If you wish to take a walk, you need only pin on your long sleeves; you will thus be clad more warmly and properly. On returning, you may replace them with a canezou, be it with long sleeves or only *à épaulières*, which will be even more dressy. Or again you may put on your neck only a light scarf or an embroidered triangular tulle shawl, or even nothing but a necklace; because this style of gown is not at all low-necked in the middle of the front, nor in the middle of the back; only over the shoulders, which renders the waist very graceful.

For this style of gown to be perfectly pretty, make it a blouse gown. You have another means of changing it by adapting draperies *à la Sévigné*, either in tulle, gauze, or a similar stuff if the gown is of plain material. If you put a trimming at the bottom of this gown, a flat trimming is preferable to any other.

The Body *à la Raphaël.*

The pattern for a laced body *en fourreau* will serve to make almost all the bodies which fashion may introduce, including a ball gown, though excepting a high-necked gown or a redingote.

The Body *à la Raphaël.* If you wish to make a body *à la Raphaël* (the name given to bodies gathered at the top and bottom and three-quarters high, more or less), fold your material double. If the material is too narrow, put a seam in the middle of the front, because for this body you need more than twice the pattern. Begin by leaving the material double, in order to cut out the front in one piece, laying on it the paper pattern for only half the front. Mark the first fold near the selvage which is on the front of the body, and then a second or a third, and so on, up to where the shoulder-piece begins, which must be two or three fingers wide, rather smaller than larger.

Finish the body at the top with a corded piping or a *demi-jarretière* (see the article below on making *jarretières*). Take care, before placing the *jarretière*, to place the gathers on a little *signet* (a little riband like a book-mark). Leave a plain space of about a finger on each side of the front seam. The gathers should be fastened at the bottom of the shoulder-piece. Do the same for the back. Put a hook at the top as for the plain body. The gathers at the bottom of the body should all be brought towards the middle of it *en gerbe*, that is, fanning out towards the shoulders. Those on the back are arranged in the same way. Then set onto the body any kind of sleeves you please. Set the skirt onto the body, following the same steps as for the previous one.

If you wish to make the body with draperies, be they lengthways or widthways, or even slantways, take your paper pattern. Pin the front to the back, pin the bosom plaits closed, and pin the shoulders together. Use a little imagination, then display your good taste: you can create with your fingers a prodigious quantity of elegant styles.

Long Sleeves. Long sleeves are prettier and fit much better if they are cut out on the bias. But as it is rare to find a suitable width of silk for this cut, content yourself with folding the material in that direction insofar as possible. If the material is plain, put the most bias side at the back; the elbow will be found more comfortable. But you cannot do the same with striped material; that would have the most hideous effect. The arms would have the air of being turned round, and the bosom would appear narrower. If, as I do not doubt, you are in a position to consider such a thing, give me your attention.

Work the sleeve seam with back-stitches if the material does not wash. In the contrary case, work a mantua-maker's hem. If the sleeves have cuffs, leave about three good fingers unsewed. Border the little slit with material similar to the gown, in such a manner that it will admit of a very thin bone. By this little expedient, the sleeves will no longer hang over the forearms; and what is still better (without it holding the slit longer) extend the bone-case twice as far as the slit. By this means the sleeves will fit as if glued to the arms. This little improvement is still unknown, but I have found it most convenient.

The cuff should be three fingers high; two hooks should be used to close it. On the other side of the cuff, work silk bars, which are much better than eyes. Do not position the hooks so as to tighten the cuff; you will prevent the blood from circulating and the hand will become red. No one likes to see a red hand, above all on a woman.

The front part of the top of the sleeve, whatsoever the style, must be hollowed; that is to say, you must cut off a little piece. Fig. 14, *qr*, will give you an idea of the quantity which you have to remove. About four fingers from the seam under the arms, begin to gather with running stitches, and stop at the same distance from the seam as you began. Make a second row of gathers an inch lower; this produces a pretty effect, and aids much in setting the sleeve onto the gown.

Here, therefore, is the sleeve ready to set onto the body. Bring the wrong side of the body towards you; enter the sleeve into the arm-hole on the right side of the body, putting the sleeve seam forwards by one finger on the front of the body. Beginning from the seam of the side-piece, pin and observe, before basting, that the sleeve is graceful, and that it does not prevent the arms from moving in any direction. The greatest part of the sleeve gathers should be at the top of the arm. If this is a silk gown, sew the sleeves on the wrong side with back-stitches, taking them without tightening. Then trim the seam evenly and over-cast it. If the body is not lined, turn it back onto the sleeve, at the place where the shoulder-piece seam is found, and take some back-stitches at the place indicated: this excellent mode is followed by only a small number of persons. By this means, the sleeve is prevented from coming over the shoulder and narrowing the width. It is all these little things, which are nearly invisible to the untrained eye, which add or subtract grace from any gown soever: therefore, this way of setting on the sleeve should be used for all kinds of gowns.

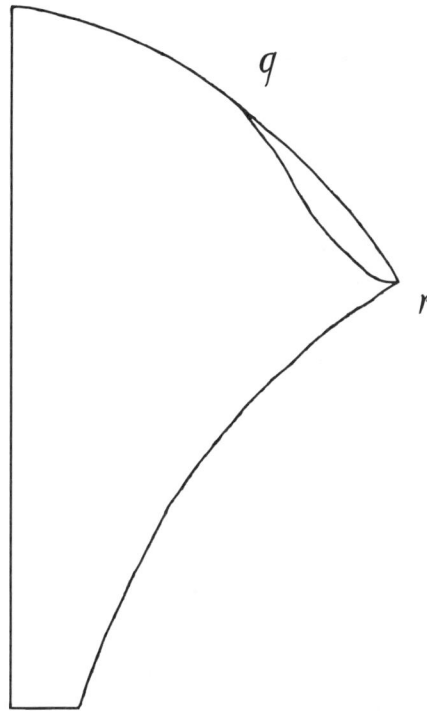

Figure 14. To hollow the sleeve.

I do not recommend any mancherons, finding them very ugly. Only, one kind is nearly indispensable when the sleeves are made of a different material than the gown. Then, around the arm-hole, add a double bias, about a hand high in the middle, and sloping to both ends; it must harmonize with the gown.

Long muslin sleeves are sometimes made *bouillonnée,* or puffed. For this cut out a sleeve on the straight-way, fitting tight to the arms. The *bouillonnée* is ordinarily made lengthways on the sleeves; the puffs number seven or nine. Trace their places with threads on the flat sleeve. The muslin which must be puffed is twice the length of the sleeve, and a little more than twice the width. As the sleeve is much wider at the top, take care to arrange the puffed material in the same way. Sometimes the puffs are made separately, and an *entre-deux* of muslin or embroidered tulle is put between each puff.

It is impossible to describe all the kinds of sleeves which may be made. Your taste will make up for that. A good model of a gigot sleeve (a sleeve very narrow at the bottom and very wide at the top) will serve to form a thousand others.

Short Sleeves. I shall begin by saying that every woman whose arms are even tolerable should wear short sleeves. This kind of sleeve gives ease; unhappily it cannot be adopted by every body.

Short sleeves are always cut on the bias. The pattern for long sleeves will serve for cutting them out, but cut them twice as wide as the others. Gather the bottom of a short sleeve flat, if it is of silk. You will do well to line it with lawn or any other clear, but starched, material.

Measure the width of the sleeve-band, and put over the gathers a narrow piping, which you may cover with a strip of satin or of the same material as the gown. Before turning the narrow band to the wrong side, insert a straw, which is used by *marchandes de modes* to support and impart stiffness to the sleeve.

You may add to these bands a tulle ruche, or even gather a blond two fingers wide. Sometimes a tolerably wide puffing (about a third of the sleeve) is added to these little sleeves. You adapt the band already placed, and finish the puff with a band similar to the first. On the band, a little to the front of the sleeve, place a riband bow alone, or surmounted by a flower if this is a ball gown. Such sleeves are very simple, very easy to make, and very pretty for young ladies.

For an elegant young woman, make the sleeve extremely short, surmounted by a flat band three fingers wide, onto which is plaited three blonds about four fingers wide. Relieve these blonds with a large bow of riband No. 12. (Ribands, as you know, are numbered like all materials.) The bow must be placed a little above the crook of the arm.

The Mode of making Separate Draperies. Take the pattern for the laced body *en fourreau*. Baste it together as if you wished to put it on. Fold on the bias the material intended to make the draperies; cut off and remove the corner which you have formed.

Cut the bands three fingers wider than half the front of the body, and five times as long as the front of the body. Form plaits about two fingers deep. These plaits should be formed on the body of the gown to closely follow the curves of the bosom. Then take, with another band, the length of the shoulder-piece, beginning where the front drapery ends, and continuing up to the beginning of the width of the back at the shoulders. Allow for this drapery about six times the length of the shoulder-piece, and make plaits like those on the front.

You therefore have two draperies for the front, and two others for the shoulders. But those of the back are not separated, and only one is formed.

This shape renders the back more square and more graceful. When the draperies are placed, always sew to the top of the body some tulle folded double, or a blond two fingers high; but only loosely. The blond is glimpsed now and then; for example, on the right side at the place where the drapery is joined with *liens* of satin or *gros de Naples,* &c. (see Fig. 15).

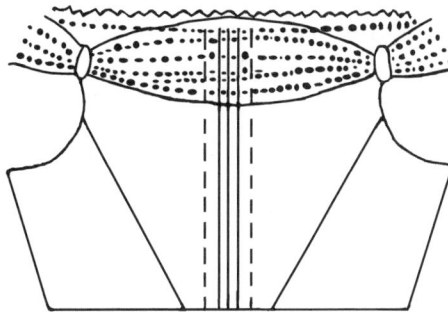

Figure 15. Draperies joined with *liens.*

The Little Accessories of which Trimmings are composed.

These include corded piping, *jarriètieres, liens,* the rouleaux called *tuyaux-de-pipes,* and turned rouleaux.

For corded piping, cut a narrow strip of material on the bias. This should be about a finger wide, according to the thickness of the cord which it must cover. The strip cut, take it between the thumb and forefinger of your left hand, and fold it double. Pass a cord between both parts of the strip; hold it quite tight with the nail of your left thumb, and then take half-long running stitches under the cord, which is thus fixed to the narrow strip.

For *jarretières,* cut a bias strip a finger wide, or wider according to your taste. Take care that the bias is perfect, or else this kind of trimming is as ugly as it is pretty when well made.

If you wish to join these strips together, take care to remove the selvages. That done, sew a corded piping on each side of the strip. Recollect to use a long needle, especially for this kind of trimming, which is made with only one running stitch at a time, the length of about a quarter of the long needle. If you follow all these steps, your pipings will have the air of being glued on.

When the two cords have been sewed, trim the seams a little. Lay one over the other, and work herring-bone stitches without crossing them, above all taking care not to tighten the stitches more in one place than another. That done, your *jarretière* is finished.

Demi-jarretières are made with only one corded piping. Therefore, you leave the satin strip much wider and without a cord, so that you may fold it on the wrong side of the one piping.

For *liens,* take a strip of satin or other material of the width you desire for this kind of *agrafe.* Form six or seven plaits on the width of the strip. Turn the former to the wrong side, as well as the latter. Take running stitches to hold the plaits, and the *lien* will be made. This kind of *lien* is used to join the draperies of bodies.

Liens for trimming are made differently. Cut a narrow strip of Chambery gauze, of the length and width you desire for the *lien.* Then lay on a narrow piece of corded piping, which must exceed the Chambery gauze, adding enough to cover the gauze. When you have arrived at the other end, take a strip similar to that used to make the piping. Sew it on its wrong side, then turn it. Next, slip in a cord similar to the preceding rows, and take running stitches across the cords. At both ends of the *lien,* tighten the thread a little, fasten it securely, and the *lien* is finished.

The name *tuyaux-de-pipes* sufficiently indicates that these rouleaux must be perfectly cylindrical. To make a rouleau of which the base is no more than the circumference of a small O, the strip of material intended to make it must be cut on the bias, and three fingers wide. These strips must be stretched; the rouleau will be found to be much more supple and crumple much less. Fold the strip so that one side is hidden by the other; repeat the same operation and sew with side-stitches, taking care not to pierce through. The stitches must be taken nimbly; a little practice is needed to work them well; then it is not at all difficult. Indeed, once you have the habit, you can do it with your eyes closed.

These narrow rouleaux are used to embellish pelerines in blond net. Ordinarily three are placed at a distance on each foot of blond; so many rows of the latter, and so many rows of the narrow rouleaux.

Turned rouleaux are made with the aid of a satin bias strip. We will suppose it to be an inch wide. Fold it on the wrong side; securely attach a narrow braid, which you put inside; once passed it will not be awkward. Take both edges of the strip between the thumb and forefinger of your left hand. Pin it here and there, and pull the strip a little to ensure that the rouleau will not pucker when it is made. Finally, begin to sew it with small running stitches, taking good care to work this seam near the edge, and not to introduce any back-stitches, because the rouleau must be very flexible. It is wise to use *écru* silk to work this seam, because thread is subject to knotting and breaking. This silk is not costly, and it is the only one used by the best *marchandes de modes* for their hats.

At each half-ell which you have sewed, pull the narrow braid with your left hand, while you take the end of the rouleau made between the thumb and forefinger of your right hand, taking good care that the seam is always under your thumb, and always turned to the same side.

These rouleaux are used to decorate a great many trimmings, and to stripe tulle sleeves, bodies, &c.

The Trimmings which are put on the Hems of Gowns. These include wadded rouleaux, *bouillons*, flounces, and divers kinds of ruches.

A wadded rouleau is a bias of satin, or any other material which is not transparent. It is most commonly four fingers wide. Cut some strips of wadding of about the same width. Fold and re-fold each strip over itself, so that it forms a roll. Fasten the wadding together with over-cast stitches, which are very long and not tightened. Next cover the wadding with the material intended to envelop it. Fasten it here and there, and sew it with running stitches. Recollect to take only one stitch at a time.

After that, it is easy to cut out leaves, triangles, diamonds, or any other shape. The rouleaux serve to decorate them and in making trimmings, be they flat, or raised by puffs of tulle, gauze, *crêpe lisse*, &c.

Bouillons are puffs sewed on the bias, a third of an ell high. Take a strip of Chambery gauze cut on the straight-way, a sixth high. This tulle must be gathered for certain trimmings, such as those which are raised by *liens* here and there. For all trimmings which are not made like the gown, pay close attention to the narrowing of the latter at the top. It will therefore not suffice to measure the width of the skirt at the bottom; it is also necessary to measure it at the place where the trimming will end.

There are also strips which are plaited *à gueule-de-loup*. I have no need to explain to my readers the manner in which these box-plaits are formed, because it is exactly that of a *collerette*: it will suffice to know what depth to give the plaits. The plaits must be four fingers wide; sometimes they are made double, that is to say, each is surmounted by another a little less wide. Make these plaits so that you may spread or compress them at will. When one side of the trimming is finished, make contrary plaits, with the middle of the first plaits being the beginning of the others, which is very pretty.

To form a heading for these *bouillons*, or *gueules-de-loup*, place a garland of flowers there. The flowers must be set on nearly flat. These trimmings are proper for young persons. I advise my young readers to employ as little satin as possible in their trimmings: only a wadded rouleau at the edge of the hem.

For some time flounces have been made a quarter of an ell high. This trimming is made on every kind of material, even on silk tulle; this simple trimming is suitable for the mistress of the house when receiving visitors. Flounces are sometimes cut into points, and the points are trimmed with piping, or a turned rouleau. Sometimes a hem is made there, with a cord put into it.

Place the flounce about a finger from the edge of the gown. The top of the flounce, if it has no heading, should be gathered, turning the material a line or two over itself with stitches *à cheval,* that is to say, the same stitch as over-casting, only a little longer. Take care to fold the trimming into eighths: at each fold pass a thread of a different colour than the flounce. Divide the skirt in the same way. Measure the skirt at the place where you will put the flounce with a piping. Set the flounce onto this covered cord; sew along it with side-stitches, and place the trimming on the gown. Pin it on the right side, turn the gown to the wrong side, and take running stitches to fasten the flounce to the gown.

Often a heading is made for a flounce. In this case, cut out the flounce plus the heading you wish to allow for it. Use a paper measure to mark the heading equally, folding the material over itself, and marking the fold with your thumb and forefinger. Then turn down this portion of the material and gather it flat. Take a rouleau of the kind called *tuyau de pipe,* which you place on the right side of the trimming, along the gathers. Sew it on the wrong side so that you may even out the gathers. That done, place the flounce on the skirt. Attach the heading at intervals of about a hand. Without this precaution the heading falls down, which does not make a pretty effect. At the edge of the heading, I recommend entering a straw of the kind used by milliners. The trimming will appear to much more advantage and will crumple less.

It is needless to explain that wash materials must be sewed more securely, which is the situation for using whipped gathers. Here is the mode of making them: take the material which you will whip between the thumb and forefinger of your left hand. Moisten your thumb a little, and roll a very small quantity of the edge of the material very tight. Next pass your needle under the roll without pulling the thread. Re-pass it on top, and then underneath. Do this seven or eight times before pulling the length of thread. You may proceed very quickly by this means, and without wearing the thread as much as if you pulled it with each stitch.

Ruched trimmings have existed for centuries, are still the fashion, and will be for a long time. To my mind, this is the queen of trimmings. Ruches cut on the straight-way are prettier than those cut on the bias. They are employed in the latter fashion when the edges of the strips are meant to enclose a straw or cord. Excepting that case, always cut the strips between the two selvages; because in the other direction, the plaits could only be very flat. I strongly advise my readers not to send out their ruches to be pinked by means of punches, since the punches do not have a pattern of points which is suitable for this trimming (see Fig. 16). Ruches pinked with scissors have the appearance of being infinitely more full. To pink a double row of ruches with scissors requires only half an hour; you will not have the trouble of conveying the strips back and forth; in short, you will not need the assistance of any one.

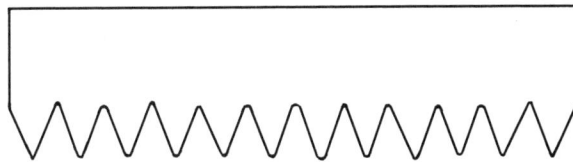

Figure 16. Material pinked for a ruche.

These kinds of ruches are only made with simple plaits; it is necessary not to make them too small. The entire plait of one ruche an eighth of an ell high must be two good fingers. You must be careful to make the plaits quite straight, and fasten them with running stitches, which permits them to spread a little if they are scant, and which requires no more material. You may spread these plaits, but not tighten them: that is very ugly when two rows of equal height are plaited. Take both of them on the wrong side between the thumb and forefinger of your left hand. Next make the two ruches fast with very long over-cast stitches. Take very little material on your needle, and do not tighten the stitches.

The height of this kind of trimming is left to the taste of the person who wears it. Sometimes one is put at the bottom of the skirt, a quarter of an ell high; the second is a little less high than the first; as you put on rows, you must diminish their height.

These ruches are sometimes made in two colours, and sometimes made to meander over the gown. Again, sometimes they are cut into pieces, which are placed in chevrons one into another, the first ones with the base at the top and the others at the bottom. Sometimes also these ruches are placed slantways at the edge of the gown, but on the gown itself. The ruche must slant in one direction beginning from the middle of the gown to the middle of the back breadth, and in the other direction beginning from the middle of the back breadth, to the middle of the front. At these two places a triangle is formed, with its bottom at the top and its point at the bottom.

You may make two narrow ruches divide at the top of the skirt which, gradually moving apart, come to rest on the trimming, the extremities being about a third of an ell apart at the bottom, and a sixteenth at the top. This kind of *tablier* must be made on the front breadth for married ladies, and on the back breadth for young ladies.

When a gown is trimmed with ruches, it is necessary only to enclose the hem in a satin bias sewed flat. The ruches will impart enough roundness to the skirt.

Well! I have said enough about the modes of making the principal trimmings. The taste of my readers will supply any thing I have forgotten.

The Mode of cutting out a Redingote. Use the pattern of the laced body *en fourreau* to cut out another with a high neck (see Fig. 13), because this style is tight like the body *en fourreau*, and only differs in rising to the nape of the neck. This latter pattern will serve to cut out redingotes, canezous, or *fichu-guimpes* opening at the back.

For the skirt, take two breadths of equal length, and place them flat across their whole width. Next take the measure which must serve you for cutting the top of the breadths. Allow something like a hand extra, which will be used to make a hem, and cross one over the other. Cut the bottom of the breadths twice as wide as the top; in short as was explained for gowns. (See Fig. 12, *gh*, for the mode of cutting the breadths slantways.)

If the redingote is lined, cut out the breadths of the lining a finger wider than the outer material, then spread the two corresponding breadths on a table: for example, the back breadth and its lining, and so on for the other parts of the skirt. Spread the lining smoothly on top of the corresponding breadth. Begin by basting the pieces together along the edges. Then fold the breadth of the outer material in a straight line, and pass your hand firmly over the fold, so that it may later serve as a guide. These folds must be spaced about a sixteenth of an ell apart. When you have thus taken up the material, until no more than the space of a sixteenth is left up to the end of the breadth, freeze the layers. That is, baste them permanently, as follows: take a needleful of thread longer than the breadth; stick the needle into the outer material and the under material, catching only the surface of each; after that re-enter the needle at a distance of a sixteenth, always catching the outer and under material, which will make a long hidden stitch.

When you have to wad a gown, cut out the breadths of wadding exactly like those of the lining. Wadding which is sold by the piece has two glazed surfaces, and has an opening only at the bottom. It is necessary to split this piece on one side, and divide it in half. On being opened out it will present a very soft fleece; it is this fleece which is placed on the lining, so that the warmth is felt more readily by the person who puts on the gown. Spread the breadth of lining which must receive that of the wadding, and fasten them together with crossways rows of long running stitches spaced a thirty-second of an ell apart. Above all, do not knot the threads used to baste the wadding, because after this operation you must grasp the top and bottom of the breadth and pull it in a straight line; if you neglect this step, your gown runs the risk of being very ill-lined.

Gowns which are wadded, or simply lined, are made up differently from others. Lay the two pieces of the outer material which must be sewed, one over another. Join there the lining of the breadth, on the back of which you work, basting these three breadths together, and working a seam composed of back-stitches and running stitches. The fourth piece is sewed onto the seam of the other three.

I advise my readers to acquire the habit, which has been followed for a long time by sensible people, of making all gowns to open in the front, excepting those for the ball; because if you do not have a lady's maid, you risk being very ill-dressed. If it is otherwise, the absurd fashion of our day can only have originated with a woman who wanted every one to be persuaded that she had people to spare her the fatigue of unhooking or unlacing her clothing. You ought to be content with wearing your stays made thus, without giving yourself the same trouble over the rest of your clothing. I know by experience that the gowns most difficult to make, fit perfectly if made to open in the front.

The Mode of cutting out Divers Mantles for Women, called Pelisses *à l'Autrichienne.*
The curve of the pieces must gradually disappear into the bottom of the mantle. (See Fig. 17; *A* is the front, *B* is the side-piece, and *C* is the back.) There are mantua-makers who cut out these mantles without giving them any roundness over the shoulders: those are far more heavy to wear. The slit for your arms must be made a third of an ell lower than the neck; its length must be a sixth. Add a small strap of the same material, which is attached on the side of the back, and comes round to button on the front of the opening.

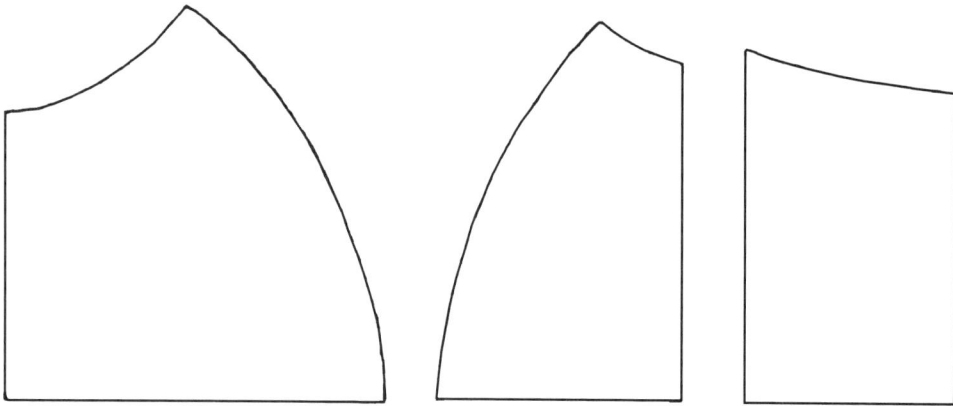

A   *B*   *C*

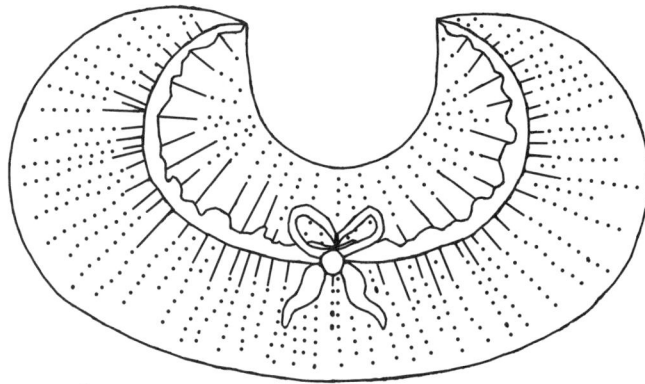

s

D

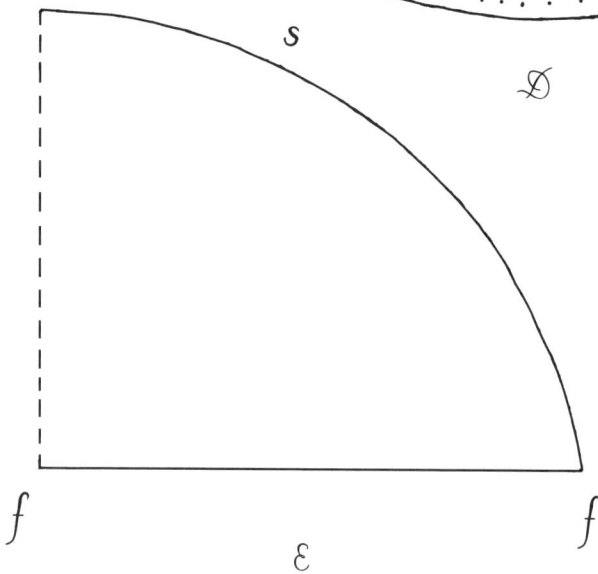

f   *f*

E

Figure 17. The pelerine and hood for the *pelisse à l'Autrichienne*.

These pelisses or mantles, when they are of silk, are wadded. It is necessary to space the rows of basting holding the wadding much closer than for a gown. You should also work them so that the stitches form little squares on the inside of the mantle.

After having made up the pieces above, put a pin in the middle of the top of your mantle. Make a plait to the left of the pin, and one to the right. Continue these plaits to three fingers from the seam on top of the shoulder. Leave the same distance on the shoulder for commencing the front plaits. The measure round the collar must be about half an ell long. You may want to tighten or loosen the plaits; have the collar measure near you.

Formerly hoods were fitted to these pelisses; now two pelerines are substituted. This fashion is much more graceful, above all when the pelerines are cut like those of a man's carrick; that is to say, forming flutes at the bottom. But there is nothing so convenient as a hood; it is for my readers to decide; they have a choice between the useful and the agreeable. If I were in their place, here is what I would do: I would put on a pelerine which descended to about a hand lower than the elbow, and add a hood to the pelerine. Such mantles succeed in being both useful and pleasing (see Fig. 17 *D*). The hood is plaited onto a narrow strip separate from the collar, and is basted when the mantle is finished. The hood is cut on the straight-way; Fig. 17 *E* shows exactly half of it; the selvage is at the bottom and is shown by *ff*.

I shall not speak of those to which a long pelerine was added; that fashion was no prettier than it was useful.

The Mode of fringing and using Ribands in making Belts.

For a belt using fringed ribands, take riband No. 16 or 22. Cut two pieces, once of half an ell, the other of five-eighths. Cut off their selvages along about a twelfth of an ell. Withdraw the threads across the riband with the aid of a pin. The pin is only used to make the end come out; then you finish the operation with the thumb and forefinger of your right hand, while your left hand is occupied in holding the riband very straight.

Next divide the threads into seven or nine strands. Knot each strand about half an inch from the end. When this first row of knots is made, take two of the strands and knot them together. Neither the first nor the last strand should be knotted in the second row. In the third row, knot the first strand with the second. Four rows of knots will suffice. The other end of these pieces of riband is gathered.

Use riband No. 12 to make four loops; that is enough. Then make a *lien* to separate the bow in the middle. Tighten it as much as possible, which will impart more grace to the bow. The band which encircles the waist must be three fingers high, and have an inner lining of coarse lawn.

The belts for the ball worn last winter were very elegant. To make one, attach four pieces of fringed riband, about five-eighths of an ell long, to a band which encircles the waist. These four pieces are placed on the front, spread apart from one another, and five are placed on the back of the band. These belts are only pretty on gowns of clear, plain material.

The trimmings are matched to the sleeves, and three of these pieces of riband are put round them, or rather at the top of the little short sleeve, along the seam. Each bow has only two loops, and the fringed ends are a sixteenth of an ell. But, though this sleeve trimming is pretty on a person whose shoulders are low and well sloped, it is ugly on a person with high shoulders.

If you wish to make a belt with shoulder-straps, pin together the pattern for the laced body *en fourreau*. Fold riband No. 16 into a roll, so that one selvage is over the other in the middle of the riband. That done, measure the length of the gown body with the riband, the front and the under-arms all along the shoulder-pieces, and extend the riband to the bottom of the back. Fasten it to the gown body and lay it over the pattern, in order to impart the necessary slant to the riband. Shoulder-straps may be embellished with a bow placed at the top of the shoulder. It is needless to say that the shoulder-straps are attached to the band which encircles the body.

Some Pretty Collars for *Fichus*. There are certain persons who cannot go without putting on a *fichu*, even for full dress; they are forced to do so by age or leanness, or perhaps by some infirmity. Blond net is preferable to blond lace for trimming these *fichus*. The collar of the *fichu* should not exceed three fingers in height. The seam at the top of the collar is enclosed in a bias strip of satin or *gros de Naples*, into which you put a cord to give it a little support. The net meant to trim the collar should be one hand high, and plaited separately. The first row is sewed on the right side, precisely over the cord. When you cut out the net, allow enough to fold it over itself two or three times. Place the second row at one finger from the first, and preserve the same distance for all the rows which you place. Add a gauze or satin bow to close the collar; however, this bow is not acceptable for full dress.

Collars puffed in blond net are dressier and prettier. To make one, cut a band of the aforementioned net a third of an ell high. Both ends of the band should be cut to almost a point (see Fig. 18 A). Then take the middle of this piece, which you gather flat at the highest place; four rows

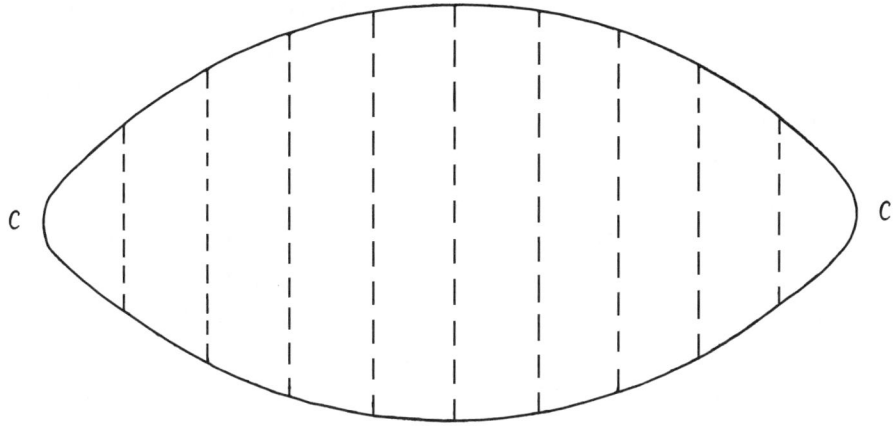

A

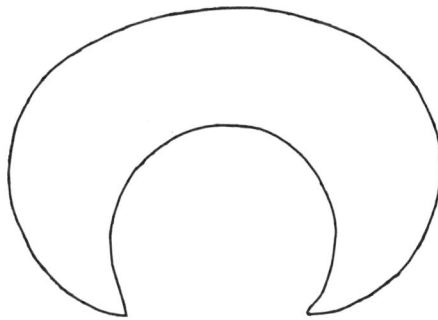

B

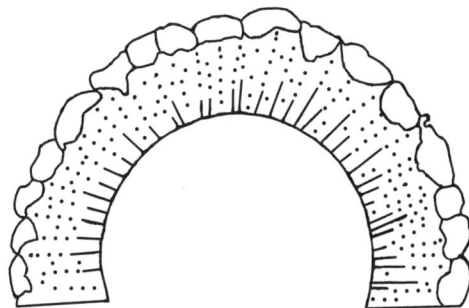

C

Figure 18. The collar *à la Médicis*.

of gathers should succeed this one on each side of the collar. You need do no more to give it the shape of a collar *à la Médicis* (see Fig. 18 *B*).

For each row of gathers, you will need a piece of straw covered with satin or other material. Cut the straws twice as high as the collar. Fix them to your pattern, and sew them one after another to the gathers of the wide band. These gathers must be brought onto the top of the collar, and sewed into the space of four fingers at the most. That done, join the two ends of each straw (bending the wide piece of material over itself) by over-casting, which must securely hold the straw by the satin in which it is wrapped.

Then take running stitches to hold the two ends of your net. Place this band on the collar *à la Médicis,* and make it take the same shape. This style of collar is very pretty in *gaze de laine* (see Fig. 18 *C*).

Attach the collar to a *fichu* (which should be of the same material as the collar), holding the *fichu* in front of you, on the right side of the material. The collar is at the back, and you attach the collar and the *fichu* together by back-stitching, being careful to take only very small stitches. Even so, trim this seam evenly, and conceal it with a rouleau of material similar to that which covers the straw supports.

These kinds of *fichus* are cut out by a redingote pattern, folding over itself the piece which forms the under-arms, because these *fichus* do not need it. It is useless, and even awkward, to put a case for a drawing-string along the fronts, because you cannot cross them and the *fichu* stays open.

I believe I have said enough to render my young readers capable of making themselves the principal parts of their clothing, and in a position to do without professional mantua-makers. The advice which I have given them permits of dressing at less expense, and often with more grace. They can thus follow their taste, themselves making what they believe most suitable to their social position, age, and appearance, instead of being compelled to follow the general fashions dictated by mantua-makers, who make so much difficulty about departing from them.

——*Art de la couturière en robes.*

Diversion 3.

Gentlemen's Night-shirts and Ladies' Night Jackets. I have not followed the art of the mantua-maker with that of the *lingère.* The same stitches are used by both. Shifts are cut out by a mode similar to that for gowns. *Fichus* and caps are subject to too many variations in style, and I cannot write a treatise solely on night-shirts and night jackets.

I shall, however, describe the manner of making these two garments in a sufficiently extensive note, viz.: to cut out a night-shirt, take some toile two-thirds of an ell wide; cut a length of about two ells. Fold it over itself so that one side exceeds the other by four inches; this will be the back (see Fig. 19 A; k is the bottom of the front, l of the back). Over-cast this doubled toile at the sides, leaving two openings on each side: one at the top for sewing on the sleeves, and an unsewed length of about a quarter of an ell at the bottom (measuring by the longer piece). Then slit the top of the shirt front in the form of a T, or a cross lacking the top part (see Fig. 19 A, m). That is to say, cut a lengthways slit about a quarter of an ell long down the middle of the front, beginning from the fold. Then cut a crossways slit along the fold to the right and left of the lengthways slit; this is where you will attach the collar.

For the collar, cut a strip a third of an ell long and a quarter wide (see Fig. 19 B). This must be folded over itself, but it will require two gussets to go round the corners of the crossways slit (see Fig. 19 C). These are square pieces which you will fold along the middle, after they have been sewed to the shoulder-pieces.

The shoulder-pieces are each three or four inches wide, and placed from the end of the crossways slit up to the selvage. Cut them out all in one piece, then slit them a little at the end closest to the shoulder slit. This will form two narrow strips which will be sewed along the collar gusset, which is placed in the middle of them. One of them will extend over the back of the shirt, and the other over the front.

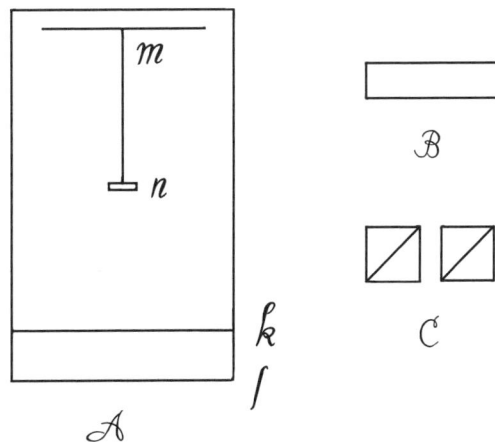

**Figure 19. The front and back of the body,
and the collar pieces, for a night-shirt.**

Then cut out the sleeves the length of the arms, and about half an ell wide at the top. As these must be cut sloping, the bottom will be about half as wide. Line the bottom with a piece of toile a sixth of an ell high. Then cut two gussets for the sleeves (which are placed at the top of the sleeve before sewing it). Cut two others, half as large, to sew to the side openings at the bottom of the shirt, for fear that these openings will tear across the end of the over-cast seam. Finally, cut a little strip about three inches long, and half an inch wide. This strip is placed crossways at the bottom of the lengthways slit to secure it, and the plaits corresponding to those for the collar (see Fig. 19 A, n).

I shall add a mode, little known but very useful, for preventing the front of the shirt from rising, and folding back or coming open over the chest. It consists of hollowing the part of the shirt front which is sewed on each side to the collar. To this end, measure an inch down from where the slits meet at the top of the T. Remove a narrow triangular piece from each side; this is an inch wide at the end next the lengthways slit but much longer, ending in a sharp point around the shoulder-piece. This operation done on both sides, sew the two front parts of the collar to the hollowed upper edge.

Night jackets are simpler. Fig. 20 A shows the shape for both fronts, and Fig. 20 B half the back; cut them out by paper patterns. Then cut out the sleeves the length of your arm, following the pattern. Cut a band five or six inches wide, and a third of an ell long, which you fold over itself, rounding the two ends; this will be the collar. That is all there is to cutting out this kind of garment.

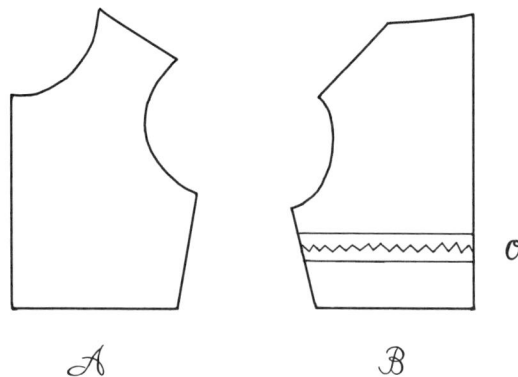

Figure 20. The front and back of a night jacket.

To make it up, sew the fronts to the back with a row of prick-stitches, making a flat seam on the wrong side. For setting on the sleeves, see my directions for the sleeves of a gown. For trimming night jackets, refer to the mode explained for flounces. To draw in the back, sew a broad linen tape, at a suitable height, over the selvages on the wrong side (see Fig. 20 *B*, *o*), through which you pass the strings.

—*Manuel des demoiselles.*

Ladies' Shifts. These directions are for two shifts, which take two yards and a sixteenth each. The best width to cut is the thirty-six-inch linen or cotton. (See Fig. 21.) The length of these shifts is forty-five inches. Divide three and three-quarters yards into three lengths. Then split one breadth into two halves. Take the gores off the other two breadths, eight inches wide at one end and an inch at the other. Put one gore on each side of the half breadths, and that will make the shift twenty inches wide at the top, and thirty-four at the bottom. The sleeves are seven inches long, and six wide, and the gussets five inches square.

—*Sectum.*

Diversion 4.

Marking. In the marking stitch, two threads are taken each way. Before the stitch is perfect the needle is passed three ways: once aslant, once straight towards you, and once across. To fasten on, the end of the thread is left out a little on the right side of the work, and worked in with the two first stitches. The thread must not be passed on from one letter to another, but must be neatly fastened on the wrong side, and cut off. Every letter is begun as at first. Every capital letter has seven stitches in height. In marking small letters, one thread each way is taken to form a stitch.

What is called the Spanish-stitch is much admired for its beauty and durability. In this, the two threads are always taken up straight on the needle, so that on the wrong side each stitch forms a small square.

——*Instructions for Needle-work and Knitting.*

Diversion 5.

To cut out a Gown. In taking patterns, you must, above all, be careful to form a correct notion of the figure to which you are to adapt the gown, and have correct measurements of the principal distances, according to which you are to shape out your pattern before cutting the stuff. Those who

One-sixteenth Scale

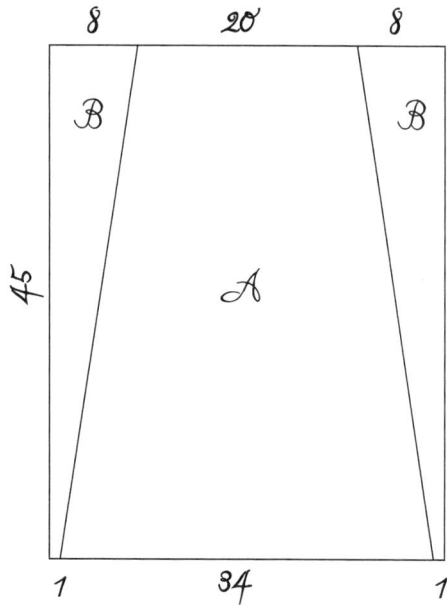

First Two Breadths

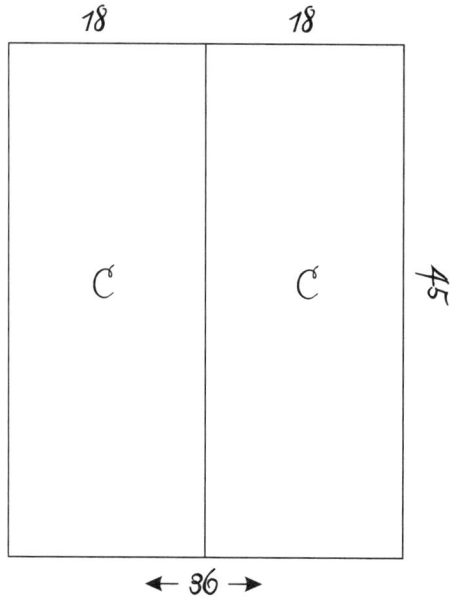

Third Breadth

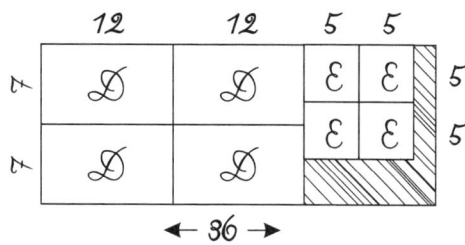

Sleeves and Gussets

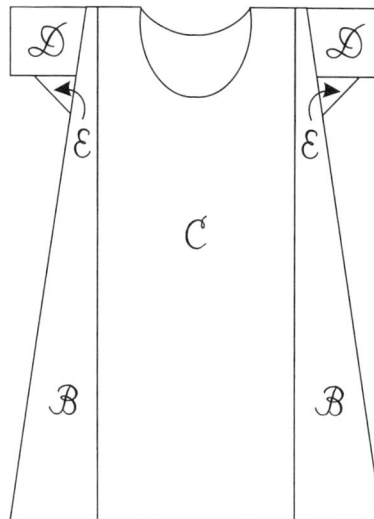

Shift with Gores

Figure 21. A tentative layout for two shifts.

have had much cutting out can guess at this very nearly by the eye; but it will always be safest to rely on actual measurements, particularly when the gown you are about to make is required to fit tight to the shape. In the case of full, loose gowns, it will not be so necessary to be very exact; yet even in this instance, accurate measurements will enable you to make a gown fit better than the best guess measure you can take by the eye alone.

When you have once procured a pattern, however, which fits a lady's shape (and this you ought to make of soft paper or cloth) you will not require to measure a fresh one for every new gown, though the fashion should change ever so considerably; for the same measurements must be kept to, how much soever the fashions may vary.

In cutting out gowns, you will have great room for the display of economy, and may, by proper attention and ingenuity, save many pounds to your employers—a circumstance which is by no means unimportant, even to the most wealthy. By trying your patterns and shapes on the stuff, before you begin to cut, you may in this manner so manage it, that you will have but few useless pieces to throw away. According to this careful plan, you may frequently save a yard or two of valuable stuff, which may be of great use for trimmings or alterations. In cutting out figured silks, and other stuffs of the same kind, it is requisite to be very attentive to the manner in which they are to hang. Otherwise you may spoil the whole gown, or at least occasion a considerable waste of the stuff before you can rectify any mistake of this description.

——*The Duties of a Lady's Maid.*

Diversion 6.

The Trade of the Tailor. The tailor makes clothes for men and boys, and riding habits for ladies. In a tailor's shop, where much business is carried on, there are always two divisions of workmen. First there is the foreman, who takes the measure of the person for whom the clothes are to be made, cuts out the cloth, and carries home the newly-finished garments to the customers. The others are mere working tailors, who sit cross-legged on the bench. Of these, very few know how to cut out, with any degree of skill, the clothes which they sew together.

The tools requisite in the business of a tailor are very few and inexpensive: the shears for the foreman, who stands to his work; for the others, a pair of scissors, a thimble, and needles of different sizes. In the thimble there is this peculiarity, that it is open at both ends. Besides these, there are required some long strips of parchment for measures, and an iron called a goose. With the latter, when made hot, they press down the seams, which would otherwise take off from the beauty of the goods. The stand for the iron is generally a horse-shoe, rendered bright from use. Before the foreman, or master (for where the trade is not extensive the master cuts out, measures gentlemen, and carries home the clothes) is an open box. This contains buckram, tapes, bindings, trimmings, buttons, &c., with which every master tailor should be furnished, and from which they derive very large profits. On the shelf is a piece of cloth ready to be made into clothes, and a pattern-book.

——*The Book of English Trades.*

The Ladies' Riding Habit. There are many in our trade whose practice is very extensive, and whose abilities in cutting gentlemen's clothes indisputable; who nonetheless consider the riding habit an object entirely above their comprehension, and have refused to take an order (I would think reluctantly) for a garment which is generally considered profitable, and when well executed no less creditable.

It would perhaps be considered superfluous, if not absurd, in me to offer any thing in the way of argument, to induce such persons to possess themselves of the knowledge of so essential a part of their business. The necessity of the thing renders it self-evident. The habit, however, it must be acknowledged, is a very delicate piece of workmanship, requiring the combination of grace, taste, and symmetry of proportion; for certainly Nature's fairest and most gracefully-finished form, demands our best exertion to supply it with a corresponding neat and tasteful covering.

However difficult the subject may at first view appear, it will be my object in the delineation of the shape, to divest it of every thing which is abstruse or obscure, and to define it in the most clear, perspicuous, and simplified manner, of which the nature of the subject will admit. The reader is aware that the female shape differs from that of the other sex in several essential particulars, both as to nature and custom; for to the rising prominency of the breast is added an artificial, though very useful appendage, viz., the stays.

Still, I must be confined to the relative proportion for the principal points; and various have been the modes devised (by different writers upon the subject) for dividing, as it were, the shape into just proportions. But in all these admeasurements, it is evident that only general notions may be formed; for in no two human shapes may the same precise proportion be discovered. The sum of the above observations

The Ladies' Riding Habit.

Lengths of Jacket.	
Measure	Inches
From top of back seam to waist of jacket	9 1/2
Length of jacket skirt (by fashion or taste)	4
From top of back to middle of front at bottom	14
From ditto to extreme point of breast	10 1/2
From back seam to elbow	17 1/2
Continued to hand	32

Widths of Ditto.
Taken quite round the fullest or largest part of breast.

Measure	Inches
Half of which	18
Waist ditto	15
Neck ditto	7
From centre to centre of breasts, half of which	6
Top of sleeve (being plaited)	7 1/4
Sleeve just above elbow	6
Sleeve at hand	5

Length of Skirt for Walking or Riding.
From about an inch higher than bottom of jacket front, to bottom of skirt.

Measure	Inches
Walking length	42 1/2
Full riding length	54
From waist of back behind, to bottom.	
Measure	Inches
Riding length	60
But turned up for walking	44

Table 1. The habit measures.

amounts to this: your measure (carefully taken) is the only criterion upon which you may depend for the proportions of the shape, aided by your own observations when taken. It may be well to observe that in taking the measures, that the lady should have on the same stays and similar gown as she intends to wear the habit over—otherwise all your care and ingenuity may be rendered abortive. To prevent repetition, the measures in Table 1, being a middle size, may suffice for both the pelisse and spencer, which follow, as they are formed on the same principles as the habit.

Of the Back. I beg to remind my readers, that my observations are first and principally directed to the standard of proportion, and afterwards to the change of fashion. The back of the habit (see Fig. 22 A) may be cut either with or without a seam; it is, however, generally made without one. The line AA is the imaginary back seam, being from the top to the bottom of the waist nine and a half inches. Mark the width of the top and bottom of the back, by the eighth of the waist measure (being for this size an inch and seven-eighths). Next mark point B eight and a half inches from the top, this being half the measure from the back seam to the elbow, after deducting the half-inch (this is the rule by proportion for finding the lowest point of the back arm-hole). From A at the top then, as a centre cast the curve BC. Next mark the width across between the shoulders, by the fourth of the waist measure (being three and a quarter inches) from D; point D is five and three-quarters inches from the top at A, this being the third of the measure from the back seam to the elbow.

Having determined the lower part of the back arm-hole as at C, you will easily complete the back by dividing the distance between the top at the shoulder, and the bottom at C into three equal parts, taking one part for the arm-hole and the remaining two parts for the shoulder, which thus determines the top of the arm-hole, or bottom of the shoulder seam. The back skirt may be cut about four inches long, and shaped as in Fig. 22 B, and may be cut either on or off. The outer lines represent the present fashionable back, being nearly twelve inches wide between the shoulders from arm-hole to arm-hole.

The Front Piece. Now direct your attention to the principal part of Fig. 22 B, namely the delineation of the front piece. First draw the line at the bottom square across, and consider the front line AA as the edge of the cloth. Next mark point B on the bottom line six inches (being a third of the breast) from the front line, and by consulting your measure, you will find the difference between the waist and breast to be three inches. Mark then an inch and a half on each side of point B, this being the quantity to

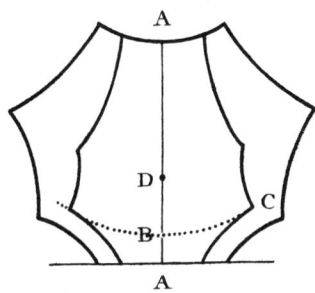

A

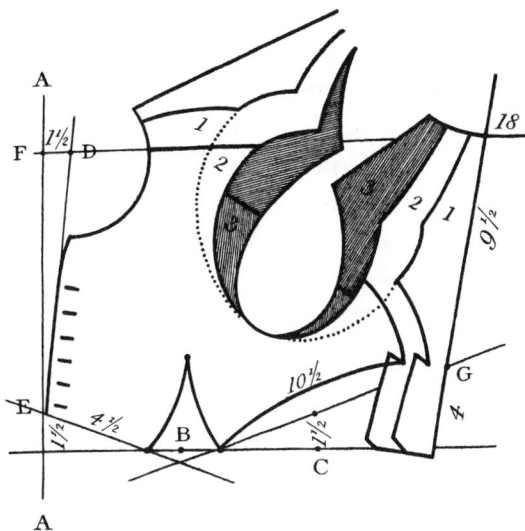

B

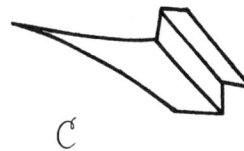

C

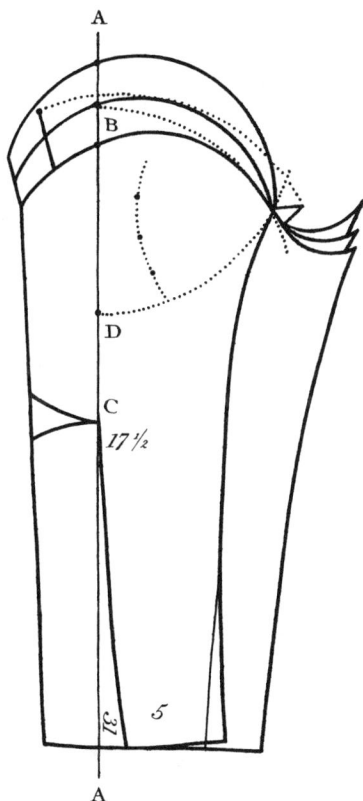

E

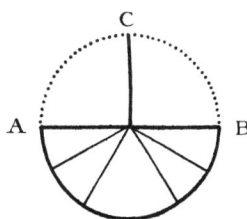

D

Figure 22. The body of the riding habit.

be taken out under the breast, and will be hereafter explained. Next mark point C twelve inches from the front line (being two-thirds of the breast). Mark also the point an inch and a half above C (this being the half difference between breast and waist). Now mark point E an inch and a half from the bottom in the front. Draw the sloping lines, passing through those points respectively, and which you will perceive, cut or intersect each other exactly under point B. This then is to be the bottom of the front piece; for when the incision or aperture under the breast is closed, it will draw this to its proper position. Now mark point F by your front length measure from the bottom at E, deducting the width of the back. You thus make the length of the front piece in this example from E to F twelve and seven-eighths inches, the whole length being fourteen inches. Mark point D an inch and a half within point F, and draw the straight line from the bottom through this point. This line is to be considered the front edge of the habit body, for when the incision at B is closed, it will draw this edge to a perpendicular line.

Proceed to the formation of the side seam, &c. as follows. Mark point G on the sloping line six inches from the point above C, thus making eighteen inches (breast measure) from the front line at E. Place now the bottom of your back seam at the waist, to point G. Extend it upwards, and draw the shoulder of the front piece from D across to the top of the back eighteen inches (or breast measure) from point D, thus making the back seam and front edge parallel to each other, at eighteen inches (breast measure) distant. While the back lies in that position, mark the side seam of the front piece by the back. Mark also the front of the arm-hole, being two-thirds of the waist measure (ten inches) from the back seam.

Next place your back in the closing position on the shoulder line of the front piece at the distance of three and a half inches from point D (this being half the size of the neck by measure). Then cast the fore-gauge (beginning from the neck at the shoulder point) by three and a half inches, and mark the length of the shoulder by the back. Thus you have obtained the three essential points for the arm-hole, namely the shoulder, front, and top of the side seam. To these may be added a fourth. Thus, from the back seam (when closed at the shoulder) to the bottom of the arm-hole, take twelve inches (two-thirds of the breast); but as the back seam lies in a sloping direction, you must take the latter measure about the third of the waist (five inches) down from the top.

Thus you have all which is requisite in practice for casting the arm-hole. But if desired, and for the edification of the curious, it may be scientifically formed by means of curves or sections of circles, as follows. Place your pivot measure or compasses at the shoulder point, extend to the front of the arm-hole, and by that length cast the curve and counter-curve, the intersection from which will cast the upper part of the arm-hole. The same operation performed between the front of the arm-hole and the top of the side seam, will complete the same.

Now we will pass on to the bottom of the front piece under the arm-hole, which you will perceive is considerably hollowed. This also may be cast by means of the intersecting curves as described above, but with this difference: you want the hollowing to be less concave or flatter. Therefore, you must cast the curves from double the length between the points, the intersection of which curves will be the position for casting the bottom of the front piece in the hollow form required. The extreme prominence or centre point of the breast is determined by the measure, being in this example ten and a half inches from the top of the back, and twelve inches across from point to point, consequently six inches from the front line.

The piece to be taken out under the breast ought not to be cut by straight lines, but by curves. These are cast by their own lengths as described above, with a view to producing when closed, that convexity or roundness so essentially requisite for this purpose. Fig. 22 C represents the short skirt somewhat hollowed at the top, where it is to be privately closed to the front piece from the bottom of the side seam.

Fig. 22 D represents a novel mode of forming the back skirt, by means of a circle, the half diameter of which is equal to the length you intend your skirt to be. The figure is cast by four inches. The crossways line AB passing through the centre of the figure, is to be folded down into plaits, proceeding from the centre, the place of which is to be supplied by the equal division of the semi-circle above the line, shown by the line which is to be cut down as drawn from C to the centre. The separated points of the circle at C are to be brought down to the points on line AB by angular plaitings, proceeding from the centre as before.

The separated line C now forming the line AB will be the edge. This is closed to the bottom of the jacket, by placing the centre of the figure to the centre of the back at the bottom, extending its widths on each side onto the front piece. When the circular skirt is adopted, you will obviously not require any plait on the front piece skirt, but merely a piece passing under the circle, cut with sufficient spring to reach the lowest plait of the back; though I generally prefer cutting it quite the width of the skirt to meet behind under the folding circle.

My observations it will be perceived, are chiefly directed to the single-breasted habit. But it is presumed that you can have no difficulty in cutting one double-breasted, by adding the required width and corresponding shape. If your front edge is required so wide as to pass the opposite breast, cut an incision, and take the same quantity out as under the breast.

The Sleeve. The sleeve of the habit is at present worn loose, but (like every thing else which is under the influence of fashion) may in a few months be entirely reversed. You will therefore see the propriety of making the standard of proportion the first and principal object of our consideration.

Fig. 22 *E* represents both the close habit sleeve, and also the loose or straight pelisse sleeve. It is to be observed that on all occasions the sleeve requires some fulness at the top both for ease and taste: it ought to be at least an inch larger than the arm-hole. But you will do well to recollect that whatever addition is made either for ease, ornament, plaiting, &c., that it is to be all given to the top or outside, for fulness on the inside or hollow part is worse than useless. I am aware that it is a very common thing with perhaps nine persons out of ten, to cut both the outside and the inside of an equal width at the top, even the loose plaited sleeve, without considering how much the gathering or plaiting must inevitably draw the points at the top out of their place, and which occasions the sleeve to have the appearance of being twisted; of being contracted, notwithstanding its fulness.

Fig. 22 *E* represents the sleeve by proportion, being cast by the breast measure instead of the waist, which produces all the fulness requisite for a close sleeve. Even in this case the inside should not be so large as the outside, for when the arm-hole is equally divided, the lower half is the exact size requisite for the inside sleeve. The line *AA* is the back arm seam, and *B* the top of the sleeve. First then mark point *D* nine inches (half breast) from *B* at the top. Let *B* and *D* be now your positions alternately from which to cast the curve and counter-curve, the crossing or intersection of which, is the point for the top of the front arm. Next cast the dotted curve from the top of the front arm by six inches (third of breast). The same distance taken from *B* at the top of the back arm falling upon that curve, will be the position from which to cast the top of the sleeve. Next mark the elbow at *C* seventeen and a half inches (including the back). Mark also the widths by measure. The front arm if required, may be scientifically formed by taking a position at double its length and equidistant therefrom; but in practice the eye is a guide amply sufficient.

I shall now direct your attention to the skirt or petticoat. The front of this we find by measure (for a lady about five feet five or six inches) a walking length forty-two and a half inches; but for riding, fancy rules, say fifty-four (see Table 1). It is usually made plain, with one plait on each side of the pocket-hole, which plaits are continued quite round the back part to meet behind. The back part is generally about an inch and a half longer than the front, when a walking length; but for riding it may be perhaps five or six inches longer behind than in the front. The extra length may either be looped, or tied up inside when walking. The skirt may be either supported by the stays, or suspended by braces over the shoulders, or loops to the jacket. Or if preferred, it may be sewed to the jacket as forwards as the pocket-hole at the side. A band about an inch wide is usually sewed across the front at the top.

Of the Pelisse and Spencer. Notwithstanding the incessant changes of form which fashion arbitrarily dictates to this article of the ladies' costume, yet all the plaits and foldings, all the curves and fulness, puffings and drawings, must ultimately be brought down to the standard of the human shape. I therefore shall repeat the observation, that to a proficient in the art of cutting, it is of little consequence what the prevailing taste may be. His business is to fit the body in the symmetry of proportion, to which may be added the taste, grace, and finish of the reigning mode.

Plain pelisses, or those which fit the body without plaitings, are formed in the same manner as the habit. The piece, however, is sometimes not taken out under the breast, but the points are drawn together by means of a thread (see Fig. 23 A). The plain back is the same as the habit without the skirt, but the loose or drawn back is shown by Fig. 23 B. The line AA is the centre of the back. Make A at the top your centre or pivot, from which extend down to the bottom of the back seam, and cast the dotted curve from that point the whole width of the back. Next draw line AB at whatever distance from A at the bottom you deem sufficient for your fulness or plaitings, and proceed to cast your figure upon line AB, as the back seam, in the same manner as for a habit. This completes the back, for you will find, when the drawing is made at the bottom, your points will all fall into their proper places. The back is at this time worn cut in the diamonded form shown by the outer lines.

The skirt of the pelisse (as worn at this time) is sewed to the top (see Fig. 23 A). It is gathered or plaited from the middle of the back, to about an inch and a half on each side, the fulness being all behind—or a double plait may be laid at each hip under the square back.

Capes are sometimes worn both on the pelisse and spencer, and are cut at the lower edge in a great variety of forms. They may be cast from a centre, both at the top and bottom. But the easiest and most simple way is to place the back and the front in the closing position at the shoulder,

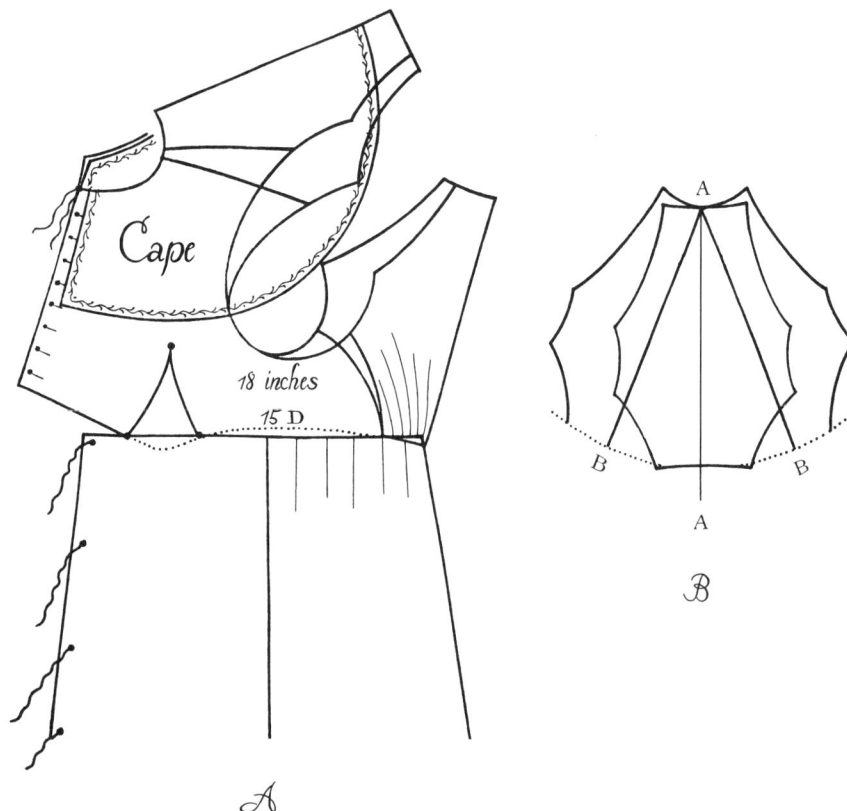

Figure 23. The pelisse.

and cut the neck of the cape by that of the pelisse &c., by which means you will make it hang well on the shoulders.

The sleeve is usually worn loose and plaited, or gathered at the top. It is cut with only one seam, and that runs under the arm. But it may be first necessary to sketch the regular sleeve, as shown in the habit, and then draw the outer lines both at the back and the front arm, at any distance you please for fulness. Recollect to give all the fulness to the top or outside sleeve, and that the points at the top of both the front and back arm, must not be suffered either to rise or fall by the fulness. Fig. 22 E (for convenience) represents this sleeve by the external lines—but it is more clearly delineated in Fig. 24 A.

The line AA is the edge of the cloth. CB is the half-width of the inside sleeve, being three and a half inches wide at the top (fourth of arm-hole)

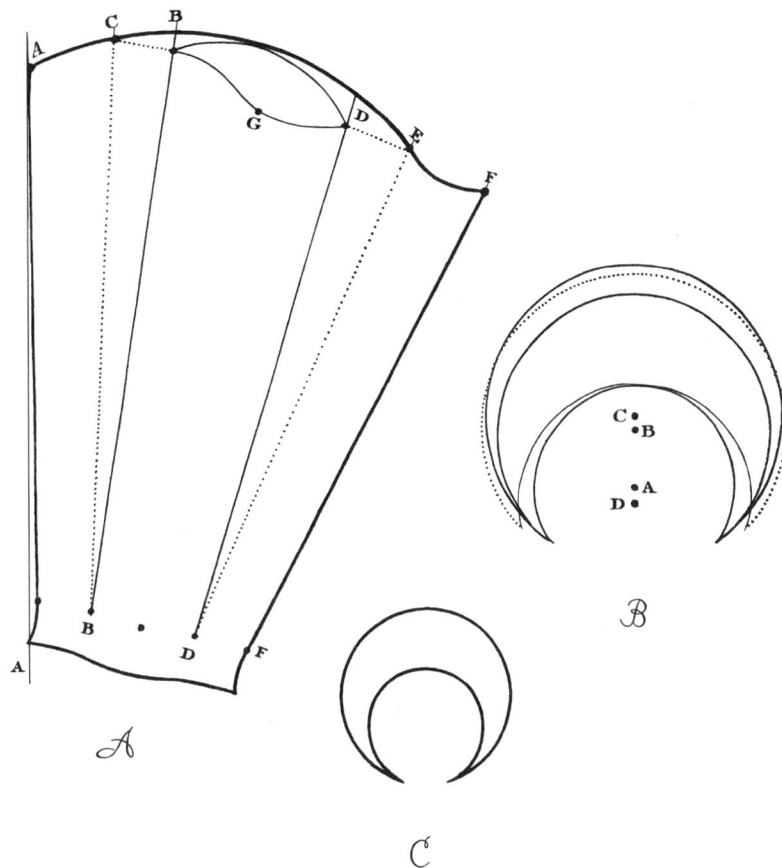

Figure 24. A sleeve and two collars for the pelisse.

within the edge, and two and a quarter at the wrist (fourth of wrist measure) from, or within the edge. The line *BB* shows the extra allowance at the top for fulness or plaiting, say three or more inches wide at the top and terminating at the wrist. Upon line *BB*, you will proceed to cast the top of the outside sleeve by the same rules as before described. Next draw the hollowing which represents the inside at the top. Make point *G* in its centre, from which point you will balance the length of the front arm across from *B* to *D* at the wrist, in width about four and a half inches (according to measure). Now place your pivot measure on point *B* at the wrist. Extend upwards to *G*, and you will obtain the exact height required for point *A* which, by being folded over, forms the back half of the inside. From *B* at the bottom, extend up to *B* at the top, and you will also obtain the true height for point *C*, being the allowance for plaiting as before mentioned. Draw the curve *AC*, and continue the same to the centre at the top. This if desired may be done by means of the intersecting curves as previously shown, but in practice the eye is a guide amply sufficient. Next place your pivot measure on *D* at the wrist; extend up to *D* at the top of the front arm. This gives the height required at *E*, the width to be determined according to the fulness required. From the same point *D* extend up to *G* in the centre, for the elevation of point *F* three and a half inches (or the fourth part of the size of the arm-hole) wide across from *E*. Now draw line *FF* to the wrist, and this completes the width of the whole sleeve. Continue the convex line from the top of point *E*, and the hollow from *E* to *F*.

Now give your sleeve whatever length the measure requires below the wrist (as these sleeves are usually made without a cuff) and spring

Height by Feet and Inches.	Half-waist Measure.	Fourth of Ditto, Being Breadth of Standard Back Between Shoulders.	Eighth of Ditto, Across Top and Bottom of Back.	Quantity for Habit, of Cloth 56 Inches Wide.	Ditto for Habit, of Cloth 27 Inches Wide.	Quantity for Pelisse, of Cloth 56 Inches Wide.	Ditto for Pelisse, of Cloth 27 Inches Wide.
Ft. Ins.	Inches.	Inches.	Inches.	Yards.	Yards.	Yards.	Yards.
5 10	18	4 1/2	2 1/4	3	6	2 7/8	5 3/4
5 9	17 1/2	4 3/8	2 3/16	2 15/16	5 7/8	2 13/16	5 5/8
5 8	17	4 1/4	2 1/8	2 7/8	5 3/4	2 3/4	5 1/2
5 7	16 1/2	4 1/8	2 1/16	2 13/16	5 5/8	2 11/16	5 3/8
5 6	16	4	2	2 3/4	5 1/2	2 5/8	5 1/4
5 5	15 1/2	3 7/8	1 15/16	2 11/16	5 3/8	2 9/16	5 1/8
5 4	15	3 3/4	1 7/8	2 5/8	5 1/4	2 1/2	5
5 3	14 1/2	3 5/8	1 13/16	2 9/16	5 1/8	2 7/16	4 7/8
5 2	14	3 1/2	1 3/4	2 1/2	5	2 3/8	4 3/4
5 1	13 1/2	3 3/8	1 11/16	2 7/16	4 7/8	2 5/16	4 5/8
5 0	13	3 1/4	1 5/8	2 3/8	4 3/4	2 1/4	4 1/2

Table 2. The quantities of material required for habits and pelisses.

out the bottom to give freedom to the hand to pass, and this completes the sleeve. Points *C* and *E* are the back and front arm of the outside sleeve, and points *A* and *F* at the top and bottom meet in the centre of the inside sleeve.

Fig. 24 *B* represents the circular collar with the points more extended than the circular collar in Fig. 24 *C*. The effect of this when on, occasions a contraction of the circumference or outer line, and consequently makes the collar in Fig. 24 *B* rise. Points *AD* are the centre of the neck or inner circles, *B* and *C* of the outer or circumferencial edge of the collar.

It remains now to say a few words on the subject of fashion, as applicable to the changes of broad and narrow backs. In this the following axiom is obviously demonstrable, namely, whatever is taken from the back (that is, reduced from the standard of proportion) must be added to the front piece and the sleeve. On the contrary, whatever is added to the proportionate back, must of necessity be taken from the front piece and sleeve, in a relative proportion both as to quantity and shape.

The spencer is so decidedly the same in form as the pelisse, or habit without the skirt, that any further description would be mere repetition, therefore superfluous.

Table 2 gives the quantities of material required for habits and pelisses. The quantities for habits are calculated for walking length. Whatever additional length is given to the skirt for riding, will require double the same in quantity to be added to the calculations in the table.

——*Golding's Guide.*

Diversion 7.

A Pattern for the Body of a Gown. Since many persons are obliged to give out their gowns to be made, because they do not know how to cut them out, I shall give a few specimens of the most approved patterns. As the extent of this work will not allow me to give all sizes, the examples are of a middle size, which may be reduced or enlarged according to wish.

Fig. 25 *A* shows the front. This must be cut on the bias of the stuff, or it will not sit well; let the straight-way of the stuff be from *a* to *b*. The letter *c* marks the plait for the bosom, which may either be cut out or tacked down after it is sewed. Fig. 25 *B* is the side-piece, which must be cut on the straight-way on the side marked five inches. Fig. 25 *C* is the back; this must be cut on the straight-way down the middle. Fig. 25 *D* is the collar, which must also be cut on the bias of the stuff.

Fig. 26 *A* is a plain sleeve; the edge *d* of the under side must be the straight-way of the stuff. These rules being observed, the rest will come

A

8 inches

6 inches

18 inches

7 inches

8 1/2 inches

13 1/2 inches

5 inches

a

c

b

5 inches

4 inches

B

3 inches

9 inches

5 inches

5 1/2 inches

C

2 1/2 inches

8 inches

12 1/2 inches long

12 inches wide

6 inches

1 1/2 inches

D

3 1/2 inches

8 1/2 inches

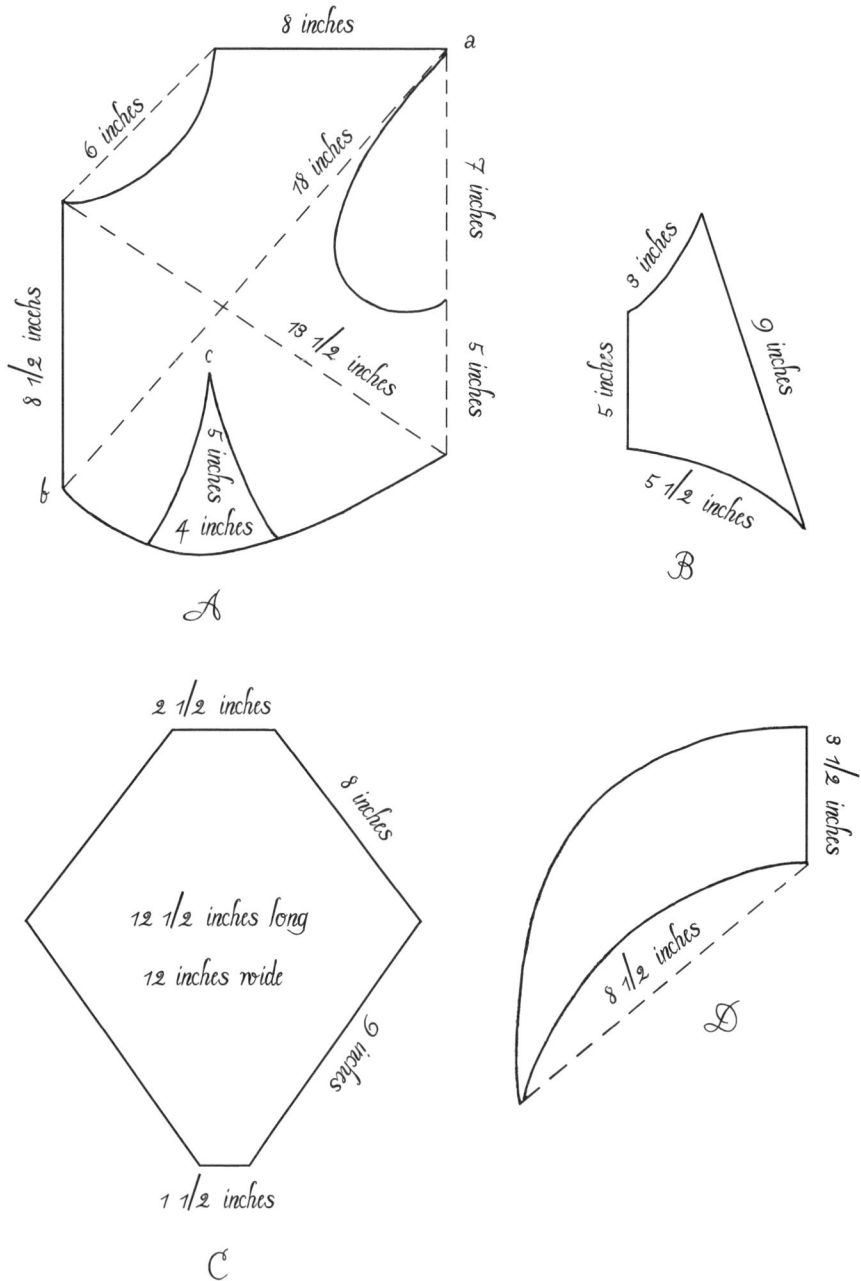

Figure 25. A pattern for the body of a gown.

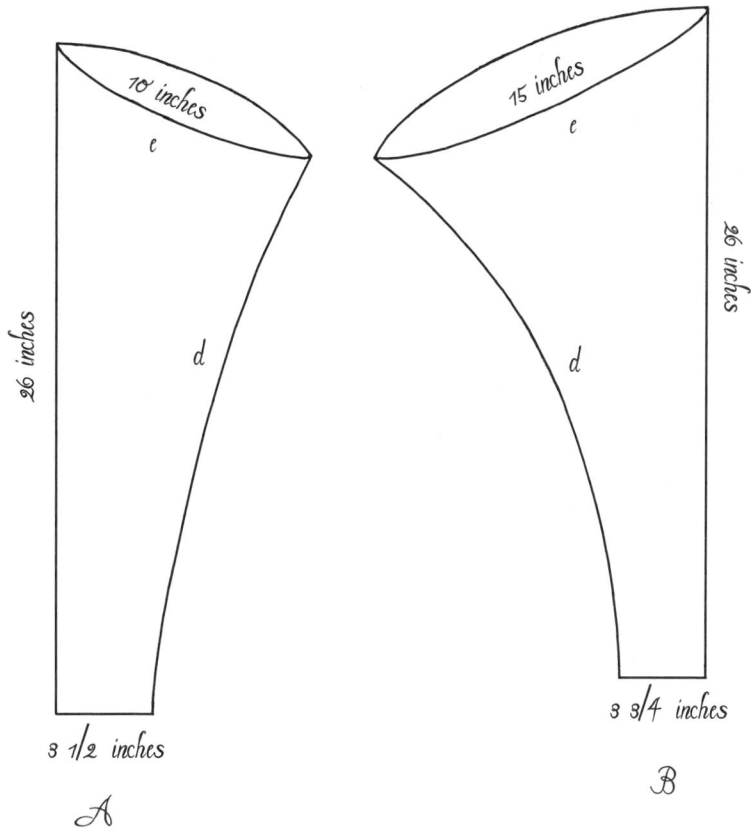

10 inches
e
26 inches
d
3 1/2 inches
A

15 inches
e
26 inches
d
3 3/4 inches
B

Figure 26. Patterns for two kinds of sleeves.

right. The letter *e* marks the line to show the curve of the under part of the sleeve. Fig. 26 *B* is a full sleeve, in the cutting of which the same rules must be observed as for the plain sleeve.

If you wear a gown, the waist and skirt of which are separate, some attention is required in regard to its adjustment; for if the top of the skirt is fastened higher in the front than behind, it will cause the bottom part of the gown to stick out, and to have a very awkward appearance. If on the contrary, the back part is fastened higher than the front, it will drag in the front, and be very troublesome when you walk. You should, therefore, fasten the front and back part of the skirt on a level, which will cause it to sit in an easy style.

With regard to the under part of your gown, unless the same rule is attended to, it will be in vain for you to try to make the outer part of your gown sit well; for the under clothing being thicker than the outer, the outer part will of course, in this respect, be governed by the clothes underneath.

The waist should have a broad tape fastened onto the middle of the bottom of the back, which is brought round and tied in the front. This holds the waist down, and draws it closely into the hollow of the back. Do not fasten the tape more than two inches along the back; if you do, it will not have the desired effect.

The best mode of fastening the front is by having hooks and eyes close under the front edge; and then let a small loop of tape be fastened at the bottom, for the tape which holds the waist down behind to be brought through. By this means, the back and front are kept in their places by one fastening. The whole are then covered by a waist riband, or waist-band. Do not line a band with any thing smooth; for with the motion of the body, it will be constantly slipping out of its place.

——*The Alphabetical Receipt Book and Domestic Advisor.*

Diversion 8.

Tambour-work. One kind of embroidery is executed at the tambour, which is a frame resembling a hoop, over which the material is placed. Another hoop, made to fit, is passed over it, both hoops being covered with woollen cloth; and the work is strained tight between them. The hoop is then placed in a horizontal position, between two upright supports, fixed in a stand, and when in use placed on a table. For large subjects, a square frame is used, the four sides of which separate, and which, having a number of holes near their ends, are united by moveable pegs, according to the size required. This frame rests on a stand, at a convenient height from the ground.

The tambour-needle is a small steel instrument fixed in an ivory handle, and has a small notch near its point, which answers the purpose of a hook. In working, your right hand, which directs the tambour-needle, will always be on the upper side of the work; and your left hand, which supplies the worsted or cotton, on the under side. The principal materials on which tambour-work is employed are muslin and net. The embroidery is generally done in coloured crewels, white twisted cotton, or gold thread.

The design is previously drawn on the material or ground with indigo, which will afterwards wash out. If it is intended to be worked in crewels, a coloured pattern will also be of service, as a guide to the selection of the worsteds, which are usually worked into very beautiful groups or wreaths of flowers, in their natural colours, principally for the bottom of gowns.

In working, the needle is passed through the muslin from the upper side. The worsted or cotton, being held underneath, is placed on the hook, and drawn through, so as to form a loop on the surface. The needle is then passed through the loop, and also through the muslin, at a few threads' distance. A second loop is then drawn up through the first; a third loop through the second; and thus the work is continued.

In a narrow or pointed leaf, it is usual to work its complete outline first, passing up one side and down the other, and filling up the middle with succeeding rows. In a round or oval leaf, the stitches should begin at the outside, and form one row within another, terminating in the centre. Stalks are worked in single or double rows, as the thickness in the pattern may require. Small sprigs are sometimes thus embroidered in gold thread on India muslin, for ladies' head-dresses.

Embroidery on Muslin. White embroidery comprises the art of working flowers and other ornamental designs on muslin, for gowns or their trimmings, pelerines, collars, handkerchiefs, &c. There are two sorts of cotton proper for this work. That which is most generally used, because it washes the best, is the dull cotton sometimes called Trafalgar, or Indian. The other sort is the glazed, or English cotton, and is only proper to be used on thin muslin. Though it looks infinitely the more beautiful of the two, previously to its being washed, yet that operation destroys its beauty, and removes all its gloss; nor is it so pleasant to use as the other.

Patterns for working may be purchased at most of the fancy-shops. But ladies possessing a taste for drawing may design their own subjects, by making sketches on paper in pencil, and afterwards going over them again with ink. A pattern may be copied, by placing a thin piece of paper over the original, and tracing it through against a window. The outline of a subject already worked, if of a thick, rich description, may be obtained by laying the muslin on a table, placing a piece of white paper over it, and rubbing the paper with a nutmeg, partly grated. The outline may afterwards be perfected with a pen.

The paper pattern for a running design of flowers, foliage, &c. should be from twelve to eighteen inches long, in proportion to its breadth, and shifted along the muslin as the work proceeds. As this kind of pattern is liable to be soon damaged, it is advisable to strengthen it by a lining of cambric muslin. The pattern for the pelerine of a gown is usually of the size of the intended pelerine. But a sketch of half the pattern (see Fig. 27 A) may be made to answer the purpose equally well, by re-tracing the design on the other half of the paper, against a window. When half the pelerine

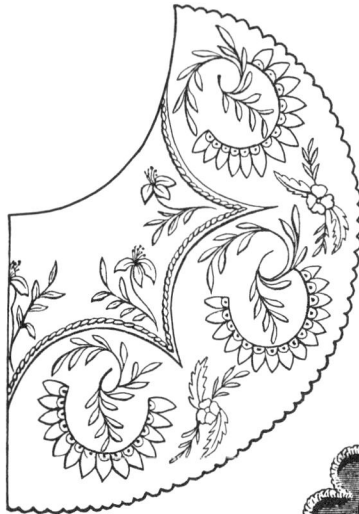

A

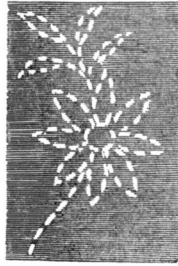

B

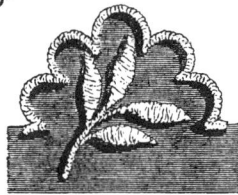

C

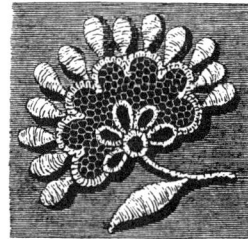

D

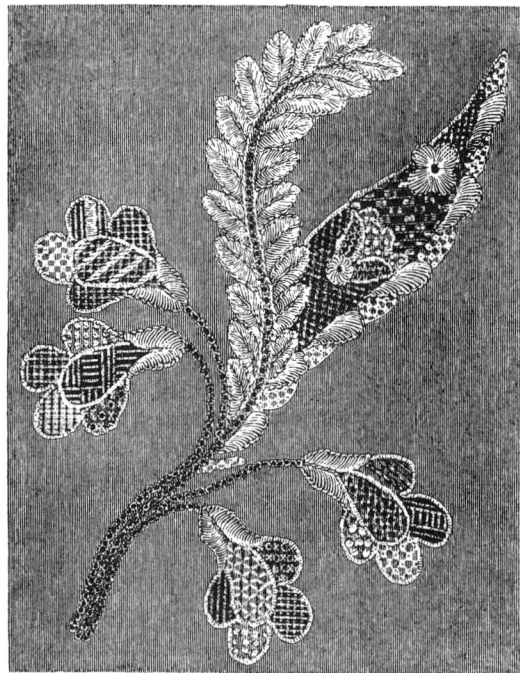

E

Figure 27. Divers designs for embroidery on muslin.

is worked, turn the pattern over to the other side; in this case the half-pattern must terminate exactly at the middle, or half of the work.

The muslin, cambric muslin, or French cambric intended to be worked, must be smoothly and evenly tacked on the pattern, so as to prevent its getting out of place. The stems, and external edges of leaves, flowers, or ornaments, must then be traced by running them round with cotton (see Fig. 27 *B*). Great care should be taken to preserve their shape and form accurately, as a fault in this stage of the work is not easily remedied afterwards.

In working the bottom of a gown, flounced pelerine, or collar, the edge of the pattern, which is usually a running scollop, a series of scollops forming larger ones, a Vandyke, or a chain, should be done first. The best and strongest way of working this part, is in the stitch used for button-hole work. The stalks leading to leaves or flowers, having been run round as directed, must next be sewed over tolerably thick (see Fig. 27 *C*). Where it appears desirable to thicken a stem, or any other part of the outline, a piece of the cotton should be laid along the running thread, and both sewed over together. Leaves or flowers are worked in what is called satin-stitch (from the length of the stitches resembling the threads in satin). Great care should be taken that the stitches do not lie over each other, but are evenly ranged side by side (as in Fig. 27 *C*). Flowers or stars worked in fine worsted or crewel of various colours, may be used with very good effect in satin-stitch. The work should be slightly pressed with your finger now and then, to assist in keeping it in shape.

Round or oval eyelet-holes, in a circle, like a star or the head of a flower, are sometimes introduced. These are first run round. Then a very little bit of the muslin is cut out in the shape of the intended hole, but much smaller, and sewed thickly round; the needle being run through the centre, and passed under the running thread (see Fig. 27 *D*). A leaf or the head of a flower is formed occasionally by placing a piece of thread net on the muslin, then running it round in the pattern required, and covering the running thread in button-hole stitch, or thick sewing. The outer part of the thread net is then cut off with fine-pointed scissors. The muslin under the net is cut out in the same way when removed from the paper pattern (see Fig. 27 *D* again).

The middle of a flower is sometimes ornamented by the introduction of very beautiful open-work, in imitation of antique lace. But the various kinds of stitch requisite, and the mode of using them, are so complex and intricate, that a practical description is scarcely possible. Nothing but personal instruction can properly convey a perfect knowledge of their application. I shall, however, endeavour to illustrate the subject by an

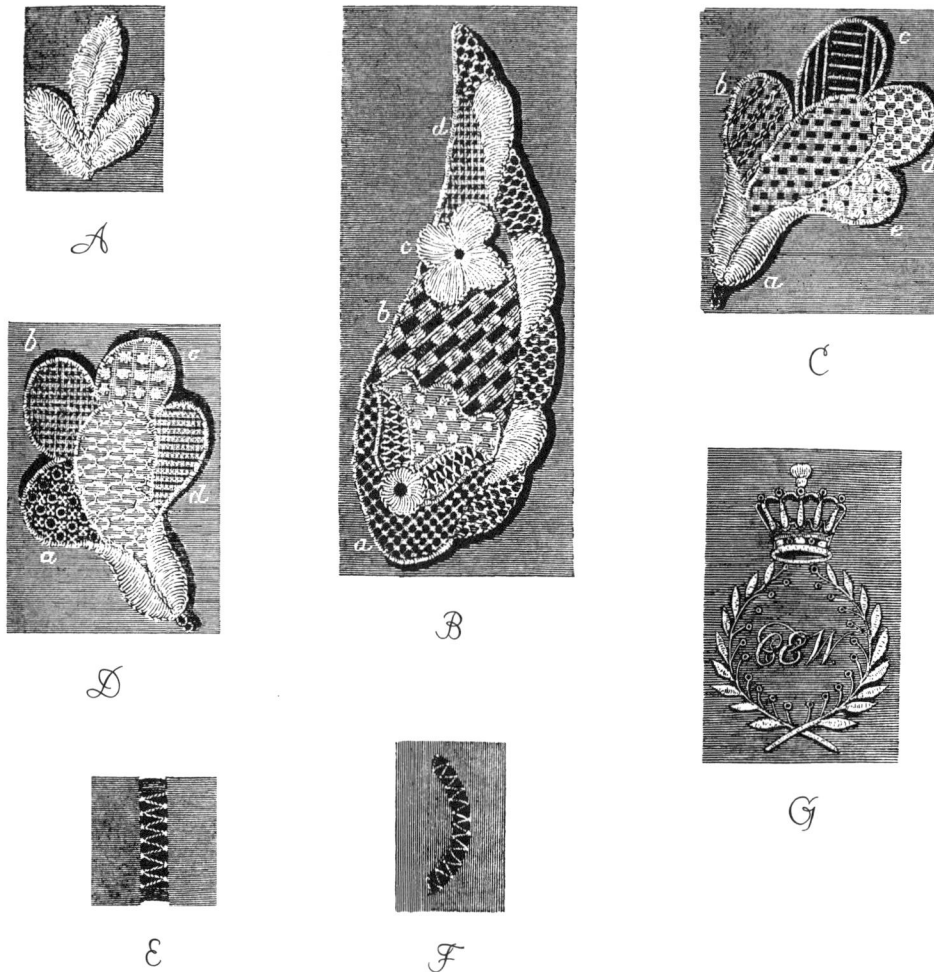

Figure 28. Additional designs for embroidery on muslin.

engraving of a fancy sprig of leaves and flowers, in the style of rich antique lace embroidery, and attempt to convey a general idea of the stitches used. Sixteen different kinds are comprised in the pattern in Fig. 27 *E*. Several portions of the leaves and flowers are shown on a larger scale, with references to the various stitches of which they are composed, in Fig. 28 *A*, *B*, *C*, and *D*.

The stalk is composed of rows of eyelet-holes, which are an agreeable variation from the usual mode of sewing stems. The running thread which first formed the outline is withdrawn; and the slight marks left in the muslin serve as a guide for further operations. Four threads of the muslin are taken on the needle, and sewed over three times; the needle being passed through the same places each time, and the four threads drawn tightly together. The next four threads, higher on the line, are then taken up and sewed over, as the last. Thus a series of bars is formed—the thread passing alternately on the right side and on the left, from one bar to another. Care must be taken to keep it at the side, and not to let it run across the apertures. Having proceeded the intended length of the stalk, the sides of the holes must be sewed down; the needle being passed through each aperture three times, including within the sewing, the alternate threads before mentioned as running between the bars.

The outline of the leaves in feather-stitch (see Fig. 28 A) being run round, each separate leaf is done with fine glazed cotton, in an elongated button-hole stitch, from the centre vein to its outer edge, the stitch being gradually shortened towards the points. The threads of the muslin will thus be divided in a line up the middle, which must be filled up in glover's stitch. This resembles the button-hole stitch, except that each stitch is taken a little higher up than the preceding one. The outer edge, and the outline of the separate parts of the leaf (see Fig. 28 B), comprising a variety of stitches, are run round. The right-hand edge of the leaf is composed alternately of feather-stitch, and a pattern worked with glazed cotton in double button-hole stitch, in which two stitches are taken side by side. Then an equal space is left, and two more are taken; and thus to the end.

The next row is formed by placing similar stitches under the alternate spaces left above, each time taking in the threads which run between each pair of stitches. The parts (see Fig. 28 B, a and d), are done in half herring-bone stitch, on the bias of the muslin; four threads being taken on the needle at a time. In forming the second and succeeding rows, the needle passes through the lower side of the first row of apertures.

The ground (see Fig. 28 B), is composed of a series of lines, each formed by drawing together, and sewing over very closely with fine thread, six threads of the muslin. Square spots are formed in the spaces, by sewing in glazed cotton over eight of the cross threads—passing the needle alternately over the first four, and under the second four. The large rosette (see Fig. 28 B) is worked in feather-stitch. All the other stitches used in this leaf are described in the succeeding flowers.

The cup of the fancy flower (see Fig. 28 C, a) is done in feather-stitch. The centre is a series of eyelet-holes, formed by passing the needle twice through the same hole; then repeating the same process at the distance of four threads; and so on in succession to the end of the row. The second row is formed at the spaces between the holes of the first row, with four threads between each as before, so that the holes of each row are perfected in the following row. Part *b* in Fig. 28 *C* is done in half herring-bone stitch, leaving four threads of the muslin between each row. Part *c* is formed by drawing together, and sewing over tightly, four threads of the muslin between each row. Part *d* is worked in double button-hole stitch; part *e* is the same as the centre, with spots in satin-stitch.

The centre of the fancy flower (see Fig. 28 *D*) is in half herring-bone stitch, worked in glazed cotton. The small eyelet-holes in Fig. 28 *D*, *a* are formed by taking up two threads of muslin all round. By the sides of them is a stitch like the cross-stitch in marking, and a short stitch passes over each end of the thread, forming the cross; then follows another eyelet-hole and a cross. The subsequent rows are done in a similar manner—the eyelet-holes in each line being invariably placed under the crosses of the line above. The series of holes in Fig. 28 *D*, *b* is formed by sewing over four threads on the cross-way of the muslin, then passing to the next four, and thus until the line is finished. The following rows are done in the same manner, until all the space is filled. The holes are then sewed over in a similar way, but in the contrary direction. At Fig. 28 *D*, *c* six cross-threads of the muslin are drawn together by passing the needle underneath, from one side to the other, and then in contrary directions, thus forming a little spot. Part *d* is formed by sewing over four threads of the straight-way of the muslin, and leaving four threads between each stitch; the same line is sewed back again, so as to form a cross over the top.

These stitches are susceptible of an endless variety of changes, by introducing spots, bars, or cross-lines, in satin-stitch; and in the half herring-bone stitch, by changing the direction of the threads, or leaving spaces, as fancy may dictate. The use of glazed cotton, instead of fine thread, will also give a very different effect to the same stitch. The edge of each flower, and of each compartment of a flower, is sewed closely over with glazed cotton. It is not expected that these imitations of antique lace-work will be practised on the extended scale here described: the separate articles may, however, be introduced, as taste may direct, to fill up the centres of modern flowers or fancy leaves.

Muslin worked with glazed cotton was formerly called Dresden-work, but is now known by the name of Moravian, from its production having formed the principal employment of a religious sect called the Moravian Sisters, which originated in Germany, and some of whose establishments exist in this country. The shops in London called Moravian warehouses were originally opened for the sale of their work; though they are now become ordinary depots for the various kinds of fancy embroidery, produced by the immense numbers of young females who, in this country, derive their maintenance from the ever-varying use of the needle.

Strips of work intended for insertion in plain muslin or lace, should have a row of hem-stitch on each side, which is thus produced: a margin of the muslin is left on the sides of the pattern, sufficiently broad to wrap over the finger. At a few threads' distance from the work, on each side, threads are drawn out to the width of a narrow hem. Three or four threads, which cross the space thus formed, are taken upon the needle (beginning at one side of the space) and sewed over with very fine cotton, about three times, when the thread will have reached the other side. At this point three or four more of the cross-threads are added, and the whole sewed twice over, so as to tie the six or eight together at that side. The last number taken up must then be sewed over three times, as the first.

By this time the thread will have reached the side from which it first proceeded. Fresh threads are then added, and tied each time at the sides as before; and so on, from side to side, to the end. Three or four threads are taken at a time, according to the width of the space formed by drawing the threads out. The whole hem-stitch, when completed, forms a kind of zig-zag (see Fig. 28 E). The muslin is joined, by its outer margin, to whatever article of dress it is intended to adorn.

Another species of hem-stitch is called veining. It is introduced to give the same appearance as the regular hem-stitch, in curved or other positions which would not admit of drawing the threads out (see Fig. 28 F). It is done on the regular direction, or bias of the muslin, by sewing over two threads of the muslin one way, then taking up two threads of the contrary way, tying them together at one side, as directed in the straight hem-stitch; then sewing over the latter two threads twice. After crossing to the opposite side, two more are sewed over; and so in continuity, according to the direction required.

Cambric pocket-handkerchiefs are generally ornamented with a row of hem-stitch, bordered by a broad hem, or with the outer edges scolloped, and a small pattern embroidered in each scollop. It is fashionable to have the corners embellished with a fancy sprig, and frequently with a different pattern in each. Embroidered initials and crests, in one corner, have a very beautiful effect. They are usually surrounded by a wreath of laurel, or some fancy device, in which the leaves and stems are worked in satin-stitch, relieved by a row of eyelet-holes. In working the letters, which are also in satin-stitch, great care and delicacy are required to preserve their proper shape, by lengthening or shortening the stitches, so as to correspond with the varying breadth of the written characters in the pattern.

A coronet or crest may be worked in satin-stitch, varied with eyelet-holes or any other appropriate stitch according to the subject (see Fig. 28 G).

Lace-work. The making of lace is not now amongst the pursuits of ladies; it will therefore be unnecessary to enter into its details. The only branch of lace-work which seems to come within my plan is embroidery on net, in imitation of Brussels point-lace, which for veils, gowns, or their trimmings is very beautiful in its effect, and perhaps exceeds in delicacy every other branch of white embroidery.

Embroidery on net is performed by placing over the net a piece of French cambric, of a size proportioned to the subject, and the paper pattern under both. Then the design (of which each particular leaf or sprig ought to be very small, though the clusters should be large) must be run twice round with cotton, the running thread sewed over pretty closely with rather finer cotton, and the external edges of the cambric cut neatly and closely off (see Fig. 29 A). In designing a veil, a small running pattern,

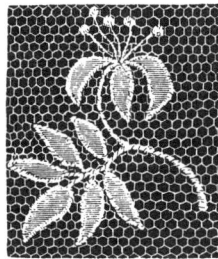

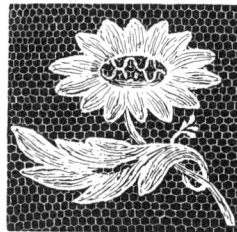

A

B

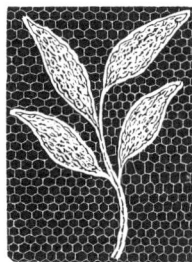

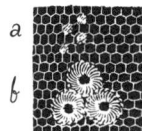

C

D

Figure 29. Designs for embroidery on net.

worked quite at the edge, is proper. When completed, a pearling (which is a species of lace edging, to be had at the lace shops) should be sewed round the outside, to give it a finish. On the lower part of the veil, within the running border, there should be a handsome pattern worked across. This style is very easy of execution, and is an excellent imitation of what it is intended to represent.

Net is also worked by running the outline of leaves and flowers with glazed cotton, darning inside the running stitch with fine cotton, doubled, and filling up the centre of the flower with half herring-bone stitch, from one side to the other (see Fig. 29 B). Instead of darning within the flower, chain-stitching is sometimes introduced, which is thus performed: having secured the cotton, one thread of the net is taken up, and the cotton being held down by your left thumb, the first stitch is taken as in button-hole work, leaving a loop through which the needle is passed, to form a second stitch or loop, and so on after the manner of a chain; until having arrived at the extremity of a leaf or flower, the cotton is turned round and worked back until the whole space is covered (see Fig. 29 C).

An agreeable variety may be introduced amongst the flowers, by filling up their centres in a stitch formed by sewing over two threads across the space; then leaving one row of threads, and taking up the next two, until the interior is completely occupied. This kind of stitch may be varied by crossing it with the same stitch. Small clusters of spots on net are very pretty; each spot is formed by passing the needle backwards and forwards through one mesh, and alternately over and under two of the threads forming that mesh, which are opposite to each other (see Fig. 29 D, a). Sprigs or branches formed by eyelet-holes, either singly along a stem, or in clusters of three, afford a pleasing variation (see Fig. 29 D, b). The eyelet-holes are worked in button-hole stitch; one mesh of the net being left open for the centre.

Book-muslin is sometimes worked into net, by placing it under the net, and both over a paper pattern. The outline is then run round; the running is either sewed over, or worked in button-hole stitch, and the external edge of the muslin cut off. This mode is not confined to small patterns, as the cambric or net which is intended to resemble Brussels point-lace.

Gold-thread Embroidery. This, in splendour and richness, far exceeds every other species of embroidery, and is principally used in court gowns, and for the ball-room. It is practised on crape, India muslin, or silk; and principally in large and bold designs. The gold thread should be fine, and it may be worked with nearly the same facility as any other thread. Where the material is sufficiently transparent, a paper pattern is placed underneath. The outline is run in white thread, and the subject is then worked with gold thread, in satin-stitch. For a thin stalk to a flower, the running thread should be omitted, and gold thread laid on the material, and sewed slightly over with another gold thread; thus giving the stalk a very pretty spiral appearance. In embroidering a thick material, the design is sketched with a black-lead pencil, if the ground is light; or with a white-chalk pencil, if dark.

The pattern is frequently varied by the introduction of short pieces of fine gold bullion, sometimes two or three of them coming out of the cup of a flower. The stitch passes lengthways through the twist of the bullion, thus confining it flat. The centre of a flower may also be finished with bullion. In this case, the stitch taken should be shorter than the piece of bullion; the under side of which will therefore be compressed, and the upper side expanded, so as to give it a little prominence.

Gold spangles may be occasionally introduced. They should be secured by bringing the thread from beneath, passing it through the spangle, then through a very short bit of bullion, and back through the hole in the centre of the spangle. This is better than sewing the spangle on with a thread across its face.

Gold-thread flowers on tulle form a beautiful embroidery, and are worked in the same way as the thread net represented in Fig. 29 *B*. This material may also be worked in gold-thread satin-stitch, or at the tambour. The whole of this kind of embroidery is also worked in silver thread.

There is a beautiful variety produced by the introduction of floss-silk, worked in satin-stitch, in any one colour which will harmonize with the gold or silver thread. The effect of green floss with gold thread is particularly good, when tastefully arranged—as for the lower part of a gown, in the combination of a wreath of the shamrock in green floss-silk, entwined with roses or other flowers in gold or silver thread.

——*The Young Lady's Book*.

Divers Embroidery Patterns. The Vandyke pattern in Fig. 30 *A*, being chiefly composed of French eyelet-holes, has a very light and neat appearance, particularly on clear muslin. Because the Vandyke pattern in Fig. 30 *B* is composed of French and English eyelet-holes and satin-stitch, it is advisable not to work it on too thin a muslin. The pattern in Fig. 30 *C* will give you an idea of the work which should always accompany hem-stitching; for if it is a large coarse pattern, it will be too heavy for the delicacy of the hem-stitching, and tear it out in washing.

The borders in Fig. 31 *A, B,* and *C,* being cloth-work, must be produced by working the muslin double in those parts which are to form the

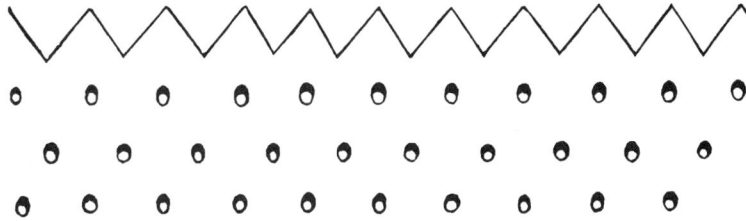

A

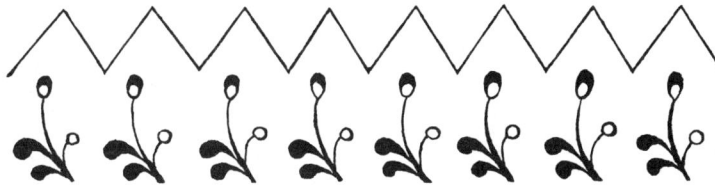

B

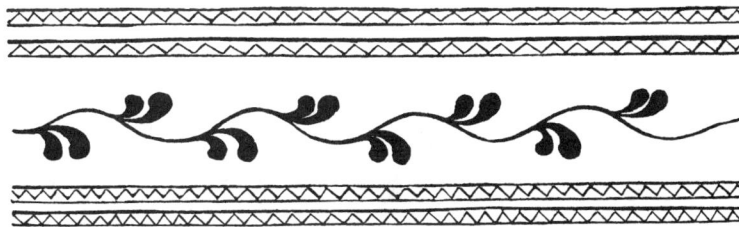

C

Figure 30. Borders for frills.

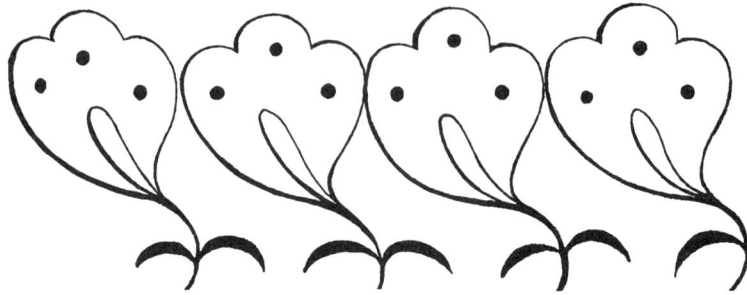

A

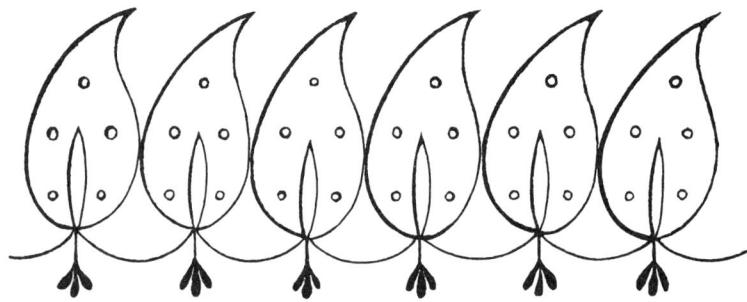

B

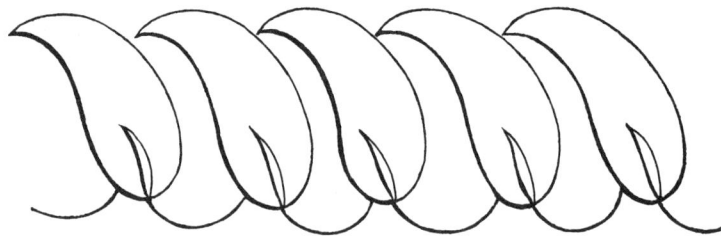

C

Figure 31. Cloth-work borders.

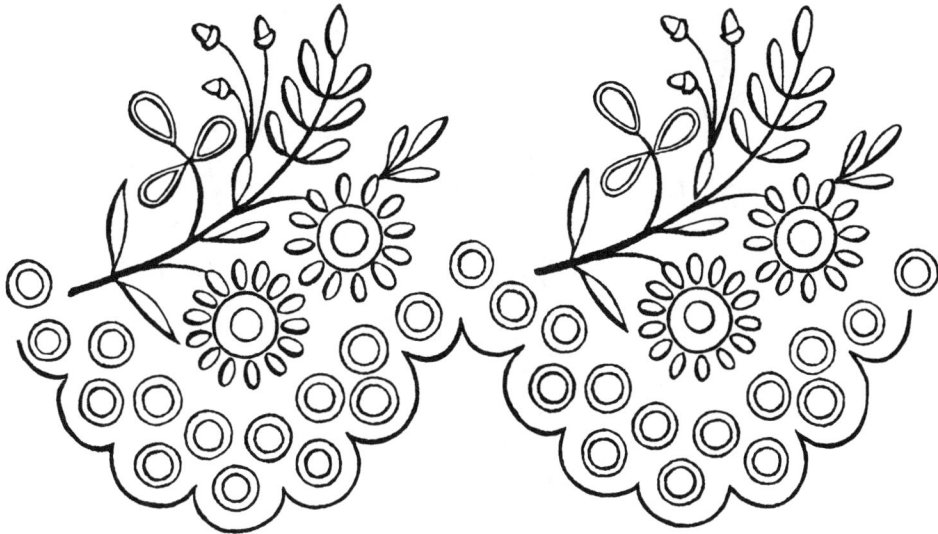

Figure 32. A genteel pattern for a flounce.

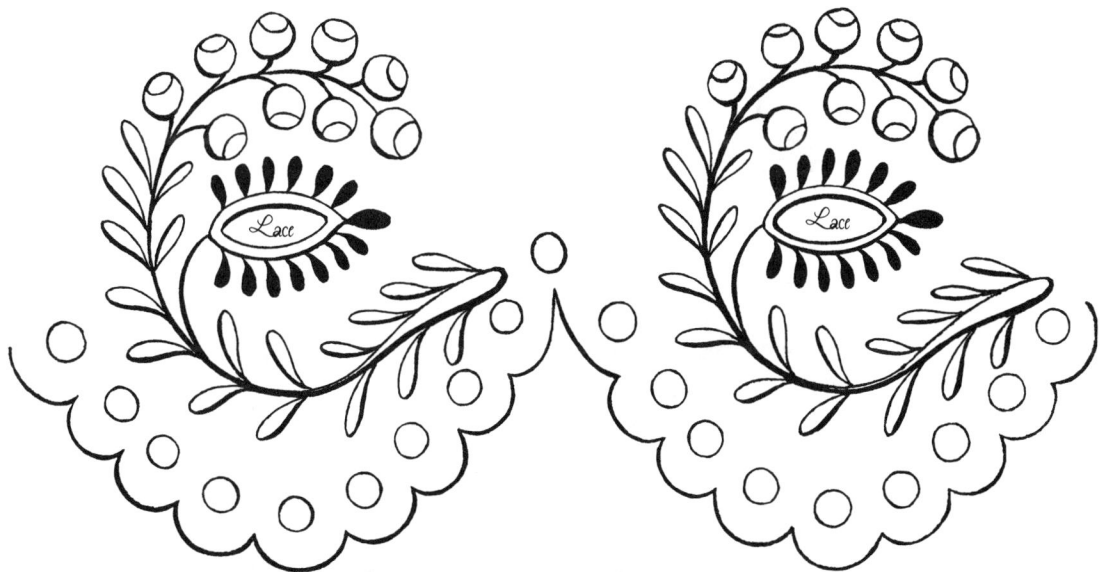

Figure 33. A rich pattern for a flounce.

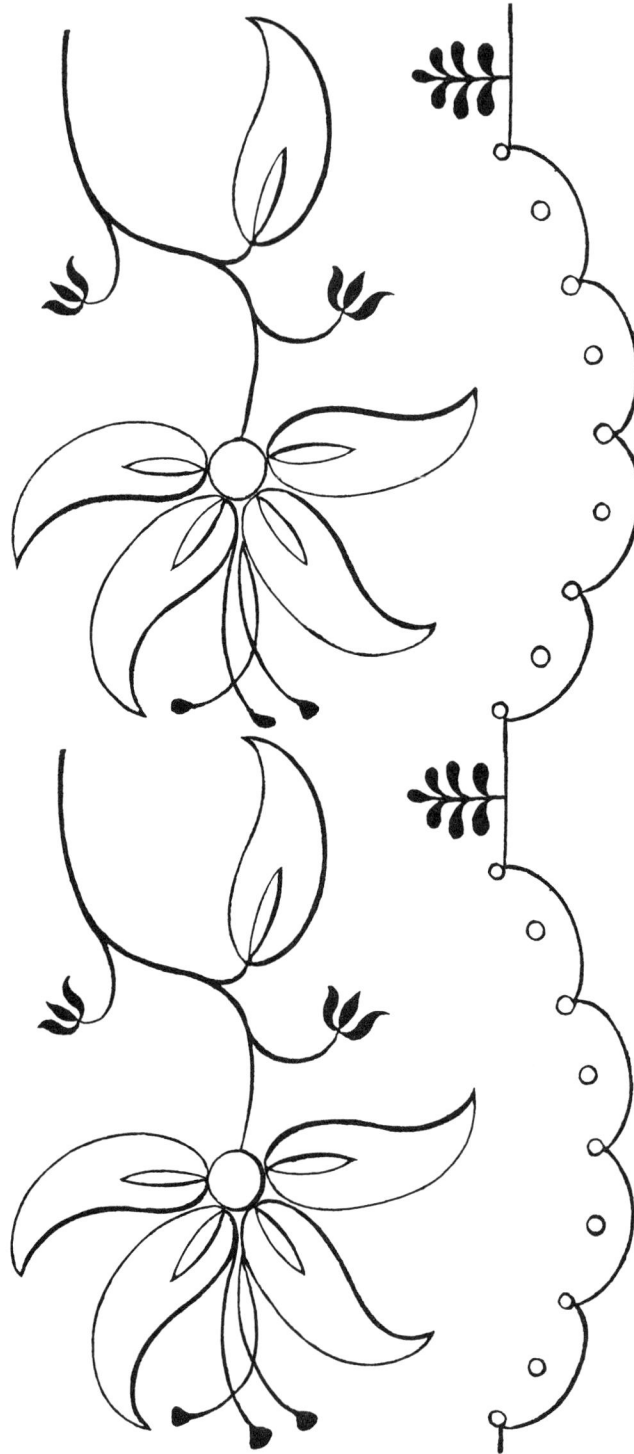

Figure 34. A handsome pattern for a flounce.

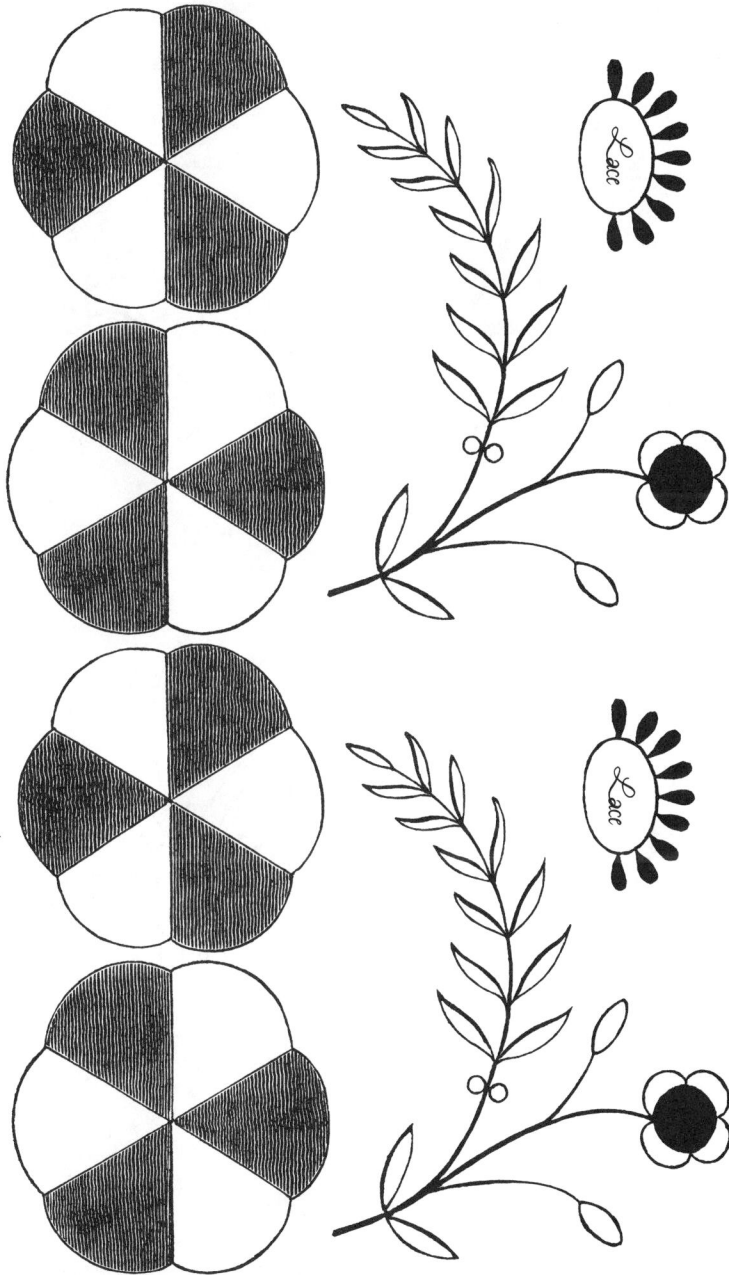

Figure 35. A bold pattern for a flounce.

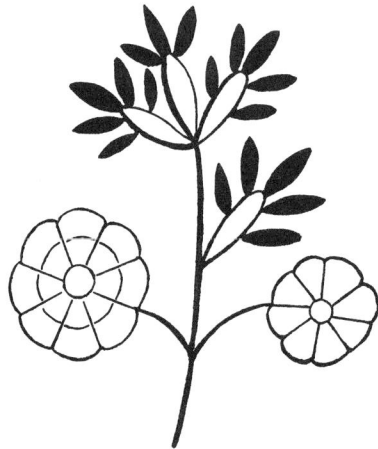

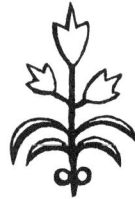

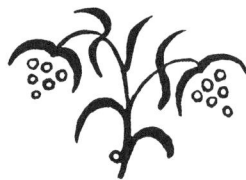

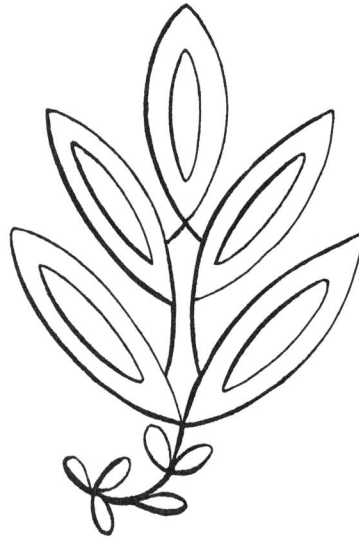

Figure 36. Sprigs, or corner-pieces.

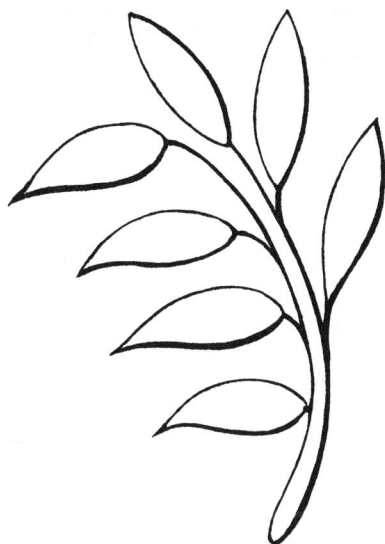

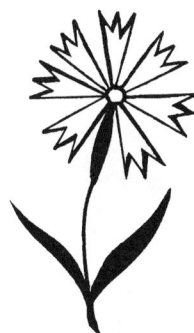

A

B

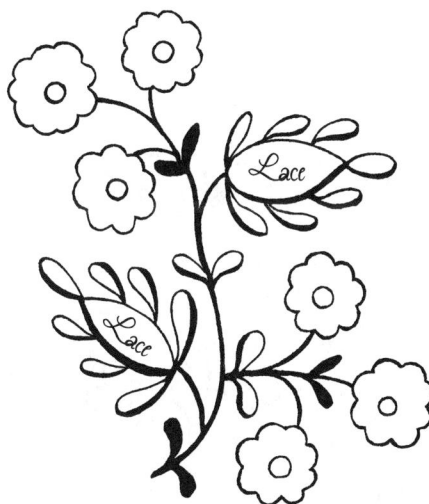

C

D

Figure 37. More sprigs and corner-pieces.

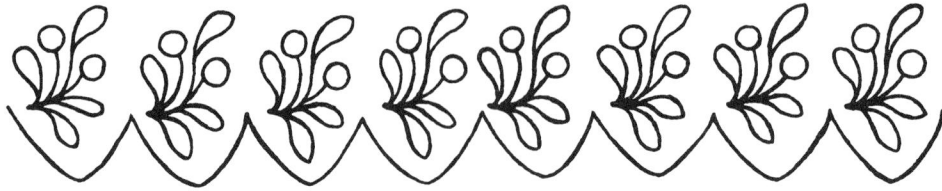

A

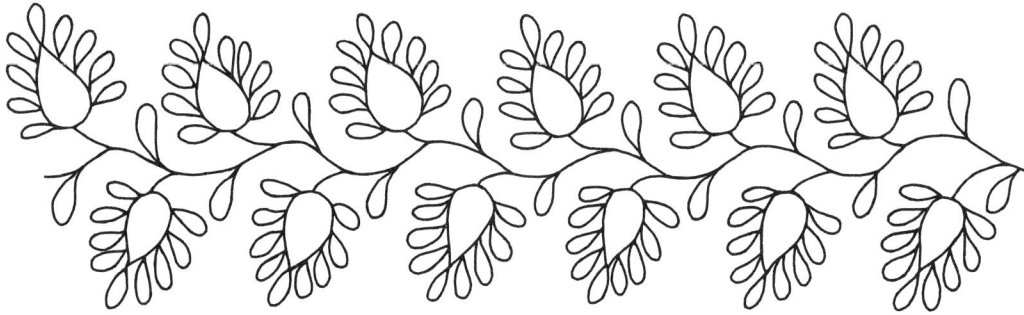

B

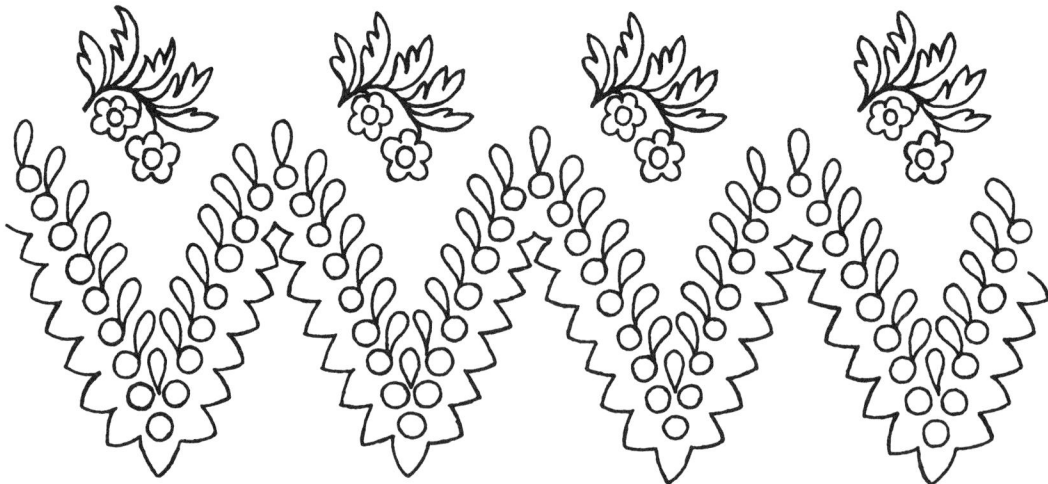

C

Figure 38. Narrow borders for muslin embroidery.

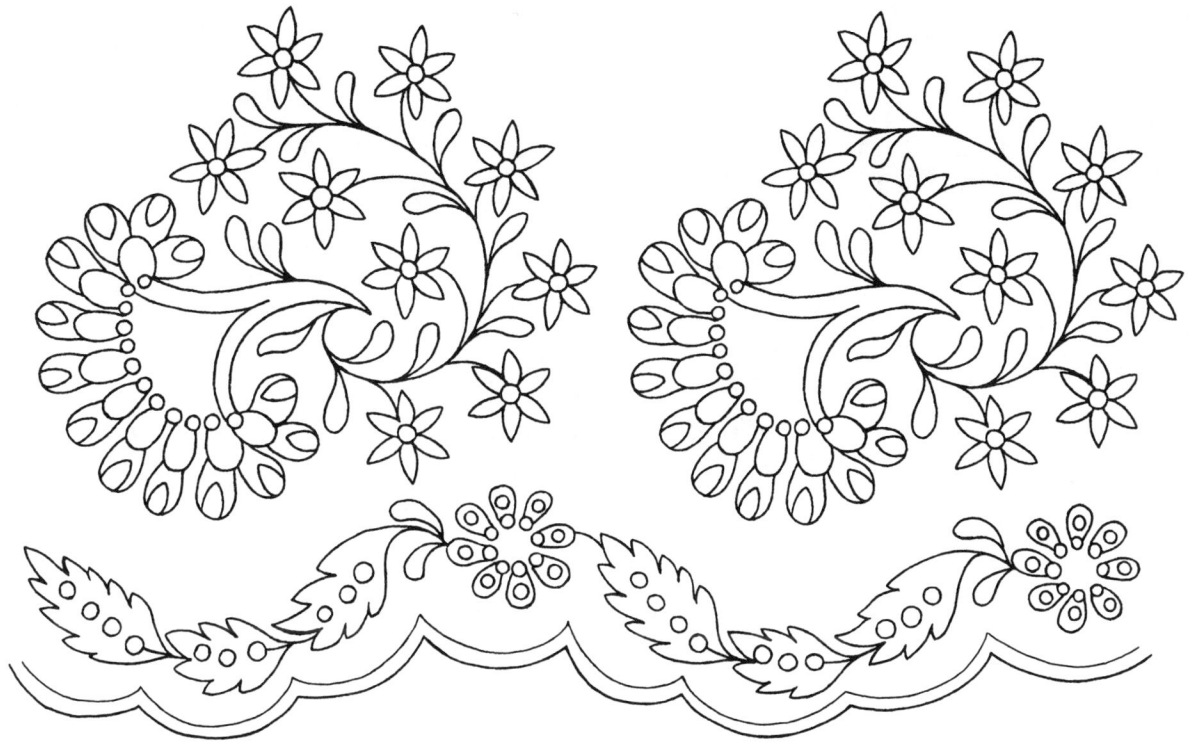

Figure 39. A wide border for muslin embroidery.

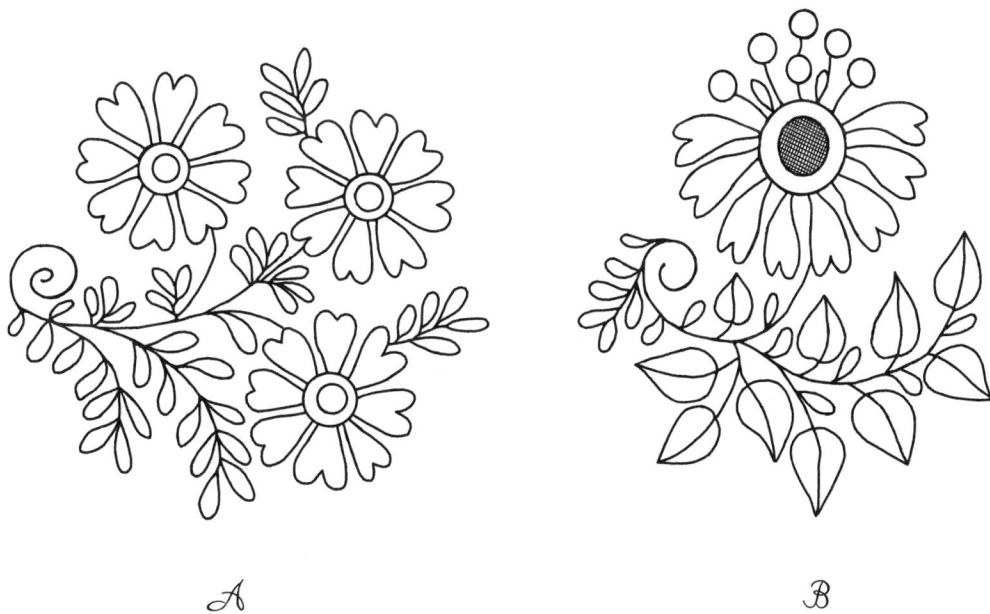

A

B

Figure 40. Sprigs for muslin embroidery.

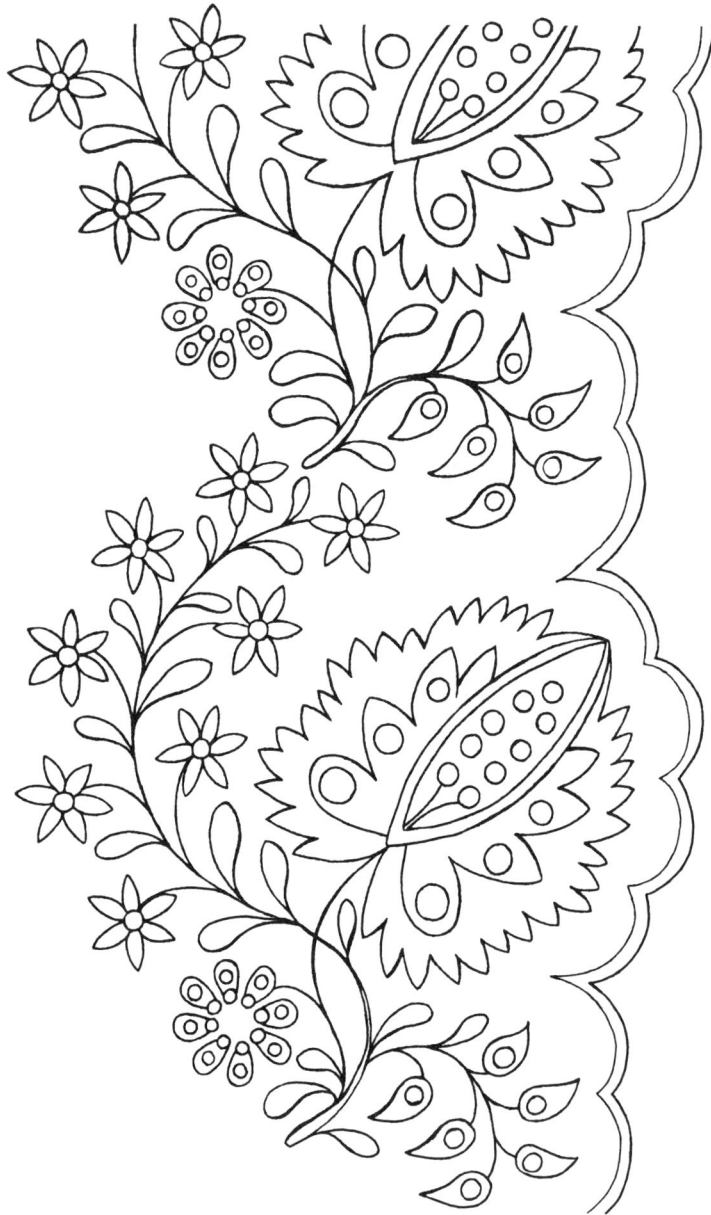

Figure 41. Another wide border for muslin embroidery.

——Ackermann's Repository.

pattern. You must observe, in this case, to let the under muslin be either jaconet or cambric, in order to give a neat effect.

The elegant and genteel pattern in Fig. 32 is particularly suitable for a clear muslin. It must be worked in satin-stitch, excepting the centre of the two flowers in each sprig, which are to be done in over-cast or button-hole stitch. The eyelet-holes are also to be worked in the same way.

The full rich pattern in Fig. 33 is to be done in satin-stitch, and when worked with ordinary care has a very elegant appearance. Observe that lace must be introduced where that word is inserted.

The fancy pattern in Fig. 34 is nearly all cloth-work, and is allowed to be very handsome. It certainly is light, elegant, and fanciful.

The bold pattern in Fig. 35 is done in satin-stitch, except the scolloped wheels at the bottom, which must be cloth-work, with every other section cut out as marked in the plate.

——*The Alphabetical Receipt Book and Domestic Advisor.*

Diversion 9.

The Lady's Maid as Embroideress. Fancy needle-work and embroidery will, for the most part, be only an occasional thing to fill up a vacant hour, when there are no other things pressing. But you should in this, as in all your services, endeavour as much as possible to excel, as it will greatly recommend you if you are capable of working a fine evening gown for your employers.

In working upon very fine gowns, such as those of white satin, &c., you must be careful not to crease or stain them, nor to injure their gloss, which will readily suffer from the slightest perspiration of your hands, and even by exposure to the heat of a fire or the glare of sunshine. As soon as you have finished a gown of this kind, it ought to be carefully folded up and wrapped in an envelope of fine paper; or what is in some cases better, hung up in a wardrobe closet, on a peg, at full length, without being folded at all.

——*The Duties of a Lady's Maid.*

Chapter XVI.
The Art of mending
and renewing Garments.

I shall first discuss how to mend holes, tears, and worn places in the material; next, divers modes of re-modelling garments and furs; and finally, those of renewing shoes. (Chapter XV describes sewing stitches; Chapter XVII describes how to mend stockings; and Chapter XXI, how to renew hats.)

The art of mending is divided into seven modes: 1st., darning; 2nd., patching; 3rd., over-cast patching; 4th., patching with button-hole or blanket-stitch; 5th., mending with laced stitches; 6th., mending *à dentelle;* 7th., invisible mending. I shall describe them in order.

Darning.

This is the most usual mode. When some material happens to tear, you join the broken and roughly-spread threads with a long series of rows of running stitches. These must be arranged so that each stitch taken underneath the material is next one taken on top of it (see Fig.1 *A* and *B*). This is called opposing the stitches.

Patching.

This kind of mending is done for round holes, such as large burn holes. It is not used for gowns, or similar articles exposed to view, but is employed on linen, principally when it is not very fine, and when the holes cannot be mended otherwise.

Take a little piece of material similar to the article which you want to mend, and lay this patch over the wrong side of the hole. Baste it; then you may work several series of six or eight darning stitches all round the right side of the hole, be it square or round, catching the patch and the edge of the hole with every stitch. The darning stitches must be made quite close together, and carefully opposed so that the patch stays in place. When you

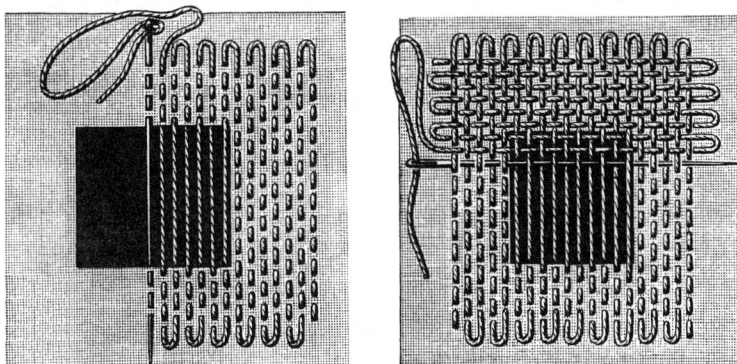

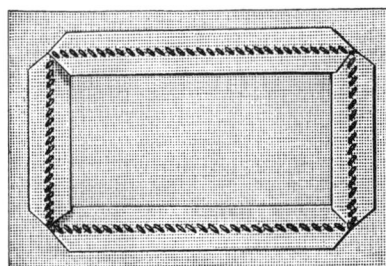

Figure 1. Darning and over-cast patching.

have thus completely joined the two, remove the basting thread; and on one side cut off the ravelled threads of the hole, and on the other side the excess portions of the patch.

Ordinarily patching is done on the right side, because of the difficulty of always catching the edge of the hole on the wrong side. However, this is contrary to the rules for darning, which is always done on the wrong side, so that no one sees the little ridges the thread makes in coming back to each row of stitches. When you mean to make a patch carefully, you must observe the principle of working on the wrong side; and to be quite sure of sticking the needle into the edge of the hole, baste on the edge. Then you will work with as much assurance on the wrong side as on the right; and if the patch is well laid on without any creases, very little of the darning will be seen, likewise very little of the patch.

Over-cast Patching.

This kind of mending is done on gowns, and all other articles where a piece of material has been caught and torn away. However, it is done to much more advantage on striped or flowered materials, because the design makes the over-casting less apparent than on plain ones.

Finish removing the piece of material already partially torn off, and cut a square hole. Make a seam fold all round the hole thus prepared. Then take a piece of similar material and cut it precisely even with the hole, except that it is necessary to leave in addition a seam fold round the patch. If the material has a design, carefully match the flowers or stripes which compose it. Baste this patch thus to the hole, on the wrong side, and unite the seam folds of the patch and the hole by an over-casting which bites only one thread. (See Fig. 1 *C*.) Above all, be very careful to arrange the corners properly, which requires the most attention. Then flatten the over-casting with your thimble, remove the basting, and your work is finished.

When the hole is longer than it is wide, you may often avoid the trouble of arranging the corners of the patch by over-casting only the lengthways sides. Then lay the material flat over your knee, and join the patch and the hole crossways with a narrow darning, or sometimes with a laced stitch, of which I shall speak below. A combination of stitches is used much more frequently than the over-cast stitch by itself. When the hole is wider than it is long, you over-cast it crossways and darn it lengthways. It is necessary to use very fine thread for both operations.

To patch with Button-hole or Blanket-stitch.

This kind of mending is another way to patch a round or a square hole without being obliged to make a seam. To that end, furnish the hole all round with closely-spaced button-hole stitches, in a sufficiently fine thread. Likewise button-hole the patch, which you have cut to fit the hole so precisely that it seems as if you wished to glue its edges to those of the hole. The button-hole stitches must be tight. The hole and the patch being thus prepared, place the patch in the gap of the hole, pin it in two or three places, then stick your needle into each button-hole stitch on the edge of the hole, and into each button-hole stitch on the edge of the patch. You may replace the button-hole stitch with a blanket-stitch. This kind of mending is much used for napkins and sheets.

To mend with Laced Stitches.

When you have to mend a hole which is not torn, but cut, such as a slit produced by a penknife or a table-knife, you must resort to laced stitches. Begin by holding the slit quite firmly, with the material folded over your left forefinger between your thumb and third finger, to form a species of cross. Laced stitches are not made through both pieces of the material at once, but through each alternately. Suppose that you have the right side of the slit resting against your forefinger, making it the under piece, and the left side on top of it, making it the upper piece. Do not knot your thread, but lay it so that the stitches you take will cover and fasten it. Put your needle between the two pieces—for more sturdiness, about six, eight, or ten threads from the edge of the slit, according to the thickness of the material. With the point up, bring the needle up through the upper piece. With the point down, pass it through the slit and then through the under piece, or right side of the slit, at the same distance from the slit as your stitch on the upper piece. This forms the first laced stitch (see Fig. 2 A).

With the point up again, pass the needle up through the upper piece just slightly below the first stitch, and so on. Take good care to always bring out the needle to the left and right sides of the slit, into the same thread of the material, so that the stitches remain in a straight line. This mending neatly makes a wide, flat *cordonnet*, divided by a slight groove.

To join on a fresh piece of thread, take three little running stitches along the slit, on the side opposite to the one where you must continue the stitch. Lay the end of the finished thread over the end of the new thread which you just fastened with the running stitches. The series of laced stitches will conceal both at once.

Sew a little beyond the end of the slit. Then fasten off the thread by passing the needle under a dozen stitches to the left, and bringing it out again underneath, fasten it on the wrong side by making a looped over-cast stitch. Take the over-cast stitch on the material covered by the laced stitches, and observe that it does not appear on top. When the mend is short, the needle is often passed to fasten the bottom and top of the seam.

When you have a very long slit in a skirt, a gentleman's shirt, or any other article, you cannot do better than to mend it with laced stitches,

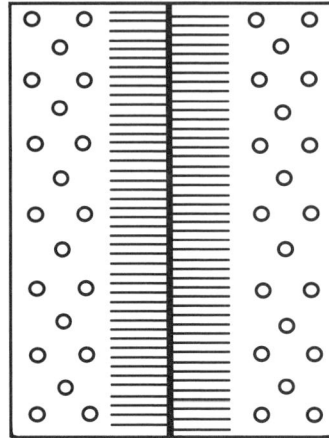

A

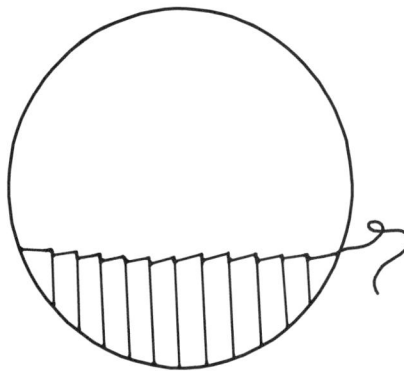

B

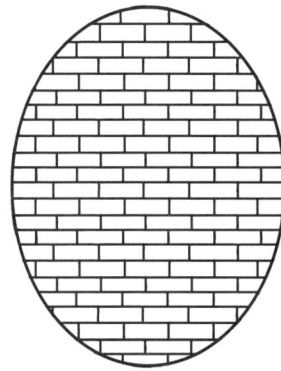

C

Figure 2. Laced stitches and tulle-stitches.

because they do not take up any of the material. You could also use it to put patches on round or square holes, but I have not seen it thus employed. It is most commonly used to mend gloves which have chanced to split; if the glove has split because it is too tight, loosen the laced stitches to leave a narrow space between the sides of the split.

This stitch is not only used for mending; it is also employed to join two pieces of material which are found to be cut too narrow to make seam folds, or when the daintiness of the work disagrees with the slight thickness of seam folds. As it takes a long time to work, a seam is made with it only when other kinds of stitches cannot satisfactorily replace it.

To mend *à Dentelle.*

If you have round or square holes in some linen (such as a sheet or napkin) which you do not wish to patch because the hole is not large enough for that, work button-hole stitches or a narrow *cordonnet* round the hole (see Chapter XIX). Then, using sewing thread, work tulle-stitches until the hole is filled (see Fig. 2 *B* and *C*). Many persons are content with that, but they should not be imitated. The net-work produced by the tulle-stitches should be only a preparation, because it produces a thin streak which does not accord well with the toile. You should completely cover it with darning stitches made with flat thread, opposed and repeated until the tissue is no longer transparent. You may also work a tissue over a round hole with darning stitches, without the assistance of the tulle-stitches.

Do not work a *cordonnet* or blanket-stitches round the hole if the material is very soft. In that case take very slanted, equally spread-out over-cast stitches. Then lay the material over your knee, pick it up between the third and fourth fingers of your left hand, and retain it over these fingers so that your thumb rests underneath the material which rests on the fourth finger, and your forefinger is placed under your third finger, parallel to the fourth. This position gives a kind of tension to the material, and helps you to cast the threads close together across the width of the hole. By entering the needle on one side, then the opposite side, you fill the interval in between. When you have thus furnished the hole crossways, turn the material around and pass the needle across its length, alternately under and over the threads.

For the second row, do the same thing, opposing the stitches; pull these lengthways rows as tight as possible, so that the darning does not spread out. But that ordinarily does happen, because you do not darn with thread that fine or take meticulous care. If you were to do so, you would have invisible mending, more or less. Unless the linen which you have to mend is very good, it is better that this darning preserve its character of mending *à dentelle,* spreading out a little, because invisible mending takes excessively long.

Invisible Mending.

Here is the *ne plus ultra* of repairs, the kind which requires the most care and produces the best appearance, since it is never visible. It is also the kind which costs most dear; the slightest repair is thirty sous, and some cost up to forty francs. Very large tears in India muslins and cachemires explain how such a high price may be put on this kind of repair.

The modes are more lengthy and meticulous than difficult. When you have to make an invisible repair in some material, begin by withdrawing all the worn threads, be they lengthways or crossways, up to the point where you must begin and end the repair. All round the place thus marked, cut off the kind of lint which is produced by the pulled threads. Then turn the material to the wrong side, and mount the right side of the hole onto green paper to impart a convenient stiffness to the material, and to spare your sight, which this operation fatigues extremely.

That done, thread a very fine, long-eyed needle with a thread of cotton cambric, or any other which accords with the material which you have to mend. Cast a thread crossways at each thread which you withdrew; do not fasten the thread by fixing it at the two opposite sides of the hole, as you have done up until now, but fasten it much farther to the right and left, by basting with very close stitches.

This lengthy operation finished, turn the material back over, and taking it lengthways, pass the needle alternately under and over the threads which you cast previously. Oppose the stitches of the second row, pressing them against the other row as close as possible, because each lengthways row must match one of the threads which you withdrew in that direction. This second row is not made by turning the needle around, unlike all other darns. When you come to the end of the first row, cut the thread and go on working from the end where you began. When you finish the repair, cut these remaining ends of thread at the beginning and end of each row, and the ends of the threads which you cast and temporarily fastened with basting stitches.

You will perceive that this operation exacts care and diligence; and muslin, batiste, and percale are not the only materials which must be thus repaired. Those materials are not twilled, and it suffices to bring together and interweave the threads which compose them. But when it is necessary to mend twilled materials, such as cachemire shawls and those called Ternaux cachemire, you must imitate the twill of the material. You achieve this by catching the threads cast crossways one by one, as if you were taking side-stitches. This naturally increases your work, because with the mode of running stitches employed for muslin &c., and for all ordinary darns, you may take eight or ten stitches at a time. To mend twills, you must not only catch the threads one at a time, but turn the needle for each stitch, because of the necessity of alternating the stitches on top and underneath.

Some workwomen who do invisible mending do not cut the thread at the end of each row, but are content to leave long loops of thread there, on the bottom and on top; they remove these when the repair is finished. This mode is quicker, but it presents the risk of cutting at the same time the material placed under the threads; furthermore, you may easily catch one of the loops, and thus tighten the mend and destroy all your work. It is therefore prudent to refrain from using this mode for invisible mending; but it is well to employ it for ordinary darning, in order to better imitate the material which you are repairing.

To make up Gowns
so that you may easily alter them.

To avoid ridicule, or spending the money required to buy new clothes, a woman must know how to alter the style of her gowns, put on new sleeves and bodies, and use the material for other pieces of clothing when any other change or repair is impossible.

When a fashion is too odd, ridiculous, or unbecoming, wait until it has become general. But if while waiting you have occasion to make a gown, try as far as possible to preserve the means of altering it to the new fashion, should you be forced to follow that. For example, when the fashion of plaits or gathers in the front breadth of a gown had arrived, I was loath to submit, and resolved not to follow it until it was impossible to do otherwise. However, I had to buy a taffety gown, and foreseeing that it might become necessary to put in those unbecoming plaits, I did not cut the front breadth gored at the top. I merely sewed on the bias line, and left the extra part at the top of each side seam, laying it beyond the gores when I made up the gown. The fashion of the plaits did not become general, so I had no need to resort to the parts which I had kept in reserve. But if it had, it would have been easy to resew the top of my seams, replacing the bias line with the reserved straight edge, and plaiting in the middle the fulness it would have provided. It goes without saying that this mode could not haven been used on a gown of transparent material.

Some mantua-makers use this mode, but for a different purpose. Because gowns are stained chiefly at the top of the front breadth, they do not make the bias cut at the top, so that in case of a mishap they may unpick it and turn it upside down. The stains are easily hidden at the bottom, but the stitch marks are unsightly. When the material is rather thick, overlapping enlarges your waist at the side. The advantages and disadvantages are about equal.

Sometimes certain styles afford means of cleanliness and economy which should be seized. For example, when sleeves consist (as they have for a long time) of both long tight sleeves and mancherons, it is very well to have two pair of sleeves for each gown, especially those of wash material. As sleeves become soiled at least twice as fast as the gown, and often force you to send it to be washed when the rest is still wearable, the soiled sleeves may be replaced with clean ones. To this end, the sleeves are hemmed at the top, and set on the gown only by a basting stitch like over-casting, which perfectly conceals the mancheron. You may undo and redo the basting in a few minutes, and not only have the pleasure of always wearing clean sleeves, but also avoid (for calicoes, printed muslins, &c.) the fading of the colours which is common for this part.

The Mode of turning Kitchen Aprons.

You may sometimes content yourself with putting the top of the apron at the bottom, and the bottom at the top, because the lower part of this garment is nearly always new, when the upper part is worn. It is therefore necessary to unpick the plaits at the top and hem it, then to unpick or cut off the hem at the bottom. Make plaits there, which you fasten by means of a doubled band, sewed on the inside, and turned down like the waist-band of a gown. (See Div. 1.)

But when the top of the apron is too worn, and it becomes necessary, or soon will, to patch it, you should, after having taken off or unpicked the top of the apron, sew it like a bag, joining the two selvages of the back with an over-cast seam. If there is a selvage on only one side, replace the over-casting with a flat seam. When the seam is finished, fold your apron double, and beginning at the top, slit it from the top to the bottom on the opposite side; that is, at the middle of the front. Then take these pieces (mend them if need be), and hem both pieces produced by the slit. These pieces are then the two backs of the apron. Make it up again afterwards, reversing it from top to bottom or not, as you prefer.

This operation necessarily disarranges the pockets, since the plaits which shape the back of the apron leave too much space in the front. You must unpick them and bring them closer together by over-casting, measuring their position so that your hand may go in and out comfortably.

All aprons, whether kitchen or not, are turned thus, even if they are cut with gores, like gowns; only you cannot reverse such aprons. When you do not wish to cut an apron gored, but you wish to make it on the bias over the hips to fit your shape, it suffices to make a bias seam on each side, from the waist-band to the base of the hip, which forms a wide fold of material on the straight-way at the top. In this manner, the fold diminishes imperceptibly, finally becoming quite lost at the end of the seam, which gives you the desired bias without cutting the material. When it is time to turn the apron, unpick the two folds, and the material regains its ordinary shape; it becomes a breadth, which you may reverse from top to bottom. Remake the folds for the bias seam, at some distance from the over-cast seam. Then mark this in the middle, if you are slitting the apron, and at the lower part, which then makes the top, if you prefer to reverse it.

The Mode of turning Merino and Silk Gowns.

When a merino or silk gown is not soiled enough to dye or wash, and you still wish to wear it as new before having it cleansed, which always discolours it a little, you must unpick it completely, and take out the lining if there is one, entirely removing the stitches. Beat it, brush it (if it is of wool), iron it on the right side (which henceforth will be the wrong side, since it is re-lined on that side) and resew all the seams. Ordinarily it is necessary to renew the hem; that is, to remove it by unpicking it all round the gown, at either the place where it is sewed, or where it is folded. The latter mode is commonly used, for fear of shortening the gown too much. This reason does not prevent removing the folded part of the hem; first because rubbing against the ground produces a thin streak which would split the first day, and second because the lining is lowered to replace the piece removed. Make amends for this by adding a narrow strip at the top or the bottom of the lining. It is better if it is at the top.

The ends of the sleeves must also be renewed. It is unnecessary to say that you will need to put on a new collar and cuffs. These parts are the most worn by use, and the scissors always fray them in unpicking them, because they are made of narrow strips; moreover, this is the final reason for replacement.

Taffety gowns rarely need these repairs because they are made into linings when they are soiled. When the body and sleeves of a taffety gown are worn, it may be made into a petticoat or an apron, always provided that the taffety is of a dark colour. (See Div. 2.)

To renew Cotton Gowns without dyeing them.

A gown ordinarily has worn out at the body, the sleeves, and the upper front part of the skirt, when all the remainder is still good. If you have similar pieces of material, you may remake the body and sleeves. But you cannot in any way repair the front of the skirt, because it is impossible to make a crossways seam which would be tolerable.

In order to be able to replace the body and sleeves, many persons always buy an ell, or an ell and a half, more material than is needed for the gown. This practice is excellent for calicoes and fast printed muslins; but however fast the colours, it is still necessary to boil the new material several times to fade them. Otherwise the new body would always stand out a little from the rest of the gown.

According to the style of the body, bands of trimming which have not worn out may serve to renew it; for example a body traversed lengthways, crossways, or slantways by braids or muslin *entre-deux,* as have been worn for the past four years. In this way you may without difficulty renew the body of a calico or printed toile gown, because flounces, having faded like the rest of the gown, do not produce the disagreeable contrast which a new body always does.

A percale gown is not in the least difficult to renew. If the body is completely out of fashion, I unpick it, and I try to cut out a cap from the different pieces. It would indeed be ill-luck, if in mixing these pieces of percale with muslin, as is the custom in making night or morning caps, I did not succeed in making use of the body. Because I may combine the percale as I wish, I make a fashionable new body, and my gown looks quite new.

Calico, gingham, and printed muslin gowns cause more trouble because of the difficulty in matching them. If I have no extra material I do not even attempt that, because it would very likely be a waste of time. I therefore make the body as simple as possible, because any trimming which is out of fashion is no longer acceptable. The body resembles a chemisette, and I wear a canezou-pelerine or a *fichu-canezou* to conceal it completely. (See Div. 3.) If the material of the gown is figured (for instance printed muslin), I replace the sleeves with new ones of gauze or lawn.

If the gown is of common calico, I cannot use the preceding remedy. A *fichu-canezou* and clear sleeves, too elegant for the calico, would have the air of a repair, and a repair in bad taste. But if the mode permits, the gown may be worn with a spencer; or as a last resort made into a lining, because a woman at all well dressed would know not to make it into a petticoat.

It is difficult to take advantage of calico gowns, but it is comparatively easy to use muslin ones. In addition to being easily matched, they may be used up to the last scrap. I have had several gowns of this kind which have worn out four different bodies. When the skirt is thoroughly worn out in the front, I cut the seams of the breadths, because it is useless to waste time unpicking them, and place the pattern of a canezou over them.

To renew Cotton Gowns.

Not only are the used parts more than sufficient, but I have even obtained various very good pieces to make falling collars and trimmings for night-caps. You may therefore make from these gowns all sorts of *fichus,* and trimmings for night jackets, night shifts, pillow covers, &c.

Trimmings afford several ways of being renewed. (Chapter XV contains directions for making them.) I had a gown trimmed with wide *bouillons* held at both edges by corded piping. The fashion of wide flounces arrived: I unpicked the *bouillons* at the bottom, hemmed them, and they became flounces quite in style.

I also had a gingham gown trimmed with five narrow flounces placed thus: three one above the other on the bottom over the hem, and after an interval of two and a half inches, two others close together. First I unpicked the two which were nearest the hem. I put one of them aside, and completely undid the gathers in the other. Next I cut off the hem of the third, leaving it on the gown. Then, matching the chequers well, I joined these two flounces with very close over-cast stitches, which seam I then ironed. After that, I unpicked the fourth flounce and joined it in the same way to the fifth. This gave me two fashionably wide flounces. I must add that seams in the middle of a flounce are proper only for coloured gowns, and tolerably dark-coloured ones at that. They would be impossible on white. When flounces are wide, and then become narrower, I divide them and place them where the new style dictates.

One of my percale gowns had embroidery with large points, which at the end of some years (fashions in embroidery last longer than others) appeared extremely antiquated. I cut it off and used it to trim pillow covers by attaching it round the cover with a line of raised satin-stitches. My gown was quite short then, but that troubled me very little; I lengthened it by trimming it with tulle *entre-deux* and bands of percale. I might equally have simply attached a percale extension, which I could then have concealed with any kind of trimming: folds, rouleaux, flounces *à la fille d'honneur,* &c.

When the wide folds with which gowns are now trimmed are no longer in use, they may easily be unpicked; but then, having cut away the extra piece which this produces, you should conceal the marks of the stitches, which are never effaced, and which would appear mean. It is the easiest thing in the world to put a new trimming there. This mode was used formerly, about fifteen years ago.

Trimmings *en coquilles* and *en agrafes,* that is, bands fastened widthways on the gown here and there, some closer together, some farther apart, do very well for flounces, ruches, and likewise folds. For these, after having unpicked the band, I have only to iron it, fold it double lengthways, and join the two edges with a coloured flat braid, which serves to hide the seam which I made to place the fold flat on the gown. This looks exactly like a tuck made in the gown, with a braid placed on it for ornament. Though bands of *agrafes* or *coquilles* lend themselves to this alteration, it is better to use bands of rouleaux or flounces, because despite ironing the stitches (which for rouleaux are in the middle of the band) the creases which they form leave a disagreeable imprint, especially if the material does not wash. Iron or wash the trimmings before using them, and see whether the imprint remains, and if it shows on the right side of the fold.

You may very well make puffed or gathered rouleaux from ruches. It is only a matter of unpicking them, ironing them, and cutting off or unpicking the edges. For trimmings with very small plaits, or a braid placed on the gown, unpicking would be a very long and perfectly useless task. Since the imprints of these little articles invariably remain, you would still be forced to cut the material. It is better to place a new trimming on top; or better still, if that makes the gown stiff, to cut it off and attach an extension which the trimming will hide.

To repair and renew Woollen and Silk Gowns when you cannot match the Material.

It is much less because gowns are worn than because they are out of fashion, that you are obliged to renew them; therefore, this necessity recurs often. As fashion, in its thousand variations, has a general rule of changing completely, it is nearly always impossible that the same body, or the same trimmings, or the same sleeves may be used. It is necessary to put on others. But it is great good luck if—after much fruitless shopping—you happen upon the precise shade of your merino, levantine, or silk *bourré*, even the most ordinary colours. (I mention these materials because they are the only woollens and silks which I advise you to have dyed. Still, levantine lends itself to the process only imperfectly.) It is therefore proper to act as I shall indicate.

Measure the material required to remake the body, the sleeves, or the trimmings of your gown, according to what needs to be replaced. Allow for more rather than less, in order not to run short. Buy material similar to your gown, of the colour which most closely approaches it. Moreover, provided there is some relation to the colour which you will impart to your gown, an exact match matters little. For example, you could have a green material and a yellow one dyed at the same time if you wanted your gown deep green, because the first two colours are necessary to the composition of the third. If you choose a light colour, be very particular when selecting material, because a shade too different shows through the dyeing, which does not happen when you choose a dark colour, because the different shades are easily lost. (See Div. 4.)

Your matching completed according to these principles, have the old gown and the new material dyed at the same time. Then make up your gown, which will appear completely new. This process may be repeated several times on the same garment.

To renew Faded or Half-worn Calico Gowns.

Suppose (as often happens) that you have several calico gowns with bodies and sleeves which have changed colour, or with worn skirt fronts, or which no longer serve because the caprices of fashion have rendered their style and the design of their materials altogether ridiculous. If you have no children to take advantage of these gowns, they may therefore be wasted. (See Div. 5.) You could, it is true, make petticoats from the bottoms, but calico petticoats are very ugly and very common. And besides, you would also be obliged to put a crossways seam in the front at the top, which would finish off the making of a wretched garment; whereas by following my directions, you may make a very suitable gown.

It does not matter if your calico gowns are of different colours. You may put them together by having all the pieces dyed a tolerably deep colour, such as dark green or dark blue. The difference in designs will not hinder you, because you will put all your calicoes wrong side out. The designs do not ordinarily penetrate to that side, or show so little that they are lost in the new colour, even when it is very light.

That understood, set about cutting out a good gown from your bad ones. First save the back breadth and the adjoining gores from the best gown, for the new one. Cut the front breadth from the back breadth of another gown, arranging things so that the slit at the top of the old back merges with the bias which you put at the top of the new front breadth. It suffices to lay, by way of a model, the front breadth of some other gown over this back breadth, and cut accordingly.

Cut out the two sleeves from the bottoms of the front breadths; ordinarily the top is worn while the bottom is good. If you like, cut out the body from the fronts instead, and cut out the sleeves from the remaining back breadth. The latter is preferable because the back breadth is always the best piece. You will easily find the trimmings in the gores and left-over pieces, even though you put all the bad ones aside.

Give the gown to the dyer before making it up. But if you prefer, you may sew it beforehand, or at least make up the skirt. This will avoid crumpling the glaze in sewing, and preserve the edges of the breadths from the holes which are made when stretching them out; but the calendering will be a little less smooth. However, this disadvantage is so small a thing that, if you have a good and fashionable calico gown, but you have found that the colour is not very fast and it has faded in washing, you may give it to a dyer made and trimmed.

To discharge the Colours from Faded Calicoes and Printed Toiles.

Some materials have only a fugitive colour, such as all the dyed calicoes called percalines, or most light blue calicoes whose colour is produced by indigo. When the gowns composed of them are faded or partly worn, you may have them bleached to be used like white calicoes; that is to make petticoats, night jackets, *serre-têtes*, &c. It suffices to soak these materials in water mixed with bleach, then soap them thoroughly.

Often the bleach is superfluous, and two or three soapings remove the colour perfectly without leaving any disagreeable stain on the material. Ordinarily, at first, the colour is weakened in one place, faded in others, and even remains in some places. But that should not disturb you; the final result will be the same. As I have said, you may hasten the process with bleach.

To repair and renew Furs.

If moths have previously gnawed on your tippets, or some mishap has worn the hair, mend it in the following manner. (Chapter IX explains how to store furs properly.)

To mend Furs. Furs are prepared with a narrow strip, at the most three lines wide, and sewed with long over-cast stitches on both edges with a light yellow, blue, or white *faveur*. The colour does not matter, since it is hidden by the hairs close to it. This inspection tells you what you must do. Unpick the strip where the pelt is eaten, and substitute a new pelt, which you sew lengthways like the first, and crossways with several stitches on the two ends which are left after you have cut to put the new pelt in. The repair will be complete and quite invisible.

Fur tippets and pelerines are lined with rose or white taffety (the latter is more elegant). Consequently the lining easily becomes worn looking and must be frequently renewed. This is easy to do, but very expensive when done by furriers; double reason for doing it yourself.

First take out the soiled lining, and cut a new one by it. Lay the new lining on the wadding with which your tippet is furnished, and baste it on one side after having marked a wide seam fold. Freeze it (see Chapter XV for directions), then baste the other side, after having also made a wide seam fold there.

Then sew all round the tippet with side-stitches, covering the ends of the riband strips well, and the wadding as well as the wool which makes up the under side. This kind of hem being finished, sew a line of small running stitches about an inch from the edge. (You may dispense with this if you wish.) This shapes the hem, and above all prevents the wadding from forming a lump on the edge. It is superfluous to say that it is proper to spread the tippet on a table to freeze it, baste it, and even to sew the running stitches. When the lining has faded on the right side, you may turn it to the wrong side, after having ironed it; it is necessary that it not be too soiled.

To change the Style of Furs. The explanation which I gave for the mode of repairing them takes care of this. Indeed, you sew furs just as you mend them; it is easy work, though meticulous. This is perhaps the greatest economy of all.

Suppose that you would like to make a tippet from wide bands of fur. Spread the tippet pattern on a table, then place a band of fur on the pattern, in such a manner that the pelt touches the paper. Because the pattern will be rounded, you must sacrifice some of the riband strips; that is, cut that part slanting, and sew it to the next strip with several stitches. That is almost never done because each pelt must be between two ribands, but this is an exception. Continue thus to cut along the pattern, and end with a riband strip. When you want to narrow a trimming or a tippet, never cut; lay down the riband at the part you mean to alter. Always put down the hairs in the same direction, preserving the natural pattern of the furs.

The Modes of renewing Shoes.

The silk braid which binds women's shoes comes apart long before the shoes are worn out, above all at the back of the heel, and this gives you an air of untidiness. Besides, since the braid supports and holds together the material of the shoe, its lining, and the drawing-string which tightens it, the consequence is an unbound shoe which soon loses its shape. A woman should prevent this misfortune, and I shall furnish you the means. (Chapter IX describes how to replace the inner sole.)

To bind Shoes. It is needless to say that you must bind all shoes with silk, whatsoever their material. When you have to bind black shoes, use the braid made half black and half white for binding, so that the white, placed inside the shoe, protects white stockings from the black streaks which entirely black braid ordinarily produces.

Begin by unpicking all the worn braid round the shoe, and remove all the stitches. (See Fig. 3.) Holding the drawing-string quite firmly, place a new braid *à cheval* over both the edge of the shoe and the string. If the string is too much in the way, first fasten it round the shoe by encompass-ing it with long stitches taken very little into the edge. Commence your work by folding the end of the braid a little, and placing it in the middle of the front of the shoe, at the place where the two ends of the string come together, or where the bow is placed. Back-stitch the braid *à cheval* only up to the hollowed part of the front; as soon as you round the corner where the band at the side begins, work with running stitches.

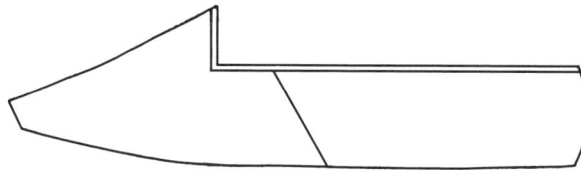

Figure 3. A shoe, with the binding represented.

The hardness of the shoe, and the necessity of making the binding firm and quite flat, require a little variation in the manner of making run-ning stitches. You enter the needle perpendicularly on the outside of the shoe and bring it through on the inside; then enter it on the inside, and bring it through on the outside, and so on. Take the stitches close togeth-er, and tighten them well.

When you reach the back of the heel, you will notice that the lining is not overlapped by the binding there, unlike other parts, but is turned down over the braid with small side-stitches, at the level of the rest of the seam which fastens the braid all round the shoe. Imitate this method, leaving that part of the lining separate, and continue to bind until you have returned to the place where you began. Then turn the lining down, allowing it to exceed the folded braid a little, so that the stitches do not pierce the right side.

To re-cover Shoes. In shoes made of material, the upper may be completely worn, when the sole and lining are still quite new. Silk shoes, above all dancing shoes, become soiled or torn in a single wearing, and in that case shoes become a very heavy expense. But skill and economy cannot fail to compensate.

When shoes of material (let us suppose it to be satin) are entirely soiled, and you think of re-covering them, commence by taking off the binding. Unpick the side seams, and allow the band to fall along the sole (see Fig. 3 again). Then, about a finger from the sole, cut off only the up-per material from the band, because you must be very careful not to cut the lining. Cut the top of the shoe in the same manner. That done, lay the cut-off pieces, which serve as a pattern, over the material with which you plan to re-cover your shoes. Place them so that the selvage is crossways to the top of the shoe. Cut along those pieces, leaving two good fingers more width to the band, and to the front parts which must be attached to the sole, in order to replace what you removed from those pieces in cutting them away from the shoe, and also to make a seam fold.

This preparation finished, pin the middle of the band, to the middle of the back of the heel. Then laying the band wrong side out round the shoe, so that it falls like a trimming over the sole, which it greatly overlaps, sew it to the lining over the finger's width of satin which you left previously, and as close as possible to the sole.

It is well to push the point of your scissors into the narrow groove at the edge of the band which is formed by the join of the sole and the finger's width of satin. Then try to sew as close as possible to the join. You must have a stout needle threaded with doubled thick thread, and take your stitches very close and very tight as indicated for binding shoes. When you come to the heel, try to follow the curve closely. You will do well to lift the band occasionally to see that you do not spread the groove.

The upper of the shoe is a little more difficult to place. Begin by sewing the end, placing the satin for the upper as you placed the band. Pay close attention so that you do not pucker the toe; to judge this lift the satin over the lining now and then, and pass your hand underneath to simulate the shoe being worn. Extend the seam to the right and left of the toe, to about the middle of the upper. Then rolling the extremity of the sole into a tight spiral, turn your work so that the satin upper is laid over the lining. You will perceive that the sole may be turned over in this way only up to a certain point, so it is proper not to sew it too much on the wrong side. Even so, you must sew it that way as far as you can, because then, to finish re-covering the upper, you must sew on the right side in the groove of the sole; also because, since the space where the needle comes out is very tight, you may pull it only with the tips of your fingers and with great effort. Happily this task is short. The shoe thus re-covered, baste the top of the upper onto the lining round the opening, matching the seams which join the band to the front of the shoe; finish by binding. A little practice will render this operation easy, but it always requires much patience and care.

——Manual d'économie domestique, Manuel des dames,
Manuel des demoiselles.

Diversion 1.

Kitchen Aprons. These are made with a toile of seven eighths. Take a dozen ells for a dozen aprons. Cut off one ell, which you then cut into a dozen pieces for the pockets. Divide the remaining eleven ells into twelve pieces. Hem them, then make them up by plaiting them onto a linen tape, the ends of which will be tied round your belt. Sew the pockets in the middle.

——Dictionnaire technologique.

Diversion 2.

A Carriage Dress consisting of a Petticoat and a Canezou-spencer. September 1829: Fig. 4 shows a petticoat of celestial blue *gros de Naples,* with a broad hem round the border, headed by two very narrow rouleaux. The canezou-spencer is of white jaconet muslin; the body is full, and the sleeves are *à l'imbecile,* with double frill mancherons. The bonnet is of white watered *gros de Naples,* ornamented under the brim by points of celestial blue satin. Two ostrich feathers, turning back over the crown, after being fixed at its base, adorn this tasteful and becoming bonnet; this plumage is white, slightly tinged with blue. The strings float loose, and the bonnet is confined under the chin by a narrower riband.

——Ladies' Pocket Magazine.

Diversion 3.

A Walking Gown with the Body covered by a Canezou-spencer. August 1827: Fig. 5 shows a gown of fawn-coloured muslin,

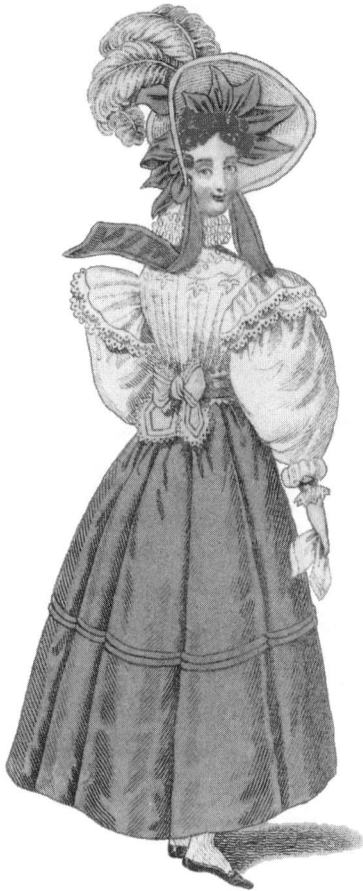

Figure 4. Carriage dress.   Figure 5. Walking dress.

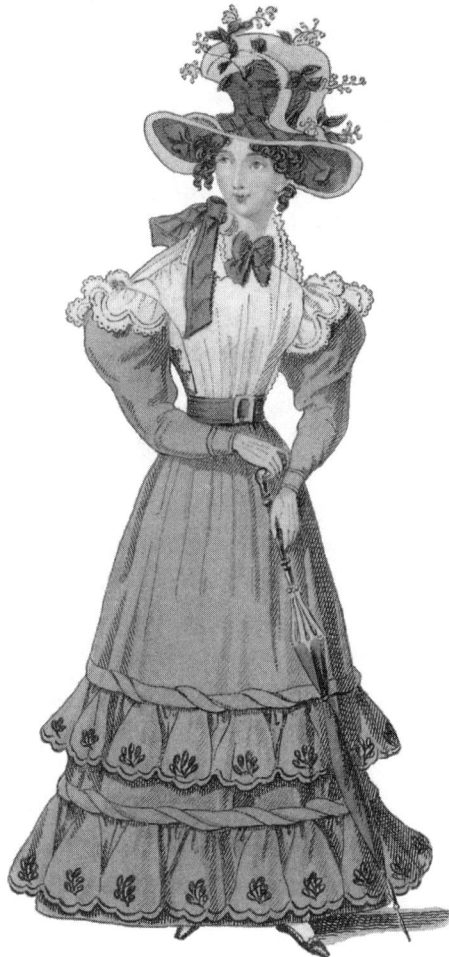

with two flounces embroidered at the edges with black, and headed by full *cordon-rouleaux*. The sleeves are *en gigot*, and the canezou-spencer is of muslin trimmed with lace, confined round the waist by a belt of spring green, fastened with a square silver buckle. The hat is of chequered green silk, ornamented with Portugal laurel and white sarcenet. The parasol is spring green.

——*Ladies' Pocket Magazine.*

Diversion 4.

Directions for changing the Colours of Garments, &c. already dyed. Upon this and other proceedings in the art, precise rules cannot well be given, as the change of colour depends upon the ingredients with which the garments have been dyed. Sometimes when these have been well cleansed, more dyeing stuff must be added, which will afford the colour intended; and sometimes the colour already on the material must be discharged and the article re-dyed. (See Fig. 6.)

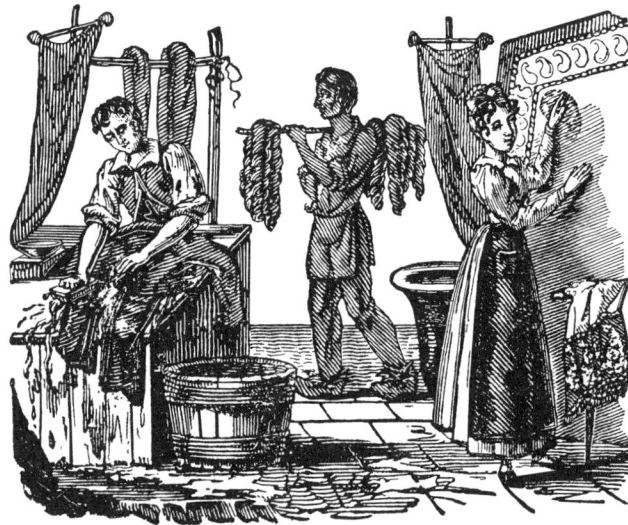

Figure 6. The workshop of the dyer and scourer.

Every colour in Nature will dye black, whether blue, yellow, red, or brown, and black will always dye black again. All colours will take the same colour again which they already possess. Blue may be made green or black; green may be made brown, and brown green, and every colour will take a darker than it at first has. Yellows, browns, and blues are not easily discharged; maroons, reds of some kinds, olives, &c. may be discharged.

For maroons, a small quantity of rock alum may be boiled in a copper. When it is dissolved, put in your goods, keep them boiling, and probably, in a few minutes enough of it will be discharged to take the colour intended. Olives, grays, &c. are discharged by putting in two or three table-spoonfuls, more or less, of oil of vitriol; then put in your garment, &c. and boil, and it will become white. If the colour is chemic green, either alum, pearl ash, or soap will discharge it off to yellow; this yellow may be boiled off with soap, if it has received a preparation for taking the chemic blue.

Muriatic acid used at a hand heat will discharge most colours. Black may be dyed maroon; claret, green or a dark brown. It often happens that black is dyed claret, green, or dark brown; but green is the principal colour into which black is changed.

For a Black Silk Gown. When your copper boils, put in half a pound of alder bark, and a gall or two, bruised. Boil (or simmer) your silks in this for an hour. Then take them out and cool them well, by hanging them up in the air. In the interim, add a piece of green copperas as big as a small horse-bean. When this is dissolved, cool down your copper by adding cold water. Put in your goods, keeping your copper on the spring for half an hour, all the while handling your goods over with a stick: this is what is called bodying, stuffing, or preparing the silks to receive the black dye. Then draw them out again, and cool them and wash them. In the interim, add to your copper six ounces of fustic, half a pound of logwood, and a quarter of a pound of alder bark. (You may add a little more fustic, or rather less logwood, than this receipt specifies.) Put in your goods, and simmer them for an hour. After handling them well, draw them out, and add half an ounce of green copperas, and two ounces of logwood. Put in your goods again, and simmer for two hours.

If the liquor in the copper, on the goods being taken out, does not appear jet-black, more green copperas must be added, and boiled half an hour, taking care not to boil the liquor with too much copperas. If the silks are to be blue-black, a little more logwood, and a small lump of blue vitriol should be added, and the silk may remain in the copper all night, if the copper is not wanted. Next morning, wash and dry.

Should the silks appear rusty, or what is known to the dyers by the name of burnt copper, or foxy, it is customary to pass them through warm water into which about half a tea-spoonful, or less, of oil of vitriol has been thrown. This will leave the silk a beautiful raven black. If the silk is a soft and thick one, you may make a thin soap lather, and pass it through; but this must not be done when it has been passed through vitriol. If care is taken to boil the silk in this process, without any of these alternatives, it will be a most beautiful black, and wear a long while. The oftener the silks are taken out and cooled, the blacker they become.

Observe bullock's gall and hot water are preferred; but the silk must be cooled from the dye-liquors before it is rinsed in gall water, that the dye may be consolidated.

——*The Family Dyer and Scourer.*

Diversion 5.

To make Good Children's Frocks from Partly-worn Gowns.

It is very disagreeable to a thrifty woman to leave off a gown which is three-quarters good, or to sell it for next to nothing. But with a little cleverness you may make very good use of it to clothe your child. Here is how to proceed:

Unpick all the seams of the gown, or rather cut them very close to the edge. Since you need to remove the narrow parts along the seams, which are good for nothing, it is useless to waste time unpicking them. Fold all the separate pieces in quarters, then successively spread them on a table. Place a child's frock, to serve as a pattern, over these spread-out pieces, and cut the small breadths of the frock from the large breadths of your gown. The worn part of the material in the front will remain amongst the surplus pieces. From the others, cut out the sleeves and the body for the child, from the surplus of the gores and the back. It is well, before cutting any thing, to lay the patterns of all the pieces for the body over the material which remains, in order to advantageously arrange all the curves which the pattern produces. It remains only to sew the frock. Very likely you will still have pieces left over.

——*Manuel d'économie domestique.*

Chapter XVII.
The Art of Knitting.

For knitting it is necessary to have silken, woollen, linen, or cotton yarn which is even and not much twisted; it must be wound off. You will need at least two steel needles; these are narrow rods, pointed at both ends, and about five inches long. To begin knitting, whatsoever the article, cast the yarn onto one or two knitting needles. For this, take the needle in your right hand, pull the single or double yarn with your left, and cast on slip-knots (see Div. 1) in the following manner. (There are several other ways to commence knitting, but this one seems sufficient to me.)

Take the yarn between your left thumb and forefinger, allowing a long end to fall over your forefinger. Wind this end round the backs of your forefinger and the two next fingers. Bring it back under your thumb, where you retain it while opening the fingers wrapped in the loop which you have thus formed. A long end must remain beyond the loop. Pass a knitting needle under this end with your right hand. Then, laying the needle over the loop between your forefinger and middle finger, pass it under the other portion of the loop, which goes from your third finger to your thumb, and is found parallel to the portion between your forefinger and middle finger when the needle is put over it. Release the loop, first removing your third and fourth fingers, then your forefinger; and the slip-knot is formed on the needle. Continue thus until you have obtained a sufficient number of stitches, each slip-knot becoming a stitch. The needle which holds all the stitches is called the stitch (or first) needle, and the needle which will pick them up is called the knitting (or second) needle.

The Mode of knitting Common Stitches.

The slip-knots made, take in your left hand the needle which you have been holding in your right hand, and turn it so that the side of the ball of yarn (opposite to that of the end), which was turned towards the left, is now found on the right. Take the knitting needle between your right thumb and forefinger. Pass the point simply under the stitch needle; and guiding it with your right forefinger, put the first slip-knot onto the second needle, holding it with your right forefinger. Thus taking a stitch without working it, is called slipping the stitch.

The first stitch taken, pass the yarn over your right forefinger under your middle finger, and pass it again over the third finger of the same hand. At the same time, pass the knitting needle as previously; but when the knitting needle is crossed under the stitch needle, instead of pushing that stitch, pass the yarn between the fork which the two needles form, and from behind the knitting needle, that is from the side opposite to you. The yarn passed, your left forefinger guides the top of the knitting needle. Your right thumb brings it from underneath the other needle, and puts it back above. Then in its turn your right forefinger, guiding the stitch needle, brings it out of the stitch, which is then found on the knitting needle.

Slip the first stitch of each row of flat knitting, and turn over the work at each row from left to right. This is how to knit garters, which are narrow strips on which people ordinarily learn to knit.

The stitches all have the same face when you knit in the round. But flat knitting with two needles produces two kinds of stitches, those worked on the right side and those worked on the wrong side. To knit a side where the stitches all look the same, put the yarn in front of the knitting needle, instead of passing it to the back as described earlier. Pass this needle over the other; wrap the yarn round it, and guiding it with your left thumb, pass it under the stitch needle with your right thumb. Guide this needle with your right forefinger, and bring it out of the stitch then passed over the knitting needle. This is called purl-stitching.

By turning the stitch, taking it thus on the needle and pulling the yarn through as usual, you obtain a turn-stitch, which produces a plain stitch in relief on the right side. (See Div. 2.) In plain knitting, the turn-stitch is used to mark the seam line of a stocking, that is the middle of the back of the leg where commercially-made stockings have a seam. Ordinarily the seam line is where you begin to make narrowing and widening stitches, which I shall discuss in their proper place. Sometimes the seam line is purl-stitched down the entire length of the stocking; sometimes a round with a purl-stitch is alternated with a round with a plain stitch. Turn-stitches are also used to form the corners of heels, and welts.

The Mode of knitting Stockings.

I shall commence by describing how to use, in one stocking, the plain stitch, the purl-stitch, and the turn-stitch. Take a set of knitting needles, that is to say, a small packet of five needles of the same length.

The needles called English are preferred, being longer and more polished. (See Div. 3.) Make slip-knots over four of the needles; arrange twenty-six to forty on each needle, according to the width of the stocking you wish to knit, and the fineness of the linen or cotton which you use. The number of slip-knots or first stitches completed, pass the fourth needle into the first slip-knot of the first needle, going from right to left. Then knit a narrow border following any model soever; be it four plain stitches and four purl-stitches; be it three rounds of two purl-stitches and two plain stitches, and three other rounds worked in the same way, of which the purl-stitches are taken into the plain stitches of the three previous rounds, and the plain stitches into the purl-stitches; or be it four purl-stitches and one or two turn-stitches. Border designs vary in a thousand ways. When you wish to knit a stocking with welts, continue all along the stocking this mixture of four, three, or two purl-stitches and two plain stitches. (See Div. 4.)

When the needle holds almost no stitches, for the greater part have been passed onto the other needle, use the fifth needle to knit the last few stitches, and place the empty needle over it. This prevents the stocking from having little stripes at the four corners, where you pick up the stitches on the end of each needle. The fifth needle ordinarily picks up the last six or seven stitches.

The stocking is continued quite straight down to the calf. The rows which compose it are called rounds, and two rounds make a seam-stitch. When you come to the calf, think of decreasing the number of stitches. This is done by narrowings; that is, you pick up two stitches at once with the same needle, and pass the yarn through. Use the back needles (those between which the seam is found, and with which the heel is knitted). It is near the seam that the decrease takes place, but so that one or two stitches come between on each side, and so the narrowings are not drawn close together. When the stocking must have a stout calf, decrease by eight to ten stitches in ten or fifteen rounds. After a round where you have decreased, knit a round without decreasing, and so on until you have finished the narrowings, which you ordinarily determine following a stocking similar to the one which you are knitting.

When the calf of a stocking is to be very stout, begin to increase the number of stitches from the back of the knee, making widenings near the seam line from one round to another. The widenings are made thus: separate two stitches from each other. With the needle, raise the yarn which is underneath, crossing between these two stitches (this is called a bar). Draw the yarn from the ball through this bar, making only one stitch there with the knitting needle, and you will have a new stitch.

There are additional modes of widening and narrowing. A second mode of widening is to divide the stitch. The cotton or linen being flat, you separate the strands, and make a new stitch in each half. This mode is not very sturdy, because the new stitch is supported by only a few strands. A better mode of narrowing than that described above is: at the place in the knitting where you wish to narrow, slip a stitch, that is take it from one needle to the other without passing the yarn through it. Work the next stitch; then enter the stitch needle into the slipped stitch. Pass this again over the tip of the knitting needle and off (which is called skipping the stitch); and as it comes off the two needles, the first one and the next one, you have only one stitch, which pulls in the stocking.

When the stocking is knitted down to the heel, it is divided into two portions: that of the front is found on two needles which are no longer worked. It is necessary to secure these needles by threading their ends into the stocking on each side and crossing them. The heel is continued with the other two needles. As this knitting, which is no longer in the round, produces two kinds of stitches, those on the right side and those on the wrong side, work a row of purl-stitches every time it is necessary to knit to the left. In this way all the stitches appear to be plain. Always slip the first purl-stitch.

In order that the heel may assume the necessary roundness, as soon as it is of a proper length, consider how to shape it. Ordinarily the heel has twenty to thirty seam-stitches, for the seam line continues to be worked to the middle of the heel. To turn the heel, make successive narrowings on each side, whose number is proportioned according to the back portion of the stocking. The stitches which remain after these narrowings (which always start from the seam line and describe a quarter of a circle on each side from that point) are ordinarily a third less numerous than in beginning the heel. This operation finished, take the knitting needle (for the heel thus decreased is all held on the other needle) and on the wrong side, on the right along the edge of the heel, pick up the stitches of the edge formed by the series of rows.

Here is how to accomplish this: enter the needle into every stitch immediately after those of the selvage, and passing the cotton over the needle, bring it out underneath the stitch, which produces a new one above a narrow ridge like that of a turn-stitch. Pick up the other side of the heel in the same way with the fifth needle, which was not used for any of the heel. Then knit with the two front needles, making small narrowings on every other round, on the sides, on the right side where the heel joins the front. (It is necessary to narrow by skipping stitches, because they make a small slanting line like a neat seam.) After about twenty rows, return to knitting in the round pretty much as you began. But now the stocking is much less wide, since it only needs to go round the foot. You no longer work seam-stitches after turning the heel.

When the foot has been knitted to the proper length (it will be necessary to measure by a model stocking), begin to narrow the two sides first. Before long, knit a round narrowing every eight stitches, then seven rounds without narrowing, then a round narrowing every seven stitches, then five rounds without narrowing, another round narrowing every five stitches, and so on. Finally, when you have narrowed every stitch, you will still narrow until there are no more than five stitches. Draw them together by narrowing and skipping stitches until only one is left. Break the yarn, pass it through the last stitch, pull it firmly, and the stocking is finished.

Stockings with lengthways welts are knitted in precisely the same manner, but they appear narrower. This is called elastic knitting, for these stockings, which look so narrow, stretch more than the others. This comes about because the yarn is not so tight as in plain knitting, and it zig-zags alternately inside and outside. You may more easily comprehend this by seeing how a stocking turned inside out stretches more than if right side out, because the stitches, like drawing-strings, tighten in that direction.

Stockings may be knitted with round welts, or with coloured corners, or without purling, or spotted. But since all these fashions are long forgotten, I shall pass over these modes in silence.

Additional Remarks.

You will rarely need to join on fresh yarn, because it does not break, or very seldom, and because a ball of yarn lasts for a long time. However, when the time comes for adding on, cross the two ends over each other, and knit with both ends. When you wish to add a strand of yarn to re-enforce the heel or the toe of a stocking, have this strand on a new ball. Then knit with both balls of yarn until you simply break the strand to remove it.

When entering, bringing out, and re-entering the needles, never let the cotton become loose on top of your right forefinger. At first this seems awkward to beginners, but it soon aids them; the knitting is more even and more rapidly done. Pull the cotton equally tight on every stitch, and pay attention to picking up all the strands of the stitch in order not to make half-stitches; that is, stitches supported by one or two strands, so that they tear when you put on the stocking.

When the knitting is full of half-stitches two or three rounds below the one which you are knitting, it is necessary to pull out the stitches which succeed it, drawing them through from bar to bar, down to the half-stitch. Spread all the bars with the needles, and try to catch the half-stitch with a needle passed through it. Collect the omitted strands which are on the wrong side, and restore each stitch from the top, passing the stitch over each bar and pulling the bar through it. Here is the mode:

Take the dropped stitch on the needle placed to the left. Lift the bar with the right needle which, passing under the bar, brings it onto the left needle, above the stitch. Then the right needle, leaving the bar, passes through each stitch as for purl-stitching, and passes this stitch behind the left needle which, guided at the same time by your right forefinger, releases the bar which is pulled through the stitch. This returns to each stitch the bar made on each round. Then bring the neighbouring stitches together with the point of the needle. A dropped stitch is raised in the same way. When two stitches are dropped at the same time it is more trouble, because the bars must skip over each stitch one after another; and because these bars, too loose on the first stitch, are nearly always too tight on the second. The stitch closest to the right is picked up first.

When tidy knitters put down their knitting, they pass the needle which remains free through it, as if they were taking running stitches. They spread out the stitches on the other needle, bring these needles close together, put them level, and bind them together by winding a little cotton on. Then they push them into their *affiquets,* narrow cases of ivory or bone, of which one end is conical and closed, and the other open and conically hollowed. A little before this end is a small round hole through which a cord is passed, which serves to hold the *affiquets* together and to spread them apart according to the length of the needles. These knitters then tie the cord of the *affiquets,* wind the cotton onto the ball, place it near the *affiquets,* and neatly roll their work over all this. They finish by fastening it with a pin. Very often, when they knit they fasten one of the *affiquets* to their belt on the left, and put the end of the stitch needle inside. This renders the knitting even; but unless you are accustomed to it, it is extremely awkward.

The Mode of knitting Slippers.

Slippers are begun with two stitches, which are immediately increased. Make these stitches into a round, and increase them again. Then knit a round without widening, then on the next increase every other stitch. After two rounds, increase each pair of stitches to three, and so on, putting after the rounds (whose number increases each time from one up to ten) as many stitches between widenings as you have knitted rounds. You will perceive that this is the toe of a stocking in the opposite direction, since you narrow to finish a stocking, in the same way in which you widen to begin a slipper.

You may also begin a slipper by working a seam line for each half of the stitches, and increasing on each side of the seam line with each round, so that there are four increases for every round. Continue thus until the slipper is wide enough, then make decreases instead of increases; stockings are finished in this fashion. The seam line may be omitted.

When the slipper is wide enough, knit the rounds simply to about an eighth of an ell, more or less, according to the size of your model slipper. After that, leave all your stitches except ten or twelve at the most, if your linen, wool, or cotton is fine, and knit these stitches only, making a narrowing on each side until the last stitch. As the knitting is no longer in the round, knit as for the heel of a stocking. This is called the strap of the slipper (see Div. 5).

After you have fastened it off by passing and looping the cotton through the last stitch, take up the other stitches, to the right and left of the strap, and knit them back and forth in plain and purl rows, because the knitting ceases to be in the round. When you have thus knitted about the length of an eighth of an ell, make a narrowing at the middle of the stitches. Then leaving the middle of the stitches aside, knit the others separately with two needles, like a heel, narrowing every round, but only on the side of the first narrowing; that is, the side where you have divided your stitches.

Work thus until no more than twenty to twenty-five stitches remain; or to say it better, the number which will make a sixteenth of an ell, because the thickness of the wool or the cotton greatly affects this number. Supposing that twenty stitches must remain, leave them on one needle, then knit the other half of the stitches in the same way; which will give you, as for the other stitches, a band narrowed only at the side of the division of the stitches. At each row, pick up a stitch from the narrowed side of the first band, and knit it with this row.

This operation, which joins the two narrowed sides, will form the heel. When no more than twenty stitches remain, as for the first knitting, turn the heel inside out and also the two pieces with twenty stitches. Join these twenty stitches by taking one into the other, and bind them off with chain-stitches. At the last loop of these, pass the cotton through the loop, knot it, break it, and the slipper is finished. The second slipper is knitted in exactly the same manner.

Some knitters, to save trouble, bind off the first twenty stitches immediately, and then knit the second part of the heel without picking up the stitches on the side of the first. They bind off the twenty stitches of this piece, and then work a seam all along both pieces, either with chain-stitches or with a bodkin. (See the article on petticoats.) It makes little difference; however, the first mode is preferable.

The Mode of knitting Gloves.

Commence your glove like a stocking, by measuring it on a model glove to determine the number of stitches which you must make. Work three rounds of purl-stitches to prevent it from curling up. Then knit uniform rounds without seam-stitches to the base of the thumb; from the edge to here you want to knit about twenty rounds. After the first ten, narrow every round, about every eighteen or twenty stitches; two narrowings in each round, one of them on each side of the glove.

The thumb which you must begin is then knitted at the same time as the rest. First make a series of widenings during the last ten rounds, in the middle of the glove. The first two widenings are separated by four stitches, the next two by eight, and so on until the end of ten rounds. To accommodate the bending of this finger, knit a little gore with these widenings, like a little heel. Next knit the thumb like a little stocking, and then knit with purl-stitches a small seam round the gore and the base of the thumb. This seam is similar to the seam which picks up the stitches on the side of a stocking-heel.

Here is the gore: with the first round work one purl-stitch, then a stitch in between, and make the next one a purl-stitch. On the second round, likewise work one purl-stitch, followed by two widenings, then one purl-stitch. Continue in this way until ten stitches have been added, and you come to between the narrow borders made by the purl-stitches. Then the thumb is knitted in the round as above. Independently of the rest of the glove, the stitches at the edge of the glove are picked up, and the thumb is finished like a very small stocking, or by binding off with chain-stitches, which takes up all the stitches and permits knitting the thumb round.

When the gore and the thumb are finished, knit ten or so rounds. Then put the glove on your hand and pass a needle between each finger to mark their places. The forefinger is begun by knitting the stitches divided for it, widening in the middle of the stitches, at the part opposite to the thumb. From this widening, knit a gore of about ten stitches, widening successively, then knit the finger in the round like a little stocking. That finished, pick up the bottom stitches of the gore, and make two widenings at the middle of the stitches marked for the second finger; then two widenings, and knit the other half of the stitches. Continue thus until you have obtained a gore on each side. Then finish this finger like a little stocking.

The other fingers are knitted separately in the same way, only they must have gores on both sides, the little finger excepted. It is needless to say that the last finger will be shorter.

Elastic, or welted gloves are also knitted. The welts are divided such that there are alternately three plain stitches and three purl-stitches. Despite the elasticity of this knitting, a gore is worked at the thumb, but not between the other fingers; several widenings replace them. (I shall discuss mitts, or fingerless gloves with a half-thumb, after the article on open-work knitting.)

The Mode of knitting Petticoats.

The wadded petticoats which were worn formerly are now replaced by knit woollen ones. These are preferable to the first because they conform better to the shape of the body, to which they cling in an elastic manner. This property gives them the advantages of retaining more warmth, and of not thickening the waist as do the wadded petticoats; so they are generally made. At first nothing was so simple; nothing is now so elaborate. I shall describe several fashions, commencing with the easiest.

A petticoat is always composed of two breadths, the back and the front. These breadths are gradually sloped on both sides up to the middle of the length; there is no need for the gores customarily put in petticoats of material. Knit petticoats are besides much narrower, since they have at the most an ell and a half, or even an ell and a third, or five quarters. The breadths are exactly alike. They are each composed of an hundred and twenty, to an hundred and forty stitches, according to the thickness of the wool. The wool must be very smooth and very white, because these petticoats yellow easily. Some persons wind it off and put it in wide loops one over the other when they begin work. The object of this is to prevent the ball of yarn from imperceptibly tightening the stitches by its weight: this precaution indicates that this knitting must be loose.

A petticoat is knitted with particular needles. They are about half an ell long, and the thickness of the shaft of a feather, more or less. Iron, box-wood, and tamarind wood serve to make the needles, which are terminated by a little knob at one end, whereas the other is tapered to a point to go into and out of the stitches. When the needles are of box-wood, ebony, rose-wood, &c., the knob is of ivory or bone. When the needles are of iron or steel, the knob is of painted wood, or even the same metal. The first are preferred because they are less heavy, and the knitting glides over them better. Also, though rarely, knitting needles are made of whale-bone.

Formerly, the bottoms of petticoats were worked with a band of wool coloured green, violet, or orange. This band was composed of ten to fifteen rows according to the thickness of the wool. Sometimes a row or two of differently-coloured wool was put above this band, such as a green border on an orange or violet band. Coloured borders were then replaced by additions (see Div. 6), which gradually have come to make up the entire petticoat.

The first mode of knitting petticoats is to alternate rows of plain and purl-stitches, which are all made to appear like purl-stitches as has been seen. The narrowings are made at the selvages of the breadths; that is, in beginning, when as usual you have slipped the first stitch, skip it over the following stitch when you have worked it. At the end of the needle, on the contrary, you slip the stitch before the last stitch, and pass it over the last.

Work a short slit in the back breadth, in order that you may put on the petticoat more easily. This is all the more necessary because these petticoats have no, or almost no plaits. When it is time to begin the slit, count the stitches which the narrowings have left. Then, taking a third needle, take onto it half the number of these stitches, and knit them up to the top of the petticoat. Bind off by skipping the stitches over each other as I have explained for narrowing; this will produce a chain-stitch. Then take up the other half of the stitches, which you knit up to the top of the piece of knitting which makes up the other half. Bind it off in the same way, and your breadth will thus be properly slit. When you wish to open the petticoat on the side, it is unnecessary to make a slit in the back breadth; but leave the upper part of the breadths unsewed, not beginning the seam which joins them until beyond the measure of the slit.

This brings me to the mode of sewing this seam: the petticoat being finished, place the breadths beside each other over your knee. Pin them to fix the edges together, of whatsoever sort. Then take a bodkin, which you thread with wool, and pass it successively through all the stitches on the sides of your breadths. It is necessary to bring both corresponding stitches together and sew them at the same time; that is better than sewing them one after another.

Since the petticoat is always knitted in the same direction, and you consequently alternate rows of plain stitches with rows of purl-stitches, without appearing to do so, the rows will tighten. The stitches at the edge will appear to be one row apart, because only the rows of purl-stitches produce an edge stitch; but that does not injure the sturdiness of the seam at all. I only make this observation to establish the difference between this seaming and that for petticoats with plain stitches, with welts, or with open-work. This seaming does not have a wrong side.

Petticoats with plain stitches are knitted like the heel of a stocking, that is to say, you knit on the wrong side every time you must work from left to right. These petticoats are otherwise knitted precisely like the preceding ones; the only difference is that you use a much finer wool or cotton, because this kind of stitch stretches much less than the purl-stitch, and the petticoat would be uncomfortably stiff. The seam of these petticoats is worked on the wrong side, picking up the stitches almost like the heel of a stocking; consequently you may work this seam with a knitting needle. The seam resembles the operation which picks up the stitches of the heel, because you pick up stitches from the sides with a single needle, and form a new stitch by only passing the yarn over the needle. But it differs in that you take the last stitch on the side without leaving any edge, picking up a stitch from one breadth immediately after the other, and unite them by passing the cotton through both stitches, which, moreover, forms a stitch with the aid of a single needle. Many persons work these seams with a sewing needle, by over-casting with slanting stitches taken through each knitted stitch on the side.

Welted petticoats are knitted like welted stockings, or like the borders of stockings; but it is well to make the welts wider, because they would tighten too much if they were narrow. These petticoats require even finer cotton than petticoats with plain stitches. They are very rarely made of wool because it is necessary to knit with wool of two strands, which does not last well. As for the dimensions and the seams, these petticoats differ in no way from the preceding ones.

Remaining, therefore, are the open-work petticoats, the stitches for which are described in the article on open-work knitting.

The Mode of knitting Night Jackets.

Night jackets are small waistcoats; therefore I shall dispense with repeating details concerning them. (See Div. 7.) Generally night jackets have a third (not of an ell) less length and breadth than waistcoats. They are often made of white wool with knitting which appears like purl-stitching, but more often still in two other fashions, one more elegant, the other more common. The most elegant fashion is to always knit plain stitches with very fine wool. This is much less warm than purl-stitching; but it thickens the waist less, which is usually a material consideration. You work the sleeves of these night jackets by knitting in the round like a stocking.

The second fashion merely consists of knitting, with coloured thick or middling wool, night jackets which do not have as much length at the bottom in front of the arm-holes, and are consequently a species of jumps (see Div. 8). These are trimmed all round at the bottom and the top with a band of a colour contrasting with that of the night jacket. This same band trims the bottom of the sleeves. Sometimes, when the night jacket is brown, black, amaranth, or grey, it is trimmed in green, orange, or violet. When it is violet, it is most often trimmed with green, red, or brown. Women of the lower orders often wear this kind of winter jacket. I describe them to my readers so that they may make them for charity.

Night jackets are made with neither welts nor open-work.

Of Open-work Knitting.

In order that holes *à jour* may be handsome, it is necessary to choose a very even, well-twisted yarn and tighten the stitches well in knitting them from one needle to another. Instead of one stitch, it is necessary to take two, as for narrowings, and to pass the yarn over the needle in front. When you have knitted a round, put the yarn found beside the subtracted stitch onto the needle, for making a new stitch.

Lengthways holes *à baguette* are worked in the same way, except that on the second round, not only the first yarn, but even the second is not picked up. On the third round, they are picked up at the same time with the needle. After having turned them, make a new stitch, which produces a lengthways hole, or the shape of a stick. You may put intervals of plain stitches, purl-stitches, or turn-stitches between the holes, and combine them to produce stripes, points, diamonds, slanting lines, or leaves. For these it will suffice to use the knitting designs found at a haberdasher's.

To work a hole of the kind called *à crochet*, commence by knitting three purl-stitches. Then when the hole is finished, the first stitch after the three purl-stitches is also worked as a purl-stitch, the yarn is passed over the needle, and the two other stitches are finished as purl-stitches together.

Now we come to knitting *varié,* which is similar to twilled muslin. This knitting lasts a very long time, and is not affected by strain; that is, it does not stretch out like welted or elastic knitting. When a stocking is to be worked in this way, cast twenty to thirty slip-knots onto each needle, according to the kind of yarn, and knit several rounds. After that, the first stitch is a purl-stitch, the second is a plain stitch, the third is like the first, the fourth is the same as the second, and so forth. Where the stocking is knitted in the round, on the second round the first purl-stitch is picked up as a plain stitch, the second stitch, which is plain, is picked up as a purl-stitch, and you continue thus. From this comes knobbed or crossed knitted work (see Div. 9). If your work is a selvage, a narrow strip, &c., where you must knit back and forth as for a heel, it is necessary when knitting on the right side to take back the last stitch on the wrong side, which is in this way already made, and continue thus to the end. In this manner, the stitch comes back to the right side.

Knitting varied with twisted stitches is called corded knitting, because of its raised ribs. It is very durable and stretches little, which makes it suitable for purses. Pass the needle through the inner side or the back of the stitch, and twist it. The yarn is a little loose, so that the twisted stitch may take up more than the other without appearing too tight when the work is finished. In this manner you twist two stitches, one to the side of the other. You may knit the following four plain. These stitches may be mixed with open-work stitches.

Knitting in a spiral, or winding, is done in the same way with twisted stitches. If you wish to knit a stocking in this manner, distribute the stitches as for welted stockings, such that there are thirty-two on each needle. First knit two twisted stitches and six plain, which must be followed by two more twisted and six plain, and so on to the end of the round. On the next round, pick up the first two twisted stitches as plain stitches, make the next two twisted stitches, and so on. In this way, the twisted stitches wind like a serpent round the foot. You may mix them with holes *à baguette* or *à crochet,* and work very pretty borders for petticoats, or even entire petticoats. Corded knitting presents the same opportunities. For petticoats, mitts, and open-work stockings, you may work one corded rib and one hole *à crochet,* alternating them for several rounds.

Mitts.

Mitts are begun at the top like a stocking, and the arm part like a sleeve, to suit the length of the arm (see Div. 7). Having reached the edge of the hand, knit a thumb gore and a half-thumb, then go back to knitting in the round for six to eight rows, and finish off. You may knit mitts entirely with combinations of the open-work stitches described. There is an infinity of others, which are very complicated and very difficult; I omit them because no one still knits open-work mitts, and it would be a useless labour. On that subject you may always consult *l'Art de tricoter,* by Netto and Lehmann. This book, by the way, has furnished me with several receipts, which I cannot vouch for as for my own.

Knit Berets.

These berets have been in existence for scarcely five or six years. They are very warm, sturdy, and made in combinations of colours. They are even pretty when they are of handsome wool, in well-harmonized colours, and neatly knitted. They are made in amaranth and black, blue and black, violet and green, violet and black, or black and yellow. The small points round the crown have a narrow border of the second colour. These berets are sometimes lined with silk material to prevent the wool from wearing away the hair. You may dispense with this step when the beret is for a woman, because women ordinarily wear a cap tied under the chin. This head-dress is very good when you have a cold, or suffer from inflamed tissues.

There are two kinds of berets: those which have points round the border, and those which have open-work instead. The crown is always the same, and is knitted as follows. The beret (see Fig. 1) is begun at the star which is found at the top, and is worked like a gore by means of widenings. Take some fine wool, in the colour chosen for the crown, and cast four stitches onto two needles, precisely as you begin a stocking. Put aside one of the needles, and pick up the four double stitches which were on it, onto four ordinary needles. That done, knit a round; then the yarn is passed over the needle, and the first stitch is finished. Pass the yarn again over the needle, and you finish the second stitch. Repeat this with the three needles. On the following round, the yarns passed over the needle are used and changed in the stitches. To make the star handsomer, on each round knit a hole *à crochet.*

The star is enlarged and continued in this manner, until you judge it large enough. When the beret is small, and knitted in fine wool, it will be sufficiently large if there are twenty stitches on each needle. The narrowings are made thus: after having passed the yarn over the needle as in the beginning, finish the first stitch. Pass the yarn again over the needle, and pull through one of the two following stitches over the other. This operation is repeated for all the stitches, and continued until the points of the star are formed.

After that, knit several rounds with the wool of the other colour, and begin the border, whether it has points or open-work. If the beret is simple, you may knit the border plain, and embellish it in the following manner. Knit the first three stitches plain; then the fourth is a purl-stitch, the fifth is plain, and the sixth is a purl-stitch; then come three plain stitches. This composes the striated welts called *de Valois*. This border is knitted with the same wool as the crown. Then take the other colour, and knit four or five rows of purl-stitches, to produce a kind of hem on the cap; you may put holes *à crochet* there. You may also work twisted stitches beside each other every three or six holes.

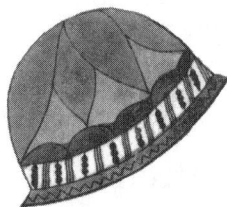

Figure 1. A design for a beret.

As mentioned above, the crown of the beret may be trimmed with small points which are raised above the edge, forming a narrow coronet round the crown. Cast on about a dozen stitches which you knit separately, while the others remain permanently apart. Knit a tab like the strap of a slipper, with the same wool as the crown. Afterwards, using wool of the other colour, pick up all the stitches round the tab, and there work four to six rows of purl-stitches. That done, bind off with chain-stitches as usual, and begin another tab, up to the end. Then pick up all the stitches below the tabs, and continue the border to the height of two or three inches. The border may consist of two rows of purl-stitches, or in the same row, two turn-stitches and two holes *à crochet*. Besides these, you may use the combinations described in the article on open-work knitting.

A Purse knitted like a Pine-apple.

This purse is begun at the round end with four double stitches, with which you work a star similar to the crown of a beret, but much smaller. At the completion of the widenings, there should be only an hundred and twenty-six, to an hundred and thirty stitches. The star is knitted in green silk, and the middle of the purse in orange silk. The star finished, work four to six rounds as follows: a hole *à jour* or *à crochet,* one narrowing, four plain stitches, another narrowing, and a hole *à jour.* Then knit two rows, replacing stitches by narrowings, and the next two rows with a widening and a hole *à jour.* Having thus come to the top of the purse, take up the green silk again, and knit six to eight rounds of ordinary stitches. After this knit a round in which every sixth or eighth stitch has a hole *à crochet* to serve as an eyelet-hole, to admit of the drawing-strings of the purse. Then above this round, with every eight stitches make a little tab, like the strap of a slipper. When you wish to make this purse prettier, when beginning you may also knit little tabs upside down before the star. The tabs finished, narrow without stopping until there are no more than four stitches, to work the small end of the purse. Only five tabs are needed; they take the place of the tassel. When the purse is closed at the top with drawing-strings, it has altogether the air of a pine-apple.

Purses knitted with Designs.

A purse, for which well-twisted silk is ordinarily employed, is begun at the bottom in a point. Take two knitting needles and some double silk, and cast on four stitches. Then put aside one needle, and pick up each of the four stitches onto a single needle. That done, add one or two stitches onto each needle, and this increase continues until the purse has attained a width of five fingers. Next knit two rows of purl-stitches, so that the work may be more durable and not lose its shape. Continue for eight to ten rounds with the holes called *à crochet.*

Next add yarn coloured according to the flowers which you wish to depict, and of which you have a model in front of you. Add this yarn by passing it over two stitches with the previous yarn, as in joining on fresh yarn when it breaks. This yarn remains suspended behind between the flowers. It is used at the beginning of the flowers and in the visible stitches. (The visible stitches are all those in the front, and the invisible ones are those whose yarn passes behind and escapes the eye.)

You are free to use as many as ten yarns of different colours, and to employ them according to the design in the visible stitches. When a yarn is no longer used, it passes into the invisible stitches, provided that it is not meant to reappear later. If it is, the little ball of coloured silk remains suspended outside the purse until the next round. This yarn skips only as much space as is required by the flowers, letters, garlands, or devices.

Purses knitted Double.

Double knitting may be done in two ways. You will need two yarns, one for knitting, the other for adding slip-knots as in knitting plush. (See Div. 10.) When the needle is full, disengage it excepting the last slip-knot; that is, knit the stitches and the knots onto another needle as you did onto the first one. In this way the work takes on a beautiful appearance, because the knots cannot lengthen or shorten.

Double knitting is done yet differently, with two yarns interlaced one beside the other inside the stitches. But you need a well-twisted yarn; and in picking up the stitches, it is necessary, if the knitting is not to have holes, to take the yarns onto the needle every time.

Purses knitted in Gold and Silk, with Spaces.

These purses are begun at the bottom like an ordinary purse, and with four doubled stitches. If these are divided onto four needles, it is necessary to immediately make widenings on each. When you have come to the gold-coloured line which ordinarily marks the design, work a hole between one stitch and the next, into which you may then interlace a little cross of gold strips. This operation is performed all round the purse. As for the width, when using silk of middle thickness, count sixty-eight stitches for half of the purse, or an hundred thirty-six all round. When you have come to the top of the purse, work a slit for placing the clasp. For this, divide the stitches in half and knit one side back and forth as for a heel, the knitting no longer being in the round. Then make the narrowings required by the clasp, until out of sixty-three stitches (see Div. 11), only twenty-four remain, which are easily fastened by passing a yarn through.

The purse finished, turn it inside out, and at the top through the stitches of both sides, pass a yarn with which you again knit a portion half as wide as the purse, which distinguishes this kind of purse on the inside. People sometimes knit on the inside with gold threads.

Sometimes these purses are knitted with gold strips, which must be flexible and ductile in order not to come loose. These are an eighth of an inch wide, or like a straw. You interlace them as little crosses, from the wrong side. To keep them from twisting so often, it is essential to thread them through with sewing needles which have crossways rather than lengthways eyes. Knit two rows with round holes or holes *à crochet;* the strips assume the shape of a double cross as you pass them in. Each cross is then cut, and the end of the strip folded over. Then it is flattened with a paper-knife.

You may also knit into silk purses pieces of fluffy yarn (see Div. 12), which give the purse the appearance of including little pieces of cut velvet. This is done in shading, and the shades are alternated according to the designs which you have chosen. To shade in knitting, collect yarns of different colours, and work only one stitch with them. When one colour must be absent in a stitch, or in beginning a motif, you must use, for example, a pink and a black yarn, in forming one stitch. Hold them carefully over your fingers as you must pass to the right or the left in the stitch. Flowers are thus shaded very pleasingly.

Beaded Purses.

These purses, which are now in such favour, are as easy as they are pretty. Sometimes they are worked in tapestry-stitch, sometimes by knitting. For either fashion, commence by separating, in a box with compartments, the differently-coloured beads which you will employ following the design you have chosen. (You may find designs entirely made and coloured at a haberdasher's. See Fig. 2, for which the ground should be white, the large leaves and the bottom blue, and the sprigs and narrow lines gold-coloured.) Place the design in front of you, and proceed as follows to knit your purse.

Take a ball of round white silk, and thread the end through a needle slender enough to easily pass through the beads. In the design, count the little squares which are at the very top of the purse; each square indicates one bead and one stitch. These squares are ordinarily white, and are meant for the white beads of which the ground is composed. For each square, thread one bead onto the silk. Note that the design shows only half the purse, so you must double it. Where the design begins to extend over the ground, the differently-coloured squares indicate the colours of the beads which you should thread on. Be careful to thread them in order and not to confound the colours of the squares, because you would find it a hindrance when knitting. Proceed thus to the end, counting all the squares in each row, and successively making rows of beads to correspond.

When you have threaded a certain quantity of beads onto the silk, slide them along to make room for more. Your ball will thus be unwound in the same measure; and for fear of tangling the silk, make it into large loops which you place gradually one over another. The end of the first must be empty, to begin the purse. When you come to the end of the design, do not slip on the beads up to the end of the ball of silk; or if much silk remains, only cut it after leaving a very long end without any beads on it: this end is meant to finish the purse and to knit the first row. Then wind

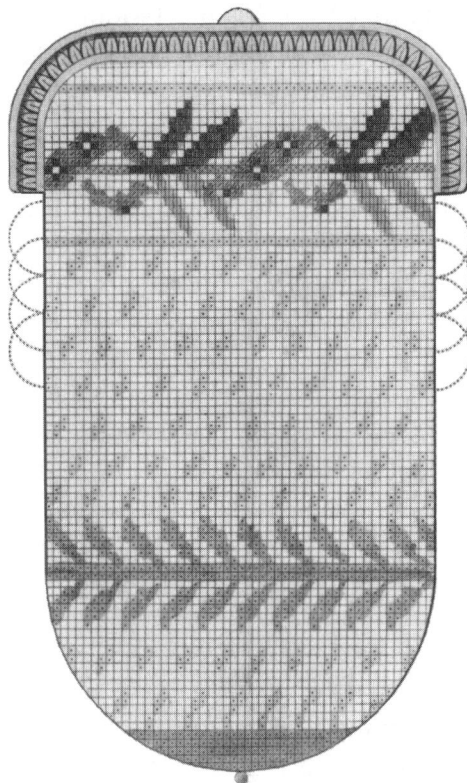

Figure 2. A design for a beaded purse.

up all the silk thus threaded with beads, beginning at the empty end. Slowly and carefully lift the large loops which you made as you wound off the silk.

When you have wound it all up again, take a set of very fine knitting needles, and begin the purse at the small end, counting the number of stitches, and widening as you advance. The knitting does not differ from ordinary knitting in the least. You have only to make sure to bring out the bead on top, in passing the silk over the needle before picking up the stitch, and to look at the design now and then to see if you are copying it properly. If you put a clasp on the purse, you must work a short slit on each side at the top.

Ordinarily no tassels are placed on beaded purses, but instead a little beaded fringe of two or three rows. First baste the finished purse lightly all round (excepting the top) onto a piece of paper cut into notches of middle size. Thread a needle with white silk. Enter it on the left side, at the top of the purse or at the end of the slit. Next thread beads all along the silk, and then raise it at each notch by a slight stitch of silk taken with another needle inside the purse: this produces pretty loops of beads. For a second row, remove the notched paper, which has become useless. Make the loops a little shorter than the previous ones, and catch them a little above the first row, so that the point of each loop is in the middle of the previous loop. A third row presents the same contrast to the second.

The colours of these fringes are mingled in all manner of ways. The prettiest is: first row, loops of white beads; second, the prevailing colour of the purse; and the third white. These purses are washed like toile.

When you wish to work a beaded purse in tapestry-stitch, cut out a piece of fine toile by the model of your purse. Count the little squares in the design; then according to each square, place a bead when working a tapestry-stitch. The purse made, join it on the wrong side with a seam of close back-stitches, and trim it as described for knit purses with beads. If the design is round, you must begin the purse at the flower in the middle.

To line Bags and Purses.

Your bag having been beaded, it is necessary to line it with white taffety. Fold the bag in half so that the embroidery touches; that is, with the right sides together. Fold the lining (which you have cut by your bag) with the wrong sides together. Place the bag over the lining and baste them together from the side of the bag, in order to see by the wrong side of the embroidery if you are basting precisely on the edge of the beads. Then sew the bag and the lining together with an unbroken series of back-stitches, excepting the top. Pay close attention to catching all four pieces (the two pieces of the bag and those of the lining) at the same time.

The seam finished, enter your left hand between the bag and the lining, and with your right hand, turn the bag so that the right sides of both materials are visible. This surrounds the entire bag with the lining, and you avoid making a flat seam or passing a thread, because the seam is between the bag and the lining.

All bags are lined thus, whatsoever their material and shape. Purses are also sometimes lined by this mode; however, their small size and their ornaments often prevent it. In that case, pass one side of the lining over the other side of the purse to surround it in a circle. A flat seam joins the two sides of the lining.

Purses knitted on a Mould.

Knitting on a mould can work not only purses, but serve for every other article, like ordinary knitting. For this it is necessary to hold the knitting firmly on a box-wood mould rounded only at the top, and furnished with closely-spaced spikes or teeth to hold the stitches. (Some persons call this a Turkish mould.) You then work with a hook similar to a tambour-needle. (See Div. 13.) If you wish to work a band of knitting, you may fix it to one side of a circular mould. This species of knitting is ordinarily quite loose. Since it is not much used nowadays except for purses, I shall only discuss it in relation to them. These purses, which are rather common, are made in thick silk of a dark colour. You may use the mixed silk prepared for netted purses.

Take a box-wood mould furnished with spikes, as described above. This mould narrows after several lines, and terminates in a square end half the width of the top opening (see Fig. 3), because it is not used to preserve the shape of the purse. The number of stitches placed after the spikes and the narrowings below are made entirely without the mould. To put the stitches onto the spikes, make a slip-knot to place on each. On the second row, take a hooked needle fitted to a small handle of box-wood or ivory for greater convenience, and pass the hook into the first stitch formed by the slip-knot. Wind the silk round the hook, and form a new stitch almost as you pick up the stitches of a heel with a single needle. This is a series of slip-knots. When you have thus reached the place where your purse must be narrowed, you will perceive from the model the number of decreases to make, and make them by taking two stitches into one with the hook.

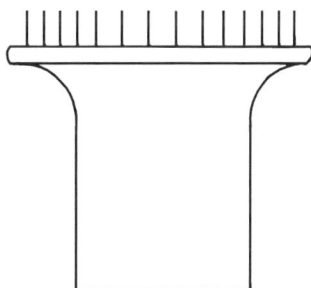

Figure 3. A knitting mould.

You may work circular rounds of different colours for your purse, as for netting. You may also work the holes called *à crochet*. Here is the mode: pass the silk twice round the hook before putting it into the previous stitch, which produces a thick stitch; but the needle having been passed into all the stitches, it is necessary that the long or thick stitches be transferred to a netting mould, on which you can work a row of ordinary netting. After or before this round, enter the hook into the long stitches produced either by the double turn or on the mould, and resume knitting.

That is all the variety of which these purses are susceptible.

The Art of mending Stockings.

Now that ladies have the good sense not only to add to intellectual labours the minor works of their sex, but also not to disdain these same works when they are not at all ornamental, I believe that I must end this chapter on knitting with the subject of mending. This is one of the most useful occupations in which a young person may be engaged, because whatever her circumstances, she is always meant to be a good housekeeper.

Repair of stockings is divided into five distinct operations, viz.: 1st., picking up stitches which have pulled out; 2nd., grafting, that is joining one piece of knitting to another by sewing the stitches together so that the seam does not show; 3rd., re-enforcing stockings; 4th., footing them; 5th., re-cutting them. (See Div. 14.)

To pick up Loose Stitches. It frequently happens, above all with silk stockings, that a loose stitch pulls through from round to round, and sometimes progresses over the greater part of the leg. It would continue thus to the end of the stocking, leaving a ladder, if you did not provide a remedy. It is necessary, therefore, to fasten the loose stitch by sewing when you become aware of its course, even if the stocking is still on your leg. When you take off the stocking, pick up the stitches as follows:

Thread a needle with coloured linen or silk if you have to pick up stitches on a white stocking, and with white linen if it is a black stocking. This thread is not permanent, and the contrast in colour will aid you. Take the stocking in your left hand, and lay the place where the loose stitch was fastened over your left forefinger, between your thumb and third finger. Then, turning the eye of the needle towards you, pass it through the stitch, and pull the thread through, but leave a long end of it, which you hold under your left thumb. Put the portion which you pulled through back under this finger to hold the stitch in back. That done, turning the eye of the needle to your side, pass it under the first bar which follows the stitch. Then, turning the point towards you, again pass the needle through the stitch above the thread which goes through it. Pull the entire thread through, excepting the end always held under your thumb, so as to bring the bar much closer. With your right thumb and forefinger, pinch the long thread and the end of thread left in the beginning, pull the stitch, and the bar will be found to have entered the stitch.

Recommence in the same way, from bar to bar, until you have restored the stitch to the place where it came loose. All this time it is necessary that the thread glide easily through the stitch, so that you may pass and re-pass it at will. To accomplish this, it is enough to carefully pick up each bar and the stitch every time, without omitting a single one of the strands of which it is composed. When all the bars have thus passed through the stitch, remove the thread, and graft this stitch to the one from which it became detached, as I shall explain.

Grafting. Stitches do not only pull out to the bottom; they separate as well by the breaking of the linen or cotton which holds them in a circle. It is necessary to replace the yarn and join the stitches; this operation is called grafting; it is performed as follows. Thread a needle with silk or cotton similar to the tissue of the stocking. Put the end of the yarn at the beginning of the crossways crack which causes the separation of the stitches, and for this time only turn the eye of the needle towards you when entering it, to fasten it in the row of unbroken knitting which delimits the crack. (It is almost needless to say that the stocking must be held at the place of the hole over your left forefinger, and retained by your thumb and middle finger.) The end of the yarn positioned, turn the needle with the point forwards, and enter it into the stitch to the right, next the first broken stitch, and into the broken stitch. Repeat this operation on the left. Then again pass the needle to the right, into the stitch previously taken on that side, and into the next stitch at the same time. Pick up the same stitches in the same way on the left, paying close attention to passing the needle only into the little loop of the stitches, and not into the bar which holds them. Stitches reunited in this way leave no sewing visible.

If stitches pull out while you are grafting, pick them up as I described earlier and continue grafting. Having come to the end, fasten the yarn by passing the needle under three or four stitches on the wrong side, so that they do not show on top.

Grafting is used to put pieces onto stockings, or to rejoin parts in a circle. For example, if you have stockings whose lower parts are worn while the upper parts are still good, and you wish to add these latter to half-stockings, sew them together by grafting. After having cut the two pieces which you propose to unite, go over every stitch with a pin in order to extract the little piece of cotton left in the stitch when cutting, and to restore the circular straight-way of the stitches, which it is impossible to preserve. Failing these two preparations, you cannot graft, because the stitches must be clean, and the yarn of the rounds perfectly free. Follow the same steps for pieces which have side grafting, which I shall describe in a few words.

Every stitch in plain knitting produces a straight lengthways line. When you graft, you unite these lengthways lines crossways. If the grafting is in the round, your task is limited to that. But if you have to graft a flat piece or band it is necessary, when you are at the end of the piece, to join the side along a lengthways line. This is equally necessary at the beginning of the piece. It is an easy task.

Make a seam fold on your piece along the lengthways line which will delimit it. Lay it along the lengthways line which borders the stocking, at the place where you have placed the piece, and where you have finished grafting. Then, stretching the lengthways line a little, pass the needle which you used to graft under two short threads or bars placed between the two furrows of the line, and which follow the crossways crack, for this is the yarn of the knitted rounds. Pick up the same two bars in the lengthways line of the piece which you are adding, and so on at one and the other line, to the end of the piece. Instead of side grafting you may over-cast on the wrong side, but the former is preferable.

To re-enforce Stockings. This work is usually performed in one of two ways. The first is by lining the heel of the stocking with pieces of similar knitting; that is, silk if the stockings are of silk, and cotton if they are of cotton. The second mode is by darning. I shall begin with the first mode.

Turn your stocking to the wrong side. Place it flat over your knee while putting the corners or the seams of the corners precisely over each other. (These seams are the stitches of the side of the heel, which form a relief on each side of the stocking below the corners, when there are any.) Then take a knitted piece four or five inches long and about three wide. Fold it lengthways right side out, and place it thus doubled on the stocking, from the part of the foot where it will lie along the width, to the part of the leg on the seam-stitches where it will lie along the length: this is the lining. Fix it with pins at the bottom. Hollow out a little of the angle which makes up the lining below the heel (see Fig. 4, *h*), so that the lining may fit the roundness of the heel. Sew both edges widthways from the hollow to the end. That done, freeze the fold (as described in Chapter XV) which was first made lengthways, at the middle of the lining, to the seam line of the stocking. Also freeze the latter seam to the fold which divides the heel. Hollow the top of the lining so that it presents a slanting line, very sloped towards the upper part, from the top of the beginning of the seams of the corners (see Fig. 4, *ii*).

Figure 4. The lining for a stocking.

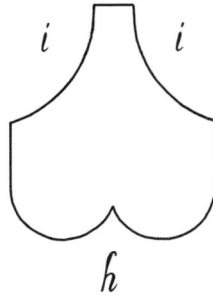

Then pass your left hand into the stocking. With your right hand, turn down half the lining to the other side of the stocking, from the seam line. Pass the palm of your right hand firmly over the upper side, without taking your left hand out of the stocking, so that it is only your thumb which will hold it folded for greater convenience. Take a long needle with a very long eye, threaded beforehand with flat silk, linen, or cotton (according to the yarn of the stocking). Holding your lining spread out over the stocking, attach it all round with herring-bone stitches (described in Chapter XV).

Next spread the stocking out over the palm of your left hand (passed inside the stocking) and enter the needle at the bottom of the heel, on the right, at a distance of eight to ten stitches from the freezing of the seam line. Take long running stitches along this freezing; but they are long only in going from one to another, because the needle must pick up only one or two bars in piercing the lining and the stocking at the same time. Take care that the stitches do not show on the right side of the stocking. (However, do not concern yourself much about this near the heel.) When you have reached the top of the lining, again lower the needle towards the right, to the same distance and in the same way as before. Continue thus to the end of the right side of the lining, then work the left side in the same fashion.

Some persons line the toe in the same way. Another mode is to freeze the piece of lining crossways onto the stocking.

Let us pass on to the second mode of re-enforcing stockings. Turn the stocking to the wrong side and enter your left hand as described above. Then thread the same kind of needle with a long thread, and enter it along the seam line from the heel, into the first, second, or third of the stitches following, according to how you wish to re-enforce the stocking. Enter the thread through every second, third, or fourth bar, according to the time and care which you propose to give to your work. From the first row made on the right-hand side of the stocking, baste to trace the distance which you wish to furnish this way. The shape of the stocking lining in Fig. 4 will guide you. However, since this second mode of re-enforcing takes a long time, it is extended over a little less of the stocking. Go back over the second row of stitches like the first, but opposing the stitches; this is a kind of darning. Since the bars are picked up on the wrong side, the stitches never appear on the right side, and the stockings are very sturdily re-enforced without it showing at all.

Work the left side after the right side, then withdraw the basting. It is needless to go round this work with herring-bone stitches.

To foot Stockings. When the heel and the sole of the stockings are too worn to repair by grafting or darning, cut the rounded end of the heel and the under side of the foot all along the stocking. The piece removed is about two inches wide towards the foot, and an inch towards the heel. Using this piece as a guide, or to say it better, cutting by the sole, cut out a new sole of tolerably stout toile. This is on the bias and wider than the model, in order to allow the seam folds which you must next make round the sole and the stocking.

Herring-bone on the seam fold of the sole, and proceed in the same manner round the stocking. Then, attaching the heel of the new sole to the heel of the stocking, likewise the foot of each, join them together all round with slightly slanting over-cast stitches. Over-cast on the edge of the stocking and right side out, so that the projection produced by over-casting will not irritate your foot. Crease the over-casting with your thimble as well.

There are stocking-menders who line the heel and the toe of the sole. This is a very sound practice, which adds almost nothing to the labour, because these linings are put inside the sole, and fastened afterwards by herring-boning. It is therefore nothing more than a small crossways seam of herring-bone stitches, or even running stitches, to hold the width of the heel and the toe. This crossways breadth must be sewed flat across the sole, without a seam fold.

To re-cut Stockings. When stockings have been footed so often that the instep is worn out, and the bottom of the back of the leg is equally bad, you can take no other course but to re-cut them while reducing their length, which you remedy by grafting a piece at the top. Proceed in this manner:

Take a model stocking to cut by. Place the stocking to be cut over the model so that the heel of the stocking exceeds the heel of the model by two, three, or four inches, according to the amount you are obliged to remove from the stocking, and consequently according to the degree of dilapidation. Cut crossways to remove the excess portion up to the corners of the stocking, or up to the place where the side seams going up from the heel would pass. If the seams are longer, cease cutting widthways, and cut a little slit starting lengthways, measuring the slits on the side seam of your model. Then cut the rest of the stocking by the foot of the model; throw away the surplus. This stocking will have a toile sole.

Here you have, pretty nearly, re-cut the lower portions of the stocking; but one essential is lacking. This is the two bands on the side which from the side seams of the heel, gradually pulled in by the narrowings, produce a slightly sloping point on each side of the stocking at the sole. Replace these bands with gores of the same shape, which you take from a piece of knitting similar to the tissue of your stocking. Place the knitted stitches parallel to the foot of the stocking, and consequently opposite to those of the heel. Take care in cutting the gores to place one over the other with the right sides of the material together; because failing this precaution, it often happens that you make a mistake, and that one of them cannot be used.

Your gores correctly cut, fold over a little of the bias side and the vertical straight side, on the straight-way; then take narrow herring-bone stitches over this seam fold. Repeat the same operation at the slit which you made at the corners of the heel, and at the bottom, up to where the gore finishes attaching to the stocking, starting at the point of the slit. You may make sure of this by measuring the gore on this part of the stocking. Then position the upper point of the gore (the point produced by the meeting of the end of the vertical side and the bias side) at the point where the slit starts. On the wrong side, over-cast the vertical side of the gore to the side of the heel, and the bias at the bottom. If you wish the work to be more pleasing, graft the stitches on the side instead of over-casting. In that case, herring-boning is unnecessary; or at least it is done only after grafting, a single stitch for both pieces. Whatsoever you choose, repeat this operation on the other gore. After that, finish herring-boning round the foot of the stocking. Line the heel, sew on a sole, and the bottom will be remade.

Nothing more remains but to work a back-stitched seam at the top of the heel and at the bottom of the seam line, in order to remove the width from the calf which has descended to the bottom of the leg. Work this seam following the model stocking. Leave more or less material outside your stitches, and finish by gradually decreasing the number of knitted stitches taken outside the seam, to nothing at the end of it. Then remove the extra material outside the seam which you just made, leaving a very narrow margin, by slitting, or by cutting along the lengthways fold in the middle of the excess material. Finally, turn down the margins to the right and left, and fasten them to the stocking with herring-bone stitches.

——*Manuel des demoiselles.*

Diversion 1.

Noeuds coulants in the original French.

——Frances Grimble.

Diversion 2.

The distinction between the *maille l'envers,* which is always translated here as "purl-stitch," and the *maille retournée,* always translated here as "turn-stitch," is unclear in the original work.

——Frances Grimble.

Diversion 3.

Knitting for the Lower Orders. Knitting is work which may be taken up and laid down in a moment. A set of needles may be bought for a penny, and a ball of worsted for another. It may be done in any light, or with a child in your arms; and when you are tired of stirring work, knitting serves very well for a rest. In summer-time, you may take a walk in your garden, and knit as you go. A pair of knit stockings, when they are done (in little odds and ends of time) are worth at least three pair of the best woven ones you can buy. A thrifty cottager's wife has no stockings for her husband or herself but what she knits, at least until she has children old enough to do them for her. A good knitter too, may generally get employment if she chooses to take it in. And if the scraps of time so employed add but sixpence to her weekly income, it is not to be despised.

Both boys and girls should be early taught to knit, and accustomed to take it up at every odd minute of time. You cannot too soon give them a comfortable notion of honest independence, and that it is very creditable to wear stockings of their own knitting, and clothes of their own earning or making. This is a good and a saving practice; even the mere habit of moving about their fingers nimbly, and not liking to be idle, is of no small value. On a winter's evening, when all are sitting round the fire, and one perhaps is reading, the rest might as well be knitting as doing nothing.

——*Cottage Comforts.*

Diversion 4.

The Trade of the Stocking-weaver. Modern stockings, whether woven or knit, are formed of an indefinite number of little knots, called stitches, loops, or meshes, intermingled in one another. Woven stockings are manufactured on a stocking loom, or frame, made of finely-polished iron or steel. Stockings of all sorts may be made on it with great art and expedition. By means of some additional machinery to the frame, turned ribbed stockings are made, as well as those done with knitting needles. These, together with the mode of making open-work mitts, a curious kind of lace aprons, and handkerchiefs, as well as a great variety of figured goods for waistcoats, &c., have sprung from the same machine, and form now a considerable additional branch of the stocking trade.

Knit stockings are made with needles of polished iron. In England, knitting is carried on as a trade in a singular manner. In many parts of the country, the wool-comber appoints a day, generally once in a fortnight or three weeks, when he will meet his spinners and his knitters, to deliver out his wool and his worsted to be spun and knit. The poor women and girls of the village meet him on the day appointed with their work, return what they have spun or knit, and take other work instead. But the money which they obtain, either at spinning or knitting, is rarely more than sixpence or eightpence a day. The wool-comber has the stockings scoured or dyed, as the colour or colours require, and afterwards dresses them by stretching them on a wooden board, the shape of the leg and foot. Then he packs them up for sale, either in a dozen or a half-dozen pairs, as in the case of woven stockings.

Knit stockings are much more durable than those made on the loom; but the time required for this work, especially if the materials are very fine, raises the price too high for common wearers. But such is their superior durability, that coarse knit stockings are preferred and worn by the common people in most parts of England, particularly by the men.

The hosier purchases stockings, night-caps, socks, gloves, &c. from the manufacturer, and sells them again. Some of them employ looms, and are, in that respect, stocking-weavers.

——*The Book of English Trades.*

Diversion 5.

Patte in the original French.

——Frances Grimble.

Diversion 6.

Joints in the original French.

——Frances Grimble.

Diversion 7.

The Mode of knitting Gentlemen's Waistcoats. Waistcoats are often composed of sleeves, and a wide piece which serves at the same time for the back and both fronts. The sleeves are commenced at the bottom. Put forty-five to fifty-five stitches there, according to the thickness of the wool which you use. Since knitted wool does not curl up at the edges, or very little, you may dispense with working a border, as is customary for stockings. These sleeves are made open. Consequently, the knitting not being in the round, you will have alternating rows of purl and plain stitches, which will all look like purl-stitches. This kind of knitting is adopted for waistcoats because they are ordinarily made of wool, and wool knits up well only in this way.

From the eighth row, make a narrowing on each side of your selvages, allowing, however, two stitches before. You will thus make ten to twelve pairs of narrowings, one pair every eight rows. Leave a lesser interval if the wool is thick; here I am giving rules proper for wool of middle thickness. These ten or twelve narrowings will give you a length of about a sixth of an ell. Then continue to knit rows without narrowing or widening until you have about doubled that length.

That done, widen every two rows as you narrowed, that is, near the selvages. These widenings, which provide the breadth of the arm-hole under the arms, must make about the extent of an eighth. Double the widenings for the last two rows. Directly after, resume narrowing twice every four rows, then twice every three rows, then every two rows, in order to obtain the hollow of the sleeve. Continue thus for the length of a sixth, and bind off the remaining stitches with narrowings in a chain. Some knitters narrow on every row, and extend the narrowings an eighth or more instead of a sixth, until finally only eight to ten stitches remain between the two rows of narrowings. But this mode has the disadvantages of rendering the sleeve too pointed, and of making the bottom of the arm-hole pull too much when the sleeve is put on, which hampers movement and immediately tears the waistcoat under the arms. The sleeves completed, lay them aside, and set about starting the body of the waistcoat.

Waistcoat all in One Piece.

A waistcoat is sometimes knitted in three pieces, two fronts and a back, which are narrowed and widened following a model; then the pieces are joined by the seam previously described for petticoats. This is more convenient and quicker to work, because you are not encumbered by such a great quantity of stitches that you must crowd them together, as when you knit a waistcoat of only one piece. The long needles which are ordinarily used seem quite short in that case. Therefore, I advise making the waistcoat in three pieces, the other mode being more suitable for commercially-knitted waistcoats. However, I shall teach both modes.

The Waistcoat all in One Piece. Make as many stitches as necessary to go round the body without being too tight. A waistcoat of middling wool requires about four hundred and sixty to four hundred and eighty, and that is for a tolerably slender man. You will already perceive the extreme difficulty of holding this multitude of stitches on the needles, and the trouble which must result. Howsoever that may be, knit uniform rows without widening or narrowing for about an eighth of an ell. Then narrow, starting from the middle of your stitches, four times. That is to say, make two narrowings every sixteen stitches, on each side of the middle. Repeat this narrowing on the third of the stitches which must shape the seam ordinarily placed under the arm. Knit a dozen rows without narrowing, then narrow in the same way until you have come to the arm-holes. Your waistcoat must then be three-eighths of an ell.

Following what I have already said regarding slits in petticoats, put a little less than a third of the right-hand stitches on one needle. Leave all the others on the other needle, which you fix with several provisional turns of yarn, to prevent the stitches from coming off. This needle must remain stationary. Then take a new needle and knit only the part where the stitches remain free, for about ten rows. After these ten rows, narrow every row on the right selvage, which makes the edge of the front of the waistcoat. This operation will gradually narrow the right piece and give it a sloping shape, while it will leave the other selvage in a straight line. This second selvage is destined to make the arm-hole. When you have narrowed down to no more than twelve or fifteen stitches for the shoulder-piece, bind off with chain-stitches. Leaving this piece of knitting which composes the first front, go to the left selvage of the waistcoat, and repeat for the second front all that you did for the first, this time taking care to narrow near the left selvage.

Both fronts being finished, proceed to knit the stitches which remain between them at the middle of the waistcoat. Knit seven or eight rows without narrowing, then make a narrowing every ten stitches, and every ten rows. You will thus knit the band in the middle, which will make the back of the waistcoat. When your knitting has grown to a length of about a quarter from the first narrowings, widen at each side of the back, leaving, from the selvage, as many stitches as for the front shoulder-piece, to which this width must be joined. Widen only two times at each edge, and make the second widening four or six rows after the first. These six rows finished, join the end of the right shoulder-piece to the end of the back shoulder-piece, with a knitted seam.

After that, pick up onto the needle for the back, all the stitches of the side of the front down to the bottom of the waistcoat, making a new stitch at each stitch with only one needle, exactly as you pick up the stitches at the side of a stocking-heel. All these stitches being picked up, knit them along the front, and continue without interruption to the back for one row. Perform the same operation for the left front. When the stitches on the side have been picked up, continue all along the back, and from the front to the bottom of the waistcoat without interruption. The row is begun on the stitches picked up to the right. Repeat this row five or six times, which will give you a narrow strip of lengthways stitches opposite to those of the waistcoat, which are widthways. The stitches on the side, which stand up to form a narrow *cordon,* add charm to this species of border, prettier still when the narrowings, continuing from the front to the shoulder-piece, present a new narrow *cordon* which follows the raised stitches. Bind off this strip by working chain-stitches all along the waistcoat.

The length of the waistcoat before the narrowings of the fronts, the length of the fronts, plus the width of the back, present a line of more than two ells. Consequently, it requires unbroken knitting along all that distance, since the narrow strip must trim the whole without interruption. You will perceive that it is impossible to work such a long piece of knitting with two needles, or to use needles with a permanent knob at the end. You will need to add another pair to the first two, when knitting the long narrow strip; and these needles, pointed at both ends, should have a knob which you may remove at will. There are besides needles of wood or iron which do not have any knob, which will answer perfectly.

Little more remains but to sew the two selvages of the sleeves together in order to give them a circular shape. Then attach them to the arm-hole, placing the top of the lengthways seam of the sleeve at the middle of the arm-hole, which begins under the arms. Use the simple seam worked with a bodkin described in the article on petticoats.

Finally, trim the entire length of the strip with a riband *à cheval.* To do this, fold the riband in half along its entire length, and place it over the edge of the knitting so that it covers the knitting equally on the right and wrong sides. Both selvages of the riband are thus found parallel. Sew them together by piercing the material with a row of running stitches, which are long underneath and very short on top. They must be imperceptible.

The Waistcoat in Three Pieces. The making of the three-piece waistcoat differs from the preceding waistcoat only up to a point. Begin with the sleeves, and knit them in the same manner. For the front, of which each half is knitted separately, cast on a third of the stitches necessary for a one-piece waistcoat. Knit both halves of the front without decreasing at all up to the arm-hole, that is for nearly three-eighths, because the narrowings which were begun earlier on the one-piece waistcoat would be relative to the back. If you wish to work your waistcoat more easily and quickly, do not trim it with the narrow strip which borders the other waistcoat, and add six more stitches when beginning each front, in order to replace the widening produced by that ornament. Otherwise, continue the front as described for the front of the one-piece waistcoat. Then, when you have come to the shoulder-piece, which you make six stitches wider if you omit the strip, fasten off and knit the second front exactly like this one.

I shall also refer you to the back already described, after you have knitted the first rows with a third of the stitches, or a little more; many persons being in the habit of putting more in the back than in each front. If you imitate them, it is needless to say that you must subtract from the fronts, the number of stitches which you add to the back. The back will also need to be longer by the height of six rows if the narrow strip is absent.

Sew the fronts to the back in the same way as the sleeves. Join the shoulder-pieces as desired, either by sewing with a bodkin or by knitting the seam.

Waistcoats are not knitted with welts, and still less, if possible, with open-work. For persons who greatly fear the cold, the waistcoat is furnished with a quilted silk lining instead of a riband *à cheval*. This quilting consists of joining two pieces with rows of running stitches in divers patterns. This kind of work, which was not mentioned in Chapter XV because it is old-fashioned and altogether discarded, was formerly in great favour. Caps, petticoats, gowns, stays, and coverlets were quilted. In the last case both materials were mounted on a frame. The worker would follow, with rows of running stitches, designs traced beforehand on the material, which had to be on the right side. Cotton wadding was put between the materials. Most often the design consisted of slanting lines crossed to produce squares or diamonds.

——*Manuel des demoiselles.*

Diversion 8.

Corset in the original French.

——Frances Grimble.

Diversion 9.

Tricotage boutonné ou croisé in the original French.

——Frances Grimble.

Diversion 10.

The Mode of knitting Pantaloons. All the great pieces of knitting which are worked in the round like a stocking are called bags. For pantaloons, it is necessary to knit two bags, eighteen inches wide and fifty to fifty-two inches long. After you have knitted about two-thirds of their length, the bags are sewed together and no longer knitted separately. You may, after these two-thirds, join the fourteen needles together, and knit both bags in one very wide band, which you continually increase every four stitches, at the middle of the stitches. These bags are knitted with seven needles; the needles are found starting with six, and the seventh is the extra. These pieces could be knitted widthways or lengthways, the same as a band; but it would be necessary to work a row of purl-stitches on both, and that mode demands too much time.

When pantaloons are made of plush, the knitting is done in the customary mode, but you use two yarns of different thicknesses. The finer serves to work the ground, and the thicker is meant for the nap, or fringe, which consists of knots worked in every sixth stitch, closely knitted, and furthermore crossed by the yarn. To render the nap warmer, make a slip-knot as in picking up the stitches of a heel; or encircling the middle finger of your left hand with the yarn, and passing the yarn through this loop at every stitch, and into the position of the new knot which must correspond to the middle of the interval of those in the previous row. Stockings of this sort are also knitted for aged persons.

——*Manuel des demoiselles.*

Diversion 11.

The original French does say sixty-eight stitches earlier, and sixty-three here.

——Frances Grimble.

Diversion 12.

Parties de mousse in the original French.

——Frances Grimble.

Diversion 13.

Gold-thread Purses and Bags. The thread is to be procured at the gold-lace shops. Form a small loop at the end of it. Then, with a tambour-needle passed through this loop, draw the thread up again into another loop; and thus in succession, until such a length has been woven as, the two ends being joined, will form the circumference of the purse. The joining is effected by passing the needle through the two end loops, and drawing the thread up through both.

Then form five loops on the continuation of the thread. Next pass the needle through the third loop from the join, on the completed circle, and draw the thread through. Form five more loops on the perfected round, as before, and so on in the same manner, until the circle is finished. The succeeding rows are formed by weaving, as before, five loops at a time, and then passing the thread through the thread, or centre loop, of the row last finished: the rounds are still continued until the desired size is obtained.

Complete the bottom by drawing the loops together with gold thread, and affixing a gold bullion tassel. Finish the top by a straight row of running loops, sewed with gold thread to a spring clasp. The lining should be of satin, and rather smaller than the net.

——*The Young Lady's Book.*

Diversion 14.

To dye Thick Silks, Satins, Silk Stockings, &c. of a Flesh-colour. Wash your stockings clean in soap and water, then rinse them in hot water. If they do not then appear perfectly clean, cut half an ounce of white soap into thin slices, and put it into a saucepan half full of boiling water. When the soap is dissolved, cool the water in the pan. Then put in the stockings, and boil them twenty minutes. Take them out, and rinse in hot water. In the interim pour three table-spoonfuls of purple archil into a wash-hand basin half full of hot water. Put the stockings in this dye-water, and when of the shade called half-violet or lilac, take them from the dye-water and slightly rinse them in cold water. When dry, hang them up in a close room in which sulphur is burnt. When they are evenly bleached to the shade required of flesh-colour, take them from the sulphuring room, and finish them by rubbing the right side with a clean flannel. Some persons calender them afterwards. Satins and silks are done in the same way.

For dyeing Silk Stockings Black. These are dyed like other silks, except that they must be steeped a day or two in bark liquor, before they are put into the black silk dye. At first they will look an iron-grey; but to finish and black them, they must be put on wooden legs, laid on a table, and rubbed with your oily rubber, or flannel, upon which is olive-oil; and then the more they are rubbed the better. Each pair of stockings will require at least half a table-spoonful of oil, and half an hour's rubbing to finish them well. Sweet oil is the best in this process, as it leaves no disagreeable smell.

——The Family Dyer and Scourer.

Chapter XVIII.
The Art of making and mending Elastic Bracelets and Garters.

❦❦❦❦

In Chapter XIV, you have already seen how to place elastics between two pieces of taffety, and how to preserve their flexibility. I have little to add here, for it is always the same mode. Yet I must return to this subject, because the circular placement of the elastics for bracelets, the leather which covers them, and the pads which terminate garters, all require particulars.

Bracelets.

Bracelets have ordinarily two rows of elastics and appear, when they are new, about half the size of the arm. Cut a small strip of leather wide enough to enclose both elastics without impeding them, and at least a third longer than these articles when they are not stretched. (Elastic bracelets are also made in black taffety and coloured ribands.) Measure the strip in half lengthways, then fold over one of the halves to the middle. Pass an elastic into the fold. Fasten it at each end of the strip, then sew it just as I described in Chapter XIV. All along the wrong side, this first stitching presents a part similar to the raw edge of ordinary seams. When tightened by the folds of the elastic, it presents a succession of little creases pressed against each other. You may easily conceal them, for to place the second elastic, you turn the second half of the strip over the previous stitching. Here you must take great care not to make the bracelet stiff. In order to avoid that, at every stitch gently pull the elastic already sewed, catch the surface of the leather lightly, and preserve all the old folds. When the elastics are placed, take a *poignée,* which is a device similar to the wooden handle of a brush, and press it to the side between the elastics to properly apply the leather on top.

Garters.

Circular garters are made like bracelets, except that you turn down at the fourth or sixth row of elastic rather than the second. Other garters with clasps are made in very nearly the same way, but there is some difference between them. It is this: after you have cut a strip of leather wide enough to contain four or six rows of elastic, make it at least an inch longer than is needed for the requirements of elasticity. The extra inch which you put at each end must be padded with cotton wadding, and sewed all round with small stitches like a little tab, when the elastics are placed. Slip the ends of the elastics over these tabs, which serve to support them, and turn down the strip at the end. In this way the ends of the elastics and the wadding are completely hidden. The tab now supports the clasp which secures the garter over your knee.

This clasp is composed of three little mortises. Two placed on the widest part are destined to receive the hook; the third narrower mortise furnishes the means of securing the clasp on the garter. Take a little strip of leather, green or yellow, but always a different colour from that of the garter. Fold it double, pass it into the third mortise, and fasten it to the tab with two rows of stitching. Repeat this operation at the other end of the garter when you put the hook there, which has only the narrow mortise. Take care that the tabs are long enough to cross under the clasp and the hook, because otherwise they would tear your stockings, stain them with rust, and finish by hurting you.

When you wish to embroider elastic garters, make the tab twice as long, and in white or pink satin. The tambour-embroidered satin is padded with wadding. The elastics, necessarily shorter, are between two pieces of white taffety. Garters are also trimmed with plush, or sewed into a slightly plushy riband.

Repairs.

After the following directions, you will see how to proceed when your garters or bracelets loose their elasticity. First determine which row is at fault. Then unstitch the piece turned down, and all the rows within half an inch, until you have reached the elastic without movement. You will see immediately whether it is unsewed, or whether it has stretched too much. In the first case you simply resew it. In the second, thread a large needle with the bottom end of the elastic, and holding the spiral very tight for several moments, you will see it regain its former consistency. In sewing it, as by the way in sewing all other elastics, take care not to fasten it only by the last ring of the spiral, for that is why it became loose. Fasten it by two or three rings, then sew it just as you unpicked it.

When the lengthways seam which holds and separates the elastics becomes unsewed, it is not too much of an inconvenience. Yet you should not neglect to resew it, because in thus coming together the elastics rub against each other, and in a short time the garter is almost completely unsewed.

——*Manuel des dames.*

Chapter XIX.
The Art of sewing Gloves.

Gloves, one of the least costly parts of our attire, are even so an object of expense because of the extreme ease with which they become soiled, and above all white gloves. Yet it is exactly these which it is necessary to wear most often. Toilets for balls, assemblies, and visits however little ceremonious, and generally for all neat attire, require white gloves, and appear incomplete without them. Now, gloves of this colour do not look well for more than three wearings, and very often for only one. Gloves of very light colours, such as reseda, straw, and rose, which replace them at need when you are not making a grand toilet, fade scarcely less quickly. Besides, these gloves, always *glacé*, tear as easily as they stain. Gloves which are not *glacé*, which are worn for *négligé* and demi-toilet, especially during the winter, are not subject to this disadvantage, but they soil even more quickly than the others. It is true that they may be cleansed; but they soon become dirty again, and cleansing is not very effective the second or third time. (See Div. 1.) From all these details it is necessary to conclude that when you often go out into society, you must renew your gloves almost daily. To economize by not doing so is impossible, because it would be uncleanliness.

However, I shall propose one economy without contradicting my advice, because its object is not to reduce the number of gloves, but only their price. First, I believe that it is important to buy them by the dozen from a wholesale glove dealer. They are matched, quite handsome, and cost much less than retail at a haberdasher's. That is not all; it is also necessary to buy them unsewed. The same dealers sell them cut out at half, or less, the ordinary price. I shall show you how to sew them, and you will see what a bargain you will get in return. (Chapter XVI describes how to mend gloves.)

Each glove consists of a number of pieces. The body, shown in Fig. 1 *A*, has three narrow tongues on each face and a wider one which, when the body is folded upon itself, form the fingers, the wide tongue being the forefinger. Because the glove body does not accommodate the thickness or

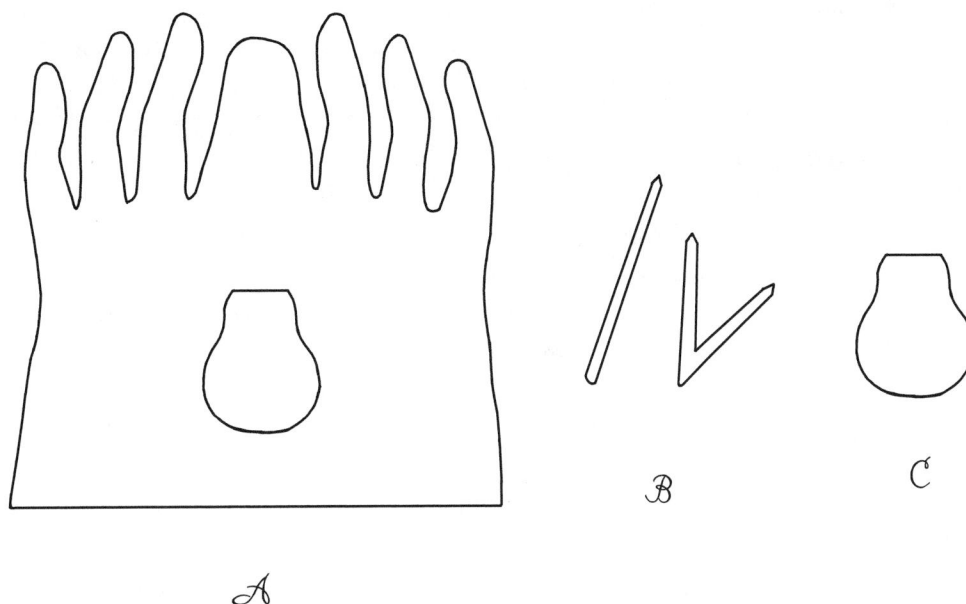

Figure 1. The parts of a glove.

movement of your fingers, where necessary you add tongue-shaped gores called *fourchettes* on the sides of the fingers, and little diamond-shaped ones called between-fingers at the bases of the fingers (see Fig. 1 *B*). The opening in the middle of the body is for the insertion of the thumb, which is cut separately (see Fig. 1 *C*).

You will commence sewing the glove with the thumb, which is the most difficult piece. Then, finger by finger, you attach the *fourchettes* and the between-fingers. Finally, you join the body of the glove. It is needless to say that both gloves are made in the same manner.

First the little pointed gore for the base of the thumb is inserted in the pointed slit at the top of the opening. Thread a needle with fine, flat silk the colour of the glove, and firmly sew the edge of the thumb and the opening together with over-cast stitches, very slanting, not very deep, and perfectly even, so that they present a narrow spiral of silk. Because this seam is made on the right side, it must be a kind of decoration. Sew the side of the thumb, taking equal care neither to tighten the thread, nor to take up too much leather. Sew all round in this way while including the bias gore for the opening, which must provide the proper suppleness for the thumb. Finish at the upper part of this digit, which you round at the end.

The Art of sewing Gloves.

Ordinarily glove cutters make the fingers inordinately long. You must trim them to fit your fingers, but leave them much longer. In stretching them to conform to your hand, the leather is taken up every where, and fingers which were cut exactly would then be found too short. Each finger is composed of two middle tongues (cut as part of the body) and two side tongues or *fourchettes* which form a V, then at the bottom the little diamond-shaped between-finger. The forefinger and the little finger, having only a single angle between fingers, have but one *fourchette* each.

For the forefinger, take two *fourchettes*, which are prepared separately from the body. They are about two-thirds the width of the tongues, and are shown by Fig. 1 *B*. Sew the lower points together in such a manner that they present a V, as shown. (The seam in the middle of this V, which is formed in joining these little points, is sewed from underneath. Ordinarily the tongues present this V at their base cut like a gore. However, it is immaterial that the same glove has a V on one seam, and the others all in one piece.) Place the point of this V in the angle produced by the double tongue of the forefinger and the middle finger, on the upper side of the glove. Try it on your hand to make sure there is no mistake. Sew one of the *fourchettes* to the forefinger tongue of the upper of the glove, and the other onto the neighbouring middle finger.

Then take a little piece of leather, and cut it into a diamond shape for the between-finger. Place this diamond with one point in the top of the V, another facing it (on the palm side), and the other two at the right and left of the *fourchettes*. Finish by sewing the *fourchette* next the forefinger, to that finger on the palm side; round it a little at the end and it will be completed. Repeat this operation for the middle finger. Then place a V and a between-finger in the angle between the middle finger and the ring finger, and so on to the little finger. Cut the *fourchette* for the little finger well pointed and a little shorter than the others. This last finger does not form an angle at the end of the glove. Wait to join it until you make the lengthways seam which unites the two halves of the glove; the little finger will then be finished.

We will now see how to embroider the upper of the glove. This embroidery consists of three rays, which begin at the three angles occupied by the three V's—the angle of the forefinger, the angle of the middle finger, and the angle of the little finger. The first and the last of these angles have a single ray; the other merits a double ray. The rays descend to the level of the base of the thumb, less about two lines. They are marked by a *cordonnet* of close over-cast stitches, by chain-stitches, or by a slightly wider *cordonnet,* but with slanting stitches like satin-stitch embroidery.

(See Div. 2.) Most often the close *cordonnet* is employed, made with the stitch with which the gloves are sewed, but straighter and closer together. The ray from the angle of the middle finger is frequently made with chain-stitches, between the other two rays of *cordonnet,* in which case the ray of the middle finger is not doubled. The rays are often doubled at all the angles, whether worked with a *cordonnet* or chain-stitches. They are closer together at the base than towards the angles of the fingers. Sometimes, about half an inch below the rays, a kind of very long half feather-stitch is made all round the glove. This stitch is becoming rarer every day.

There is nothing more to work on but the edge of the cuff. The cuff may be untrimmed or trimmed, as gloves *ordinaire* or gloves *de blouse.* For gloves *ordinaire* the cuff is circular, and simply hemmed with a single fold and very large stitches. For gloves *de blouse,* make a small slit about an inch and a half long, at the middle of the palm of the glove, to part the edge. Slightly hem this slit, and sew on one side a silk button similar to the glove, and on the other a button-hole, both very close to the edge. As for the border of the cuff, fold it to the wrong side as if you meant to hem it; but instead turn the marked hem back to the right side, and work a very close over-casting there instead of the ordinary side-stitches for hems. Then pull it straight, which produces a kind of piping. Finally, the trimmed gloves are cut into little points at the edge of the cuff. This is commonly done with a punch, or you may buy the gloves with the points ready cut.

The fashion of cuffed sleeves, called *de blouse,* which has spurred the invention of trimmed gloves, has also produced elastic gloves. These are extremely convenient. You know that in putting gloves on and off, you enlarge the cuff so that it gapes round the hand. This has no disadvantages when the ends of the sleeves extend down over the gloves. But at present the gloves go, on the contrary, over the sleeves, and nothing could be uglier. The button which is placed to prevent this annoyance is soon an inadequate resource, because the glove is not slow to enlarge despite the slit of which I have spoken. But elastic gloves always keep their firmness, as you may easily understand. This is the way to sew them:

Take two pieces of elastic, as if you meant to make bracelets, and place them permanently round the glove in a circle. These elastics must be six or seven lines from the lower end of the rays; one should suffice for each glove: it is necessary that they be very slender. The leather must be perfectly supple, for otherwise the elastic will not work.

Long gloves are prepared in the same manner as short gloves. When the hand is sewed, work the arm seam. I shall observe that the top of the arm receives a very long gore which, instead of being sewed on the outside as usual, has a seam on the inside. Without doubt, it is made on the wrong side to appear like a glove all in one piece. The stitches are longer and more slanted than ordinarily. Long gloves have a narrow string-case at the top, and when sewing it you pass a very narrow riband or *faveur* through it. Sometimes the case is replaced by a *faveur à cheval,* which serves to hold the other *faveur.* Half-long gloves, that is to say those which go only to the elbow, are neither hemmed nor embroidered. They are cut quite simply on the edge.

For very grand toilets, the tops of long white gloves are trimmed with blond lace ruches and garlands of riband loops. This is especially proper for ladies to be presented at court.

——*Manuel des dames.*

Diversion 1.

To wash and tint Gloves. Wash them in soap and water until the dirt is got out. Then stretch them on wooden hands, or pull them out in their proper shape. Never wring them, as that puts them out of form, and makes them shrink. Put them one upon another, and press the water out; then rub the following mixture over the outside of the gloves. If wanted quite yellow, take yellow ochre; if quite white, pipe-clay; if between the two, mix a little of each together. By proper mixture of these, any shade may be produced. Mix the colour with beer or vinegar.

Let them dry gradually, not too near the fire nor in too hot a sun. When they are about half dried, rub them well, and stretch them out to keep them from shrinking and to soften them. When they are well rubbed and dried, take a small cane and beat them; then brush them. When this is done, iron them rather warm, with a piece of paper over them, but do not let the iron be too hot.

To cleanse Gloves without wetting. Lay the gloves upon a clean board. Make a mixture of dried fuller's earth and powdered alum. Pass them over on each side with a common stiff brush. Then sweep it off, and sprinkle them well with dry bran and whiting, and dust them well. This, if they are not exceedingly greasy, will render them quite clean.

But if they are much soiled, take out the grease with crumbs of toasted bread, and powder of burnt bone. Then pass them over with a woollen cloth dipped in fuller's earth or alum powder. In this manner they may be cleansed without wetting, which frequently shrinks and spoils them.

To dye Gloves. Take the colours suitable for the occasion; if dark, take Spanish brown and black earth; if lighter, yellow and whiting, and so on with other colours. Mix them with a moderate fire. Daub the gloves over with the colour wet, and let them hang until they are dry. Then beat out the superfluity of the colour, and smooth them over with a stretching, or sleeking stick, reducing them to their proper shape.

To dye Gloves to resemble York Tan, Limerick Dye, &c. Steep saffron in boiling-hot soft water, for about twelve hours. Then having slightly tied up the tops of the gloves, to prevent the dye from staining the inside, wet them over with a sponge or soft brush dipped into the liquid. The quantity of saffron, as well as of water, will of course depend upon how much dye may be wanted, and their relative proportions on the depth of colour required. A common tea-cup will contain sufficient in quantity for a single pair of gloves.

——*The Alphabetical Receipt Book and Domestic Advisor.*

Diversion 2.

The Straight Over-cast stitch or *Cordonnet*. This stitch is worked from left to right over a single line of outline-stitches (see Fig. 2 A). To give it greater relief, a round, well-twisted thread may be laid along the outline and covered with straight stitches set side by side.

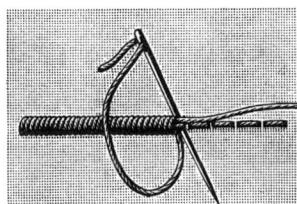 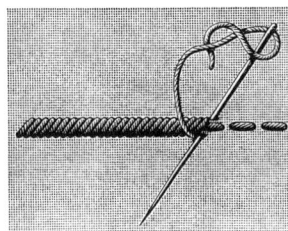

A　　　　　　*B*

Figure 2. Straight and slanting *cordonnets*.

The Slanting Over-cast stitch or *Cordonnet*. This stitch is also worked from left to right over a single line of outline-stitches (see Fig. 2 B). The needle enters above the outline, and emerges below it. When a very fine and delicate line is to be made, the needle must take up only those threads of the material which lie under the outline thread.

——*The Complete Encyclopedia of Needlework.*

Chapter XX.
The Art of the Haberdasher and Lace-woman, or the Art of preparing Belts, *Fichus,* Caps, &c.

At Paris this art is that of the haberdasher or *marchande de nouveautés* (such as are seen all along the rue aux Fers); in the provinces it is combined with that of the milliner. Their connexions are indeed numerous, because certain styles of caps and trimmings for *fichus* require a hand as skilled as that of an inventor of fashions. However, the tasks of the haberdasher and lace-woman include some very simple ones. Far from omitting these, I shall begin with them.

A Round Braid for Gowns.

Nothing could be simpler to make than the round braid for gowns, which is now sold in such great quantities. Take some flat cotton, three times as long as the braid which you want. Double or triple the cotton depending upon the thickness desired for the braid. Fix it at one end with a pin, over your knee if it is short, or to an arm-chair or the wall if it is long.

Taking the other end between your right thumb and forefinger, twist it from right to left, rolling it between these two fingers. Then, putting your left forefinger at the middle of the cotton, pass the cotton, still held between your right thumb and forefinger, on top of the pin, letting the end slip down to near your left forefinger, which holds it in a long loop. You thus divide the cotton into three parts, which you twist together in the same manner as before, but from left to right. It is essential to twist in the contrary direction the second time, because otherwise the braid will not be formed.

Instead of the flat cotton, you may use two narrow round silk braids, twisting them as described above, to obtain a very pretty braid.

Covered Cords.

Round cords called covered cords are put at the bottom of gowns, at the top of flounces, and are used as bell-pulls, &c. These cords are made by the following mode.

Take some coarse cotton or thread the desired colour of the cord. Double, triple, or quadruple the cotton, according to the required thickness of the cord. Roll it a little between your hands; then wind off some flat silk. Fasten the end to one end of the cotton; fasten the opposite end (of the cotton) to a chair or a nail. Then, holding the end of the cotton where the silk is fastened between your right thumb and forefinger, wind the silk round in a spiral, bringing it from left to right over the cotton with your left thumb and middle finger. The work is more conveniently done if you wind off a very long length of the silk into a ball; it is easy to pick up the silk when working with it.

The cotton must be entirely covered; then detach it from the chair. Take the end which was fastened there, and substitute the one which you were holding. Then take a very long length of very narrow round braid, the same colour as the cotton and silk. Wind it in a spiral, moving from left to right over the cord, and finish it with a knot. This produces a very agreeable effect, and affords as much strength as beauty, provided that you knot each piece when cutting it off.

A Cord for Watches, &c., made with the Fingers.

Take six to seven ells of braid, cord, or narrow riband, to make a cord an ell long. Divide this quantity into four equal parts. Roll each one onto a card, where you fix it with a pin, leaving only about half an ell for the work.

These four ends, joined by a knot in the other part, are held between the thumb and forefinger of your left hand. Then taking one end at the right, pass it under your left middle finger. Bring it back, thus forming a kind of loop, over your left thumb, underneath which it is held by your fourth finger. Take care, in passing it, that the end which follows it is confined under it. Then taking the second end, pass it under the third, which is brought in its turn over the fourth, which is made to enter the loop which your middle finger is holding open. By pulling all four ends equally, two in each hand, tighten the interlacing which has just been formed; and recommence the same process, up to the end.

This mode produces a sturdy cord of the kind used for gentlemen's and ladies' watches, eye-glasses, scissors, &c. When the cord is made with a narrow flat silk braid in solid black or pale yellow, it is a perfect imitation of hair-work. Using narrow strips of leather, you may make cords for walking-sticks.

These cords are made in pretty nearly the same way on a little mould, which serves to hold them open. This requires a little less material, and simplifies the interlacing.

Plaited Ribands.

Since last year, plaits of ribands have been worn at the bottom of *douillettes* and silk gowns. They are made as follows: take some satin riband No. 6, that is, riband about half an inch and a few lines wide. Redouble the riband over itself, and fold it in thirds, passing a common flat braid inside, to raise it somewhat. Take at least double the length of the plait which you desire, and thus prepare four pieces of riband. Pin all four, close together, over your right knee. It is necessary to number them to recognize them; therefore, beginning on the right: the first is 1, the next is 2, the one following it is 3, and the last is 4.

Pass 2 over 1, then 3 over 4, then cross, between the ribands 2 and 3, 4 under 1. Then pass 4 over 2, and 1 over 3, then 2 over 3, 3 over 4, 4 over 1 and over 2, 1 over 3, 2 over 1, and so on up to the end.

A Round Lace, made with Bobbins.

To make this lace, take four bobbins filled with thread. Join and attach the ends at some distance from them, either with a hook, or any other thing. Take two of the bobbins over the forefinger of each hand, and cross them, always bringing them back to the sides. Also cross the other two bobbins, but in the contrary direction, bringing one round to itself, while moving the other away to face it. Then pick up the two sides, and so on. By this mode cords are made to serve as chains for watches, &c., and in general all cords and braids with four strands.

The Mode of tagging Laces.

Laces are pieces of flat braid of silk, floss-silk, or linen which have tags at one or both ends. Take a thin strip of copper about an inch long, and four to five lines wide. These strips are called tags and are sold already prepared. Lay the strip over the end of a plain table, or on the edge of a window-sill. Roll the end of the braid, and place it lengthways over the strip so that it exceeds the latter a little. Fold the strip lengthways to the left over the braid, by striking it lightly with a hammer. Then fold it to the right in the same manner, and the end of the braid will be securely enclosed in this kind of case. If a few threads of the braid escape the inside of the tag, cut them off with scissors. The tag must be pointed at the end and a little wider at the top, where there is a rather marked groove produced by the union of the two parts of the strip. The two parts are rolled one over the other at the end of the tag.

When a lace comes apart, that is, it comes out of the tag, you may easily remedy this. Gently spread the wider part of the tag with small pliers, and insert the end of the rolled lace as far as you can without un-rolling the pointed end of the tag. Then re-fold the tag over the braid with a hammer, as I have just explained. You may always remove the tag by opening it with pliers.

The Mode of preparing Woollen Garters with Slip-knots.

Take a large ball of the white wool which is used to knit petticoats. (For knitting petticoats and garters, see Chapter XVII.) Unwind a needleful about an ell, or an ell and a quarter long. Spread this needleful on a table, and double and redouble it, until it forms a flat cord an inch and a few lines wide. Be careful that no part of the wool is tightened. Then cut off this white wool and put it aside. Take a little ball or skein of wool coloured blue, red, or green. Take one end of it and use it to tie the end of your cord. Then make a slip-knot with the coloured wool, and pass your cord through the knot, which you tighten only as much as is necessary to en-compass the cord without puckering it. The slip-knot must be made very near to the end of the cord, but henceforth it is necessary to repeat it at a distance of about two inches, and so on up to the end of the cord, where you finish it as you began. Then the garter is completed, and you make the second of the pair.

These garters have the advantage of supporting your stockings with-out being too tight on your leg. When you have the bad habit of wearing your garters below the knee, and wish to correct it, for some time you should wear these garters both above and below your knee.

The Mode of pinking Ruches and Flounces of *Gros de Naples, Crêpe Lissé,* or *Crêpe Gaufré.*

The bands which form these trimmings are not pinked with scissors, because the points would be unequal, and you might waste much time at it. Instead, spread out the material which you wish to divide into bands on a clean, but plain, table. Measure the proper height for the band, place a guide at this measure, and draw lightly along the guide with a pencil. Then take a punch which has the kind of points you wish to cut out, and apply it on the straight line which you have just drawn (the end of each point on the line). When you lift it, you will find that the band which you have just measured, and the edge of the material on which you will measure a new band, have been pinked at the same time. The concave parts of the points are found on one side, the convex ones on the other. The two bands are alike, and not a thread is wasted.

If the band is to be pinked on both edges, immediately repeat the operation. If on the contrary, the band is to be pinked on only one edge, measure the proper height from the pinked edge of the material, and cut along the straight-way at the final position of the measure. It is prudent to measure here and there across the band, in order to be quite sure that you do not cut higher or lower. Then resume punching until you have obtained all the bands necessary. As you separate the bands, fold them over themselves, and arrange them in a box or on a large piece of paper. When the bands are to be cut on the bias, you must position the guide and the punch in that direction.

If the points are to be large, and you do not have a punch, you may replace this instrument with a strip of rather stiff paper on which you have traced and cut out the points. Place this strip on the pencilled line exactly as you would place the punch. Pin the strip here and there so that it does not become disarranged, then lightly trace the undulations of the points with a pencil. Remove the paper and cut them out with scissors. To avoid tracing with a pencil, you may sometimes cut directly along the paper; but its stiffness is awkward, and the pinking is not so neat.

The Mode of Preparing Veils.

The easy operations of the haberdasher include the preparation of both veils with string-cases, and veils with tassels.

Veils with String-cases. These are square pieces of the white, green, or black silk gauze which is quite incorrectly called *gaze de laine* (see Div. 1). The string-case is marked by a groove and a raw edge across from the border. It is necessary to fold the raw edge over the groove, pass a *faveur* under the fold, and sew with small running stitches a little above the raw edge and over the groove. Since the material is clear, you may easily see whether you have stuck the needle into the *faveur,* which it is most necessary to avoid because the *faveur* must be able to glide through the case. It is all too easy to catch the selvage of the *faveur* without noticing; so it is well to pull it from time to time, to see if it has become caught. You could indeed sew the case in advance and then thread the *faveur* through it with a bodkin, but that operation crumples and dulls the gauze. Allow about an ell and a half for the *faveur,* so that the ends will come together to be fastened over the front of your head.

Veils with Tassels. Tasselled veils are also made for brides, in this way: cut out a square of tulle or gauze, of about five quarters in every direction. Make a hem all round, which is only basted, and put a thick, round, white silk braid over the edge of this hem, or a bias satin rouleau (the mode of preparing the rouleau is described in the article on *fichu* collars). Then take four thick white silk tassels of the kind called *glands à oeuf.* Thread a thin, round, white silk braid through a bodkin, and pass the bodkin through the fringe of the tassel. Try to make it come out at the hole which traverses the head. Your bodkin pulled though, make a strong knot at the end of the braid; pull it up to the knot and let a length of about an inch and a half come through the head of the tassel. This braid is a kind of tail for the tassel and makes it graceful, for without it the tassel would be stiff and heavy. Finish by sewing the end of the braid to one corner of the veil, under the satin rouleau or the thick braid, so that the stitches are not seen. Do the same for the other three tassels.

The Mode of making Riband Bows.

Riband bows may be single, double, triple, or quadruple. The loops of which they are formed are called *coques.* These loops are made over the fingers, or with a needle, with a band and a stay, according to their number, their size, and the firmness of the riband.

Small and Middle-sized Bows. A bow with two loops is made over the fingers by a particular mode. Take a piece of riband, whose length depends upon the width and size which you wish your loops to have. Fold the riband in half, and pull a little more of the folded piece to the left.

Then ask someone to extend both of her forefingers (folding her others) distanced from each other according to the size of your bow, and to keep her fingers stiff. Put the middle of the riband over her forefingers, letting it fall a little more to the left. Then take the left end, pass it under the right end, and bring it to the exact middle of the riband placed between her fingers. Again pass it under, and tie it tightly between her fingers with the right end. The bow is formed, and you may take it off her fingers, each of which is now found to hold a loop. You will perceive why I have said that you should allow more length at the left end of the riband. As it makes all those turns and re-turns, it would be much shorter than the other end without this preparation.

When the bow is small and of narrow riband, do not cut off, according to the piece or the quantity of the riband which you have, the portion which you must use to make it. Merely take the end of the riband, fold it in the middle lengthways, and lay only your left thumb over the fold, letting hang an end of riband two, or two and a half inches long. After that take the opposite end of the riband, and fold it as I have just explained, but with your right thumb and forefinger, and join it to the folded part of the first end, which your left thumb is still holding. Your left thumb and forefinger then likewise hold this new fold which you have made for about an eighth of an ell, according to the size of the loop which is formed. Furthermore, that is not measured; your eye suffices to estimate the size and justness of bows when they are of small or middle size. This loop finished, make a new one by again folding the riband at a distance equal to that of the first loop, bringing back this new fold between your left thumb and forefinger, and under the knot which these fingers are already supporting.

Then take a needleful of strong thread in your right hand, and wind it several times round the knot between the loops, and precisely at the point where your left thumb is pressing. Pull firmly and tie both ends of the thread. Release the bow then, because it is finished, and you have only to detach it from the piece of riband, cutting to the measure of the first end which falls from the knot. The more the thread is tightened, the more gracefully and firmly the loops will stand up.

Bows with several different loops are made in exactly the same way. Re-fold the riband four, six, or even eight times, instead of twice. Observe that you progressively make the loops a little larger so that they are staged; otherwise they will be confounded with each other and have no charm.

Large Bows. When the riband is broad and the bow large, you must measure the first loop. You may still do so by approximation, but it is essential that you measure the following loops by the first. This mode of measuring is so easy that the person who sees you make the bow does not notice that it is being measured. Indeed, it is but a matter of bringing the riband to the level of the first loop, supporting it a moment with your left forefinger, for which then the third finger on the same hand rapidly does the office of holding the first loop, next of forming the second fold parallel to the first. At a pinch there is not even any need to move your forefinger. Besides, the third finger replaces it with the greatest ease, even from the first loop; so that you may, if you wish or if you use gauze riband, support it from then on with your forefinger.

To fasten a large bow securely, it is advisable to thread a needle and alternately wind and sew the thread. Underneath, at the junction of the loops, some persons apply a small doubled piece of the straw which is used in mounting hats, or even a little pasteboard stay. This practice is very sound for large bows of wide *gros de Naples* riband, and for all very stout ribands. Save for these it is unnecessary.

Large bows which have a stay ordinarily have also a band. This is an inch-long piece of the riband used to make the bow. Fold this piece in thirds, baste it underneath so that the stitches do not show above, and make it encircle the point where the loops are joined after they have been securely fastened. When the riband has a certain stiffness, it is unnecessary to baste the band.

Half-bows. A bow with a single loop, or half-bow, is begun like all the other bows. But as soon as the loop is held between your left thumb and forefinger, rather than making another turn to the right, turn this loop still more to the left. Take the end of the riband which is held separately, and wrap it round your forefinger. Then cutting it rather close, put it into the little round loop which your forefinger, which had been wrapped round it, left on being removed. Tighten it well, and the loop is held by a true knot which requires only to be supported with thread.

In discussing the single bow after the compound bows, I appear to reverse the order which I have followed until now. But otherwise, I would have had too much trouble making myself understood. Moreover, bows with a single loop come almost at the last because for some time they have only been put in coiffures *en cheveux,* or amongst the trimmings of caps.

Excepting doubled loops, which require separate measures, here are the ordinary measures for riband bows. For a small bow, a quarter; for a medium bow, a third; for a very large bow, half an ell. Half-bows require a quarter. Sometimes bows are fringed at the ends; I shall explain that when I discuss belts.

The Mode of making Belts.

Belts are made in several fashions: 1st., belts fastened at the back with a bow of several loops. 2nd., belts *à chou* (this outmoded fashion may return). 3rd., belts with sewed loops, without a knot or ends. 4th., belts lined with taffety or gauze, with or without gummed toile or buckram. 5th., belts with buckles of steel or any other metal. 6th., belts with shoulder-straps (a pretty fashion which has already been revived several times). 7th., belts bordered with corded piping. 8th., elastic belts.

Belts Fastened at the Back. These are composed of a front (waist riband) and a bow, because the front of the riband is not made so wide as the bow. Since it would be necessary to fold it over itself in the front, that would be a waste. The bow must be made beforehand, because if you were to tie and untie the riband every time that you dressed and undressed, it would quickly become crumpled and stained. Besides this disadvantage, the bow would never have so much grace and elegance.

The width of the riband used to encircle the waist is Nos. 7 and 9, and that of the riband for the bow is Nos. 12 and 16. Ordinarily five-eighths of an ell of riband is required to go round the waist, because it is customary to cross the ends over each other a little; however, that depends upon the size of the person. As for the bow, use three-quarters of an ell, but fashion varies the measure for the bow a great deal; sometimes the ends are nearly an ell long. Bows are sometimes placed in the front of the waist, which is quite charming; but whether they are placed in the front or at the back, whenever the ends are long, it is elegant to fringe them by ravelling. Here is how to accomplish this:

First cut off both selvages of your riband lengthways for the space of about two to three inches, according to the length of fringe which you desire. If you are arranging a simple fringe, two, or two and a half inches will suffice. If you plan to make a deeper fringe, three and a half inches will not be excessive. Whatever the size decided upon, when your selvages have been removed, take a strong pin and pull the crossways threads of the silk, so much on the right, so much on the left, to avoid puckering the riband. At first this operation is extremely easy; but as you advance it will prove more difficult, because withdrawing the crossways threads is hampered by the length of the ravelled lengthways ones; you must also pull the thread in the middle, and that several times if the riband is very wide. When the ravelling is finished, go over it and even it out with either the pin or the point of your scissors, and cut the end crossways, so that no thread exceeds the others. This is the simple fringe.

If the fringe is double, divide the threads into several parts, and tie them on a netting mould so as to form a mesh. Work one or several rows according to your taste, but two rows are good enough. Let very long ends fall to make the threads of this kind of fringe.

When the riband is all of the same colour, you may match a silk fringe to it, and attach it to the end of the riband with very small over-cast stitches. However, I do not advise this; the effect produced by this fringe is not half so pretty as that of the previous one.

Belts fastened at the back sometimes have the bow sewed to one end of the waist riband. This practice affords more strength than beauty, because in fastening the belt, you must inevitably handle and crumple the bow. It is better to begin by putting on the waist riband, and then place the bow.

Belts *à Chou.* These are no longer made, but probably they will return; let us occupy ourselves with them for a moment. Cut out, as usual, a riband to encircle your waist; or instead cut a band of material crossways, fold it double, and sew the two edges together with running stitches or side-stitches. Then take a little square of similar material, or of wide riband. Round it by cutting off a little to the right and left, top and bottom, but principally on top. The piece thus prepared ought to be five or six inches wide, and about an eighth of an ell high in the middle, and a sixteenth at its edges. Gather it all round on the wrong side of the material or riband; then crossways, while leaving a third of the *chou* (as this shaped piece is called) from the bottom. Gather it again (see Fig. 1, *s*).

Then place the bottom of the *chou* at the half, or the third, of the length of the waist riband, according to whether you wish to fasten the riband at the front of your chest or under your arms. Ordinarily the latter position is preferred. Mark the *chou* in the middle, and fix this point with a pin at the position chosen on the waist riband. Over-cast the wrong side of the *chou* to one edge on the right side of the riband, bringing the

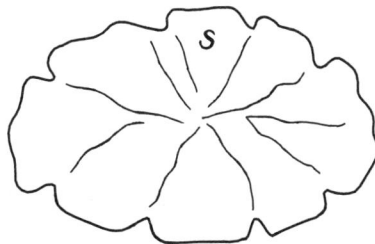

Figure 1. A *chou.*

gathers of the *chou* towards the pin which marks the middle. This seam finished, raise the *chou* over the riband and sew the second crossways gathering flat in the way you would place a rouleau trimming; that is, by making it puff out over the riband, evening out the gathers of this second seam, parallel to the first. Finish by sewing the top of the *chou* underneath to the wrong side of the riband, again evening out the gathers and making them puff out. As this part of the *chou* is very much rounded, the two side parts spread out in a circle over the riband, whereas just a little is sewed underneath. The side parts must, as far as possible, be sewed inside before the upper part is sewed underneath. When the *chou* is too small, sew the side parts across the riband, and prick-stitch it underneath. Then you may raise it with your finger-tips.

Belts with Sewed Loops, without a Knot or Ends. This kind is now the fashion, and though it has the disadvantage of making your waist appear larger (especially when the loops are large and numerous) it is necessary to discuss it with my readers. For this kind of belt, as for the first ones I described, measure the waist riband, then arrange the loops to the right and left, either over the right end of the riband or over a stay, holding tight the point where you are sewing them. This especially concerns satin belts.

I have yet to speak of another kind of belt with loops, but it has also metal buckles and a partial lining. So that you may comprehend it more easily, I shall explain it in a separate article, after those kinds of belts.

Lined Belts. The lining of a belt is sometimes made of gauze. In that case the belt is a satin riband supported by a band of gummed gauze, sewed with running stitches, long on the wrong side and extremely short on the right side, which you invariably prick-stitch to the selvage of the riband. This lining may also be of taffety, and then it is placed behind a gauze riband, whether this is plain white, white with coloured stripes, or any other. Whichever it is, the taffety is always the background colour. Most often both linings are found together in the same belt, as follows:

To add some firmness to the gauze, satin, or taffety riband of which the belt is composed, cut a band of starched toile or buckram the width and length of the waist riband. Line this with a taffety band, which you baste on the inside of the toile in such a manner that the stitches will not be seen on the taffety. That done, place the waist riband (if it is not transparent) directly over the toile, and sew it by its selvages to the lining as I have just explained. But if it is of gauze, apply a band of Chambery gauze or *gaze d'Italie* to the toile or buckram, on the side opposite to the taffety, so that the toile is not seen through the material of the riband.

Belts with Metal Buckles. These have no need of full linings because they are made of strong moiré riband. They do, however, need two little partial linings. The buckle is fitted to the belt by means of a double tongue, which passes lengthways through a crossways button-hole. So that it will be firmly held, fold the end of the riband over itself for nearly an inch and a half, and work the button-hole in the crossways middle of the lining. The folded riband must be sewed with side-stitches, so that the two parts which follow the button-hole do not hinder placing the buckle. This is the first little lining.

The button-hole made, encircle your waist with the riband, and mark the point through which the prongs of the buckle must pass. Because the prongs will not fail to tear the riband after a certain time, it is well to place a piece of taffety on the under side of this point. The taffety should be of a colour similar to that of your belt. It is useless to sew this second lining vertically on the riband, because the stitches would be seen and have an ugly effect. It is enough to make a wide seam fold on each edge, and to sew this second lining with small running stitches onto the selvage of the riband. When you tighten the belt forcefully, the buckle will widen, so it is proper to put this piece of lining a little to the back of the point which you measured.

This belt must exceed the waist measure by at least an eighth of an ell, so that you may easily insert the riband into the buckle and fold it one, two, or three times under the buckle, which results in flat loops to the right of that ornament.

If you also want flat loops to the left of the buckle, take a quarter, or a third of an ell, or more, than the measure of the toile, according to the number of loops which you desire. Then sew them securely, one over the other, commencing with the largest and diminishing them gradually. Sew them to the precise point where the waist riband joins the buckle. Pull yourself in well to obtain this measure; otherwise the buckle, which continually pulls on the belt, will render it too loose. The prongs must pass directly beside the last loop. Those which you will make with the end of the riband to the right of the buckle, must be of the same number and size as those to the left. You understand that the piece of lining put to withstand the strain of the prongs must be very narrow; all the same it is necessary to use one.

Belts with Shoulder-straps. This kind of belt is the prettiest and the most becoming to the figure. It has been fashionable for a long time, principally for balls. (See Div. 2.) This fashion differs a little from those of the belts which I just described.

Take some satin riband No. 12, or better still satin by the piece, because you must cut the riband, which being wide only at one end, would cost dear in waste. A quarter, or a third at most of satin will suffice to make a belt. Cut two bands crossways the height of ordinary waist riband, but terminating as shown in Fig. 2 *A;* these are the belt pieces. Cut as well two shoulder-straps similar, in part, to those of a pair of stays; but differing a great deal in the lower part; see Fig. 2 *B.* Place the pointed end of the shoulder-strap over the pointed end of the belt; baste them together.

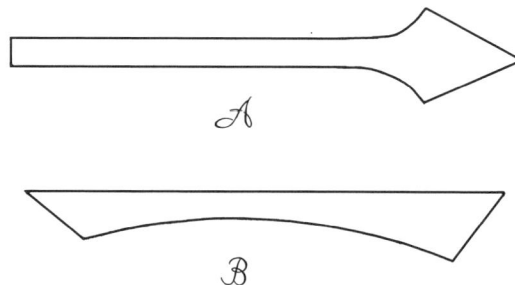

A

B

Figure 2. The pieces for a belt with shoulder-straps.

Then cut out a lining exactly like this and apply it to the joined ends, basting along the entire length (it is better to apply the lining before basting the ends together, but you may still do it afterwards). Prick-stitch with very small stitches along the basting, catching the lining which you have also basted underneath, making there a seam fold. If the stitches have not pierced all the way through, turn it down lightly underneath with side-stitches. Then sew all round the shoulder-strap, and the upper and lower edges of the belt, where you have already made a seam fold. The side-stitches which serve to make the false hem will be hidden by a silk braid which you sew all round the edge of the belt, on the right side. It will be necessary to take some stitches inside the twist of the braid underneath, so that it seems in some sort glued. This half of the belt finished, make the other in precisely the same way.

Unless you have the exact measure of the shoulder-straps, it is well to try on the belt before finishing it, while it is still basted. It goes without saying that the length of the shoulder-straps varies according to the hollowing for the arms. Pass your arm through the shoulder-strap, so that the place where it is attached to the belt is at the back. This belt goes round the back and will be attached in front of the chest. The other belt piece is placed in the same way, so that the shoulder-strap which belongs to the left arm passes under the right arm, and that which belongs to the right arm passes under the left arm. This crosses the two pieces in the front becomingly, and you pin them to the belt at the bottom of the back, one over the other.

When you wish to embellish one of these belts, add the tops of sleeves matched to the trimmings of the gown. This kind of sleeve top is called an épaulette or mancheron.

Belts bordered with Corded Piping. These are quite modern. They are now used all the time when the belt is of a material similar to that of the gown, which is even more elegant than a riband. Cut a band to replace the waist riband; then cut narrow strips on the bias for the piping; wrap a cotton cord in this bias strip. Then turning over the cord thus wrapped onto the waist-band, sew it with back-stitches, tightening it well over the piping. When the waist-band is trimmed with this piping all along both crossways edges, turn down the two excess pieces which fall from the covered cord, and put it over the band which lines the belt, which you sew all round the piping with side-stitches. If you wish the belt to be stiff, put on a band of buckram at the same time as the lining which covers it, as I explained earlier. Make a seam in the middle to fit the shape of your waist.

Proceed in the same way for the bow or the loops without ends. This style of belt is in the domain of the mantua-maker, but I did not wish either to omit it, or to write a separate article for it.

Elastic Belts. These are so in whole or in part. They are formed with elastics which you sew between two ribands, sometimes at the waist for all the width and length of the belt; sometimes only under the bosom, leaving an interval in the middle of the front. I shall say no more, because the mode of sewing elastics is the same as described in Chapter XVIII.

Riband *Fichus.*

The ribands arranged as *fichus* which are now worn confirm what I have already often had occasion to repeat: fashions become new when they are very old, because it is quite eighteen years since riband *fichus* were in style. What is new is only what is forgotten.

Nothing is simpler to make, and even to describe (which does not always follow). Take a piece of wide riband, whose length depends upon the size which you desire in the front. Fold it double crossways, wrong side out. Keeping the riband folded, make a bias line in the middle with another fold, which begins at the point where the two selvages are placed together. Pass a thread over this line, then sew with back-stitches along the thread. This operation gives the right side of the riband a conical shape, which is called the point of the *fichu* (see Fig. 3).

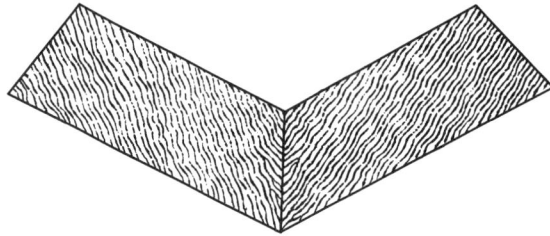

Figure 3. The point of a *fichu*.

The backs of all *fichus* of this kind are made thus, but the fronts vary much. Some have a bow at the level of the neck, such as the *séducteurs*. Others have long ends, which are crossed and fall to the knees, or are put on like a stole or scarf. Others have a new *fichu* point to the right and left at the level of each shoulder, or the riband which passes flat over the shoulder is trimmed at that part with little bows or riband points. The last are most often produced by cutting an end of riband about three inches long, and folding both edges of the selvage slantways to one end, so that this end presents a *dent de harpie*. (See Chapter XV.) The other end is gathered and sewed under the riband of the *fichu*. Three or five points prepared thus are put there: it depends upon the manner in which you tighten or loosen the gathers, and still more upon the width of the riband. The belt must always be matched to the riband of the *fichu*.

I have nothing to say about *séducteurs* because earlier I described every kind of bow in detail. I shall only add that it is well, in this case, to make the bow beforehand on one side of the riband, and to fasten both ends of the *fichu* (that which holds the bow, and the other which is nothing but the ends), with a brass hook and eye. This practice is also very sound for the strings of a hat or cap, because it preserves the riband. But you must avoid dividing the bow; that is, putting a loop at the end of one string, and a loop followed by its end on the other, because the hook and the split in the bow may easily be seen, which is altogether without grace. I do not advise using a hook for bows on belts, because the waist riband, needing to be well tightened, must be entirely free.

The riband *fichus* worn formerly were *séducteurs* without loops, which were trimmed all round with narrow, pointed tulle.

The *Fichu* or Belt *à la Duchesse.*

Since the last Carnival a very elegant kind of *fichu* has been worn, which is also in the domain of the haberdasher (see Fig. 4). This is a wide bias band of light-coloured satin or gauze, which begins from the belt at the middle of the back, is fastened in a point over the shoulder, and goes on to make a new point at the belt, at the middle of the chest. It goes without saying that there is a similar band on the other side. This band must form three or four large plaits, fastened to each other with running stitches. As the stitches of each plait are hidden by the next one, they are not seen. At the place where the *fichu* back and front begin, as well as on each shoulder, there should be a gauze bow or puff. If the *fichu* is of satin, it is trimmed all round with pointed blond lace, or plain tulle folded double lengthways.

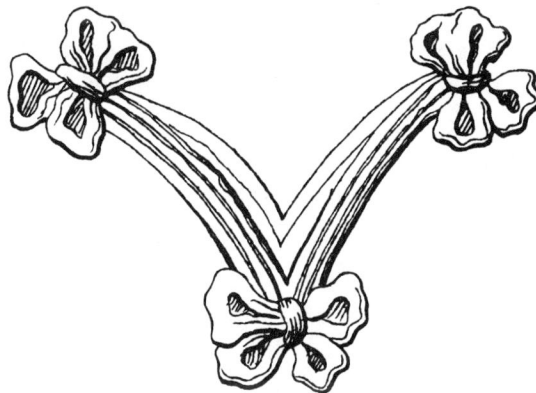

Figure 4. The *fichu à la Duchesse.*

This *fichu* is also very simply made with wide riband which is made to go flat from the belt to the shoulders. Bows are placed there, and there is always a similar belt. Gauze riband, being the most elegant, is properest for this kind of ornament. The end of this *fichu* sometimes falls nearly to the knee.

The Mode of making Fancy *Fichus.*

Richly-ornamented *fichus* are made of *gaze de laine*, *crêpe lissé*, *crêpe gaufré*, plain or embroidered silk tulle, white satin rouleaux, white silk braid, matching buttons, and blond. They are often in the same style as percale or muslin *fichus;* but whereas *lingères* deal in those, elegant haberdashers make only the first.

My purpose is not to describe all possible fashions of *fichus.* I wish only, while indicating the principal shapes and ornaments, to put my readers in the way of following all the caprices of fashion without effort. For example, *fichus* are trimmed with single or double ruches, box-plaits *en coquilles,* and blond with satin rouleaux. They are made with puffs, plaits, *entre-deux,* and standing or falling collars. These last are single, double, or triple; round or square; with points of several kinds. All this is infinitely varied, but should not frighten you in the least. Once you are acquainted with the cut of *fichus,* the principles of trimming, and the mode of cutting out collars and staging them, you have only to look at the new styles or procure models to imitate them easily, since you know their unvarying principles.

Of cutting out and making up *Fichus.* A *fichu* is always composed of a back and two fronts (see Fig. 5) unless it is a *guimpe,* which on the contrary has one front and two backs (see Fig. 6). When the *guimpe* is *à la Vierge* (this old style is returning), it is much more low-necked and has no collar. Sometimes the fronts are joined to the back of a *fichu,* under the arms, like the body of a gown. This practice, which requires more material, is quite unnecessary except for *fichu-canezous* meant to be worn over the gown. These are presently very much worn. I shall discuss them later; for the moment let us occupy ourselves with *fichus* to be worn underneath, which have the greatest number of variations.

When you have cut out your *fichu* by a full-sized pattern, make a seam fold on the crossways bias of the back, which is called the shoulder bias. The seam fold must be marked on the right side: you will see why.

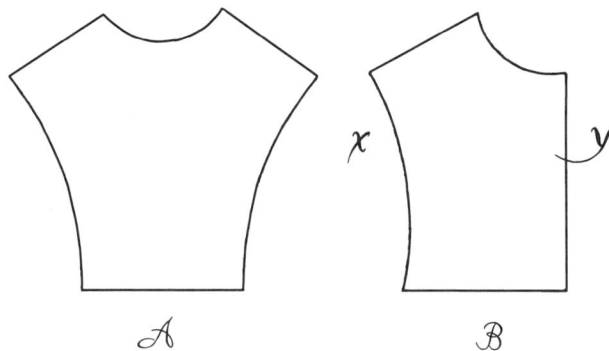

Figure 5. A *fichu* opening in the front.

Making *Fichus*.

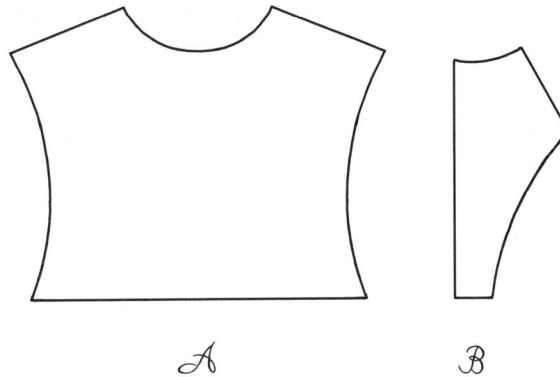

Figure 6. A *guimpe* opening at the back.

Then make a seam fold on the wrong side, on the shoulder bias of the fronts, and lay this seam fold on that of the back. In this way the seam which you will work for these two pieces will be completely turned down on the wrong side, and without any raw edges. Baste these two pieces; then prick-stitch them along the basting (when the *fichu* is made of percale or muslin, prick-stitch two rows). If it is of very light gauze or silk tulle which does not wash, you may be satisfied with working this middle seam by herring-boning very closely on the wrong side. The *fichu* being made up, that is, the two fronts joined in this fashion to the back, hem the side parts, marked by *x*, and those of the front, marked by *y* (see Fig. 5 *B*). Then make a string-case at the bottom of the fronts and the back, and pass a linen tape through it to fasten the *fichu* round the waist. That is a good mode; the following is even better:

Put the string-case only on the back; or prick-stitch the back, gathering it onto a wide linen tape two, or two and a half inches long. Pass a narrow linen tape or a braid about an ell and a half long through the case; or cut the tape into two parts and sew them to the two ends of the wide tape which you sewed to the bottom of the back. That done, hem the bottom of both fronts, which must be at least two inches longer than if you were making an ordinary string-case. The reason for this increase is that when you put on the *fichu,* you cross both fronts over your bosom, and fasten them there by means of the tape or braid which begins at the back. You will perceive that if the fronts are not long enough to exceed the tape which holds them by two or three inches, they will not fail to come open at the slightest movement which you make. This fashion is preferable to the first, in that crossing the fronts imparts more grace to the collar. Besides, you are not obliged to use a pin to prevent the fronts from opening, which constantly happens to *fichus* with ordinary string-cases, and this prevents many little tears.

It is often customary to place buttons in the front; but these buttons are there for show rather than for use, because it would be too much labour to work button-holes, or to put on braid to re-enforce them all (they must be placed very close together). Therefore, be content to button one at the top of the *fichu*, one or two in the middle, and as many at the bottom. More frequently still, none are buttoned at all, and the *fichu* is crossed as I have just explained.

It is now necessary to concern ourselves with making the *fichu* collar, which may be either standing or falling. The first style has always been more general.

Standing Collars for *Fichus*. Standing collars are single, double, round, or square, fastened in the front or at the back. The first kind is rarely seen. However, there are haberdashers who cut out collars in a single piece (see Fig. 7), and furnish them all round the top and bottom with a fine, narrow strip of wood, called a straw, such as milliners use together with brass wire to furnish hat crowns. (See Chapter XXI.) More often only the top is so furnished. The haberdasher places the edge of the collar on the straw, sews them together with running stitches, then conceals the straw with a white satin rouleau. Here is the way to place the rouleau. I beg my readers to pay attention to it, because it must often recur.

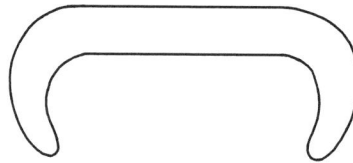

Figure 7. A standing collar all in one piece.

Cut a little bias strip of white satin, about ten lines to an inch wide, according to the size you wish to give the rouleau. The rounder and smaller it is, the prettier it is. Put the satin strip onto the collar, on the right side, and on the edge of the straw which is farthest from the edge of the collar. Sew it with back-stitches. Next turn down the satin strip so that it envelops at the same time the edge of the collar, and that of the straw. Roll it up well, fix it here and there with the fine pins called camions, then sew it as follows.

Raise the edge of the rouleau as much as possible; slant the threaded needle downwards; enter it on the edge of the straw and on the part of the rouleau which is found on top; then again enter it through the straw to make it stand out. This kind of sewing requires much care, but you will easily become practiced in it, and perform it afterwards with facility. Moreover, it is well to put the right side of the rouleau on the inside of the collar, that is to say, the side which must touch your neck. As this side of the rouleau is always the prettiest, it is better that it be in view; the other will be sufficiently hidden by the trimming.

When you furnish the compass of the collar with a fine brass wire, you may place there a satin rouleau made beforehand. This rouleau, which is much used to hide all kinds of seams, and to make ornaments for fancy *fichus,* is also within the domain of the milliner. Cut a narrow strip of satin as I explained for the first kind of rouleau; roll it over itself, turning one edge down. Finish by sewing the last edge underneath the rouleau, onto the corresponding part at this edge. Sew with running stitches, at the same time sticking the needle into this edge and into the corresponding part, but never into the upper part of the rouleau, because it is essential that no stitches be visible when the rouleau is placed onto the material. It must have the air of being glued. When the rouleau is finished, place it on the part which it must cover, then sew it lightly underneath, so that the stitches are invisible. When you wish to put a rouleau of this kind on the edge of a collar furnished with brass wire, it is well to place beforehand a very narrow *faveur* on the edge *à cheval,* to prevent the situation where the rouleau allows the brass wire to be seen.

You may also replace the strip of straw and the brass wire with a very supple narrow white whale-bone. If you wish to avoid applying a satin rouleau, as well as the straw, wire, or whale-bone, you may encircle the collar with pretty brass wire trimmed with white silk in very tight spirals. This sells for 4 to 5 sous per ell, and that is for the very best. To give collars some stiffness, you may also use a kind of muslin riband into which is woven very light metal threads.

Double standing collars differ very little from single ones. Cut two collar pieces instead of one, baste them together in the middle, and enter the straw, whale-bone, or brass wire between the two edges. For all else, follow the rules for single collars.

For square standing collars, make upright cases for little white whale-bones at the two side parts, at the middle, and half-way between the sides and the middle. Enter the bones into the cases, after having wrapped the ends with a little tuft of cotton wadding to prevent them from piercing the gauze and pricking your neck. It is equally necessary to place the cotton before closing off the case, fastening the whale-bone at the place where the collar is joined to the *fichu.*

These supports are called stays. They are also put on round collars when the crape or gauze of which the collar is made lacks firmness. You may instead make them of a straw, covered at the top and bottom of the collar with a very narrow satin rouleau. This is rarely done because the material of the collar ordinarily holds up by itself, but stays may become necessary when the *fichu* has been worn several times. Furthermore, the shape of these collars forbids placing stays in the front.

Avoid making standing collars too flared; that would have a common and affected air. Also avoid tightening them too much, because then they lack grace, and the trimming produces no effect at all.

Standing collars are fastened at the back for *guimpes,* and in the front for *fichus.* In the first case, they are joined by little hooks or light buttons. The mode of cutting them out is always the same. It is only necessary to divide them in the middle, and to make the part hollowed out several lines longer, in order to overlap the two hollowed ends at the back. When you wish to make the collar fall over itself a little, make it a little higher, and do not put stays or a straw at the bottom. When a collar closes in the front, absolutely nothing is done to fasten it because the *fichu* brings the two edges sufficiently close together in crossing over the chest, as I described above.

A standing collar is set on by placing the *fichu* over the lower edge, and sometimes this seam is covered by a narrow satin rouleau. When the rouleau is absent, the seam is made on the inside. That is, you sew at the same time the bottom of both parts of the collar with the *fichu,* straighten these parts, and the seam is found to be hidden. But in this case you do not need to furnish the collar with the straw and satin until it is set on. This practice, though excellent, is little used for *fichus* of crape, tulle, or gauze. It is enough to set on the collar on the right side, save for then hiding the seam with the final trimming.

Trimmings for Standing Collars. These consist of ruches—single, double, triple, or *à coquilles*—in a single or folded band. Ruches are strips of clear material, such as blond, gauze, or tulle, which are disposed in box-plaits. They are ordinarily made on a very narrow cotton tape, or on a narrow flat white silk braid, or likewise and most commonly on the folded selvage of a piece of gauze. If they were made directly on the *fichu* they would crumple it too much where the plaits were sewed; it is better to sew the middle of the ruche lightly to the *fichu* after it has been made.

Moreover, this mode may be used with all kinds of plaited trimmings. But now I shall describe the mode of making trimmings with box-plaits, which are called ruches or *chicorées*.

The piece of braid must be the length of the article to be trimmed. Fold it into two equal parts. Fold the strip likewise, and attach the middle of the one to the middle of the other. Put the braid over your knees, and the strip (let us suppose it to be blond) at its lengthways middle onto the braid. Make a fold to the right on the blond; fasten the fold with a stitch, then make a fold to the left and fasten it likewise. *Voilà,* a box-plait. Begin another right next to it, taking good care to make it neither deeper nor shallower; and so on. The deeper the plaits, the closer the two edges of the band approach each other and give an agreeable effect.

That is a single ruche. For a double ruche, choose a braid which is a little wider, but only by a few threads, because it is essential that the double ruche does not spread apart. Take a strip similar to the one you have just arranged as a ruche. Lift one side of the first ruche, and place the new strip on the edge of the braid which already supports the ruche. This second strip must be arranged exactly like the first. Proceed delicately in order not to crumple the preceding plaits. (See Fig. 8.)

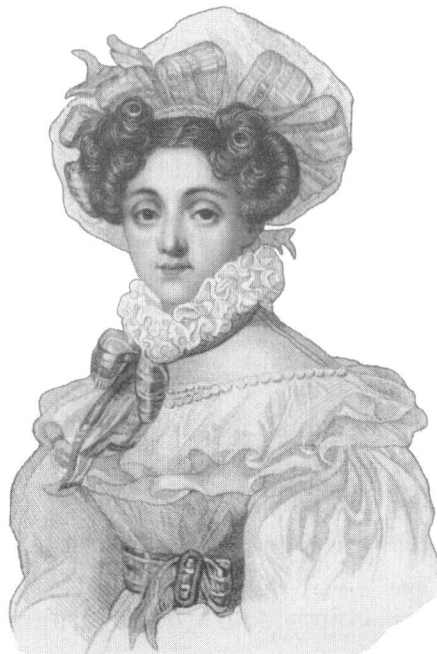

Figure 8. A lady wearing a clear *fichu* with a ruched collar.

The triple ruche is obtained by placing a half-strip between the two doubles.

Box-plaits are redoubled two, three, four, or even five times on each side. This makes a very large plait, which stands up and curls in such a manner that it is called a box-plait *en coquilles*. The ruches formed by these latter plaits are always in a single row. These trimmings have been worn for ever.

But one kind of ruche which dates solely from our time is the one made with bias strips of *gaze de laine*, which you fold double lengthways, and arrange in box-plaits by sewing both edges of the strip at the same time, so that the crease of the fold forms the edge of the trimming. You understand that these strips cannot be arranged in the middle. When you wish to have a folded edge on both sides, you must necessarily put a new strip at the same place where you sewed the preceding one, and arrange the plaits face to face. Then cut very close the short ravelled threads which may remain along the seam of the box-plaits. But this step is usually superfluous, given that the plaits, which meet up in being straightened, completely hide the middle of the ruche where you have sewed. Besides, these strips are hardly ever placed opposite to each other except on caps. They are staged one over another on *fichus*, to the number of three, five, or six rows, according to the size of the plaits, the height of the strips, and that of the collar. The seam which you work at the bottom of each strip, to fasten the box-plaits, is hidden by the top of the next strip. Place a narrow white silk braid or a narrow satin rouleau over the bottom of the last one; or even better trim the collar separately, then set it on inside the *fichu*.

Often trimmed collars are made without setting them onto a *fichu*. Then it is always necessary to put a straw in the bottom, and to edge them with a *faveur* in glossy white taffety, placed *à cheval*. These collars are pinned to the standing collars of high-necked gowns, or basted to a muslin *fichu*, which is infinitely better.

Standing collars trimmed in this fashion (in strips of gauze lined with black) are very elegant for mourning *fichus*. Box-plaits are used to trim standing collars of plain or pointed white silk blond, silk tulle, and cotton tulle. Standing collars of *fichus de lingère*, which are of percale, muslin, or cotton gauze, should always have gathered trimmings. These trimmings are composed of muslin and muslin gauze, or tulle attached to a narrow strip of gauze. However, cotton gauze *fichus* trimmed with cotton tulle should have ruches of box-plaits.

Falling Collars for *Fichus*. Falling collars of *fichus de mercière* have recently been infinitely varied, so I shall describe only the principal styles. (See Div. 3.) They are little pelerines, square (see Fig. 9 *A*), rounded (see Fig. 9 *B*), Vandyked (see Fig. 9 *C*), or double (see Fig. 9 *D*). Take a paper pattern of the collar which you have chosen (it is enough to have the shape of half the collar). Fold the material on the bias or the straight-way, following the model (it is nearly always on the straight-way). Fix the paper pattern on top of the material with pins, and cut all round.

Falling collars are set on the right side of the *fichu,* by means of a mantua-maker's hem worked with running stitches. This seam is made on the right side because the collar hides it in being turned down, and it would be visible all round the neck if it were sewed on the wrong side. Falling collars are trimmed in a thousand ways: with ruches, plaits, gauze rouleaux, satin rouleaux arranged in points, goffered puffs, plain puffs, and puffs divided by rouleaux and by bands of tulle or blond *entre-deux.*

If the collar is entirely composed of puffs crossed by blond *entre-deux* or satin rouleaux, you must cut them out differently than I explained previously. The entire pattern, not just the half, must be spread out on the table where you are working. As you gather, fold the strip into small box-plaits to form a puff. Lay the pattern over it, fixing it at the bottom, the top, and the middle with camions in order not to disarrange it. Then make a new puff near the last one, in the same way, leaving between them the space required to receive the *entre-deux.* (If the puffs were only divided by a rouleau, you would proceed quite differently.) When the pattern is entirely covered by a succession of puffs and *entre-deux* placed alternately, fix them together lightly with camions. Remove the paper pattern, then sew on the wrong side.

I have created the impression that you do not divide the material for making puffs which have satin rouleaux, and that is indeed the case. Take a square piece which should be a little less than double the model, be it in width or length, and separate the puffs only by gathering, beginning at the middle of the collar. Then cut out the piece in the front as required, and apply a satin rouleau over each gathering.

These two kinds of collars are then trimmed with blond or pointed silk tulle, which you gather only a little. Place them flat with running stitches on the edge of the collar, on which you have marked a seam fold on the right side. A satin rouleau hides at the same time the seam fold, the stitches, and the gathered selvage of the tulle or blond.

When fancy falling collars are smooth and all in one piece, hem them on the wrong side, always with small running stitches. The light materials of which they are composed, such as gauze, crape, or silk tulle, will not wash, so it is needless to use more secure stitches. Moreover, those would

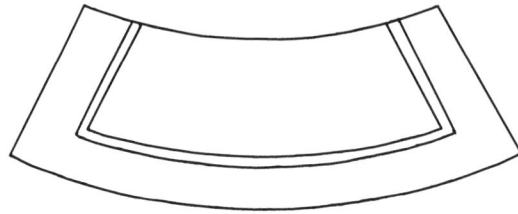

A

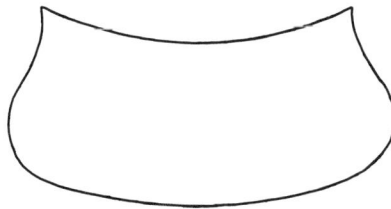

B

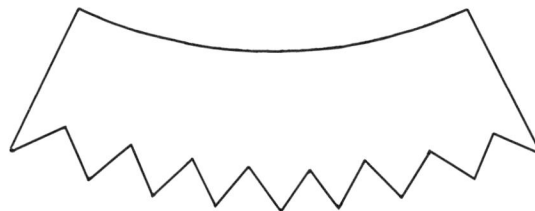

C

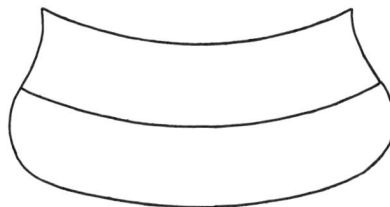

D

Figure 9. Divers shapes for collars.

injure the charm and freshness of these articles, which must be handled as little as possible and have the air of being untouched.

Then you trim them, be it with a blond or tulle ruche, or plaited strips of gauze; be it with plaited strips of *crêpe lissé* or *crêpe gaufré;* but placed a little loose like the bias trimmings of gowns. These strips should be wide, tolerably full, and closely fit the shape of the collar. Sew a braid or a narrow rouleau over the seam which joins the two edges. Ordinarily two rows are put close together, or separated by one or several satin rouleaux. For the latter, the strips are a little less wide. As crape has some firmness, the upper fold of the strip naturally leaves between itself and the lower fold a small and graceful interval, which it is important to preserve while sewing.

Gaze de laine biases are also placed in this way, but these biases and the preceding never trim any thing but round or square collars. It would be too difficult to make them follow the contours of Vandyked collars properly. These last have a trimming which is, as it were, particular, though sometimes it is used on square collars. I shall explain it, after having said that the styles of *fichus* which I just described are also made in black *gaze de laine* and black *crêpe lissé* for mourning.

The Vandyked collar receives a wide seam fold all round on the right side. (This is on the turned-down part, since with all these collars it is never a matter of the hollowed part, which is set onto the *fichu*.) This collar of *crêpe lissé* (not *crêpe gaufré*) or *gaze de laine* must be trimmed with similar material. Cut several little strips on the bias, about two inches wide, and make them into flat rouleaux. Sew them underneath in the same manner as the satin rouleaux described above. The rouleaux made, place the first on the edge of the collar, fixing it with camions here and there, and making it follow the indentations closely. Then turn the collar to the wrong side, to sew the rouleau from that side. The material being clear, you may see the join of both edges of the rouleau, and you must sew at that seam, avoiding entering the needle into the upper part of the rouleau, which may be done without difficulty. The first rouleau sewed in this fashion, place four, six, or seven others likewise (but the last number seems excessive to me) close together (see Div. 4), leaving between them an interval of only a few lines; unless you put a very narrow satin rouleau between each gauze rouleau, which necessarily requires that you space them a little wider and lessen the number of rows.

Whichsoever you choose, when your rouleaux have been placed, take flat buttons of very glossy white silk and apply them on every gauze rouleau at the very edges of the points, which will produce several lengthways rows of silver-white buttons on the crossways rows of flat white gauze rouleaux.

Vandyked collars are also trimmed, first with unplaited pointed blond, then with five, seven, or nine rows of white satin rouleaux close together, which follow the contours of the points.

Double falling collars are composed of a large collar, and a smaller collar which falls over the first. These collars are trimmed like all the others; only, the trimmings must not be too wide, since they are necessarily doubled: a single ruche of tulle, or plain or pointed blond, only lightly attached, suits them best. Baste the two collars one over the other, and set them on the *fichu* at the same time. Ordinarily a gauze riband matched to the toilet is passed between the collars, and tied in a bow in the front.

When you find that falling collars leave your neck too much uncovered, you may put a tulle ruche on top. However, this ruche, though very becoming for flat collars, becomes heavy and unbecoming on puffed collars, double collars, and collars whose trimmings are too spread out.

As I promised, I have spoken of all the fancy *fichus* which the haberdasher prepares. However, in order to leave nothing to be desired, I shall encroach a little upon the domain of the *lingère-couturière*, so that my readers may choose amongst all kinds of *fichus*.

Double and Single Three-cornered *Fichus*.

Nothing is so simple as these fichus, and yet nothing is more graceful when they are of very clear material. Take a square of *gaze de laine* or very fine lawn, double it like a shawl, and place it in the same way, fastening it in the front: this is the double *fichu*. The single *fichu* is a double *fichu* cut in half slantways. When the single *fichu* is of *gaze de laine*, it scarcely needs a hem. When it is of lawn or organdy, it should be trimmed with pointed tulle. Made of cotton tulle embroidered all over or only round the edge, it is at the same time simple and elegant.

Fichu-canezous.

Canezous properly speaking have long sleeves, and are really spencers of transparent material; I shall not discuss them. But sleeveless canezous are *fichus* to wear over gowns, and consequently within the plan of this chapter. Three things make a *fichu-canezou* different from an ordinary *fichu:* 1st., it is wider and longer; 2nd., it is sewed under the arms and has arm-holes like the body of a gown; 3rd., it is set on a belt like a gown. Furthermore, it has trimmed mancherons and a fan of plaits in the front. It is absolutely a body with no skirt or sleeves. The collar is like a *fichu* collar. *Fichu-canezous* are made of tulle with similar ruches, in lawn gauze, organdy, or starched muslin, always with very elegant trimmings. Haber-dashers rarely deal in them.

Somnambules and Shawls of Blond or Tulle.

The *somnambule,* so called after the *fichu* which plays an important role in the pretty play with this title, is a double pelerine which is long in the front, sometimes falling as far as the knees. There are small ones, which I advise you to make of cotton tulle which you may easily embroider, or of gauze, organdy, or lawn. Properly speaking, these small *somnambules* are *fichu-pelerines.* The grand *somnambules,* always of tulle, or white or black silk blond, are made commercially. You may, however, embroider the first, as well as the tulle shawls which are nothing but a veil embroidered all round, with a slightly raised garland. It goes without saying that these have no drawing-strings, and that they are folded like a shawl.

The Mode of making Cornettes and Fancy Caps.

The caps which are in the domain of the haberdasher, though of elegant materials such as *gaze de laine,* silk tulle, *crêpe lissé,* or *crêpe gaufré,* are perhaps the simplest of all, because caps embellished with ribands and trimmings, other than those round the edge, belong to the *lingère,* and mounted ones to the milliner. (See Div. 5.) Haberdashers therefore scarcely make more than the pretty cornettes which are worn under hats, or in the morning. I shall describe them precisely, then I shall add some details on the manner in which elegant Parisian *lingères* embellish the head-dresses which emerge from their hands.

Cornettes are ordinarily made of *gaze de laine,* cut in either three pieces like an infant's cap, or in two pieces, which fashion is called *à casque.* Another style is called *à la folle* or *à la jolie femme.*

Three-piece Caps. This kind of cap is sewed and trimmed as follows: make a seam fold on the right side around the rounded part of both side-pieces. Place the lengthways edges of the middle piece flat on top of it. Apply a white satin rouleau over this seam, sewing on the wrong side, after having fixed it to the right side with camions. Take care that the middle of the third piece is a little plaited, but imperceptibly. If you wish to put a blond *entre-deux* between the pieces, border them with a narrow corded piping of white satin; then place them onto the *entre-deux* from the wrong side. Plait the third piece as I have just said, trimming it with the piping. Be careful to reduce the width of the pieces according to the width of the *entre-deux.*

That done, put a circular string-case on the cap two and a half inches from the edge, using a white taffety riband about eight lines wide, which you sew to the wrong side of the cap. Pass a braid or a narrow riband through the case. The braid must come out at the back, in the middle of the lower part of the third piece. To hide it, place a pretty little bow of white satin riband above the eyelet-holes from which the braid emerges. In a pinch, you might well place a folded riband in the case and tie it at the back; but you know that you always place bows permanently, to preserve the freshness of the riband. Trim this cap with pointed blond, a silk tulle ruche, or a ruche *à coquilles* made of plaited *gaze de laine,* as I described for trimming *fichus.*

Yet another kind of trimming is prepared for cornettes. Allow much more fulness than is customary for a cap, and make it a little longer. Then cut all round in shallow scollops, and make a narrow roll, similar to that for gathers, round the scollops. Next take either some blond with very small points, or a little strip of silk tulle about half an inch wide, and place this strip round the edge of the scollops with single box-plaits made close together. If you wish, then place a very narrow round white silk braid over the seam of the plaits; however, this braid is not essential. The circular case being all round your head, the cap puts the borders in play, which being wavy and delicately trimmed, are much more becoming to your face than voluminous ruches.

Cornettes *à Casque.* This style is only the two side parts of a three-piece cap enlarged to replace the middle piece (see Fig. 10 *A*). The pieces are made up exactly like a three-piece cap. Do not put a circular string-case in the middle of the crown. Put it all round the cap, but trim the edge of the case with any ruche you please.

Caps *à la Folle.* This kind is cut in a square piece, a third of an ell in each direction, with hollowings arranged to make strings, to which you add long bands similar to the cap (see Fig. 10 *B, d*). So that the piece thus cut be may kept on your head, make a circular string-case, *e,* about two and a half inches from the edge, which forms the trimming, *f.*

Caps *à la folle* are trimmed especially with the pretty trimming which I just described in speaking of three-piece cornettes. Indeed it is to them that we owe this fashion; their flared border and circular case first provided the idea. Some persons place the little half-ruche round the cap without making it first follow the scollops, but in my opinion they should not be imitated; this trimming then becomes too mean.

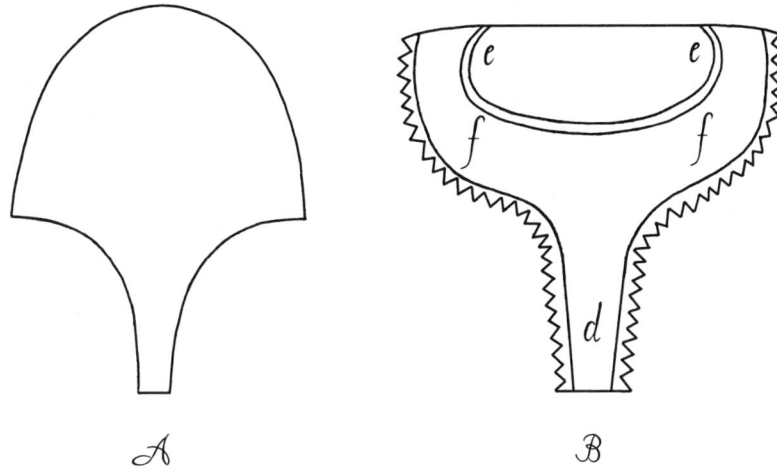

Figure 10. Shapes for the cornette *à casque* and the cap *à la folle*.

Additional Remarks. All these caps have strings of white ribands, or barbes (bands eight to nine inches long and three to four inches wide), trimmed with unplaited blond, and similar to the trimming of the cap. When the cap is trimmed with *gaze de laine,* it is better to have strings of riband, because you would not know, in that case, how to trim the barbes. The ribands are either tied or sewed to each string of the cap, without being cut. If they are tied, you will do well to make the bow beforehand on one side, and to hook it as described in the article on riband bows.

Haberdashers also make caps of *gaze de laine,* or silk tulle whose trimming is a plaited bias, and without any plaits in the front. This bias is enhanced by large riband bows; but as it is principally in the domain of the milliner, I shall treat of it more in detail in Chapter XXI.

Trimmings *de Lingère.*

You will recognize the usefulness of these directions when after washing caps of gauze, embroidered muslin, or cotton tulle, you want to take care of replacing the ribands.

Lingères ordinarily put two trimmings in the front of the cap. These trimmings, sewed with gathers, form large, slightly flat flutings. Between these two trimmings it is necessary to insert coloured ribands, but not ordinary bows; that would be extremely common. You ought to cut the riband in pieces long enough to make an ordinary loop and attach it inside by each end, above and below the second trimming.

That is the general picture; let us pass to the details. Cut three similar loops, and two other pieces of riband which may make a loop and one end of a bow. These pieces are destined to be put on the sides of the cap. Here is the way to arrange the whole: a loop is placed by its end on the right side, letting the end on the side of the string fall. This end is attached under the trimming, and the loop, slanting a little, is attached on top. The next loop begins by being attached underneath, then on top. However, as you have repeated this operation to the left, two loops are found on top in the middle of the cap. Then you delicately cross them over each other; or rather, you unpick several stitches of the trimming, and pass the end of one loop underneath while keeping the other above. This fashion of placing the riband seems to make it wind round the trimming. You will perceive how pretty it is to see a spiral of celestial blue or pink round a very clear, very white tulle.

When the cap has a crown *à étoile,* with rays descending in pointed trimmings on the front, place a riband half-bow in the convex part of the points. These half-bows or single bows are more elegant than whole bows. It is above all necessary to employ only rather wide riband gauze, satin riband having become common.

A very pretty fashion of placing the riband is to form on the left side of the front of the cap, between the two trimmings, a series of loops pressed one upon another (four, six, or eight, according to your taste), roll it in a loose *torsade,* then repeat the little mass of loops on the right side.

Another time you may vary the riband trimming by making a double half-circle like a coronet above the ruche of the cap. With this object, begin to make an end of the riband fall towards the string. Next form the half-circle to the left, laying the loops over each other and turning their folds to the right. You thus come to the middle of the cap, at the front part. Fasten it there, and taking the opposite end of the riband, repeat the same operation to the right, turning the folds of the loops to the left so that they face the first ones. Arriving at the front part of the cap, rejoin your other half-circle with a bow, with its ends spreading over the trimming. If you do not wish to put the riband strings separately on the cap, you may take your measures so that the strings will fall directly from each side of the half-circles. Fold the riband in the middle, leaving both selvages visible, and spread it along the string of the cap. You may very well replace these half-circles of loops with half-circles of *torsades,* only the bow in the front must be rather large.

When the cap is decorated with bows, it is proper to place them between the trimmings two by two, with a half-bow underneath, or three by three without a half-bow. Often the bows are placed under the trimmings, so that they touch the hair. This practice has the double disadvantage of soiling the riband very quickly, and of appearing affected.

It is very elegant to surround the cap with a *torsade*, which comes round to be looped on the right side. It is also quite pretty to join the bows placed between the trimming with *torsades* in this fashion: bow on the first trimming on the left; *torsade* placed on the bias beginning from this bow, passing over the trimming, fastened to the bow underneath, placed a little more to the right; interval of several lines; repetition of the *torsade* and the two bows. Double bow in the middle of the cap, on the front; two other *bow-torsades*.

The ribands which are passed through the string-cases, producing the appearance of a coloured rouleau owing to the transparency of the material, are ornamental as well. Also, crossways cases are often arranged close together solely for decorating the cap; but never circular ones, because those are very difficult to make.

Caps with puffed crowns are also made. The puffs are separated by *entre-deux* of tulle or blond, braids, or string-cases. These puffs are placed either crossways or lengthways. In the second case, they terminate in a cone on the summit of the head with a large riband bow.

When a cap is simple, it is enough to pass a folded riband under your neck, which will form a bow on the summit of your head. This bow must be of a very pretty, very wide riband, and made beforehand. A *marmotte* is also placed on these caps; this is a small triangle, rounded at the back, trimmed all round with tulle, lace, or pointed embroidery. The *marmotte* is always of very light material. It is also worn alone over the hair; then it is always of tulle or *gaze de laine*, trimmed with narrow blond in small box-plaits, or gathers. This style is becoming and very elegant, but it looks affected.

Howsoever you may have placed the ribands on your caps, always put a bow at the back which appears to be the tied riband of the string-case.

To omit nothing, I shall say that you should attach and adorn percale caps with bands and bows of similar material, or of hemmed muslin. It is also well to fasten *négligé fichus* in the same way.

——*Manuel des dames, Manuel des demoiselles.*

Diversion 1.

Literally "woollen gauze."

——Frances Grimble.

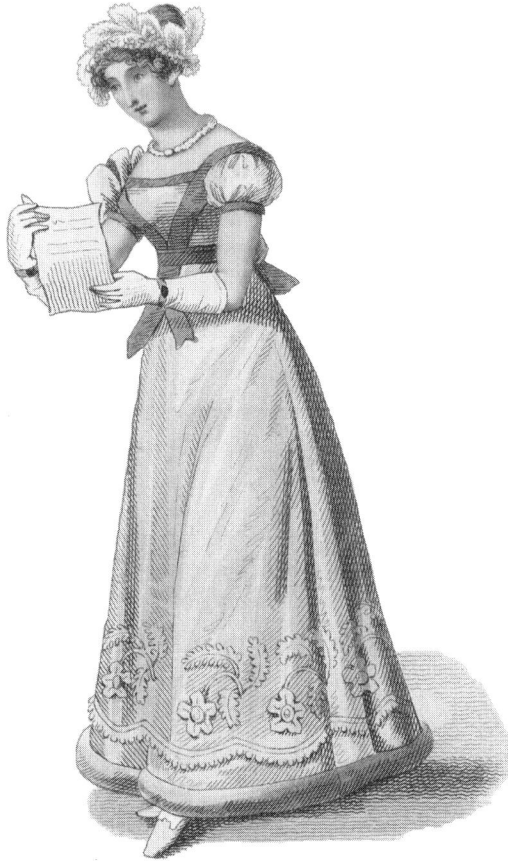

Figure 11. Ball dress.   Figure 12. Evening dress.

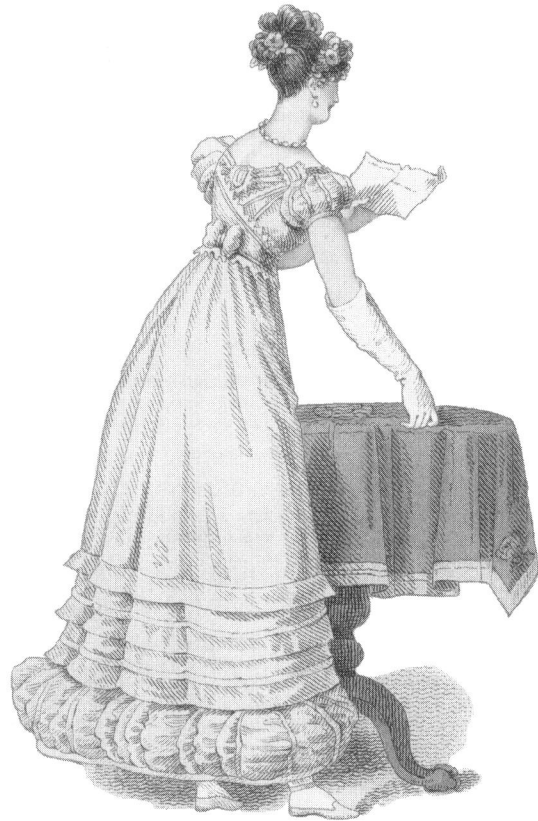

Diversion 2.

Belts worn with Evening Dress. For June 1824: Fig. 11 shows a ball gown of tulle richly embossed with a border of flowers, over pink satin, with a broad pink rouleau next the feet. The body is made quite plain, of pink satin, and short sleeves of white figured tulle. The hair is simply arranged in light curls, with a diadem bandeau of cameos on white satin, and the diadem surmounted by very short plumes of white marabouts, encircling the head in the Mexican style. The necklace consists of one row of very large pearls. White satin shoes and white kid gloves.

August 1824. Fig. 12 shows an evening gown of white gauze over white satin, with a rich puckering of tulle at the border, divided by ornaments of blond; three broad bias folds surmount this puckering, each headed by beading. The short sleeves are of white satin, surmounted with white beads. The body is of white satin, with Spanish bracers edged with narrow blond, and a white satin belt encircling the waist, which terminates behind in a bow without ends. The hair is arranged in the Lesbian style, and ornamented with full-blown roses. The necklace is composed of one row of large pearls.

June 1829. A ball gown of apricot-coloured *crêpe aerophane* over a white satin slip. Two flounces, scolloped at the edges, ornament the border, the scollops finished by three rows of dark purple or apricot-coloured satin, in bias-rouleau binding; and the upper flounce is surmounted by three narrow dark purple or apricot-coloured satin rouleaux. The sleeves are short and very full, with cleft mancherons. The body is made plain, and over it are Iberian bracers of apricot-coloured satin, with a belt of the same encircling the waist, finished by a rosette behind, with very short ends. The hair is arranged in light curls next the face, and bows of hair on the summit of the head, ornamented by a wreath of large full-blown Provence roses.

——*Ladies' Pocket Magazine.*

Diversion 3.

Ladies' Collars. Those shown in Fig. 13 have been selected from the most approved patterns, and when worn their shapes are calculated to sit well, provided you always cut them on the exact bias of the material. Fig. 13 *A* gives the dimensions for one of moderate size. This pattern is adapted for a narrow frill round the edge; for frilling will not sit so well, when it has to surround a sharp corner.

The pattern in Fig. 13 *B* is allowed to be very handsome when worked with a sprig at each point. The pattern in Fig. 13 *C* will look well with tatting, or a narrow edging of lace round it, and a sprig worked in each of the front corners. Fig. 13 *D* is for mourning. It is not any particular shape which constitutes a mourning collar, unless the hem is very wide.

Gentlemen's Collars. All the specimens in Fig. 14 have been approved of by the wearers as patterns which sit well. The pattern in Fig. 14 *A* is very much approved of, on account of its being whole in the front; the corners, therefore, cannot move from each other. The collar in Fig. 14 *B* has the same appearance when on as *A*, and is used by those who do not like that which ties behind, but wish for the same pattern.

The pattern in Fig. 14 *C* is a very neat one, and is used by those who do not wish to run into the extreme of fashion. Fig. 14 *D* is a French dress

5 1/2 inches

14 1/2 inches

A

5 inches

B

C

D

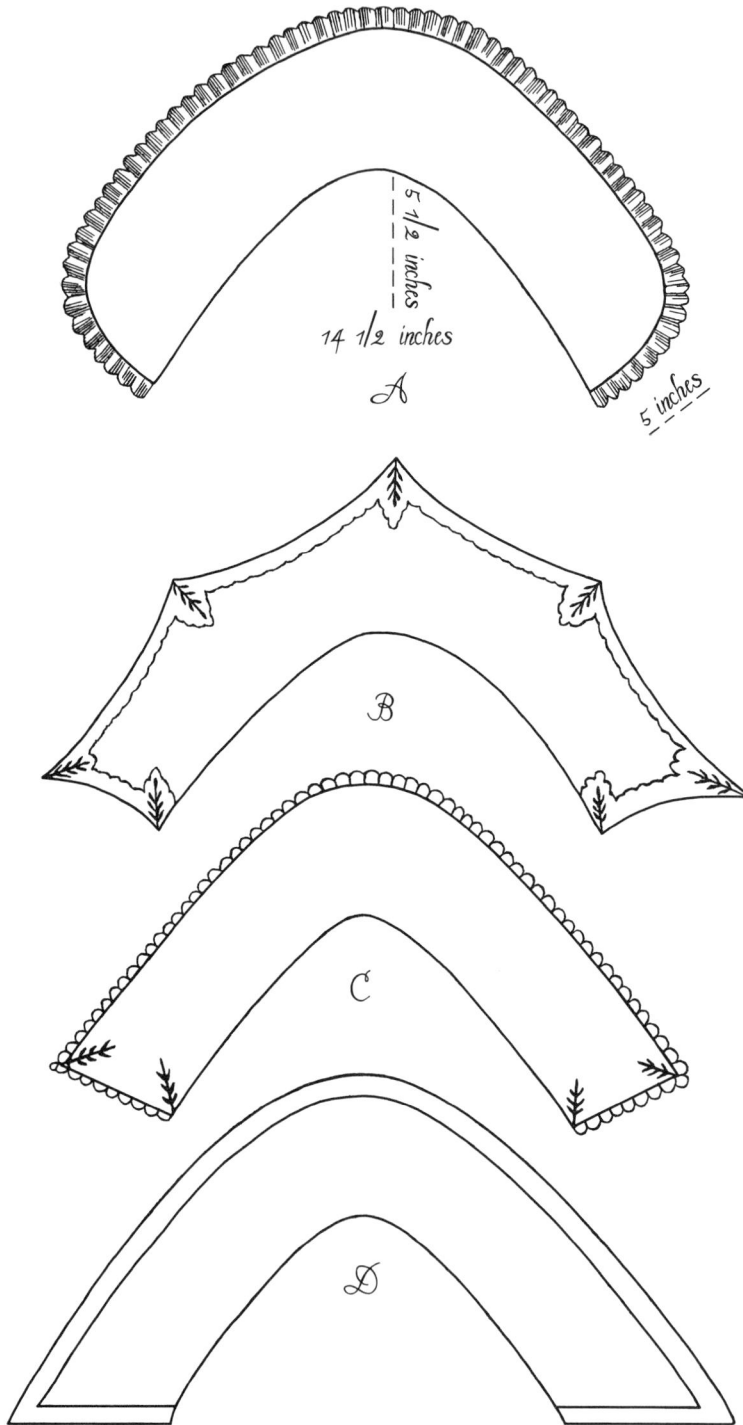

Figure 13. Patterns for ladies' collars.

Gentlemen's Collars.

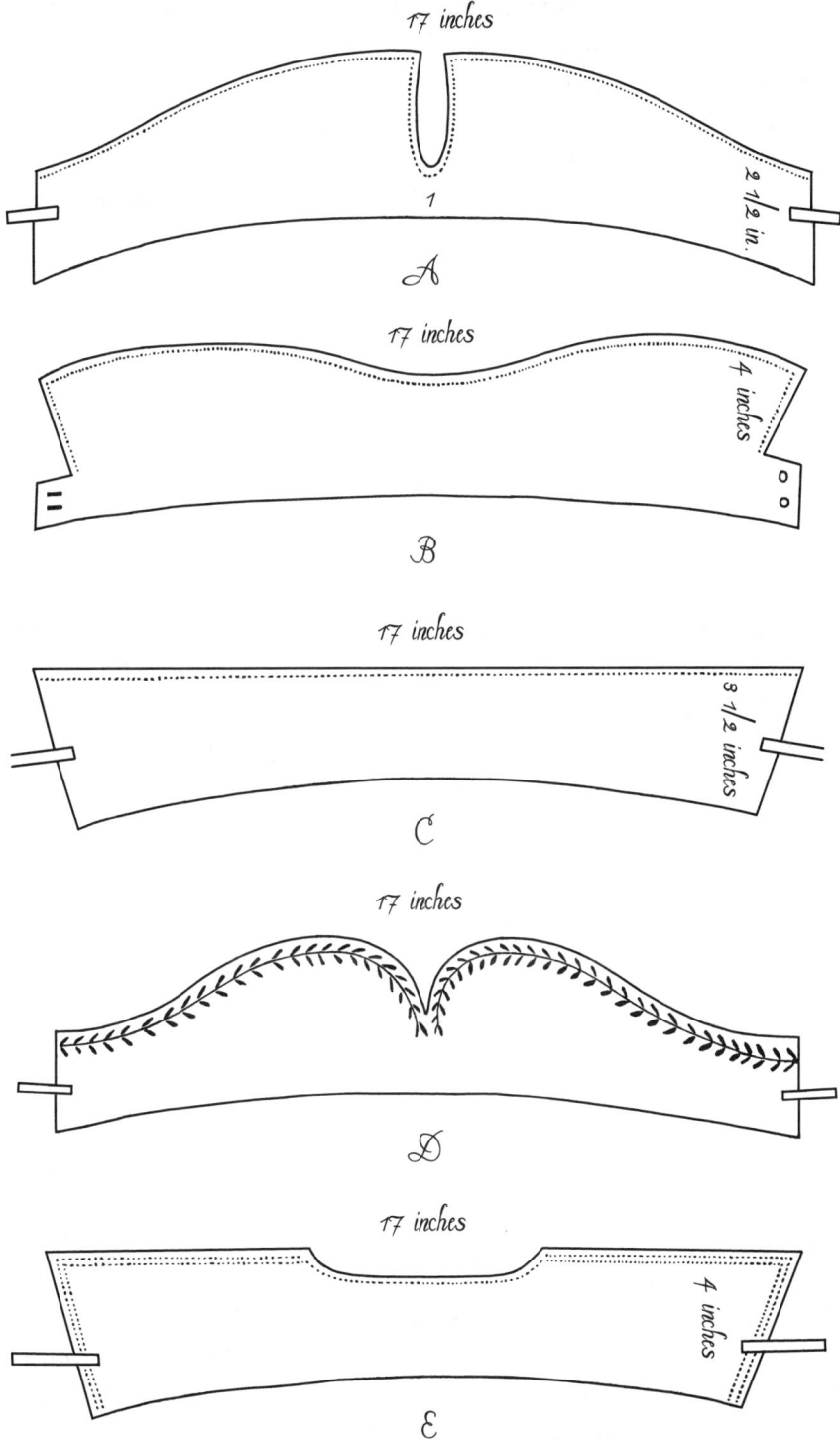

17 inches

2 1/2 in.

1

A

17 inches

4 inches

B

17 inches

3 1/2 inches

C

17 inches

D

17 inches

4 inches

E

Figure 14. Patterns for gentlemen's collars.

pattern, and is certainly very handsome, and a great favourite. The sprig may be worked proportionately small or large, at the option of the maker. The depth is two and a half inches, the same as Fig. 14 *A*. Fig. 14 *E* is used by those who like collars to sit high above the neck-cloth, being hollowed out behind for that purpose.

—*The Alphabetical Receipt Book and Domestic Advisor.*

Diversion 4.

This may be a typographical error for either "four, five, six or seven"; "five, six, or seven"; or "four, six, or eight."

—Frances Grimble.

Diversion 5.

Ladies' Caps. The cottage cap in Fig. 15 is mostly worn by those who wear their hair in a bow on the crown. The dimensions and shape you will find in the illustration. The horseshoe or crown must be whipped from the top, drawing Fig. 15 *A, a* round to the same on the other side, and gathered a little as shown in the illustration of the finished cap in Fig. 15 *D*. The piece shown in Fig. 15 *C* is whipped on each side and gathered into the length of the head-piece, and then sewed onto the crown and head-piece. You must run a wire riband in the inside of the front of the head-piece, and the top of the gathering, which will keep the cap in shape. To make a neat finish, it is piped round the top and bottom of the gathering, and over the top edge of the lace, which is gathered or plaited on the front of the head-piece, as in Fig. 15 *D*.

Morning Cap. The kind of cap in Fig. 16 is usually made of muslin, and sprigs worked round the head-pieces. Fig. 16 *A* is the shape of the head-piece, and the size is there given in inches. After you have worked the sprigs along the head-piece, the two straight ends (marked by *es*) are sewed together. The crown, Fig. 16 *B*, must be whipped round, and gathered into the size of the head-piece, and then sewed onto it. Fig. 16 *C* is doubled, and the two circular edges whipped together, and gathered, to form a puffing. Two of these are placed in the front of the crown, as in Fig. 16 *D*; before the two puffings are put on, a frill of fancy-work is tacked round the crown, two and a half inches wide. The frilling, or borders round the front, must not be more than two inches wide, and of the same pattern as the one round the crown. This forms a very handsome cap for the afternoon, if worked in net.

12 inches

a ——— a

8 inches

A

3 1/2 in.

8 in.

21 inches

B

1 in.

4 feet

4 1/2 in.

C

D

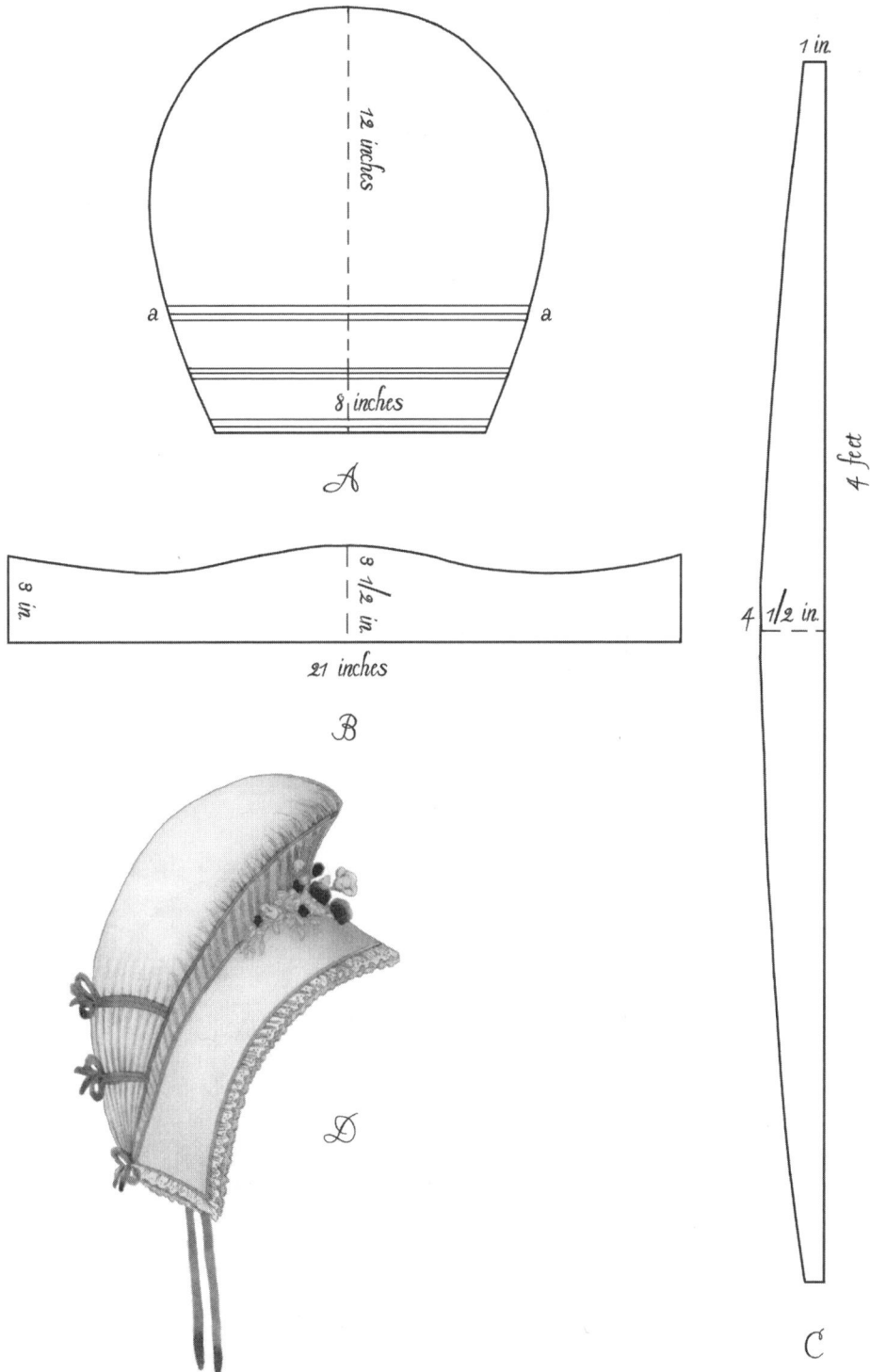

Figure 15. A cottage cap.

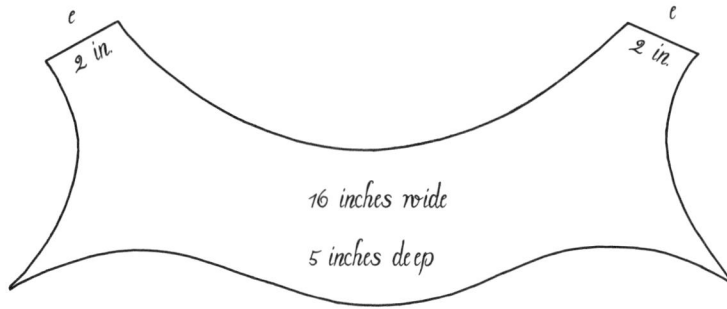

c   2 in.   c   2 in.

16 inches wide

5 inches deep

A

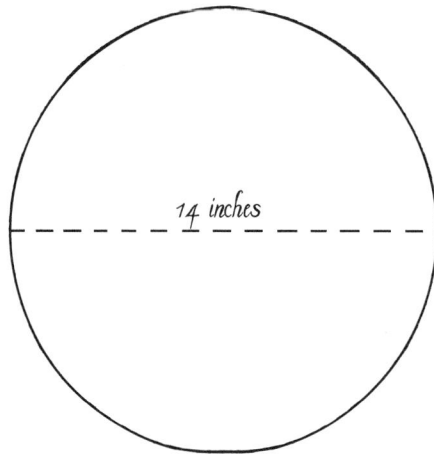

14 inches

B

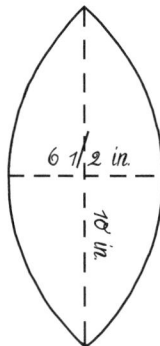

6 1/2 in.

10 in.

C

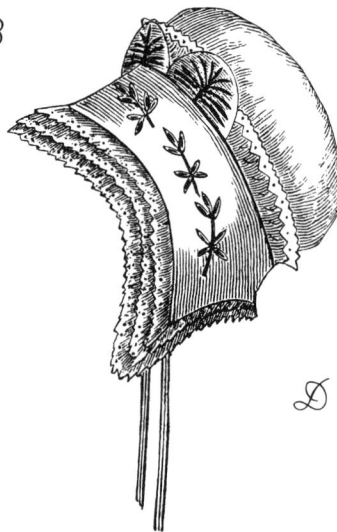

D

Figure 16. A morning cap.

Dress Cap. The cap in Fig. 17 is one very much admired for its neat and handsome appearance, though the pattern is very simple, being made of one piece, excepting the small lace crown. Fig. 17 *A* and *B* show the pattern and the size of the pieces which form the cap. Sew the main piece Fig. 17 *A* together at *b*, then whip the top and gather it a little to the size of the crown-piece, Fig. 17 *B*, which is then sewed in, and a gathering or plaiting of lace put round it, over which a piping is added. When the straight sides of Fig. 17 *C* are run together and piped round, they will form Fig. 17 *D*, which is the trimming which the flowers are placed into. This trimming should be made of satin. Five of them are placed round the front of the cap, as shown in Fig. 17 *E,* the finished cap. The lace which you put on should be nearly plain in the front, but very full at the sides. These caps are generally made of net.

Dress or Mourning Cap. Fig. 18 *A* is the straight piece which is drawn in behind. The *es* show the string-cases; on account of their width, you must make an allowance for them when they are cut out. Fig. 18 *B* is the head-piece; in the cutting of which you must allow for a wide hem, as all the hems in this kind of cap are wide. After you have hemmed it, sew each end of Fig. 18 *A* onto it at *dd*. Next draw it up with strings of white love-riband to the size of the head you intend it for. Then take the crown, Fig. 18 *C*, and whip it round, and gather it to the size which will fit into the head-piece and back gathering; see Fig. 18 *D*, the finished cap.

The border is two inches wide; the hem must be wider than for other caps, and is put on plain in the front, and full round the other part. It is trimmed round the top edge of the border and round the crown with white love-riband, twisted and tacked on, and bows of the same on the head-piece; see Fig. 18 *D*. These caps are invariably made of plain muslin; the strings are made of the same, with a wide hem or love-riband.

Turban Cap. Caps like the one shown in Fig. 19 are made on a shape which is cut out of foundation muslin. The pattern gives the size in inches, together with the shapes of each piece. First take the head-piece, Fig. 19 *B*, and fasten the two ends together. Next put a wire round the bottom and top. Then take the crown, shown in Fig. 19 *A*, and plait it all round to the size of the head-piece, and tack it onto it: this forms the foundation.

After this is done, cut a piece of white satin, or any other colour you choose to make it of, and plait it onto your shape. Then cut a piece of the same to the size of Fig. 19 *B*, allowing for whatever number of plaits you may wish to have round the edge of the head-piece, and for the seam fold; then put it onto the shape.

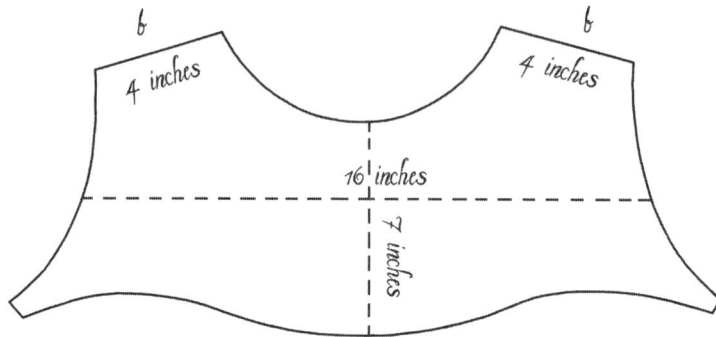

b   b

4 inches   4 inches

16 inches

7 inches

A

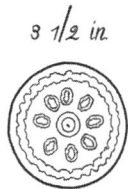

3 1/2 in.

B

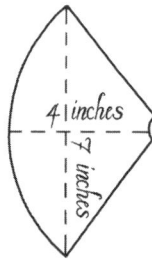

4 inches

7 inches

C

D

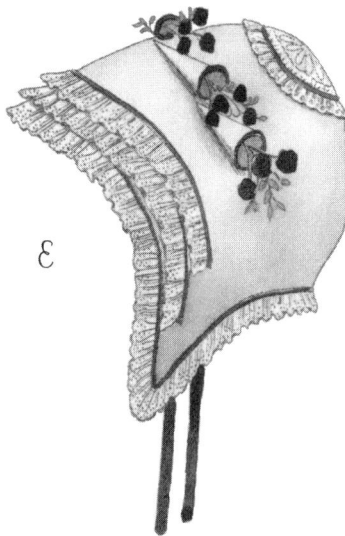

E

Figure 17. A dress cap.

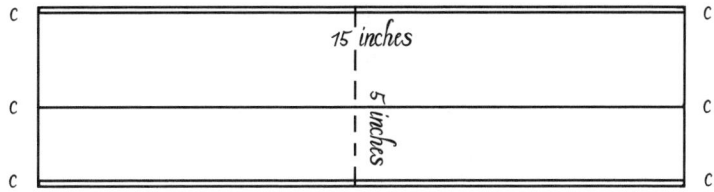

c   15 *inches*   *c*

c   5 *inches*   *c*

c   *c*

A

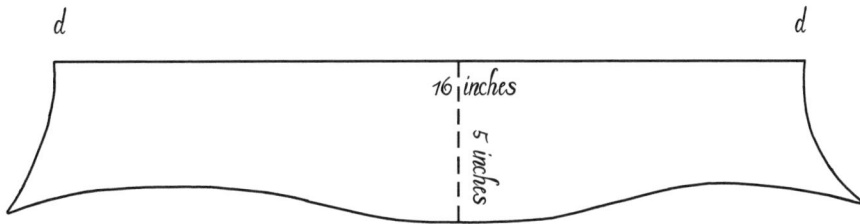

d   16 *inches*   *d*

5 *inches*

B

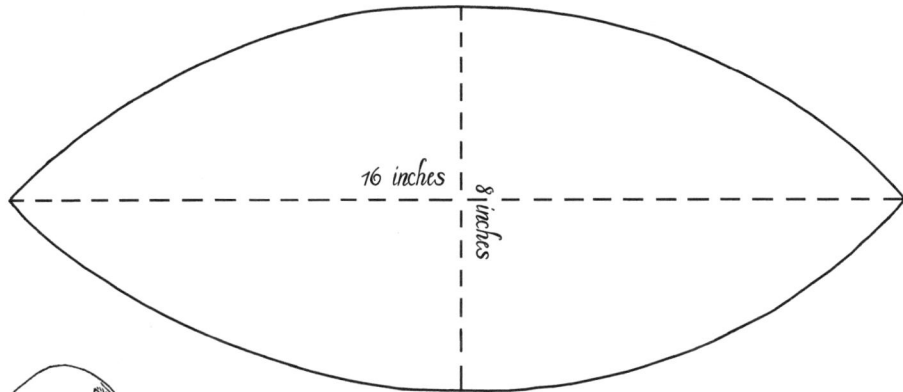

16 *inches*   8 *inches*

C

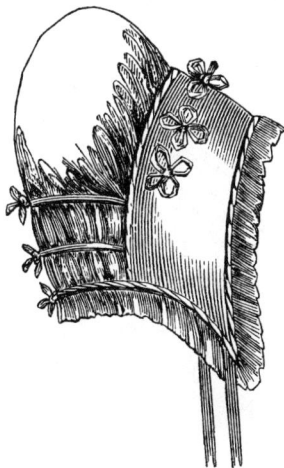

D

Figure 18. A dress or mourning cap.

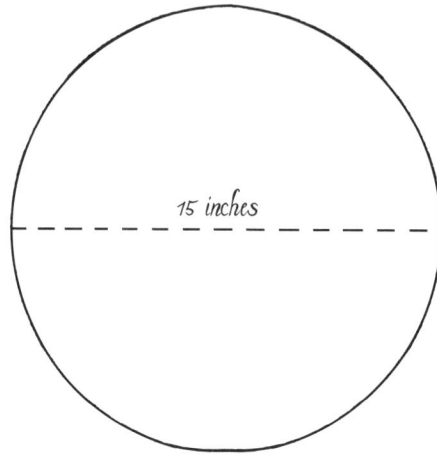

A

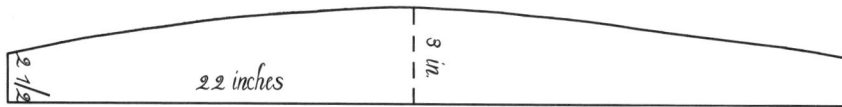

B

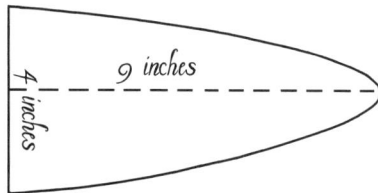

C

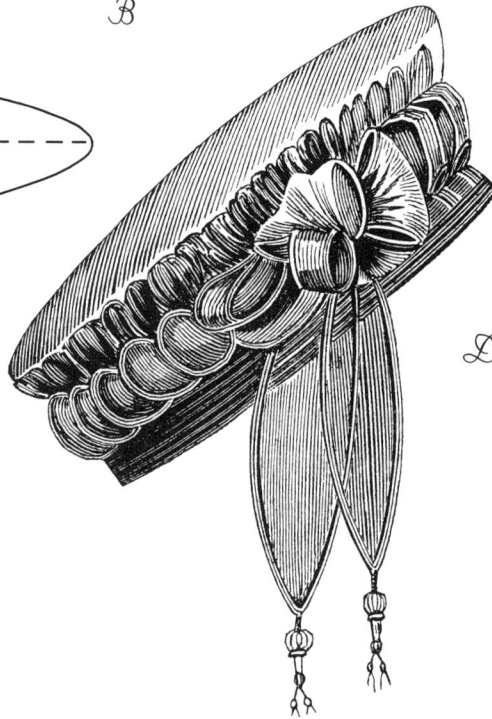

D

Figure 19. A turban cap.

The trimming round the head-piece is made of silk gauze, the doubled way of the stuff, which is twisted and tacked on, bringing the ends to the right side, where the bow is to come. Fig. 19 C is also silk gauze, piped round with satin, which forms one of the two pieces of trimming to which the tassel is suspended, as in Fig. 19 D. These pieces are gathered in a little at the top, and tacked onto where the bow is to come, one a little forwarder than the other; see Fig. 19 D. Then four or five satin stripes are placed in the front, over the gauze trimming: see the front of Fig. 19 D.

Widow's Cap. This kind of cap is of various shapes, and the only peculiar feature in them, is the form of their trimmings. The one given in Fig. 20 is much approved of, for its plain and sable appearance. Fig. 20 B is the head-piece; the two ends which are to be run together are marked by ds. Fig. 20 A is the crown, which is whipped all round and gathered up to the size of the head-piece, bringing rather more of the fulness in the front; then tack it into the head-piece. Then place two single borders, one in the front, one close above the other, as in Fig. 20 C, a. Over these a double border is placed, one part being brought closely over the two single ones, and the other side placed towards the crown, as in Fig. 20 C, b. In this kind of cap, the hems must be very wide for a round mesh to be run through after it is made up.

A single or double border must be placed round the bottom of the crown, similar to those in the front. The mob, Fig. 20 C, c, is a double frill with wide hems, gathered or plaited onto a piece of tape six inches long. All the borders must be twice the length of whatever part you intend them for before you whip them, or the meshing of the hems will not look well.

Night-cap. The general aim of this article being comfort, the pattern in Fig. 21 has been selected, as it is allowed to be the most comfortable. This kind of cap may be made to fit any one, by taking one measure, which is round the crown, for that must be the size of the head-piece. The crown being made with string-cases, as shown in Fig. 21 B and E, it can be drawn to any size. The dimensions of a moderate one are therefore given in inches; in Fig. 21 B the cases are marked by fs. Fig. 21 C is for the bands which are fastened at each end of the head-piece, Fig. 21 A. The crown must be whipped from the top on one side to the same on the other, and then gathered and sewed onto the straight part of the head-piece. You must sew the part with the string-cases first, which are to be sewed on quite plain. You will then see what space you have left to gather the part which is whipped into. Fig. 21 D is the string to tie under the chin, and is fastened as in Fig. 21 E.

———*The Alphabetical Receipt Book and Domestic Advisor.*

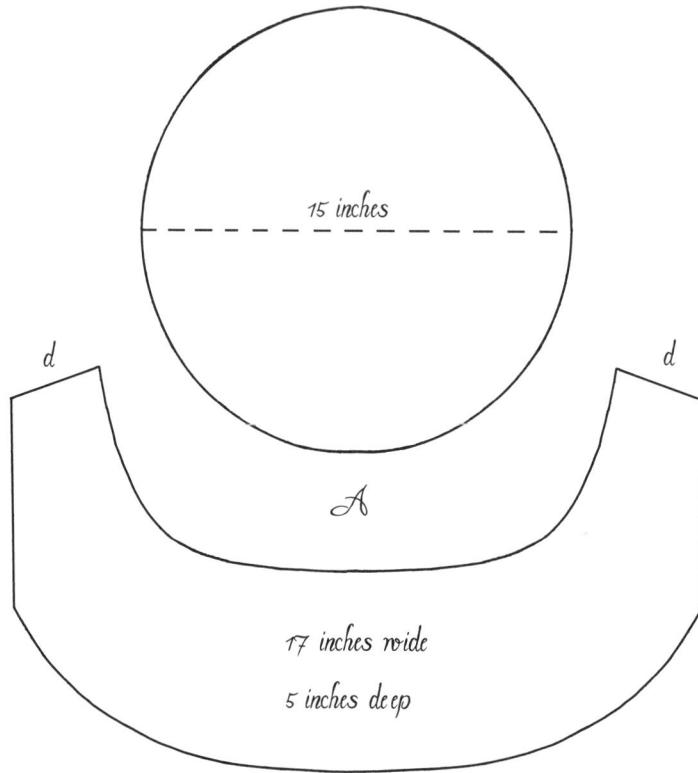

15 inches

d   d

A

17 inches wide

5 inches deep

B

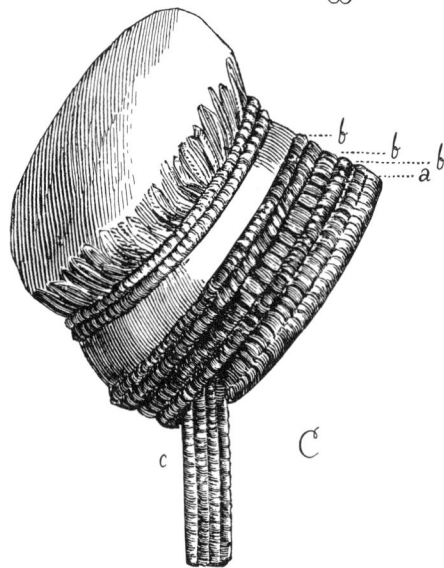

b

b

b

a

c

C

Figure 20. A widow's cap.

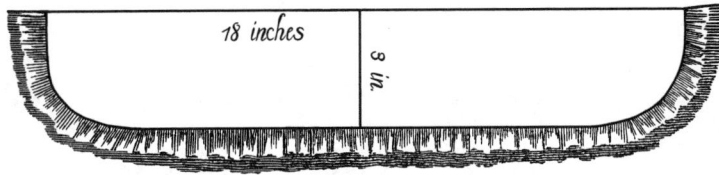

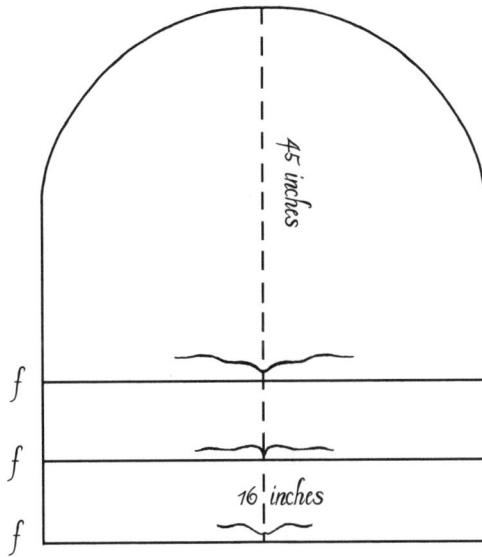

18 inches

3 in.

A

45 inches

f
f
f

16 inches

B

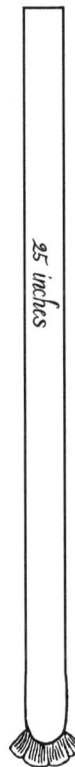

25 inches

C

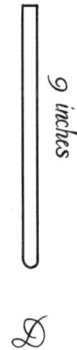

9 inches

D

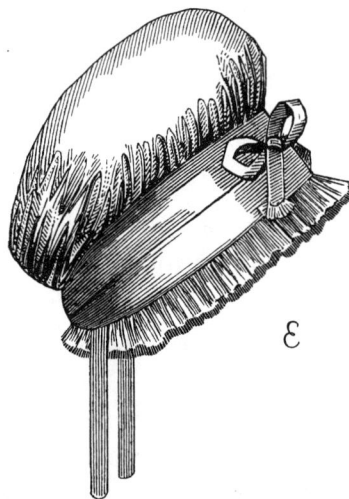

E

Figure 21. A night-cap.

Chapter XXI.
The Art of the Milliner, or the Mode of making Hats, Toques, &c.

Millinery is the most agreeable and the least meticulous kind of needle-work. The nature of the articles which are employed, the speed with which results are obtained, the ease of judging your work with the first glance, and the grace and variety which distinguish this art, at the same time amuse and capture the attention. Ordinarily I think of other things while doing needle-work, but when I touch a hat, my thoughts are nearly all on my work. This, therefore, is a diversion; it is also an economy, because if it is not exactly possible for you to make all your hats, you may at least turn and change those which you have—and repairs of this kind are always the most expensive. (See Div. 1.) You may remake those which have been cleansed, and finally you may make those which are worn for *négligé* and demi-toilet. If you are deft and patient, after some practice you will be equally able to make all your other hats.

Kinds of Head-dresses.

Six kinds of head-dresses are made by milliners: 1st., hats; 2nd., bonnets; 3rd., toques; 4th., turbans; 5th., caps; 6th., berets. (See Fig. 1 and Div. 2.) For these they use marquetry, marli, coarse silk tulle, heavily-gummed tulle, brass wire, and strips of straw or wood tissue: those are the materials for constructing hats. Satin and all sorts of sturdy silk materials, tulle, crape and all soft silk materials, gauze, and cotton tulle: those are the materials for covering hats. Ribands, bands of tulle, blond, feathers, artificial flowers and fruits, pearls, all kinds of cotton braids, silk, straws (likewise the fibre), satin-finished brass wire, supple whale-bones, tassels, silk fringe, *agrafes*, and metal lozenges: those are the materials for decoration. A great quantity of the fine little pins called camions, middle-sized black pins for hats of that colour, moulded plaster heads for trying on head-dresses as they are made, very high wooden hat-stands to place them on when finished, and finally large boxes in which to keep them: those are your tools.

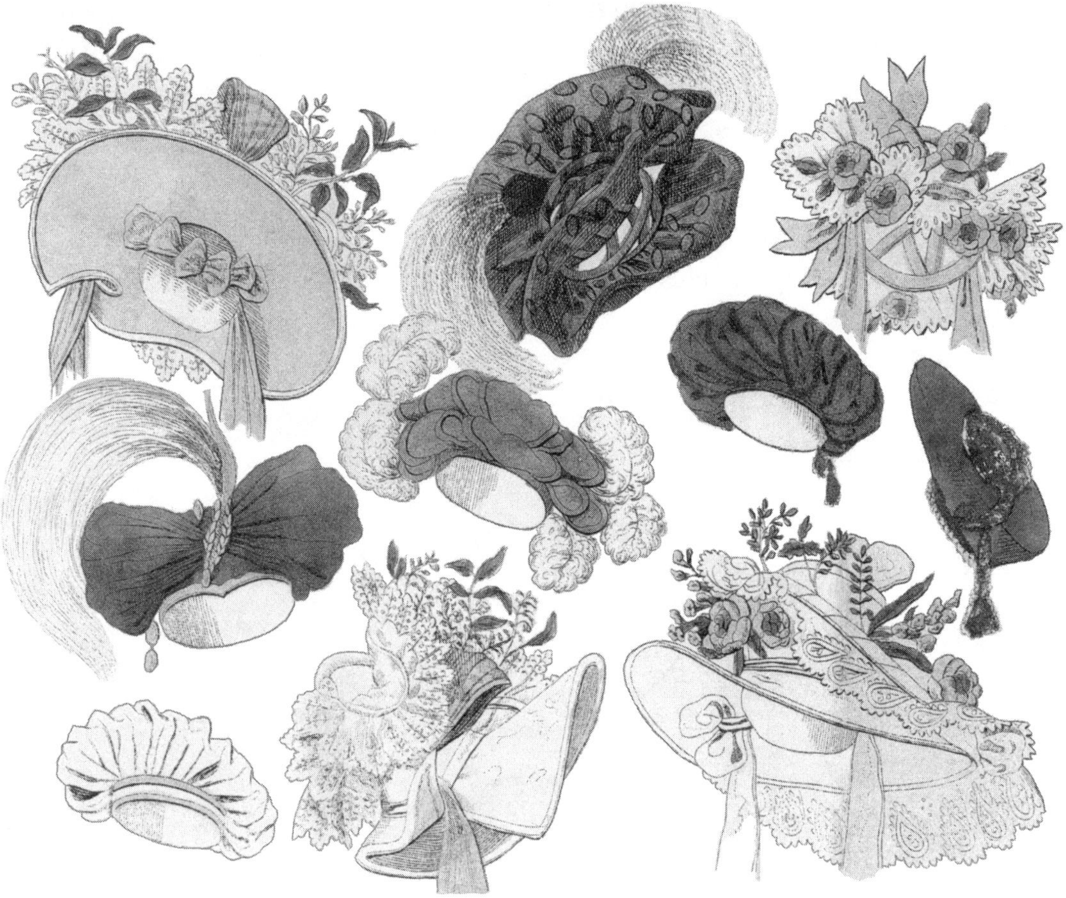

Figure 1. Divers head-dresses.

I have not included in this list hats of the wood called rice straw or chip; Leghorn, Swiss, or Monaco straw; esparto; gauze woven with straw; decorated marli; stitched straw; or cotton or silk tissue imitating straw, because those articles are sufficient in themselves, and are not constructed like all other hats. I shall discuss their preparation after that of hats covered with material.

The Body of the Hat.

A hat is first composed of a crown and a brim, on which you then put the trimmings. I shall begin by explaining how to cut out and make up this first part, which might be called the frame-work of the hat.

To cut out and prepare the Body. Take a pattern for the brim, according to the received style (see Fig. 2). This model varies in height or width, but the cut is always the same. The pattern of tolerably thick paper, whose two ends are not joined, is placed on a breadth, or piece of heavily-gummed toile, or on some close marquetry (marquetry is a wood tissue). Toile is preferable in that it does not break. The brim is ordinarily too wide for the breadth of the material to suffice for it; therefore you lengthen the hollowed part which makes the back, with the scraps yielded by the part rounded in the front.

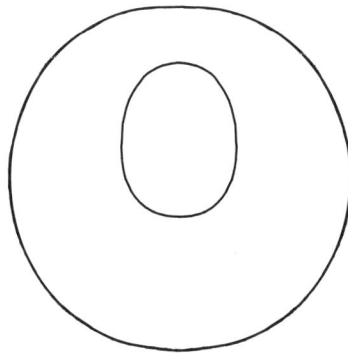

Figure 2. The shape for a hat-brim.

This operation finished, set about cutting out the crown: it may be cut rounded or flat. In the first case, cut a side-band half an ell wide and about seven inches high. Then cut a circle of three or four inches in every direction; this depends more or less upon the height of the side-band. Sew the side-band with large plaits round the circle, underneath, so that the edges of the circle are flat on the right side, over the plaits whose edges are on the wrong side. Join the two ends of the side-band, standing it upright, by a slanting seam which traverses the bias, or even simply by a lengthways seam: the first is much better in that it contributes to the sturdiness of the hat. The plaits of the side-band, in spreading round the circle, enlarge it to the measure of your head.

The circular part of a flat crown cannot be enlarged in this way. You directly give it the proper size relative to the size of the summit of your head, and consequently cut the side-band about two inches larger at the base. It is, therefore, unnecessary to make plaits in it, since it is found to be exactly as wide as the circle. It is well to cut the side-band two inches longer than needed to fit round your head. First, it will not then be necessary to expose an extension there if it does not fit easily round the circle; next, it is essential to cross the ends of the side-band in seaming them. Both rounded and flat crowns prepared thus serve to make all kinds of bonnets and hats.

The brim requires a little more care in its sewing and preparation. Border it flat all round, using running stitches, with a very narrow strip of straw, in the middle of which you place a brass wire, which you fasten by alternately entering and bringing out the needle over and under the brim. Always use a coarse thread to sew the crown and brim, as well as to assemble them. Some persons join the two ends of the brim when these have been furnished with a straw; others join them after having placed the brim lining. You will see if the brim has a good cut by trying it on the plaster head.

If you intend to make a hat, cut by the pattern of the brim, a new brim of the material which will cover it. The hat-brim, without exception, is always plain, and it is decorated with ornaments not found in cutting it; whereas for most bonnets the material of the brim is used to make adornments. Also cut out the lining of the bonnet or hat by the pattern of the brim. The lining and the upper side must be several lines wider than the pattern, in order to cover the edges of the brim.

To cover the Brim. Let us now concern ourselves with the mode of covering the marquetry brim with the upper side, which I shall suppose to be in velvet, and the lining in satin. There are several ways of doing this; I shall begin with the simplest.

First, spread out the satin lining on the wrong side of the brim, carefully placing the corresponding parts of the brim and the satin together. Temporarily pin them with four or five camions placed here and there, where they seem most useful. Turn the edge of the satin over the straw which furnishes the outer edge of the brim. Sew over the straw with rather long running stitches, only on the edge, because no stitches must be apparent. That finished, again spread out the satin, while pulling it the proper amount, neither too much nor too little; because in the first case, the brim would puff up; in the second, the lining would pucker horribly. Then border round the stretched part where the brim will join the crown, the same as you did for the outer edge. When the lining is thus sewed, it produces a rather wide border at the stretched part, which because of the bias, pulls disagreeably. Therefore, do not fail to slash this border all round with scissor-cuts, about half an inch deep and half an inch apart. (Sometimes the base of the crown is slashed in this way.)

Then set about placing the velvet upper side. Apply it on the right side of the marquetry brim, with the steps indicated for the lining. Make a seam fold there all round the outer edge beforehand, and sew at several lines from the seam fold, which you put over the edge which has formed the fold of the lining. Take good care that the stitches do not show at all underneath. The upper side matters less because you cover the line of stitches which holds the seam fold with velvet, or a beaded braid, or a little *torsade* of narrow riband, or better yet a satin-finished brass wire. All these things are sewed from underneath, by sticking the needle into the twist of the various *cordonnets* which they form, because it is still indispensable that the stitches be concealed. It is necessary that these articles never have the air of being sewed. Finish by stretching the upper side in the same way as the lining, joining the two over the straw, at the edge of the tightened part. However, make a seam fold on the upper side and put it over the straw of the edge covered by the lining, after the edge of the lining has been slashed. Before sewing, also slash the upper seam fold here and there.

I said before that you place a braid or a satin-finished brass wire at the outer edge of the brim, and I did so to put more order in my description. But this edge is so embellished only when the brim is completely covered. To join the two ends of the lining, sew a slanting seam beforehand. For the upper side fold one over the other, making a seam fold on the end found on top. A braid, a piece of riband, or any similar thing hides the seam fold.

I have declared that there are several ways to border the front of a brim: here they are. Cut a narrow strip of satin on the bias; put a braid or string in it, in order that this kind of piping may be rounder. Baste along the braid, then put the folded part of the piping over the edge of the brim, which the lining borders as I have explained. Sew the piping over the edge of the straw with large stitches; or even, if you are practiced, sew it at the same time as the edge of the lining. Then place the front over the piping, and finish as I have just explained.

When you wish to make several rows of these braids, place one above another. Often a corded piping of the same material as the hat is seen—especially if it is made of *gros de Naples*—then a bias satin fold, then another braid, and so on, according to how much you wish to increase or decrease the amount of this kind of trimming. You may also sew a corded piping at the edge of the brim on the upper side, before placing it over the straw, then sew it in the groove formed by the braid and the material, in such a manner that the stitches are entirely imperceptible.

To cover the Brim.

When you must put a tulle ruche round a hat, or a wide blond as a half-veil, it is equally necessary to be careful at the edge, because the transparency of these materials permits the edge to be seen. But you are exempted from so much trimming of this edge; it is underneath the brim that you put corded pipings. However, oftentimes these are replaced with a very narrow round braid of tightly-twisted white silk, which you put half an inch from the edge. Sometimes the braid is put under the brim, but more commonly on top. It performs the office of the satin-finished brass wire, and is sewed in the same way by the twist. Try the lined brim on the plaster head.

The upper side of a bonnet brim is cut out, as I have said, much larger than the marquetry brim, with the effect of adding gathers or plaits. You may easily obtain this pattern. If you lack it, plait the material here and there when putting it on your pattern; fix these plaits with camions, and then cut. Be careful to allow a little extra length to the material at the place where each plait will be, because in next opening it you will find there a jagged edge, which occurs every time you cut across a plait. You may then neatly even out the material.

You have seen that the upper side of a brim without plaits is always placed by starting with the outer edge. Quite the contrary is true when it has plaits. These are first arranged at the top—where, incidentally, there is no need to slash the seam fold on the upper side of the brim, considering that the plaits prevent tightening the bias, which that operation is intended to avoid. Then work on the outer edge; and if the bonnet must be trimmed with a ruche of similar material, content yourself with basting the upper side on the edge, with large slanting over-cast stitches, very often made with white thread on a dark background. If the bonnet is not destined to receive this trimming, you proceed pretty nearly as I have explained for hat-brims. However, never make a seam fold apparent on the upper side; the plaits would render it heavy and crude. It would be better to use this edge to wrap a strip of wood straw, which you sew by hemming. The line of hemming stitches is then placed on the edge of the brim; the straw stands up, and produces an agreeable raised effect.

When you wish to make a crossways case in the middle of the brim, again use a straw. Pass it underneath from the upper side of the brim, and sew it with running stitches, precisely like the cord in an ordinary string-case; tighten it a little as you advance. Then stretch out the upper side of the brim as usual. The straw-case is tightened, draws up the plaits which fall from the tightened part, and prepares for the arrangement of those parts of the edge. Later I shall discuss still another use of this straw-case.

This kind of case is used when there is only one on the brim, and when it must be wide, and the material is not transparent. In the contrary situation, use supple white whale-bone, cotton cord passed through narrow cases, or simple gathers on the wrong side, over which you put a braid of silk, beaded or much twisted, or a riband *torsade*, &c. If the brim must have very large puffs, such as the *bouillons gonflés* or *tuyaux d'orgue*, do not cut it by a pattern. Take a very large piece of *gaze de laine*, muslin gauze, or tulle (since this kind of bonnet necessarily requires light material). Then form it into very large plaits, by approximation, making them much inflated; each plait is fixed by a camion, and crumpled and puffed as much as possible in the middle and on both edges of the brim. Then cut all round without troubling with the ragged edges. Baste on both edges, withdrawing the camions there; but leave them permanently in the middle. Conceal the edge with a satin rouleau, which a twisted braid divides in the middle. Those are the bonnets *à bouillons gonflés* which were worn six years ago.

The bonnets *à tuyaux d'orgue* worn formerly were a little less odd, the plaits having at least a definite shape. This style has enormous box-plaits, parallel from top to bottom of the brim, and only a little wider on the outer edge. The plaits are held, along their length, by means of unseen camions. Satin rouleaux are often placed between them, lengthways from the top to the bottom of the brim, which is extremely long. (This ornament is also permitted on the preceding bonnets.) Camions hold these rouleaux, which ordinarily number seven, nine, or eleven, according to the amount of separation, or the width of the brim. They are close together at the top and a little more spread out towards the bottom, which gives them, towards the crown, some resemblance to the top of a fan. The gauze puffs rise to the right and left of the rouleaux, which flatten them.

All the other possible brims differ only by divers ornaments.

To cover the Crown. When the crown is plain, the thing is simple. Cut out a circle of material like the circle of marquetry (this applies to the flat crown), but more than half an inch larger. Lay it over the foundation of the crown, fixing it with pins to the top of the side-band. Baste it, removing the pins.

Then cut out a side-band in material by the pattern of the marquetry side-band. Sew a corded piping, similar to that on the edge of the brim, to the upper edge of the side-band. Then place the side-band material flat on the edges of the circle, commencing at the middle of the marquetry band, which is found in the front of the hat, in order to hide, under bows or ornaments, the place where the two side edges of the band are joined.

Just as for the edge of the brim, and an hundred times more easily, you may make a seam fold in place of the corded piping, then put a beaded or twisted braid on top. Or, if the crown is very high and decorated with three narrow *cerceaux,* and one of them hides the join of the crown and the side-band, do not trouble to make a seam fold, nor even to sew with thread matched to the material. "That is not seen," and "That will not last," are the milliner's mottoes. The *cerceaux* in question are veritable cuffs trimmed with corded piping, bias satin folds, and little *torsades* or decorated braids, which last year were placed in a circle round the hat-crown, one at the place where the crown joins the brim, another at the junction of the side-band and the circle, and the third between the two. When the crown is much raised, the *cerceaux* or strips sometimes amount to four. Whatsoever their number and extent, they always meet front of the crown, for the same reason that the ends of the side-band are joined there.

The rounded crown is dedicated to hats which are plaited and puffed in a thousand fashions, of which I shall indicate a few, as well as to brims *à tuyaux d'orgue.* Sometimes the hat material is placed in very large hollow box-plaits all round the crown; but this material does not require to be transparent. The plaits are made at the base of the crown, then their "pipes" are raised up quite stiff, at least two inches above the circle, and drawn down together in the middle of it. This makes a kind of hemispheric hollow, agreeably puffed up. This effect is produced by gathering, at the end, the material placed in box-plaits, and pulling it as close as possible, placing it at the middle of the foundation. A collection of eight or ten rows of corded piping, or a rouleau of cotton wadding, covered with satin (these two articles about an inch and a half long), forms a ring which covers the gathers. This ring is made by sewing both ends of the assemblage underneath, and by giving it a slight curve. There are many milliners who open the material, pass the two ends underneath, then sew them from inside the hat, to the marquetry circle. This mode is more graceful and sturdier.

At other times, the plaits are not placed all round the crown, but only half-way and on the front. Then this part is crowned by very large puffs, which are brought together in the middle. Sometimes a *torsade,* obliquely thrown across the middle of the crown, marks the back of these plaits. Sometimes they are gradually lost in a bundle at the back of the crown, whose upper part is surmounted by a straw-case, which stands up round the little ring, and serves to agreeably distribute the plaits in the front. Place a bow in the middle of the ring which encircles the straw-case.

It goes without saying that you have previously covered the corresponding circle on the crown, with a little round piece of material.

Sometimes you cut out a very large circle of material, about a foot in every direction, and put the centre point on the corresponding part of the circle forming the crown. The circumference is fitted at the base of the side-band, and you fix it there by various folds. This kind of crown is especially suited to fancy caps, toques, and berets—whose crown, by the way, is nearly always rounded.

The other kinds of crowns of hats, or rather of bonnets, are puffed. To this end, before placing the upper side round the crown, cut it double in width and height. Make cases there from top to bottom, and insert cords, straws, or supple whale-bones, which you pull to make crossways gathers. The cases having been made all round the upper side, putting the last over the seam which joins the two ends (this seam may be made in the front or at the back as desired), pass the crown into the material thus puffed up. Dispose the puffs gracefully, inflating them more in the front of the crown. Then pulling and tightening the gathers in the upper part as much as possible, collect all the puffs at the middle of the top of the crown. These puffed foundations are placed on a rounded crown. A bow of riband, or an *agrafe* of corded piping, is placed where the gathers meet. Sometimes you simply gather instead of placing the cords, and when the upper side is laid on the crown, spread *torsades* or satin rouleaux over these lengthways gathers. The corded gathers, or to put it better, the puffs which they form, sometimes swell up in a circle round the crown, instead of being formed lengthways as this explanation indicates.

All the other ways of covering a hat-crown differ from the preceding only by outside ornaments.

The *Coiffe*, or Crown Lining. This part is composed of a band of material cut on the straight-way, about half an ell wide, and half a foot high. It is made of *gaze d'Italie*, satin, or fine silk taffety. Do not use ordinary marli to make a *coiffe* for a hat, whatsoever its purpose. Marli is in the worst taste, and it is one of the signs by which common hats are recognized. *Gaze de laine* and silk tulle are too light. The best material is lightly-gummed muslin, because it is durable, and absorbs the sweat from your hair. Make a sufficiently wide case at one edge of the width, on the wrong side of the material, and pass the first braid which comes to hand through it with a bodkin. All the same, it is better that it match the colour of the *coiffe*, which must be that of the hat. Mark a wide seam fold at the other edge of the width, on the wrong side.

Then apply the right side of the *coiffe* over the lining of the brim, and sew this seam fold to the edge of the straw at the narrow inner circle of the brim. The *coiffe* must fit this circle exactly. If it is too large, join the two ends by a seam on the wrong side and cut off the excess portion; this seam must be at the back of the crown. This shows you that it is there that you must begin to sew the *coiffe* to the brim. When the hat is assembled, the raised *coiffe* will be positioned round the inside of the crown, and will prevent the marquetry, or the gummed toile, of which the crown is composed from rumpling your head or pulling your hair. Tighten the *coiffe* as needed when you put on the hat, and it will contribute to its grace.

This fashion of placing the *coiffe* is very well, in that it hides the stitches which have fastened this part, those which you made in assembling the hat, and the edge of the curve of the brim. It serves also to preserve this edge from the sweat which collects principally at this place on the hat. However, there are milliners who attach the *coiffe* to the crown, extending it a little to the outside. This mode is not bad, but the first is still better.

The *coiffe* is put on after the entire construction of the hat only when it is a matter of renewal, or of trimming an uncut straw hat, because the operation is then quite awkward. You must pass the needle alternately over and under the base of the crown, taking care that the stitches do not show. I shall repeat some of this when speaking of straw hats. When you place ornaments on the hat, always turn down the *coiffe* on the brim, in order to avoid sewing it, or catching it with the pins which hold the bows, flowers, &c.

To assemble the Hat. The *coiffe* sewed, keep it turned down on the lining of the brim. You may then put the edge of the crown over that of the brim. Find the middle of each with the aid of a string, and fix them together with a pin. After these preparations, sew the crown securely to the brim, passing the needle over and under. Use a very coarse thread, which is sometimes doubled, and take several rows of stitches. This mode of assembling hats never varies. You should, before permanently assembling the hat, try it on the plaster head.

The brim has sometimes a notable variation: on some straw hats and many bonnets, the marquetry brim has no back. It is cut to the right and left at the level of the ears, and in place of a back you put a band of material cut on the bias, about three or four inches high. This band, or rather this back, is sewed on the side parts cut from the brim. It is here of the same height, but narrows towards the middle. Gather it or plait it a little when placing it on the back of the crown. This kind of back must be bordered at the sides and across with a rouleau of similar material, which serves as a hem. Some milliners replace the gathers with an ordinary string-case through which they pass two ribands which, when tightened, pull the back of the material, and are tied in the middle, at the base of the crown.

Cover the join with a narrow hoop or band of the hat material, bordered by a corded piping, or with twisted braid, placed all round the seam fold of the band. You may substitute a satin-finished brass wire, a *torsade* of rather wide riband, or a riband folded through the middle. Or more often, a satin rouleau, or one of material similar to the hat; a wide riband put on flat, and tied at the back or on the side; a bias of material bordered by corded piping; a thick beaded braid; a succession of corded pipings (seven to eight); and other like things, serve to conceal the join of the brim and the crown.

Toques.

A toque is the crown of a hat without a brim, because its brim is rather a bandeau, since it is composed only of a two-inch band on which the crown is mounted. This crown, ordinarily rounded, is made exactly like a hat-crown. Sometimes, however, a toque has a brim which merits the name. This is a rim similar to that of a man's hat, but more flared and more rolled up: such were the toques called Bolivar.

To make this brim, cut a square piece of marquetry, and round it off into a ring two or three inches wide (see Fig. 3). Then cut a bias band in marquetry, three or four inches wide, according to the size of the rim. Double it like a gauze bias band, and sew it to the outer edge of the brim. Sew it on top of the brim, flat, and in such a manner that it accommodates the curve by forming imperceptible folds. This seam must be sturdy, with several rows of stitches, because you must sew at the same time the marquetry brim and both edges of the folded band. If the band is well placed, it will produce a border rolled up in half, which is called a turn-up. If, as sometimes happens, the border must be more rolled and more turned up towards the ears than in the front or at the back, you must take it in more round the sides. (When you wish to roll or turn up the edge of a hat, proceed precisely as just described.)

To cover this border or turn-up, first put on a bias band of material which encompasses it entirely on the wrong side and the right side, in such a manner that you may sew both sides at the same time, entering the needle alternately over and under. Keep the border from rolling, and hold it as flat as possible.

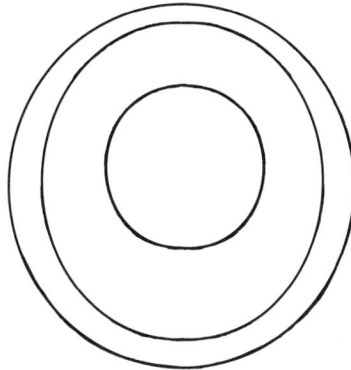

Figure 3. The shape for a toque brim.

Then place, over and under the marquetry brim, a brim of material which is applied over the seam of the bias band of the border. Make a seam fold which is hidden by a twisted braid, and attach a corded piping, as I have explained at length for the borders of hat-brims. Then join this brim to the crown. As to the mode of covering and decorating it, refer to the articles on hat-crowns and ornaments.

Turbans.

Head-dresses of this kind have no brim at all excepting a bandeau. (See Div. 3.) The crown is rounded, and made of two pieces, a top and a bottom. It is covered with a square of material. The middle of this is placed on the middle of the crown, and plaited on the base of the side-band; trim off the surplus. (For the front see No. 19 in the article on trimmings; and for the ornaments see *esprits*, feathers, rich floral decorations, chains, &c.)

Sometimes, over the marquetry bandeau, you place a bias band, or rather a turn-up which encircles the crown and rolls to the other side. This turn-up is covered like the preceding one, or rather you commence by covering it with material. As soon as it is cut and lined, mark the imperceptible plaits which it must have, and sew it round the covered crown; this turn-up must be plaited rather than taken in with little folds. In order to fold over well, it is sometimes given the form of a diadem. Whatsoever its shape, the base is covered with the edge of the band of material which conceals the bandeau. This edge receives a corded piping, or is beaded. Sometimes the other edge of this band has also a braid; more commonly it turns underneath the turban or toque. This band is always on the bias, without folds. Put the *coiffe* on the turned-down edge, proceeding in the same way as you sew a *coiffe* to a hat-crown.

Berets.

The name beret comes from the Italian *berreto,* or cap. This kind of toque is made for very young and very elegant married ladies. There are two kinds: *négligé* berets and fancy berets. The first are made of velvet, barége, or *écarlate.* The front is a narrow bandeau formed from a bias band, or often a single braid; the crown is rounded and covered with material forming enormous puffs or flutings. The base of the crown is nearly always like that of a turban; that is, all in one piece. But sometimes it is composed of two; one is a very wide band, and the other is a little circle an inch and a half, or two inches in all directions, trimmed with corded piping. The band is a little lower at the back, and puffed round the crown, and pulled with close gathers to the base of the crown at the back, under the little circle. Sometimes the circle is centred at the middle of the crown, and then the band is of equal height every where. Because this circle is so small, you do not ordinarily trouble to cut a wide band; you proceed as if you were making a turban, only you fold the material to the right side where you must place the circle.

There are also flat berets with a large circle, but they are less elegant. If you have a black velvet hat which is out of fashion, you may make it into a flat beret. The brim makes the front, and you put the outer edge round the crown. The seams of the other pieces are lost in the flutings. The crown serves the same purpose, and the band which conceals the side-band just makes the little bandeau.

The fancy berets also called *toques aérienne* are composed of gauze, silk tulle, or blond. The flutings make the circumference of the crown at least four times that of your head. That is not all; you add there a coronet of marabouts, or *esprits* perched on the band, or sprays of round feathers placed crossways, to the right and left, and separated by a gold, steel, or diamond clasp. This last ornament is placed on the bandeau; it is the most beautiful. Generally berets are quite becoming, but they are very near to laughable exaggeration. Plaids are completely ridiculous.

Caps.

Caps are toques of gauze or tulle without any turn-up. (See Chapter XX for cap patterns.) Often strings are used in making ordinary caps, and then they no longer resemble toques, excepting the crown, which is always rounded. The crown is never made of esparto, which would be seen through the gauze, but of fine marli, silk tulle, or coarse gummed muslin. This crown is mounted on a very narrow bandeau. Caps are covered with puffed gauze, satin Vandykes, and folded biases. They are ornamented with *torsades,* flowers, &c., but never with feathers: those are proper only for women of a certain age, or persons of modest rank.

The Mode of making Hats of All Kinds of Straw, cutting them, trimming them, &c.

These hats, which I listed earlier, in the description of styles, are much less complicated and less difficult than those preceding. According to the plan generally adopted, and with reason, it seems that I should have taught their easy modes first. But their trimmings are for the most part the same as for hats made of material, and that is the most meticulous part. Moreover, making and preparing straw hats is a mixed art, which is practiced by the haberdasher and the milliner at the same time; it is at the border of their respective functions, which each one exceeds a little. At Paris, milliners only cut hats of Leghorn straw, trim them, and make chip hats; haberdashers make and sell all the rest. But first, this is not every haberdasher; then Paris excepted, milliners are responsible for every thing. This is quite relative to their usual work, and I believe that I must present this article as part of the milliner's art.

Chip Hats. These hats are made of little strips of wood stuck together and formed into narrow flat braids. It is easy to see that they are not very durable: indeed nothing is so fragile, but also nothing is prettier. Men who ordinarily do not know the value of fashionable things, judging the price of this material by its charm, believe it superior to Leghorn straw: but without trimming, the most beautiful chip hat is worth from twelve to fifteen francs, whereas the others go for twelve hundred francs and more.

These hats are ordinarily ready-made by the workman; that is to say, the crown and brim are prepared and put together. But sometimes the brim is bought separately, along with a circle and a wide band which it is necessary to cut and assemble. These latter are a little less charming; but thanks to the attentions of a skilled milliner, they acquire nearly as much grace and much more sturdiness, than the first.

When the hat is ready-made, or complete, you have only to line the brim with white crape or *gaze de laine* (in order to support it), then to sew on the *coiffe* and place the ornaments. In order to leave nothing to be desired regarding lining the brim, I shall say that very often two or three rows of straw are left unlined on the edge. A narrow twisted braid, or any other, hides the seam, as I have explained. When the hat is composed of several parts, line the brim separately with crape and the circle with Chambery gauze; then measure the band just to fit your head. Subtract the excess, leaving about an inch extra, in order to cross the two ends. This completes the side-band, which is also lined with Chambery gauze. Baste a corded satin piping to one edge of the side-band; this may be the colour of the trimming, but more often it is of white satin. Then sew the side-band, thus making a border round the crown. Conceal the seam of the two side ends with a rice straw, a satin rouleau, a braid, &c. The hat is mounted after that as usual: the trimmings depend upon taste or general usage.

When chip hats are half faded, it is possible to cover them with white *crêpe gaufré.* Cut the back of the brim of a chip hat as I shall describe in the following article.

Leghorn Straw Hats. These beautiful hats are always complete, and as large in the front as at the back. When you wish to wear them thus, there is nothing more to do; it is only necessary to be careful to put at the back, the part where the two ends of the straw produce an unevenness where they are joined. Then sew in the *coiffe,* taking care that the stitches do not appear on the outside, because you do not ordinarily put any thing at the base of the crown. To succeed in hiding them, place the *coiffe* into the crown of the hat as it must always remain, mark it with a seam fold at the base, and sew it with long stitches underneath, and imperceptible ones on top. Then occupy yourself with the ornaments.

However, this brim, which droops at the back as much as in the front, covers your shoulders, crumples your *fichu,* and is extremely annoying. To obviate these difficulties, some persons fold it back upon itself. That is a poor remedy, which only increases the awkwardness at your neck and the pulling on your *fichu.* Therefore, many ladies are in the habit of cutting their hats, that is, taking a portion off the back of the brim. Here is the way to do it:

Take a paper pattern of the shape shown in Fig. 4, and apply it to the back, placing the middle of the pattern, on the middle of the back of the brim. Fix it with pins, letting it exceed the edge by two, three, or four rows of straw (according to the fineness of the hat), which you separate by unpicking them very carefully. This is because the tissue of Leghorn straw is formed of straw plaits sewed together without the thread being perceptible. Unpick all along the lower edge of the pattern, and even an inch or more to the right and left. Then cut the straw of the hat along the upper edge by this same pattern; put aside the cut-off part. Bind the whole edge which you have cut, with a *faveur* the colour of the straw. The binding being finished, place upon it the narrow band of rows which you previously unpicked. This band will be too long; cut off the surplus parts and cross the two pieces. Be careful to bind both ends with a straw-coloured *faveur*. The band of rows must be sewed in such a manner that the stitches are not at all perceptible on the right side. To decorate it, you may put a row or two of twisted straw braid over the seam. This braid conceals all the seams which can possibly be made in this hat. As it flattens out in washing, you must renew it every time you have the hat cleansed.

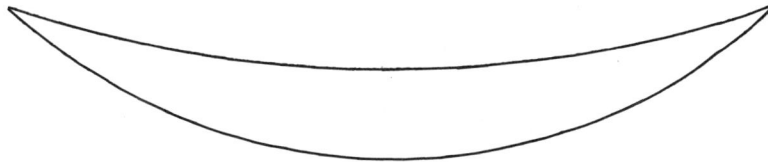

Figure 4. The shape for the brim of a straw hat.

The portion cut off may be used to make a *recoquillage* in the middle of the bows, on top of the crown, or in the front at the base of the side-band. You must border it with a flat satin rouleau, over which you place a twisted straw braid.

No doubt a hat thus cut is more convenient, but the fashion changes every year. It will become necessary to re-cut the hat, or to lengthen it. Happily the very beautiful Leghorn straw is permitted to defy custom: when narrow brims are worn, these hats may retain all their width. When you have committed the folly of cutting a hat in this fashion, you might then lengthen the brim with a bias of marquetry which is covered with straw-coloured *gros de Naples,* or with a riband similar to those on the hat: this is not very pretty.

For a time the back of the brim was trimmed so much that the cut-off part formed the front of another hat. The crown was made of green or yellow taffety, and the back of the brim similar to the backs of bonnets where no marquetry has been put.

A few years ago, fashion decreed that strings attached on top, on the side, or at the beginning of the brim, be fastened about three inches lower and pass underneath. It seemed that it would be necessary to pierce the brim, and some persons were clumsy enough to do so. The fashion passed, and their hats were found to be hopelessly spoiled. They should have acted as I shall explain: at the place where the string ends, cut the riband, make a wide seam fold underneath, and sew it underneath as well, so that it is evident that the riband has been cut and sewed; then turn the hat and sew the loop under the brim at the same place where you just fastened the riband on top.

Hats of Swiss straw, cotton tissue imitating chip, or silk tissue imitating Leghorn straw, are cut and furnished as I have just described.

Hats of Sewed Straw and of Monaco Straw. These hats are never cut; first, because having little durability, they are renewed with the fashion; second, because they are rarely made too large; and finally, because once the thread is cut, the straw becomes unsewed all round the hat. They are never lined, and are very simply trimmed. Such hats are, especially at Paris, the work of the haberdasher.

Hats of Esparto.

Esparto, another wood tissue, but not in distinct braids, makes hats which are very light and nearly as common. There are three kinds: white, straw-coloured, and a mixture of divers tints. These are sold in pieces by straw-hat dealers. Each piece, composed of a great square, costs from two francs to two francs ten, and suffices to make one hat. Cut the piece by an ordinary hat pattern. Line the parts, then assemble them as I have taught you to do several times. The edge of the brim is bordered by brass wire and is trimmed with a silk braid, but more often with a similar rouleau. There are no kinds of bows, *recoquillages, torsades,* puffs, or flutings which are not imitated in esparto. Sometimes all this is mixed with riband bows and edgings. Plaids do best on these hats, which moreover are always *négligé.*

Hats of Gauze Woven with Straw.

This tissue, worn two or three years ago, is transparent, lustrous, light, and very becoming to the face. Little pieces of glistening straw are woven into the gauze, forming little ribs like rather smooth dimity. It makes pretty bonnets. The brim is nearly flat and trimmed with a rouleau nearly two inches wide; a narrow one would be more becoming. On the edge of the rouleau, put a silk braid or a twisted straw one. The bows are similar. When you see a woman's profile through the hat, she looks twice as pretty. The only fault of these sweet head-dresses is their fragility: they do not cost much more than nine or ten francs.

Hats of Decorated Marli.

Here is a hat material which may at the same time serve to amuse my readers, and procure them an agreeable head-dress.

Take some marli, rather fine and well gummed. Cut out a hat by an ordinary pattern; fold the pieces and wrap them well. Take little stalks of glistening straw, which you will easily find at the shops which sell straw hats.

Take one of these straw pieces and thread it, as if you were taking back-stitches, into the slanting line which forms the tissue. Omit the next line, and pass another piece of straw into the third, opposing the stitches. That is, arrange them so that the stitches passed underneath on the first row, are found to be opposite to the stitches passed above on the second, and *vice versa*. Then make, from one space to the other, a little cut with your scissors on the meshes of the intermediate line. This will make little projections, which look agreeable with the rows of straw. In this way you may make nice enough hats at very little cost, but you must expect to see them soon broken.

The Mode of making Hats of Cotton Tissue, Silk Tissue, and Straw Braids.

You may, following the mode described below for crocheting flat braid, prepare narrow lengths of cotton or silk, which you assemble in the shape of a hat, as I am going to teach you. But perhaps it would be better to buy the braid ready-made, because of the difficulty of making sufficiently long pieces by hand; besides, this braid is cheap.

Flat braid *au crochet* is made by a kind of knitting, or rather a chain-stitch, since a new loop or stitch is always formed by the cotton or silk drawn through the previous one. Begin by turning the cotton between the thumb and forefinger of your left hand, as if you wished to make a double bow. Take a hook, which is an iron instrument two or three inches long terminating in a curved point, and fitted into a wooden handle. Pass the end of the hook at the middle of the two loops and draw through the cotton, which will catch underneath the loop; then raise the hook to tighten them a little. Pass it through the loop just formed and the one which directly precedes it, below which you then re-take the thread to make another loop or stitch; and thus one after another.

Here is how to use the braid: take a rather large pattern of a hat, because the braid tightens in washing and during the work. This pattern or model is composed of a brim and a crown; it must be of straw or pasteboard. Begin in the middle of the crown. Fasten the end of the braid there and wind it round itself in a spiral, describing progressively larger circles. As you make a certain quantity of circles, fix them together with pins, then baste them. But as soon as the circles become a little larger, it is better to baste them immediately, not only to each other, but also to the model.

You thus encircle the entire crown of the model. Then, threading a needle with fine white cotton (if the braid is of cotton) or straw-coloured silk (if the braid is of silk), sew the braids together with slanting over-cast stitches, catching the little loops on the edge of the braid. Take the stitches close together, for fear they will spread apart and become unsewed in washing. This operation finished, remove your work from the model, turn it right side out, and set about making up the front or the brim.

You proceed pretty nearly in the same manner, save for the difference required by the model. Measure the brim in the middle; it is according to this middle that you divide your braid to the right and left on the edge of the brim, in order to see where to cut on the side to obtain the curve of the brim. Before basting, measure each row of braid on the brim, so as neither to lose too much in trimming off the edges, nor have to begin again if by chance a piece is found too short.

Thus place about twenty rows, basting them firmly to the brim of the model, and then basting them to each other. When you reach this point, you must make the narrowings; that is to say, cut the braid at the end of the row, and tuck the end between the braid of the preceding and following rows, in such a manner that no crease forms. You achieve this by biting both selvages rather deeply. As you work on the wrong side, the portions which exceed each other will not show. The number of narrowings cannot be prescribed; it depends upon the shape of the hat.

You sew the brim like the crown, then join them together. When the hat is washed and dressed, it will have the appearance of chip if your braid is of cotton, or of Leghorn straw if your braid is of silk. (See Div. 4.)

Straw braids are sewed differently. They are not sewed to each other, but on each other with running stitches. They are not assembled on a model, because they have more firmness, and you cannot turn the crown right side out without breaking the straw. You may only make hats of this kind by following a model. For the rest, you begin with the middle of the crown, as I have said. You make the narrowings in the same manner, passing the excess portion of the cut braid underneath, and covering it little by little with the neighbouring braids.

Ornaments for Hats.

Ornaments for Hats.

We have finally arrived at the innumerable ornaments, at this bugbear of the milliner's art. Let us see if it is so fearsome, so indescribable as is commonly thought. In order to prevent confusion, I shall divide them into fifty-two kinds, and I admit that these are not all. However, when I have described them, each in accordance with the amount of detail it requires, you will understand all possible ornaments, because they can be nothing but combinations of these.

1st., Bows of Riband. After the long and detailed explanations which I gave on this subject in Chapter XX, it might seem that I have nothing more to add. But there are so many variations of them, that I still find important observations to make.

If you wish, at the same time, to widen and vary the bow, sew two ribands on the wrong side at one selvage. Combine them thus: white ribands, one moiré and one satin, or satin and taffety, or taffety and moiré, or gauze and satin. You may equally mix ribands of similar colours, and also those of different colours: straw and lilac, blue and straw, blue and white, yellow and ponceau, rose and white, lilac and white, &c. But ordinarily one of the ribands is satin, the other taffety. Sometimes two taffety ribands are seen, but rarely two satin ones.

If it is a matter of giving firmness to the bow, apply a straw. This straw is sewed to the wrong side of the riband, at the lengthways middle, with long running stitches underneath and very small ones on top. Always insert it before making up the bow, whose loops it holds securely. It goes without saying that you begin to place it only after having allowed enough riband to make the ends of the bow, and that it supports only the loops. Moreover, a straw thus placed is very effective for restoring firmness to silk materials which have been made into puffs, when they have been softened by use. When turning hats it is often necessary to resort to it. To support bows of gauze riband, sew an extremely narrow rice straw to the wrong side on each selvage. There are also bows decorated with straw braid; but the braid is placed on top, as an ornament, whereas the straw serves as a support.

2nd., Bows of Material. Take some material similar to the body of the hat. Cut a bias band about two inches wide: this is the band of the bow. Then cut a little strip about an inch, or an inch and a half wide. This is commonly similar to the hat trimming when there are two colours. When the hat is of *gros de Naples,* the strip is of satin. When the hat is of satin, which must always be bordered, the strip is of *jaspé* or *broché,* like the taffetys called granite. Sometimes the strip is similar to the hat material, but rarely.

Whatsoever the materials, sew the two bands together all round with back-stitches, placing them like the two parts of an ordinary seam. The seam finished, lift up the edge, and fell it to the wrong side of the band of the bow, taking good care that the stitches do not pierce through to the right side. To manage this, be careful to enter the needle only on the previous seam. It is well to work this seam by sewing from the side on which the border lies, in order to take it in imperceptibly, so that it turns over like a rouleau without tightening.

Bows of material are rarely arranged like those of riband. Mark the places for the loops, and at each measure fix the material on the hat with rather strong pins. However, from time to time collect the loops together on a little stay, and pass a little band there.

I have not spoken of the length of the long band for the bow, because nothing is more arbitrary. When this band, after having supplied the bow at the front of the hat, goes on to form *agrafes* (flat loops) at the back, it is clear that its extent cannot be estimated. It would, however, be disagreeable to waste time and material preparing it longer than need be. To avoid this difficulty, it is sufficient to take a wide faded riband, and temporarily imitate the loops and *agrafes* on half the hat. Note the measure which the riband requires to this point. Double it, and you are prepared to cut the real band for the bow.

A singular ornament is often mixed with these bows, with which it is frequently confounded. Take about an eighth of an ell of the unbordered band for the bow. Cut it crossways, after having doubled it: this is not ordinarily done, because the band is left whole, without being divided. This doubled piece is placed so that the two right sides of the doubled material touch. Stick a camion through the middle of the doubled pieces to keep them equal, than sew to the right and left along their length. The lower part which faces the fold remains unsewed. Put your hand there, between the two doubled pieces, and turn them to the right side.

3rd., Gathered Bows. Fashion demanded for a time that hat ornaments display kinks reminiscent of calf innards. To obtain these effects, bias bands are bordered like those of the preceding bows, sometimes with a twisted braid introduced in the same edge of the band, in order to make it curl better. Other times it is bordered by piping or a rouleau, according to taste. The band, more or less wide, is either bordered on one side (that is, a half-band) or all round. In the first case, the side not bordered is gathered; in the second the gathering is made lengthways in the middle of the band, which is folded when sewing it to the crown of the hat. Other bands or half-bands placed near these complete the bow; or arranged in arches or festoons, they produce intervals where flowers are placed.

4th., *Recoquillé* **Bows.** These are always wide bias bands of material like the preceding ones, but bordered by a flat rouleau. When making the first seam on this border, you insert a straw in the rouleau to impart enough stiffness for the folds to form loops. Or, the band is partly lined with light marquetry, covered in its turn with either *gaze de laine* or satin muslin the colour of the hat, according to whether the wrong side of the loops will be seen.

This fashion is at its height. Sometimes the band is placed so that it crosses the crown, from where it falls to form a coronet over the front, at the edge of the side-band. Or, place it round the side-band and double the volume in the front. Or, place it beginning on the left side of the hat, at the side-band, traverse the side-band in the front, and fasten it on the right side of the hat. Much folded, the band produces large box-plaits which form as many loops, in the midst of which you set *esprits,* flowers, and riband bows of a colour which contrasts with the hat. Often, in place of these divers ornaments, lined pieces of esparto are used, as I have explained. These pieces may be hearts, circles, diamonds; all kinds of shapes.

5th., Cockades. These bows are made of heavily-gummed satin riband, and are pinked by means of a punch, as explained in Chapter XX for ruches. The riband, pinked on both selvages, is placed lengthways on top of the front of the crown. There along the middle, make triple and quadruple box-plaits. Make them close together, not very deep, and take care to round them so that they give the bow the aspect of a long cockade. This band is commonly accompanied by another: at the end of the bow bring both ends together, folding the riband upon itself so that the selvages meet, and the line of points does not appear interrupted. These bows, which were worn about ten years ago, returned to fashion last year. They are put on hats with a flat crown, which have several *cerceaux* (as described earlier), and on plush or velvet hats, principally for very young persons. The cockade is never accompanied by an ornament.

6th., Fringed Bows. On this subject, see the mode of fringing belts and bows in Chapter XX. These bows require very stout, wide riband. Satin riband is not ravelled. When the bow is made of material, it should be on the straight-way if it is to be ravelled. However, it may be on the bias if the ends are cut slanting, which divides the bias and consequently gives a straight-way. Otherwise, or when you wish the bow to have rounded ends, you must sew on a ravelling or fringe of similar silk. Ravelling the bow is incomparably more elegant. You should use plaids, that is, materials with several colours.

7th., Trimmed Bows. These are composed of ribands or bias strips of material, trimmed with real or false blond with little points, without any plaits. The blond is sometimes placed quite simply on the selvages of the riband, or on the seam fold of the material. Sometimes, and more frequently, a corded piping, a pretty twisted silk braid, or a satin rouleau serves as a border. Though united, the materials must be imperceptibly loose. There should be a large fold at each end of the bow; this fold, wide underneath the selvage, disappears towards the opposite edge, and produces a slanting line on top.

Trimmed bows are arranged at the whim of fashion and in different ways, but are seldom arranged to receive feathers and flowers, unlike *recoquillé* bows, biases, &c. That mixture would make too heavy a mass. Thus hats with trimmed bows are simple, though elegant.

These bows are sometimes bordered by a very narrow double bias of *gaze de laine;* but this practice is extremely rare for hats, where it produces little effect. It is more suitable for caps.

I must not pass silently over one kind of ornament which has much in common with trimmed bows. This consists of rectangles, triangles, and diamonds of material trimmed in the same way, which are placed round the side-band of the hat. These divers articles are rather wide, so that they may be nicely folded.

8th., Bows with Pompons. These are bows made of satin, gauze, or any other riband. Very pretty little silk pompons, the colour of the hat, or instead of its borders and trimming, are sewed onto the ends. These decorations are sold by haberdasher/lace-women; they are expensive and very elegant. For some years milliners have used them especially to ornament crape and gauze hats.

9th., Bows with Thick Braids and Flattened Pompons. These are just like the bows which ornament the shakos of the Hussars and Lancers. Each thick, twisted braid is passed negligently to the base of the hat-crown. It is then fastened on the right, over the side; the pompons fall to the edge of the brim. These bows are always matched to the colour of the hat. Like the preceding ones, they are devoted to winter headdresses, and are even more restricted to young ladies. They are especially used on beaver hats.

10th., Bows Decorated with Flowers. It may seem that I have only to review the preceding bows, amongst which, according to my directions, the curves leave intervals in which bouquets may be placed. However, besides these, there are gauze bows mixed with flowers, which are so pretty and graceful that, without fear of being accused of exaggeration or affectation, I may say that they seem to be the work of a zephyr. Indeed, ladies, imagine a wide *gaze de laine* bias, which elegantly folded, forms several light loops, amongst which rosebuds may be glimpsed. Some, more slender, are at the level of the fold of loops; others, half hidden by the gauze, show crimson through the transparent tissue.

Because the gauze will stretch as you wish and the stalks of the flowers are passed under the loops, you ordinarily place the bouquets after the bow, in order to judge the effect of the whole.

11th., Bows Decorated with Feathers. This description will be less poetic. Take a wide satin riband, or the band of a bow suitably bordered by braid or a rouleau. When there is comparatively more riband, arrange one or two loops on the hat, then place an *esprit* or marabouts. When feathers dominate, place them first, prepare the bows separately, then attach the bows between the feathers and over their shafts.

12th., Bows with Metal Clasps. These are large bows of material or riband, in the middle of which is applied a steel or gold clasp rather like the kind used for belts, if it were not for the absence of prongs. They do very well on black hats; this is chiefly a head-dress for young persons. This simple and elegant ornament is seen especially on winter hats, such as those of plush, velvet, or beaver.

13th., Biaises. Ordinarily of *gaze de laine,* these are similar to those with which haberdashers decorate *fichus* and fancy caps. On milliners' caps and white hats, arrange them like *recoquillé* bows, but without folds other than those which are necessary for the bias to turn and curve according to the chosen shape. The bias is ordinarily sewed beforehand to a corded piping of white satin or riband edging, giving it the proper length, then applied to the hat. In general this mode of making the ornaments separately and then affixing them, permits you to work more easily and crumples the hat less. The first four bows described may be used, although (above all for *recoquillé* bows) a skilful milliner prefers to place the bias on the crown at once, in order to judge the effect. Riband bows, flowers, and other ornaments also decorate the intervals produced by the curves of the bias.

14th., Ruches. Blond or plain tulle ruches are placed on the outer edge of the brims of hats which are white, or not dark coloured. They are very small flutings. Ruches of similar material serve to trim bonnets of *gros de Naples:* the bands are pinked with a punch. These two kinds of ruches are doubled, and mounted on a flat braid or a very narrow riband. They are then placed round the brim; they should be touched as little as possible. These trimmings are pretty; the last are very elegant, but they have the great disadvantages of becoming crushed very quickly, of being pulled out of shape, and of making the hat or bonnet appear extremely faded when they are still tolerably new. (Ruches whose colour varies here and there are called *boiteuse* ruches.) This trimming frequently goes in and out of fashion.

15th., *Torsades.* You have seen how small *torsades* of narrow riband form borders for hats. Large *torsades* of wide riband play another role well: placed at the back, over the side-band, the *torsade* rises over the crown, where it ends in a bow. Or, encircling the side-band, it holds the feathers and flowers on the front; it again crosses the crown from one side to the other. *Torsades* are also made of white *gaze de laine*, alone or twisted in a more or less long spiral, with light-coloured riband or *gaze de laine*.

16th., Vandykes. Large rounded or pointed notches are cut in the material of the hat when it is sturdy, such as *gros de Naples*, satin, or velvet. These notches are trimmed with a rouleau, a braid, a pointed blond, or a ruche. They are placed round the base of the crown over the side-band, sometimes with the points at the top, sometimes with them at the bottom. In the first case, which is the most frequent and produces the most beautiful effect, the points lie over the crown. Other times they are lowered just a little and bows, flowers, or marabouts are put in the spaces. In the second case, the trimming is fastened on the top of the crown and cut into notches round the bottom, over the side-band.

17th., *Agrafes* of Material, Gauze, or Riband. These are rather large loops, which, instead of joining the folds which are formed, spread both ends over a space more or less narrow, according to whether you wish the *agrafe* to puff out. When they are made of material, the band used is cut on the bias and bordered like the bands of bows. Gauze *agrafes* are also composed of a bias band folded into overlapping plaits, and lined underneath. *Agrafes* encircle the hat as I explained for *torsades*. At each point where an *agrafe* ends, make a *coulant* of silk, straw, or corded piping, according to the trimming of the hat. This *coulant* is similar to the little folded piece which is put in the middle of bows.

18th., Tulle or Satin Panes. Panes of the first sort are placed flat on the part of the hat which they decorate. They are gathered all round and surrounded by a braid of twisted silk, a narrow satin rouleau, or a piping. The second are passed under the material by means of a gap through which they are slipped by the end. They are simply folded underneath and have no border. They were formerly the same colour as the trimmings of the hat, of which they were a part. They were mixed with flowers; they were especially common on toques: gauze panes on silk toques, satin ones on velvet toques; the ornaments being sometimes the colour of the foundation, sometimes of a different shade; such as rose, deep yellow, or celestial blue on black velvet.

19th., Turbans. I am not speaking here of the turban as a particular head-dress, but solely as an ornament. It is ordinarily a wide bias band of *gaze de laine,* which is arranged in lengthways plaits round the hat, at the base or at the middle of the side-band. It is in some sort two great *agrafes,* since the plaits are not tight and are fastened on the under side but twice. A tuft of feathers or flowers on the front is the only thing joined to a turban.

20th., Blond Half-veil. This charming trimming, which has been the fashion for a long time without interruption, decorates only very rich and very elegant hats. It is composed of silk blond about a quarter of an ell wide, either pointed or plain, but always of the first quality. White silk blond decorates white hats, or those of a very light colour. Black silk blond trims black hats, and sometimes hats which are dark blue, deep yellow, or bright pink when the rest of the trimming is black.

The blond is placed round the brim when the hat is finished, so that you do not crumple the brim by turning and re-turning it. For this, secure the hat on the plaster head with two or three large pins, which pierce at the same time the plaster and the hat. The blond must be applied loosely; gather it and sew it lightly round the brim, placing it on top so that its right side touches the upper side of the brim. The seam is thus made from underneath, because when the blond is allowed to fall, it conceals the seam. You may also—and this mode is better—sew the blond to a narrow white silk braid, and apply it afterwards on the edge of the brim. Or, you may sew it in a flat seam with running stitches, without letting them be seen from underneath. Sometimes a blond ruche surmounts the half-veil. Then the blond is first placed on the narrow riband which serves as a base for the ruche. This is then placed on the gathered selvage of the half-veil, and both are sewed together flat at the same time.

The two ends of the half-veil are joined at the back by means of a slanting lace seam (see Chapter XV). A lengthways seam *à la reine* would be quicker, but it would be visible and very ugly. Milliners usually unite these two ends without using either seam; they place a narrow satin corded piping between the two pieces, which they then sew together.

When the hat is on your head, you raise the half-veil on one side of the front, so that the blond is reversed over the brim. Thus partly raised, it is in exquisite taste, and thoroughly becoming. In case of sun, it is lowered and serves as a veil; but it is rarely worn for this purpose. Such a superb hat is unfrequently worn for the promenade, and certainly cannot dispense with the aid of a parasol.

21st., *Fichus* **on Hats.** For a time, people took a coloured gauze *fichu* of about three quarters, and spread it diamond-wise over the top of the crown, with the middles of each more or less together. To arrange the *fichu,* bring the fulness to the side-band in the front, leaving no more over the bottom than a little of the front point. This fulness serves to make large round plaits. The back point of the *fichu* falls from these plaits onto the right side of the brim. The two side points serve as strings. Prepare them by folding them upon themselves, then divide them from the top fulness at the side-band, fastening them there with a strong pin. These *fichus,* ordinarily plaid and trimmed with a short fringe, have a very agreeable effect. Some are made of light taffety. This trimming is often suitable for straw hats.

For straw hats which you wish to be extremely simple, cut the *fichu* slantways in half, forming two triangles. The first is placed over the crown with one point at the back; the other two points are tied below your neck. This is called a *pointe en marmotte.* The second triangle is put round the *collerette,* and tied in a large bow in the front: this last style is still in use. Hem the bias of the triangles with running stitches; the hem will be concealed by the plaits.

22nd., Marabouts. Marabouts, also called *follettes,* are, as every one knows, small round feathers, so slender and fine that they might be called a glossy little cloud. They are white, rose, blue, lilac, or black; sometimes only one colour, sometimes mixed. (See Div. 5.) They are always placed in clusters or bunches of two, three, or four; and these clusters are repeated as many as six times. Bows of *gaze de laine,* blond, gauze riband, or satin riband mix with them agreeably. When you put the marabouts on in a single mass, you need seven, nine, or eleven. Their joined stems are hidden by a full-blown rose, or a very small cluster of sessile ears of grain, that is to say, ones without any stem.

Marabouts are a very dressy and very expensive ornament: they are worn only by young married ladies. Hats for full dress and toques *de salon* are very often trimmed with marabouts; white ones are the most elegant. They are mingled with ears of grain, currants, and gold grapes.

23rd., *Esprits.* These are aigrettes of feathers, sometimes straight and about half a foot long, sometimes curved and at least a third longer. The stem, of about an inch and a half, is surmounted by several overlapping circles of small feathers with soft and flexible barbs, forming a setting rather like the calyx of a flower. A long aigrette with barbules resembling bulbous horsehairs rises from this setting. The base is often black or yellow, whereas the aigrette is a beautiful white. When curved *esprits* have long uneven barbs, they fall like the branches of a weeping willow. Other times the aigrette is composed of soft feathers, to the ends of which are attached little globes of gold, silver, or steel. These ornaments enrich black *esprits* especially. Toques and hats trimmed with *esprits* are still more rich than the preceding: this is a head-dress for married ladies, and for elegant ones. You may put up to three straight *esprits* on the same hat; you place only a single curved one on a toque or turban. *Esprits* are especially meant for these last two articles.

24th., Weeping Willow Plumes. So are called the great beautiful white ostrich feathers which decorate the richest toques and hats. Ordinarily they are three in number and are placed on the right, one over another. The first one placed must be at least a third longer than the others, because it is meant to fall as far as your shoulder. No other kind of ornament should be mixed with this opulent decoration, on which the oddities of fashion are very rarely exercised. Whatsoever their circumstances, young ladies must not use them.

25th., Plumes Decorated with Gold or Steel. See what I have just said about the *esprits* from which shining metal globes are suspended. The feathers are not only laden at the end of the barbs, but also mixed with long gold or silver threads.

26th., Bird-of-paradise. A little while ago, a particular oddity in fashion was a stuffed bird-of-paradise spread over the front of turbans and toques *de salon*. It was also an ornament for balls.

27th., Bouquets of Feathers. It is one of the most singular caprices of fashion that the leaves and the petals of flowers are imitated with feathers. Sometimes the flower, called a *fantaisie*, is made entirely of peacock feathers or other naturally vari-coloured feathers. More often the leaves are made with green parrot feathers, and the petals with other feathers, coloured by Nature or by art. In the midst of these strange flowers coloured barley grains are often put, resting on long stalks, and forming a ball like virburnum blossoms. Each grain is surmounted by a long horsehair or barb resembling the bristles on true ears of grain. These ornaments are for demi-toilet: they are used on crape or silk hats.

28th., Mixed Flowers. The bouquets which adorn hats are often of a single species, but still more often they are of two, three, or four; and sometimes they unite a quantity of many different flowers, which is called a *jardinière*. Different mixtures have different purposes. In a bouquet with two kinds of flowers, the aim is to contrast small flowers to large ones, in order to better bring out the elegance of their shapes. It is thus that roses and dropwort, or pomegranate blossoms and jasmine, are sometimes mixed. At other times the purpose is to soften and blend their colours, such as deep red China asters joined with pink, rosy, and white ones.

You are still supposed to match the flowers to the season. Thus in the spring you may make bouquets of corn-flowers and poppies, of daffodils and narcissuses, &c. Women of fashion are in the habit of changing the flowers in their head-dresses as the season produces new ones. This custom is charming, but costly. During the winter it is neglected; then, however, the bouquets of early spring are not worn, such as violets, lilacs, and the flowers already mentioned. Only roses are for all seasons. Daisies are seen only in autumn, when they bloom. Also persons who, through sense or necessity, economize on their toilets, guard well against choosing flowers which must be left off at the end of a month. *Jardinières* are not subject to this disadvantage, but that kind of ornament is common and not very pleasing.

29th., Flowers and Fruits. It is not enough to mix flowers with each other. They are mixed with grapes; or red, white, or black currants, artificial or gilded.

30th., Flowers and Feathers. Flowers combined with marabouts, small *esprits*, and the round feathers called *queue-de-chat* make up this kind of ornament.

31st., Flowers and Tinsel. These flowers have leaves of silver or gold, and even part of the petals. Recently fashion has thought of imitating bladder-sienna pods in this way: the long bulbous capsule of this bush is made of red or dark blue batiste decorated with a line of silver. The leaves are also of this metal, and long barbes like the husks of ears of grain, finish this odd creation. This description will give an idea of the flowers decorated with tinsel, and show how they imitate Nature.

32nd., Veiled Flowers. These take their names from the large loop of *gaze de laine* which spreads over the flowers. The flowers must be combined with *gaze de laine* bows, so that one of these appears to conceal the flowers while revealing them. They are always in rather strong colours. Thus common flowers may be used, but not faded ones, as you might think.

33rd., Velvet Flowers, for Winter. Velvet flowers imitate flowers whose corolla is velvety, such as pansies and lamb's ears. These flowers are beautiful, but they need assistance from other flowers which are more flexible and lighter. Thus it is well to mix them with jasmine, anemones, or gillyflowers. These last must be white, or at least of a soft colour. Jasmine and heart's-ease, with their brilliant colours, blend very well.

34th., Chenille Flowers. These are very rarely employed, but they are still put amongst the stalks and foliage of artificial flowers. They are heavy, lack grace and flexibility, and are much dearer than the others.

35th., Straw Flowers. These flowers, composed of tufts of straw, have come into fashion several times, but they have never caught on. I mention them solely to omit nothing. They are too heavy and common for toilet, like other flowers, and for *négligé* they are not worth the riband bows. Extreme sturdiness is their sole advantage. They are decorated with leaves and circles of scarlet or any other coloured wool; and this ornament succeeds in making them ugly.

36th., Herbs. Bunches of herbs, ferns, or heather, either alone or strewn amongst flowers, are much used on straw hats in summer.

37th., Sticks. Dry wood, twisted and curved in a thousand ways, and sometimes bristling with thorns, is an ornament for straw hats and silk ones, as fashion dictates. Sticks are often mixed with riband bows; more often a single flower is placed amongst the dry twigs.

38th., Pearls. False white pearls adorn toques and turbans very agreeably. Small, and arranged in several rows close together, they make bandeaux which partly cover the narrow brims of this kind of head-dress. Larger, and in one or two rows, they are twisted in spirals round the multifarious plaits of gauze, or *torsades* of white satin riband, with which the base of the crown is decorated.

39th., Steel Ornaments, such as Bees, Crescents, &c. These shining and varied ornaments are a species of buttons which are placed right side up, or sewed to the riband *agrafes*, gauze loops, curves, and plaits of all kinds, which I have described in the course of this article on trimmings. They are pierced with two holes in order to pass the stitches, or furnished underneath with a crude little ring, like all metal buttons.

40th., Chains and Gilded Circlets. These are usually gilded and silvered braids which enrich the brims of richly-decorated toques and turbans. The most remarkable of this kind is that which depicts a serpent biting its tail. The join is placed in the front. The symbol of eternity applied to ephemeral fashions is curious enough.

41st., Buttons. For a time buttons matched to the hat trimmings were placed at the extremities of points and panes, and at the point where the folds of *agrafes* were sewed. They were also used to attach strings, by means of a button-hole. This fashion is old; the more reason to revive it soon.

42nd., Circular Garlands. Until now, I have spoken only of flowers arranged in bouquets; I must now say that they are often in unbroken garlands, like the ones put on the hair. These garlands are placed on the hat in several ways. At the base of the crown, or at the place of the side-band, they form a circle of flowers fastened at the back with a little riband bow similar to those on the strings. Nothing is more simple, more graceful, or more truly elegant. When the garland is equally thick every where, it is composed of large sessile flowers such as roses, China asters, buttercups, or anemones. When it forms a diadem on the front, the flowers have short stems, and are mixed. They are principally used on Leghorn straw hats. Garlands are also placed as a half-coronet, on the side-band or the crown, as I explained in the article on *torsades*.

43rd., Garlands of Foliage. Our ladies seem to be decorated with civic crowns, because they are wearing garlands of oak leaves. These are principally used on hats of white *gros de Naples*. Olive leaves, and leaves of various exotic trees are also seen, but more rarely.

44th., Garlands of Bows. These are little riband bows placed close together so that they form a garland arranged like the *torsades* and garlands above. In order not to risk placing the bows badly, you will do well to mark the path you wish them to follow with a brass wire.

45th., Garlands of Loops. Similar to garlands of bows, they require the same method. You may fix the loops with camions before sewing them, and even let the camions remain.

46th., Garlands *en Casque*. These sometimes cross the hat from the end of the middle of the brim in the front, to the end of the brim at the back. They are never in a straight line; they are made to describe a slightly slanting line in order to be more graceful.

47th., Ornaments under the Hat-brim. Until now, people were content to trim the upper side of the brim in a thousand ways, but now the trimmings are on its lining. It is not as though there were fewer above; on the contrary, they are every where.

These ornaments are riband bows or loops which are put at the beginning of each string; then large bows are placed to the right side of the edge of the brim. Sometimes a riband which begins from a bow, or any other article placed on the crown, crosses the brim; and bows, or bunches of feathers or flowers, are attached under the edge. Many milliners fasten a few flowers under the side-band, so that they mingle with the curls of the hair. These flowers are always matched to those which trim the hat, from which they appear to be escaping.

That fashion is elegant, but affected; the following is scarcely less so: it consists of sewing a row of riband loops similar to the strings all round the lining under the side-band, to become the neck and the curls of hair. The custom of trimming the side-band in the front with box-plaited blond, which extends along the strings and forms a cornette, is much more sensible and prettier. Unhappily this trimming has the disadvantage of aging the features.

48th., Riband Strings. These are looped on top at the place where they are sewed, or at that where they are tied. The one on the left side is a little shorter, because the one on the right side will join it to make the bow. Recently they have been made equal and left loose; then they may not be divided.

49th., Strings with Corded Piping. These are formed from two bias bands of the material of which the hat is made, bordered by piping, and terminating in points. Make up the bow beforehand, and fasten it to the left as for riband strings.

50th., Gauze or Blond Strings. The first are very wide and very long bias bands of *gaze de laine*, bordered by a satin rouleau. The rouleau is rose or white, according to the colour of the hat; sometimes it is trimmed with a very narrow pointed blond edging; the edges may equally be finished with a twisted silk braid. The most beautiful strings in this style are composed of two bands of blond, sewed at the selvages in such a manner that they have points on both sides.

51st., Strings Trimmed with Box-plaits. This kind, which I have already mentioned, serves as a cornette. When you wish the strings to float and to become your features, use at the same time the kinds above and the strings with box-plaits.

52nd., Double and Triple Strings. The preceding article serves for half of this one. It is enough to add that you may also put at the ends of ruched strings, others of *gaze de laine*, because these being attached only by an imperceptible knot, are rather forwarder on the cap than the strings. Then you do not divide the strings intended to float. This very late fashion is a true mark of affectation.

——*Manuel des dames, Manuel des demoiselles.*

Diversion 1.

To wash Straw Hats. First remove the *coiffe* and all ornaments from the hat. Choose a form of very clean white wood which fits the inside of the crown; then place the hat flat on the table. Rub it all over with a weak solution of pearl ash or very white potash, which comes from the United States. All the stains should come off quickly.

Sulphur afterwards, then give it the finish. To this end, moisten a sponge with rice-water and starch, and pass it over the hat. Then iron the hat with an ordinary flat-iron, first putting a sheet of brown paper over the entire surface, so that the hat will be ironed only through the paper. During this operation the hat should be on the wooden form.

——*Manuel des demoiselles.*

Black Varnish, for Old Straw or Chip Hats. Take half an ounce of the best black sealing-wax, and two ounces of rectified spirit of wine. Powder the sealing-wax, and put it with the spirit of wine into a four-ounce phial. Digest them in a sand-heat, or near a fire, until the wax is dissolved. Lay it on warm, with a fine soft hair brush, before a fire or in the sun.

This gives a good stiffness to old straw hats, and a beautiful gloss, equal to new, and resists wet. If the hats are very brown, they may be brushed over with writing ink, and dried before the varnish is applied. Spirit of turpentine may probably be used in place of the spirit of wine.

——*The Alphabetical Receipt Book and Domestic Advisor.*

For dyeing Straw and Chip Bonnets. Chip hats, being composed of wood shavings, are stained black in various ways. The first is to boil them in strong logwood liquor three or four hours, taking them out often to cool in the air, and now and then adding a small quantity of green copperas to the liquor. Continue this for several hours. The saucepan or kettle in which they are dyed may remain with the bonnets in it all night. The next morning take them out and dry them in the air, and brush them with a soft brush. Lastly, dip a sponge in oil, and squeeze it almost to dryness. With this rub the bonnets all over, both inside and out, and then send them to the blocker's to be blocked.

Others boil the bonnets in logwood; and instead of green copperas, use steel filings steeped in vinegar; after which the bonents are finished as above.

For dyeing Straw Bonnets Brown. Take a sufficient quantity of Brazil-wood, sumach, bark, madder, and copperas, and sadden according to the shade required.

For dyeing Straw Bonnets Black. Wash the bonnet in a little warm chamberlye and water, and rinse it in cold water. Take for one bonnet about a quarter of a pound each of alder bark and logwood. Boil the bonnet in this liquor for an hour or two. Then take it out, and add a small piece of blue vitriol, as big as a small tick-bean. Enter the bonnet, and boil it for half an hour longer. Then take it out, cool it in the air, and add two ounces of fustic chips. Boil these half an hour, then put in the bonnet again; and put in, at the same time, a piece of green copperas, as big as a small bean. Boil again for an hour, take the bonnet out, and cool it in the air. If the liquor remaining in the boiler or copper is jet-black, you may put in the bonnet, and let it remain all night; but if the liquor is not quite black, add a handful more of bark, and a little logwood and green copperas.

The next morning take out your bonnets and dry them in the air. When they are dry, brush them with a soft brush, and afterwards rub them with an oily cloth (called by the trade an oily rubber). Lastly, send them to the blocker's to be blocked.

If this receipt is attended to, the bonnet will be a most beautiful raven black. It is customary with some hat-dyers to steep them in oak saw-dust one night previous to their being dyed, which is a good mode, and generally esteemed. More copperas may be used than is here specified: it may be used in the copper before the article is dyed.

——*The Family Dyer and Scourer.*

Diversion 2.

Divers Head-dresses. For November 1827: several fashionable head-dresses are illustrated in Fig. 5. *A* shows a hat of stiffened cream-coloured net, trimmed with broad plaid ribands and white marabout feathers.

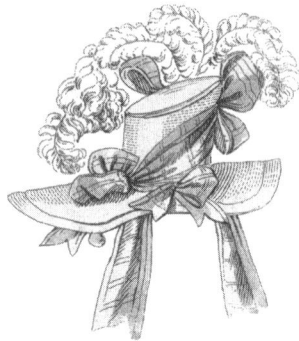
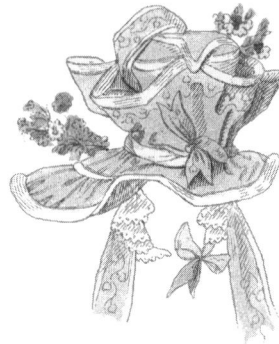

A

B

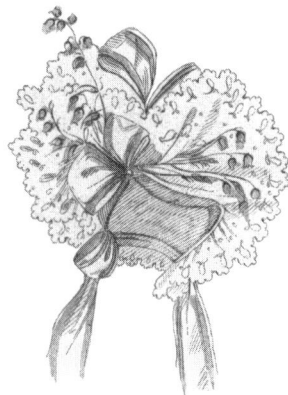
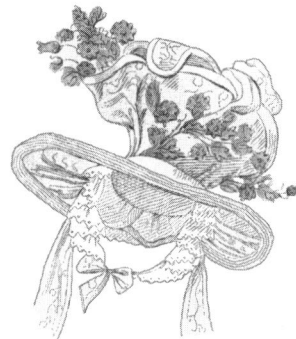

C

D

Figure 5. Fashionable head-dresses.

Fig. 5 *B* shows a bonnet of pink satin, bound with white, and fluted ornaments standing up at the crown, of the same material. Bouquets of differently-coloured ranunculuses adorn this bonnet. Fig. 5 *C* shows a cap of the turban kind, in blond, ornamented with sprigs of green oats, and slightly trimmed with white and green riband. Fig. 5 *D* shows a hat of white crape, with striped satin or riband under the brim. The crown is ornamented *en pattes* with yellow satin, and an elevated scroll in the front, with a profusion of blue corn-flowers.

April 1827. Fig. 6 *A* shows a turban of blue *gros de Naples*, striped with black, and ornamented with two black osprey feathers. Fig. 6 *B* shows

Figure 6. More head-dresses.

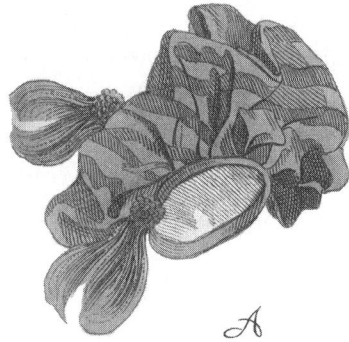

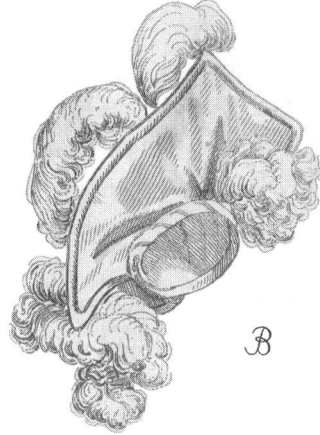

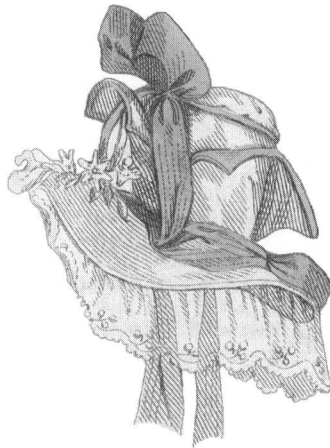

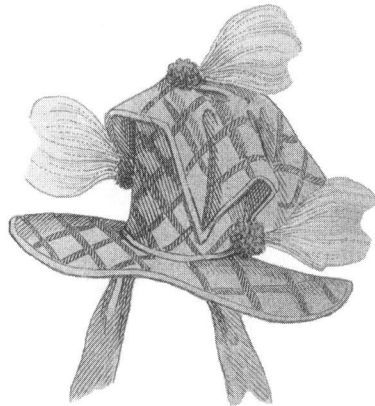

a diadem toque of white satin; under the diadem part, on the right side, is a bunch of marabouts. Full ostrich plumage towers over the head, and one long feather droops over the shoulder. Fig. 6 C shows a hat of white *gros de Naples,* bound and ornamented with celestial blue riband, and a sprig of blue hyacinth. Fig. 6 D shows a hat of bird-of-paradise yellow, chequered with black, with three white aigrettes, black at the base, and disposed in contrary directions.

——*Ladies' Pocket Magazine.*

Diversion 3.

Kinds of Turbans. There are divers modes of forming turbans, and there are turbans of many kinds. There are turbans *à la asiatique, à la greque, à la turque, à la circassienne, à la bayadère, à la egyptienne, à la juive,* &c. Those sold by milliners are ordinarily suitable only for ladies of a certain age. Such an ornament should be made only by an experienced hair-dresser, who knows better how to understand the whole of the person's face.

Turbans may be made with all kinds of materials: with silk, cachemire, merino, barége, muslin, gauze, &c.; with shawls, scarves, &c., &c. Turbans made of several pieces of material, and of different colours, are very elegant. But the changes in hue and the intertwinings must be skilfully managed: a turban in which the differences are not well understood, and the contrasting shades are very marked, most often lacks harmony and charm. In general, I believe that the most beautiful turbans are those made with a scarf of several colours, though sometimes plain ones are made which are not devoid of grace.

Turbans can suit all faces: all depends upon the arrangement, the dominant colour, and the shape chosen. A head-dress which leaves the face bare does not become a woman whose face is round or too prominent, nor even one whose face is oval; yet it is also not unfavourable to that shape, which is ordinarily combined with delicate features and a smooth complexion. In that case, the colours which are preferred are red, in its various shades, pink, and white. Yellow agrees very well with all women, above all brunettes, to whom light blue, black, and all dark colours give radiance and whiteness; delicate green, blue, and lilac are the province of blondes.

When you know how to make any kind of turban, with intelligence, taste, and a little practice, you will easily succeed at varying the shapes for new combinations.

To make a Turban with a Scarf. When you propose to make a turban with a scarf, you must have a riband about an ell and a half long, with which you encircle your head, above and very close to your ears. Knot the riband above your right ear and let it fall beyond the ear on that side. Then take the scarf: the longer it is, the more ample the turban will be. Fold it with your fingers near one end, so that it forms a section of drapery a quarter of an ell and five inches long, which you separate from the rest of the scarf by tying it with string of the same colour. That done, pin a riband at the end of the drapery, so that it hangs to the left, along your temple, and pass the whole scarf over your head, making several graceful plaits. The scarf thus set up, you must spread it out so that it wraps all round the upper part of your head. Then gather it while twisting it round at the nape of your neck, and attach it there with the end of the riband, making two knots for more sturdiness.

When the knots are made, have some one hold the riband straight in front of you, so that it is taut and horizontal. Fold the scarf in your fingers as if you wished to begin a spiral round the riband; pass it over and, having brought it back under, form it into the first loop. Repeat the same operation six or seven times, according to whether the scarf is more or less long, and your head more or less large. These loops, contiguous to each other, present the aspect of a garland, which encircles your forehead and is disposed like a diadem above your curls; this garland is finished on the left side, by means of the riband which supports it.

With the rest of the riband and the rest of the scarf, finish the turban by making several loops at the back. For a riband *à la juive*, pass the end of the scarf under your chin, so as to attach it on the opposite side. You will observe that, for more elegance, the loops must be unequal and become increasingly small, while going from left to right.

Plumes, marabouts, *esprits*, birds-of-paradise, crescents, pearls, diamonds, and precious gems of all sorts may be employed to ornament turbans (see Fig. 7 A). A crescent is placed on the forehead, either very much in the front, or more over the turban. Pearls are disposed in rows, which are made to meander so that they describe agreeable curves; ordinarily they are only put round the front.

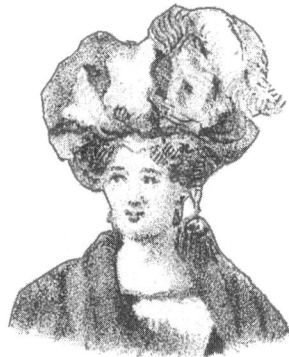 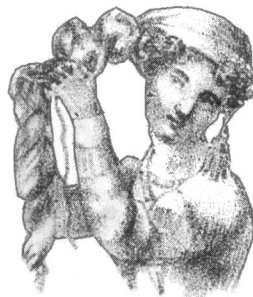

A   *B*

Figure 7. To ornament and wind turbans.

Another Turban made with a Scarf. You must have a flat cord; pass the cord into your hair, which you part with the first tooth of the comb, and pass half your hair over the cord, and half under it. Tie the cord round your head, above your ears, where you knot it rather tightly. Take the scarf by one end, and collect it by folding it. Tie it so that you let about five inches pass; re-attach the end of the scarf with a pin. Tie it on the left side, above your ear: take care that the end of the scarf falls becomingly by your face. Pass the whole scarf over your head, letting fall in the front all which is necessary to fix it to the riband with a pin. Then take the whole scarf in both hands; fold it, and attach it above your right ear with a cord.

Either you or your maid must hold the long end of the cord which was first allowed to fall. Pick up the scarf to refold it; have it passed over the cord, then between the cord and your head, to form a loop (see Fig. 7 *B*). Form several loops thus round the cord, the second being larger than the first, the third smaller, and the fourth smaller yet. When the loops are placed, arrange them in the form of a garland. Temporarily fasten the cord near your left ear, while you round and arrange the first loops. When they are finished, pick up the rest of the scarf and make new ones until no more is left but the end of the scarf, which you tuck under the first loop.

To make a Turban with a Shawl. The turban which I shall teach you how to form, is made with a square cachemire. First take it by one corner, then bring down your left hand at a distance of eight inches below the point, fold the shawl in that part, and tie it with a cord. Place the shawl on your head, the tied corner falling in the front. The tie being made, with the thumb and the two first fingers of your left hand, hold the shawl suspended by the corner under which the tie is placed. Then with the thumb and forefinger of your right hand, grasp one edge of the shawl about fourteen inches from the knot, which you fold until it goes up the other side, loosening your two first fingers, and picking it up in turn with your other three fingers. As soon as the folds are thus collected, pass the shawl over your head, the point falling over your forehead, and fix it with a pin. Collect it at the back, always folding the shawl in both hands, and twist it so that it remains held, or tie it if you think that more suitable. When you do not tie it, insert a pin to secure it, taking care to leave the base of the hair on your nape uncovered, unless you have some reason for not allowing it to be perceived.

When the shawl is sufficiently attached, pick up the rest, then pass the shawl over the point which is held. Put a pin at that place, and place one loop forwarder than the one formed on the right side, so that they will not be regular. Then make another larger one on the left side and lower than the one on the right; insert a pin, and leave the shawl as it is for the moment. Now it is necessary to return to the point in the front, to form a half-slanting loop which must impart grace to the turban. You must hide the point behind the other loops, or the back of the loop which you formed; and for that, bend the point before pinning it.

Pick up the shawl, with which you form only one twist, which you turn gracefully behind your head. If the shawl is long, you may encircle your head a second time and form a new row of loops on top of those which you already placed, constantly opposing them. Turning to the right, fold it for six inches, to form one loop, which you fix with a pin, on the portion of the shawl which covers your head. Fold again as you did previously, to form a second, larger loop, and fix it with a pin. Finally, form a third, even larger loop. If the shawl is not long enough, finish the turban behind the loops which you formed in the first place.

To adapt the turban to the look of your face, it will be well to touch it up, always without disarranging it. The loops must, as far as possible, be long and placed on the bias. It is essential to observe that the right side of the turban must always be higher than the other. The last piece of the shawl is used to form a bias loop on the summit of your head; this must dominate all the others.

———*Art de se coiffer soi-même.*

Diversion 4.

Dressing for Hats of *Écru* Silk imitating Leghorn Straw. These new hats are lighter than those of Leghorn straw, and may be washed and re-dyed divers colours at will.

The dressing consists of ten parts of gum-dragon, one part of alum, and nineteen parts of water. When these materials have arrived at a state of mixture by calorific action, immerse the tissue until it is saturated, then leave it, not until it is entirely dry, but until it has lost its excess moisture, so that it may be put in press and ironed immediately.

Dressing for Hats formed of Braids of Cotton or Silk Thread. The shaped hats are dressed with the following composition, sufficient for a dozen hats: four ounces of fish-glue, two ounces of gum-arabic, four ounces of potato-starch, a pint of spirit of wine, and about half a gallon of water.

To render hats water-proof, use a paint-brush to apply Venetian varnish on top (for white hats) or copal varnish (for coloured hats), after which pass the hats to a warm cylinder.

———*Manuel complet des fabricans de chapeaux en tous genres.*

Diversion 5.

To cleanse Brown, Fawn-colour, and White Feathers. All these colours are cleansed by the same mode. Suppose a plume of three feathers is to be done. Take a large-sized wash-hand basin, cut two ounces of pure white soap into thin slices, and pour boiling river-water upon it. Add to these a piece of pearl ash, as big as a pea. When this soap solution comes to a hand heat, keep passing your feathers through it, and draw them gently between your hand. When this liquor is spent, a second must be made of half the quantity of soap, but an equal quantity of ashes. As at first, you must run your feathers through this liquor, and at last rinse them in cold water, and beat them across your left hand, holding the feathers in your right. After you continue this for ten minutes, the feathers will be nearly dry. Next, with a fruit-knife, or any other round-edged knife, take one or two of the fibres at a time, and scrape them with the knife, turning them round as you wish the curl to be. Then, if you want them flat, put them in a large book to press.

To cleanse Black Feathers. Pour a pennyworth of bullock's gall into a wash-hand basin. Pour warm water on this, and run your feathers through it. Rinse in cold water, and finish them as you would other feathers.

For dyeing and cleansing Feathers. Feathers, to be dyed, must first be cleansed by passing them through, or between your hands, in warm soap and water, and by giving them fresh liquors of soap and water, and at last rinsing them in warm water. Previously to their being dyed, it is necessary that they be soaked in warm water for several hours. The same degree of heat should be kept up, but the water must be but little more than blood-warm. For yellows or reds, you must alum the feathers in cold alum liquor for a day or two, according to the body of colour you require them to imbibe; then immerse them in your dye-liquor.

For some drab colours, it is necessary to use the alum water at a blood-heat: its being too hot would injure the feathers. For dyeing browns, archil, &c. are used instead of woods, barks, &c.; cudbear is also used. After a feather has been dyed any dark brown or other dark colour, its nature is lost, and consequently its texture. It is unprofitable for the wearer to re-dye it, and difficult even for a dyer to perform.

A feather by being beaten across your hand soon dries; by this means feathers are as easily dyed as silk or woollen, and there is a greater certainty of obtaining the desired shade. The only difficulty in dyeing feathers is in compounding the dyeing materials, and making a homogeneous liquor of them, so as to produce the desired shade, after being saddened or made a dark colour by means of green copperas, which is generally used to darken brown-greys, blacks, slate-colours, &c. Sumach and fustic, or sumach alone, is the general ground of browns. The red is obtained by archil; and the black hue by green copperas, in warm water. After the feather has been put into the copperas water, you may return it to the dye-liquor, and back again into the copperas. But care should be taken each time that the feather is rinsed from the copperas water, before it is again returned into the dye-liquor; otherwise the copperas would spoil it. Also take care not to use too much copperas in saddening colours, as it injures the texture, and prevents the colour from appearing bright; and if the ground-colour is not of a sufficient body, the saddening or copperas will make it uneven.

The same preparation as would dye silk of the same colour, will dye feathers. In short, feathers as well as silk, being animal substances, are more alike in nature than any other two bodies, either animal or vegetable. You must remember, that though in dyeing silks the water is used hot, or on the simmer, for most colours feathers must always be dyed in cold liquors, excepting black; the dyeing materials being first boiled, and then suffered to cool. Then put in your feathers; and when this liquor is exhausted add a fresh one, pouring off the old liquor.

For dyeing feathers black, use the same liquor as for silk, but with this difference: for feathers, the dyeing materials must be boiled for two hours, and then used as warm as the feathers will bear, heating the liquor four or five times. It often happens that a feather is four or five days dyeing black; but violets, pansies, carnations, light purples, light blues, greys, &c. are dyed in ten minutes. Light blues are dyed in chemic blue; the greys in galls and green copperas; the violets in warm archil and water; the greens with ebony wood, in warm water and chemic blue. Finish these by gently beating them out over your hand, and this will dry them. Just before they are dry it is requisite to curl them, which is done with a round-edged knife.

The Finest Blue on Feathers. This is obtained by means of the silk blue vat. You should cleanse the feathers well in soap and water, then rinse them in warm water. By these means the feathers will be sufficiently soft. Next, boil as much water as will serve to dye it, to which add (for one feather) half a tea-cup full of purple archil. Simmer the feather for twenty minutes, until it is of the full violet colour; then take it out of this dye, and immerse it in the vat. According to the shade required, so deep must be the shade of the violet; a full violet, by remaining in the vat long enough, will dye a full blue.

There are various other ways of dyeing blue on feathers. For instance: cleanse the feathers as described in the preceding receipt. When your water boils, throw in a tea-spoonful of tartar, and as much chemic blue as will dye the desired shade of blue. Cool down the copper by means of cold water, put in the feathers, and keep the water much below a hand heat. You will have a blue of the brightest dye, more or less full, but of the false dye.

Another Receipt. Use blue vitriol and logwood, as for silk and woollen, at a blood-heat; this also is a false colour, but very bright.

Brown Feathers. Neither camwood, barwood, nor the other woods will do. Madder, archil, walnut root and rind, and green copperas are used; brown being a shade of black. Such a number of combinations enter into brown that you must dye it like black, only do not add the copperas until the feathers have been a day or two in the liquor. The copperas, in the brown, serves to blacken them. Galls and sumach are always used for browns. For red or brown, madder, archil, &c. are mostly used, and saddened by copperas. In fawn-colours, bright root-colours, &c. fustic is also used; but for chocolate, coffee, &c. yellow is omitted; and consequently fustic, or other yellow dyeing materials are not requisite. If the stem or quill is required to be stained, the feather must remain longer in the dye-liquor, and a little heat may be applied.

Chocolate and Full Rich Brown Feathers. These are produced by archil, logwood, and sumach, boiled together, and the liquors heated at different times. The feather must be dipped as hot as it will bear, without injuring its texture. Fustic is also used for chocolate brown, and copperas; and sometimes, pearl ash in the saddening.

For Orange, Madder, &c. Feathers. These colours are very simple, and are produced by annatto and pearl ash, which dye the feathers a buff-colour. They are reddened or oranged by means of acids, such as vinegar, cider, lemon-juice, tartar, and bran-water.

Oil of vitriol, &c. are also used, and especially vinegar, being the simplest. Green copperas is also applied as a corrective. Thus annatto and turmeric are used in dyeing bright reds and scarlet, as they redden by means of the acid liquor, and at the same time add beauty and fulness to the colour.

——*The Family Dyer and Scourer.*

Part III.
Etiquette.

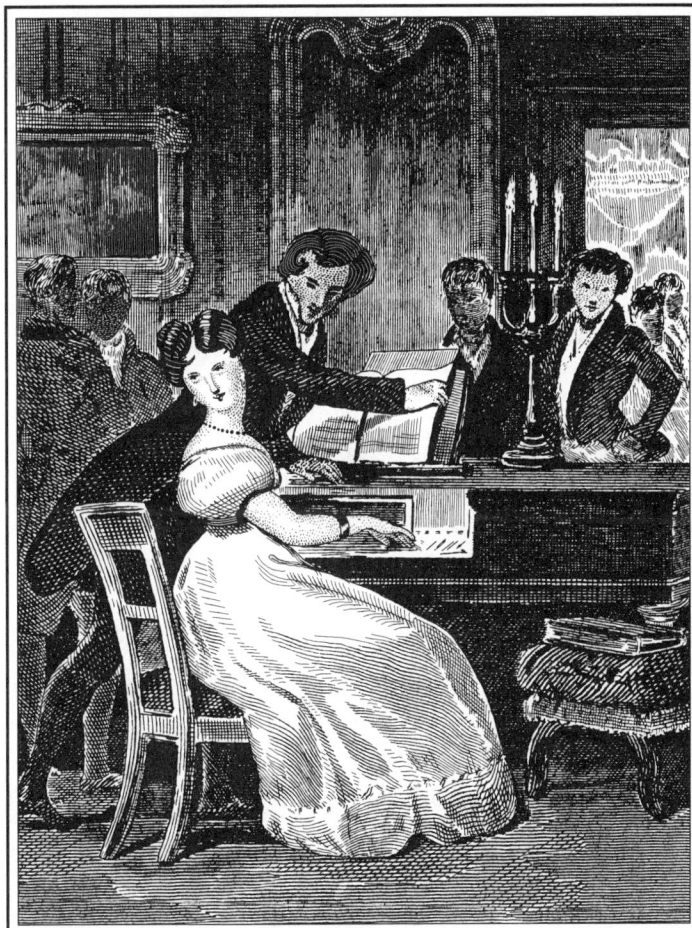

Chapter XXII.
Of Propriety, and its Advantages.

Propriety, or politeness, is a happy union of the moral and the graceful. It should be considered in both points of view, and ought therefore to direct you in your important duties, as well as your more trifling enjoyments. When it is regarded only under this last aspect, some contend that mere intercourse with society gives a habit and taste for those modest and obliging observances which constitute true propriety; but this is an error. Propriety is the valuable result of a knowledge of yourself, and of respect for the rights of others; it is a sense of the sacrifices which are imposed on self-esteem by social relations; it is, in short, a sacred requirement of harmony and affection.

But the customs of society are merely the gloss, or rather the imitation of propriety; since instead of being based upon sincerity, modesty, and courtesy, they rest on nothing. It is permitted to play on the feelings of others by ridiculing their faults and virtues, as long as this provides amusement, and is never carried so far as to wound the self-esteem of any one. Thanks to custom, in order to be recognized as amiable it is sufficient that the subject of a malicious pleasantry may laugh as well as the author of it.

The customs of society are therefore often nothing more than a skilful calculation of vanity, a frivolous game of wits, a superficial observance of forms, a false politeness which would lead to frivolity or perfidy, did not true politeness animate them with delicacy, reserve, and benevolence. Would that custom had never been separated from this virtuous amiableness! Then we would never see well-intentioned and good people suspicious of politeness, nor victims to the deceitful bitterly complain, and with reason, "There is your man of politeness." Nor would a distinction ever be made between politeness and the fixed principles of virtue.

The love of good, in a word virtue, is therefore the soul of propriety; and the feeling of a just harmony between personal interest and social relations is indispensable to this agreeable quality. Excessive gaiety, extravagant joy, great depression, anger, love, jealousy, avarice, and generally all the passions, are too often dangerous shoals to propriety. Moderation in every thing is so essential, that it is even a violation of propriety itself to affect too much the observance of it.

It is to propriety, its equitable and kind attentions, that we owe all the charm of society, I might almost say, the ability to live in it. At once the effect and cause of civilization, propriety avails itself of the grand spring of the human mind, self-love, in order to purify and ennoble it; to substitute for pride and all those egotistical or offensive feelings which it generates, benevolence, with all the amiable and generous sentiments which it inspires. In an assembly of truly polite people, all evil seems to be unknown. What is just, estimable, and good, or is called proper, is felt on all sides; and actions, manners, and language alike indicate it. If a person who is a stranger to the advantages of a polite education is placed in this select assembly, he will at once feel all the value of it, and will immediately desire to display the same urbanity by which he has himself been pleased.

If propriety is necessary in general, it is not less so in particular cases. Neither rank, fortune, talents, nor beauty, may dispense with this amenity of manners. Nor can any thing inspire esteem or friendship, without that gracious affability, that mild dignity, and that elegant simplicity which render the name "Frenchman" synonymous with "amiable," and make Paris dear to whoever has understanding and taste (see Div. 1). If all the world feels the truth of the verse which is now a proverb, "That grace, which is more beautiful than beauty itself," every one also is sensible that grace in conferring a favour includes more than the favour itself, and that a kind smile, or an affectionate tone, penetrate the heart more deeply than the most brilliant elocution.

As to the technical part of propriety, or forms alone, intercourse with society and good advice are undoubtedly useful. But the great secret of never failing in propriety, is to have an intention of always doing what is right. With such a disposition of mind, exactness in observing what is proper appears to all to possess a charm and influence. Then not only do mistakes become excusable, but they become even interesting from their thoughtlessness and naïveté. After the manner of St. Augustine, who said, "Love God, and then do what you wish," I shall say to those just making their debut in society: be modest, be benevolent, and do not distress yourself on account of the mistakes of your inexperience. A little attention, and the advice of a friend, will soon correct these trifling errors.

Such a friend I wish to be to you. In undertaking to revise, and almost entirely reorganize, the *Manual of Good Society,* I have wished and have engaged to be useful to you. A more methodical arrangement of the work, more precise and varied details, in short, important applications to all conditions and circumstances of life, will, I venture to believe, make this treatise worthy of its design.

——*The Gentleman and Lady's Book of Politeness,*
Manuel complet de la bonne compagnie.

Diversion 1.

Differences between French and American Etiquette. The present work has had an extensive circulation in France, the country which we are accustomed to consider as the genial soil of politeness; and the publishers have thought it would be rendering a useful service on this side of the Atlantic to issue a translation of it.

Some foreign visitors in our country, whose own manners have not always given them a right to be censors of others, have very freely told us what we ought *not* to do; and it will be useful to know from respectable authority, what is done in polished society in Europe, and of course what we *ought* to do, in order to avoid all just censure. This object, we are confident, will be more effectually accomplished by the study of the principles and rules contained in the present volume, than by any other of the kind.

By persons who are deemed competent judges in such a case, this little work has been pronounced to be one of the most useful and practical works extant, upon the numerous and delicate topics which are discussed in it. We are aware that a man can no more acquire the ease and elegance of a finished gentleman, by any manual of this kind, than in the fine arts he could become a skilful painter or sculptor by studying books alone, without practice. It is, however, equally true, that the *principles* of politeness may be studied, as well as the principles of the arts. At the same time, intercourse with polite society, in other words *practice*, as in the case of the arts, must do the rest.

The reader will find in this volume some rules founded on customs and forms peculiar to France and other countries, where the Roman Catholic religion is established. But it was thought better to retain them in the work, than to mutilate it by making such material alterations as would have been occasioned by expunging every thing of that description. In our liberal and tolerant country, these peculiarities will give offence to none; while to many, their novelty at least will be interesting.

——*The Gentleman and Lady's Book of Politeness.*

Chapter XXIII.
Propriety as regards yourself.

❧❧❧❧

Care for your person and reputation is an important duty of propriety. If vanity, pride, or prudery have frequently given to these attentions the names of coquetry, ambition, or squeamishness, that is a still stronger reason why I should endeavour to clear up these points.

The Toilet.

Propriety requires that you always be clothed in a clean and decent manner, even in private, on quitting your bed, or in the presence of no one but your family. It requires that your clothing be in keeping with your sex, fortune, profession, age, and shape, as well as with the season, the different hours of the day, and your different occupations. (See Chapter XI.)

The dress for a gentleman on his first rising is a cap of cotton or foulard, a dressing-gown, or a waistcoat with sleeves (see Chapter XVII). For a lady, it should be a small percale cap, and a night jacket or a gown of common material. It is well that half-stays should precede the full stays (see Chapter XIV), which last are used only when you are dressed; for it is most unseemly for a lady not to be laced at all. The curl-papers which cannot be removed on rising (because the hair would not keep in curl until evening) should be concealed under a bandeau of lace or formed of hair. They should be removed as soon as may be.

In this dress, you may receive only intimate friends, or persons who call upon urgent or indispensable business; even then you ought to offer some apology for it. To neglect to take off this morning dress as soon as possible, is to expose yourself to embarrassments often very painful, and to the appearance of ill-breeding. Moreover, it is well to impose upon yourself a rule to be dressed at some particular hour (the earliest possible) since tasks will present themselves one after another to prevent you from being presentable all day; and you will easily acquire the habit of this. Such disorder of the toilet may be excused when it occurs rarely, or for a short time, as in such cases it seems evidently owing to a temporary difficulty.

If it occurs daily or constantly, if it seems the result of negligence and slovenliness, it is unpardonable; particularly in ladies, whose dress seems less designed for clothing than ornament.

To suppose that extremely hot weather will authorize this disorder of the toilet, and will permit you to go about in slippers, or with bare legs and arms, or to adopt listless or improper attitudes, is an error of persons of a low class or ill-breeding. Even the weather of dog-days does not excuse this; and if you would remain thus dressed, you must give directions that you are not at home. On the other hand, to think that cold and rainy weather excuses like liberties is equally an error.

You ought not to be in the habit of wearing vulgar shoes (this is addressed chiefly to ladies) such as list slippers and similar articles; much less noisy shoes, such as galoches lined with fur, wooden shoes, shoes with wooden soles, clogs, &c.; this habit is in the worst taste. When you go to see any one, you cannot dispense with taking off your clogs or over-shoes before you are introduced into the room; for to make a noise in walking is entirely at variance with good manners.

However pressed she may be, a lady of good *ton* should not go out in the dress she wears on rising, neither with an apron nor cap, even if it is made of clear material and trimmed with ribands. Nor should a well-bred man show himself in the street in a waistcoat only, a jacket without sleeves, &c. I said before that dress should be adapted to the different hours of the day. Ladies should make morning visits in an elegant and simple *négligé,* all the details of which I cannot give, on account of their multiplicity and the numerous modifications of fashion (but see Chapter XI). I shall only say that ladies generally ought to make these visits in the dress which they wear at home. Gentlemen may call in an out-door coat, in boots and pantaloons, as when they are on their ordinary business. In short, this dress is proper for gentlemen's visits in the middle of the day. As for ladies, when visiting at this time they should arrange their toilet with more care. Ceremonious visits, evening visits, and especially assemblies, require more attention to the dress of gentlemen, and a more brilliant costume for ladies. For the latter there are head-dresses particularly designed for such occasions, and for no other, such as rich blond caps ornamented with flowers, and brilliant berets and toques called *de salon* (see Chapter XXI).

The handsomest cloth; very fine and very fresh linen; an elegant but plain waistcoat; a beautiful watch, to which is attached a single costly key; thin and well-polished shoes; and an entirely new hat, of a superior quality—is a dress at once *recherché* and rigorously exact, for a gentleman of good taste and *ton*. Your profession requires very little modification of this costume. I should observe, however, that men of learning, letters, and law should avoid wearing a fashionable or military costume, which is generally adopted by students, shop-keepers, and dandies, for the sake of *ton*, or for want of something to do.

A lady's position in the world determines those distinctions which, though otherwise well marked, are becoming less so every day. Every one knows that whatsoever the fortune of a young lady, her dress ought always, in style as well as ornaments, to be less *recherché* and showy than that of married ladies. (See Chapter XI.) Costly cachemires, very rich furs, and diamonds, as well as many other brilliant ornaments, are forbidden to a young lady. Those who act in defiance of these sensible conventions lead people to believe that they are possessed of an unbridled love of luxury, and deprive themselves of the pleasure of receiving these ornaments from the man of their choice.

All ladies cannot use indiscriminately the privilege which marriage confers upon them in this respect, and the toilet of those of moderate fortune should not pass the bounds of an elegant simplicity. Considerations of a more elevated nature, such as good domestic order, the dignity of a wife, and the duties of a mother, support this law of propriety, for it concerns morality in all its branches.

Beware of a shoal in the following situation: frequently a young woman of small fortune, desiring to appear suitably in some splendid assembly, makes sacrifices in order to embellish her modest attire. But these sacrifices are necessarily inadequate; a new and brilliant article of dress is placed beside a mean or old one. Her toilet then wants harmony, which is the soul of elegance as well as of beauty. Moreover, whatsoever the opulence which you enjoy, the desire for luxury is so strong, that no riches are sufficient to satisfy its demands. Happily propriety, always in agreement with reason, encourages social and sensible women by the following maxim: dress neither too high, nor too low. It is alike ridiculous to strive to display the most magnificent attire in an assembly, or to resign yourself to wearing the meanest.

The conventions for age resemble those imposed by a mediocre fortune. Thus aged ladies ought to abstain from gaudy colours, *recherché* designs, too late fashions, and graceful ornaments, such as feathers, flowers, and jewels. A lady in her decline coiffed *en cheveux,* in a low-necked gown with short sleeves, and adorned with necklaces, bracelets, &c. offends against propriety as much as against her interest and dignity.

The rigorous simplicity of the dress of gentlemen establishes but very little difference between that of young and old. The latter, however, ought to choose dark colours, not to follow the fashions too closely, to avoid garments which are too tight or too short, and not to have in view in their toilet any other object but ease and neatness. Unless the care of their health or complete baldness requires them to wear a wig, it is more proper that aged persons should show their white and noble heads. Aged ladies, whom custom requires to conceal this respectable sign of a long life, should at least avoid hair too thick or too full of curls.

If they do not wish to appear ridiculous and clothed in a disagreeable or unhealthy manner, ladies should adopt in summer light materials and delicate colours, and in winter furs, thick and warm materials, and full colours. Gentlemen were formerly almost free from this obligation; they were constantly clothed in broadcloth in all seasons. But now, though cloth may form the basis of their toilet, they must select materials for winter or summer, as may be suitable. It is in good *ton* for gentlemen to wear a rich cloak; an outer coat over the suit (especially a silk redingote) is left for men of a certain age. Only septuagenarians and clergymen wear *douillettes* or redingotes of wadded silk.

It is superlatively ridiculous for a lady to go on foot with her head dressed *en cheveux*, and attired for the drawing-room or a ball. If you dwell in a provincial town where it is not customary to use carriages, go in a sedan chair. Who does not perceive how laughable it is to see a lady who is clothed in satin, blond, or velvet laboriously walking in the dust or mud?

It would be extremely uncouth to carry filth on your shoes into a decent house, especially on a ceremonious visit. When there is much mud, or when you cannot walk skilfully, it is proper to go in a carriage, or at least to call for a shoe-scraper at a short distance from the house.

Vary your toilet as much as possible, for fear that idlers and malicious wits, who are always a majority in society, will amuse themselves by making your dress the description of your person.

Certain fashionables seek to gain a kind of reputation by the odd choice of their attire, and by their eagerness to seize upon the first caprices of the fashions. Propriety tolerates these fancies of a spoilt child with difficulty. But it applauds a woman of sense and taste, who is not in haste to follow the fashions, and asks how long they will probably last before adopting them; and finally, who successfully selects and modifies them according to her size and shape (see Chapter XII).

Reputation.

Reputation.

Amongst the cares which propriety obliges you to take of your person, to please is but incidental. The principal object is to indicate by your cleanliness and suitableness of apparel, that good order, a sense of what is right, and propriety in all things direct your thoughts and actions. In this point of view, you will see that caring for your reputation is an essential part of the duties of propriety towards yourself.

To inspire esteem and respect is therefore the great object of propriety; for without these treasures, social relations would be a humiliation and punishment. Esteem and respect are obtained by the discharge of your familial and professional obligations, by your probity and good manners, and by your fortune and social position.

Reputation is not acquired by speeches. An article so precious demands a real value; it requires also the assistance of discretion. You must begin by fulfilling exactly your duties towards your relations. Beware of making public those petty quarrels and little differences of interest, ill-humour, or opinion, which sometimes trouble the most closely-united families. These momentary clouds, soon dissipated by affection and confidence, would be engraven on the memory of others as a proof of your domestic discords, and in the end of your faults.

Probity, a powerful means of obtaining reputation, is by its elevated and religious nature outside my investigation of the principles of propriety. Though the word "gentleman" encompasses both courtesy and honesty, I believe it superfluous to remind you of the eternal principles of justice. This is not the case with the reputation attached to purity of morals. The proof of probity lies in probity itself. But thanks to the delicate shades of reputation in regard to chastity, there exist, independently of good conduct, a multitude of cares and precautions, which however minute and troublesome at times, ought never to be neglected. Ladies, to whom the following advice is particularly addressed, know how the shadow of suspicion debases and torments them. It is necessary to avoid this shadow at all costs, and on that account to submit to all the requirements of propriety.

Up to the age of about thirty, a young lady must never go out unaccompanied. When she does errands in town, shops, visits intimate friends, or goes to church, she must go with a maid. When she pays ceremonious visits, promenades, or goes to assemblies or balls, she must appear with her mother, or instead a married lady of her acquaintance. (See Div. 1.) This lady, or chaperon, thus conducts several young persons. She does not permit them to play cards, or to walk round the room, and in a word does not let them out of her sight. Often negligence of chaperones in this regard injures the reputations of their charges.

Young married ladies are at liberty to do errands and visit their acquaintances by themselves; but they cannot present themselves in public without their husband, or an aged lady. They are at liberty, however, to walk with young married ladies or unmarried ones, whereas the latter should never walk alone with their companions. Neither should they show themselves except with a gentleman of their family, and then he should be a near relation or of respectable age. It is very improper for young cousins of opposite sexes to be habitually together.

Except in certain provincial towns, where there is excessive rigorism, young married ladies receive the visits of gentlemen. They permit their company in public promenades without suffering the least injury to their reputation, provided it is always with men of good morals, and that they take care to avoid every appearance of coquetry. Young widows have equal liberty with married ladies. (See Div. 2.)

A lady ought not to present herself alone in a library, or a museum, unless she goes there to study or work as an artist.

A lady should have a modest and measured gait; too great hurry injures the grace which should characterize her. She should not turn her head to one side and the other, especially in large cities, where this bad habit seems to be an invitation to the impertinent. If such persons address her in any flattering or trifling terms, she should take good care not to answer them a word. If they persist, she should tell them in a brief and firm, though polite tone, that she desires to be left to herself. If a man silently follows her, she should pretend not to perceive him, and at the same time hasten her step a little.

Towards the close of the day, a young woman would conduct herself in an unbecoming manner, if she walked alone. If she passes the evening with any one, she ought to see that a servant comes to accompany her; if not, to request the person whom she is visiting to allow some one to do so. But however much this rule may be considered proper, and consequently an obligation, a well-bred married lady will disregard it if circumstances prevent her from finding a conductor without trouble. If the gentleman of the house wishes to accompany you himself, excuse yourself politely from giving him so much trouble, but finish by accepting. On arriving at your house, offer him your thanks.

It may be well to instead request your husband, or one of your relations, to come and wait upon you. In small towns, where malice is excited by ignorance and idleness, people frequently censure the most innocent acts. It is not uncommon to hear slanderous and silly gossips observe, that Mrs. Such-a-one goes to Mrs. Such-a-one's for the sake of returning with her husband. The seeds of such a rumour, once sown, very quickly germinate. (See Divs. 3 and 4.) But if you have recently been apprised of it, and the gentleman offers to accompany you again, resign yourself for this once. Take good care to refuse the defence of your habitual guide in making the incident known to him, because in society there is no more ridiculous *rôle* than that of a woman who thus defends a virtue which has not been attacked. It is prudery, foolishness, or a game.

In other circumstances, a woman's situation may become delicate and distressing. A man of your acquaintance, a friend of your husband's, pays you attentions which are no more than polite, but which threaten to become so. It is therefore necessary to be reserved; watch for the moment the change takes place, but take good care not to appear to expect it. It frequently happens that men whose intentions are not at all questionable, seeing you move to foil them, pretend to change their tone, with the object of embarrassing conceited and thwarted prudery, and taking a malicious pleasure in making a poor woman look ridiculous.

When a man addresses you with exaggerated compliments, seizes your hand, or approaches you too closely, withdraw your hand, and move away in a very dignified and cold manner, but without displaying any anger. Nothing more clearly displays ill-breeding. If vanity does not make you secretly take satisfaction in these misplaced compliments, if it does not lead you to smile when your look should be glacial, you will soon be relieved of these troublesome attentions.

After having attempted to show the delicate distinction between propriety and prudery, I shall describe the distressing situation where propriety is found in opposition to kindness, mercy, and perhaps even justice. (See Div. 5.) Unhappy victims of slanderous misinterpretations or foolish overtures are singled out by public scorn; every when and every where blows are lavished on them. At the promenade no one returns their friendly salutations; at spectacles, no one responds to their obsequious kindnesses. You know how often a word suffices to tarnish a spotless reputation. Therefore, you may pity these unfortunates deprived of respect, and plan a generous project to rehabilitate them in public opinion, to surround them with your personal consideration. . . . Do not yield to this touching, but imprudent generosity. Unless you have the influence of age, or can impose it by a high social position, you also risk moral contagion. Be well assured that instead of saving the reputation of such unhappy women, you will lose your own. Therefore abandon them, do not think of them, be deaf to their timid overtures; but without any stiffness or disdain. After having satisfied the rigorous demands of propriety, think of those whose needs oppose it. Do not refuse a salute or a gracious word to these poor women, display benevolence to them in particular, and pity their lot, making a firm resolution to avoid gossip as a crime.

Gossip (too often slander under another name) is for some persons a means of preserving their own reputation intact. In severely condemning the frailties of others, it appears to prove that the gossiper is exempt. Others seek social success in gossip: they are always looking out for scandalous adventures, provided these are piquant. For them the dishonour of an attractive woman, the despair of a whole household, is merely an excellent opportunity to display their wit. Who knows if they make a mistake in their false reluctances and inventive remarks? All this may be tolerated, even licensed by the habits of society; but it is nonetheless detested by any one with moral and wholesome propriety. Therefore, far from uniting with these wretched story-tellers, take the side of the accused; or if the scandal is too notorious, maintain a disapproving silence.

A lady's care for her reputation further demands a modest deportment. She should abstain from forward manners and free speeches; she should not welcome flatterers. (See Div. 6.) I shall return to flattery in Chapter XXXI. Just at present, I shall end by asking my readers not to mistake the spirit of my advice, or let it give rise to prudery.

——*The Gentleman and Lady's Book of Politeness,*
Manuel complet de la bonne compagnie.

Diversion 1.

Chaperons. The material on chaperons was omitted from the original American translation.

——Frances Grimble.

Mrs. L.—How should a young lady behave in society?

Mrs. B.—Not only appearances, but the comfort of a young lady in public, depends upon her having an unexceptionable escort or chaperon, to whom she may have recourse upon any dilemma, and whose experience and greater knowledge of the world may be useful to her in assisting her out of her difficulties. Her mother is, of course, the best escort she can have; but if circumstances prevent her from accompanying her daughter, a near relation or an intimate friend should supply her place. A young lady venturing into public without a proper chaperon, is a thing scarcely known. Indeed, without such a sanction, she would be shunned by the circumspect part of her sex, and perhaps too much noticed by the amusement seekers of the other.

——*Domestic Duties.*

Diversion 2.

Conduct of a Widow. I shall now endeavour to give you a few hints respecting the conduct of a young woman, who may be unfortunately left a widow. When time has healed the wound which her husband's death has inflicted, and when the season has elapsed which decorum has appointed for retirement from public amusements, and from scenes of gaiety (supposed to be incompatible with the state of feeling of one recently bereft of the most intimate of human ties) the widow will probably be again seen in the world, and will again mix in her usual societies. She should now bear in mind that from the circumstance of her being left entirely to her own conduct, many eyes will be upon her; and from various motives, many will curiously examine into the circumspection and prudence of her conduct. If the breath of slander ought not to reach her as a wife, it is even more essential to her, that as a widow it should be completely suppressed. She has no longer a protector to shelter her when reproached, nor to sanction with his approbation her future steps. She has to screen the name she bears from the very shadow of disrepute; because besides belonging to her children, he who owned it and bestowed it on her can no longer defend and rescue it from calumny and disgrace.

——*Domestic Duties.*

Diversion 3.

The material on female reputation, from here nearly to the end of the chapter, was omitted from the original American translation.

——Frances Grimble.

Diversion 4.

Gossips and Scandal-mongers. Mrs. L.—Independent of those whose characters are tainted by vice, what other circumstances of conduct and character should prevent a newly-married woman from seeking, or accepting, the acquaintance of her neighbours?

Mrs. B.—It would be well in young married women to avoid the company of such as habitually indulge in the foibles of scandal, ridicule, or gossiping. Over these society has little control, and nothing can be opposed to them but example. These contemptible propensities occasion much mischief and vexation. Happy would it be, if an intolerant spirit were never evinced in any other cause, than in that of expelling those who are addicted to them beyond the precincts of good society. Contemptible propensities they are, and seldom found carried to any great excess, except by those whose frivolous turn of mind has prevented the employment of their faculties in nobler and more enlightened pursuits.

Mrs. L.—But as scandal is not confined to the weaker sex, how is a lady to discriminate the characters of the gentlemen who may visit at her house?

Mrs. B.—By the chosen pursuits of the men who visit in her family, a woman may form some judgement of their characters. Is any portion of their lives spent in benefiting their fellow-creatures, or in the acquisition of knowledge? Then their moments of relaxation and amusement are not likely to be employed in retailing or in enlarging upon the scandals of the day; nor in wounding by satire the feelings of their fellow-creatures, in whose frailties they know themselves to be participators. Are frivolous pursuits their delight? Are they employed in administering pleasures to the senses rather than to the mind? Then it is not judging them too severely to suppose that they are unworthy to form a part of enlightened society, or incapable of adding either to its amusement or improvement.

Mrs. L.—How is a gossiping woman to be known before she has fixed herself upon a newly-married woman? Is not such a character sometimes rather amusing than dangerous?

Mrs. B.—The same criterion by which the characters of men may be tried, will enable a lady to select her acquaintance amongst her own sex. Many women, either for want of sufficient employment in their families, or from deficiency of intellectual energy, occupy themselves in prying into the affairs of their neighbours, and in spreading every report which is disadvantageous to their credit. The habit of even listening to the gossipings of such busy-bodies is like the contagion of disease. It gradually propagates a morbid sympathy in the mind, and engenders the same evil in those who would never otherwise have become susceptible of its influence.

Such an acquaintance, therefore, should be shunned as a pestilence. If the duties of a family are not sufficient to occupy the leisure hours of a married woman, she ought to seek for the society of those who can communicate instruction of a general and interesting nature, free from local and family tattle or domestic politics, which can neither add to her own happiness, nor increase the pleasure which is derived from forming a good opinion of those around us. Much danger results from such acquaintances. For example, it often happens that those who are not prone to such kind of conversation themselves are led inadvertently to give an opinion of conduct or character, on the information communicated by some gossips. As this is always conveyed, by the same channel, to those from whom it ought most particularly to be concealed, a coldness and reserve, if not an entire breach of friendship, are produced where no real injury was intended. The fiend who has lighted up the feud escapes with impunity, while the innocent victim of the delusion which she has practised must bear the calumny of injustice and insincerity.

Women who are gossips are also generally flatterers. They discover the weak side of every one with whom they associate; and in administering incense to self-love, obtain the possession of secrets, under the mask of confidence, which they are impatient to impart to the whole circle in which they move. Such women are dangerous in proportion as they are insinuating; like the Circean cup their obnoxious qualities are not discovered until the poison has touched the vitals.

———*Domestic Duties*.

Diversion 5.

Means of avoiding Moral Contagion. Mrs. L.—Are there not some points to be observed in the formation of an acquaintance, which should always be firmly adhered to?

Mrs. B.—There are several. Thus it is evident that those whose characters and conduct stand impeached of any thing dishonourable should never be admitted into good society. This should be a rule with every one, of which neither interest, policy, nor even the pleadings of pity, should induce the neglect. As general security and good order require that the transgressors of the law of the land should pay its penalties, so the purity and comfort of society depend upon the banishment of those who have proved themselves unworthy of its sanction. It is true, the observance of this rule may sometimes banish from our circles wit and talents equally amusing and instructive; but wit and talents, unaccompanied by moral worth, allure to danger. If the young view the vicious with approbation, in their minds half the barrier between right and wrong is broken down; by which inlet, more serious attacks may be made on innocence and virtuous principles.

———*Domestic Duties*.

Diversion 6.

Means of avoiding Censure. Mrs. L.—To observe and censure the manners of individuals in public, is the favourite amusement of some ladies; and young married women are especially considered as fair subjects for the study and satiric remarks of these keen-eyed observers. Can any magic veil be found which will protect me from these?

Mrs. B.—The best protection I can suggest is to act with propriety in public as well as elsewhere, which will render the remarks you dread undeserved. Acquire also the capability of bearing censure, especially if unmerited, with indifference, or at least with as little disturbance of mind as possible. To be too sensitive of blame is a great weakness; and it is yielding up our comfort to the mercy of others. Deserved censure is more difficult to endure than that which is unmerited; but in this case we should receive it patiently, and as a just infliction which we have brought upon ourselves.

Impropriety of manner in company, though it does not bespeak a very correct mind, may be attendant on an innocent one. A woman may have too much levity of manner, laugh and talk too loud, give herself many fantastic airs, or be too familiar with some of her acquaintance, and too haughty to others. Yet she may mean nothing wrong to any one; and perhaps her sole view may be to attract momentary notice, or to endeavour to render herself a person of consequence in the eyes of others. These are weak, but not criminal motives; and yet they render her liable to derision, and to just censure, even from the lenient in judgement.

Propriety is the union of every desirable quality in woman, by which her conduct and manners are influenced under every circumstance. Propriety never desires a deviation from any of the laws of good society, and neither seeks notice nor admiration which, from their natures, would be incompatible with its own characteristics. Improper familiarities, haughtiness, intrusive forwardness to superiors, and insolence to inferiors; the indulgence of any whim by which our conduct to others may be influenced, are all equally unknown to propriety.

Unless a woman desires it, she seems but little called upon in public to bring herself and her actions into a prominent point of view, or to render herself a mark for sarcasm and ridicule. At home, when entertaining guests, she cannot pass altogether so unobtrusively; though the manners of the present period allow of more ease and latitude of deportment than formerly was deemed correct in a lady hostess, when thoughts and time were condemned to the strictest attention to the comforts and pleasure of her visitors, often to the entire destruction of both.

Ease of manner in a woman is very pleasing, when the self-possession which gives it is unaccompanied by masculine courage, or by an undue value for herself. In general, the manners will be free from any painful degree of constraint, when the mind is not engaged upon the self, or occupied with the idea of exciting attention and admiration from those around. Affectation has its origin from these sources; and this, besides being a symptom of a weak mind, is entirely destructive of good manners. Good sense and simplicity of manners are generally companions, forming a natural gentility which is far preferable to any artificial politeness, inasmuch as the one is part of the individual herself, and the other only a garb worn when occasion calls for it. However, those who possess this natural gentility may, by mixing in good society, have the additional polish given to it, which afterwards distinguishes it as the perfection of good manners.

——*Domestic Duties.*

Chapter XXIV.
Propriety in Domestic Duties.

The most sublime, the most touching lessons of religion and of Nature unite in commanding us to love and honour those from whom we have received life. I shall not offend my readers by supposing it requisite to insist upon the necessity of fulfilling a duty which is felt by all with sound morals and good hearts.

The prevailing custom is to address your father and mother in the familiar form. (This is an allusion to the idiom of the French language, and is inapplicable in English.) This mark of great confidence and affectionate freedom ought never to degenerate into an offensive familiarity. Always address them in a respectful and kind tone; anticipate them in every thing; ask their advice; receive their reproofs submissively; be silent with regard to any errors they may commit; show them a lively gratitude on every occasion. In short, whatever advantage you may have over them, let it be forgotten, and consider them always your superiors, your benefactors, and your guides.

Besides the daily marks of deference which you should lavish on your parents, there are particular occasions on which you should express your affection. At certain times, such as the new year, their birth-day, or their name-day, you should offer them tender congratulations and ingeniously-devised presents. You are not allowed to dispense with these delicate attentions. If you have had success in the sciences or arts, pay your respects to those from whom you have derived the benefits of your education.

If you are separated from your parents, write to them frequently. Let your style be impressed with a devoted affection; repeat more particularly at the end of your letters, the sentiments of respect and love with which you should be inspired.

As to what your uncles, aunts, brothers, sisters, and cousins require of you, you will know what are the duties of propriety in that regard, if you respect and cherish family ties. Show towards some a respectful, and towards the others a friendly politeness. They should claim on every occasion your first visits and your first attentions. Identify yourself with them in all their prosperity or adversity. Invite them above all others to fêtes and assemblies at your house, except when you assemble a select party to whom they would be entire strangers. Always take care to invite your relations by themselves from time to time, to prove you have no intention of slighting them. You may be more intimate with some of your family, and give them particular proofs of affection; but at these gatherings you will do well to abstain from every mark of preference.

Without being at all wanting in cordiality, use a little more ceremony towards your relations by marriage, to whom you indeed owe as much respect as to your own.

Propriety in Conjugal and Domestic Relations.

If any thing can render politeness ridiculous, and even odious, it is the disposition of certain persons, who in society are reasonable, amiable, and gracious, but in private show themselves morose, rough, and ill-natured. This all-too-common fault is one of the greatest inconsistencies of the human mind. You exert all your powers of pleasing in society, which you see only in passing, and where you have only the power to procure a few moments of pleasure; and you neglect to be agreeable to your husband or wife, from whom you expect a lifetime of happiness! Perhaps it would be better to be continually capricious or harsh, for the contrast of your politeness in the drawing-room with your impoliteness at home makes you appear even more odious. Conjugal intimacy, it is true, dispenses with the etiquette established by politeness, but it does not dispense with its consideration. In the presence of your spouse, you ought never to satisfy those needs which arouse disgust, nor perform those duties of the toilet, which before any one but yourself offend decency and cleanliness. (Such as washing your feet, cutting your nails, quitting your bath, &c.) Never permit disorder in your attire under the excuse that you are just up, or in your own house. To dress with neatness and elegant simplicity is important, even at home.

The conversation of husband and wife cannot be elegant, and sustained in the same manner that it is in society. (See Div. 1.) It would be superlatively ridiculous that it should not have interruption or relaxation; but it should be free from all impoliteness and indelicacy. If at any time the society of your spouse causes you ennui, you ought neither to say so, nor give any suspicion of the cause by abruptly changing the conversation. In all discussions you should watch yourself attentively, lest domestic familiarity raise itself by degrees to the pitch of a quarrel. It is especially to women that this advice is addressed; and to the impressive words of Scripture, "Woman was not created for wrath," may be added these, "She was created for gentleness."

To entertain your wife's friends with a particularly affectionate politeness; to respect inviolably the letters which she writes and receives; to avoid prying into the secrets which she conceals from you through delicacy; never to act contrary to her inclinations, unless they are injurious to herself, and even in that case not to oppose her, but to endeavour to check them with address and kindness; to beware of confiding to strangers or servants the little vexations which she causes you; to dread like poison marks of contempt, coldness, suspicion, and reproaches; to apologize promptly and affectionately if you have allowed yourself to run into any ill-humour; to receive her counsels attentively and kindly, and to act on them as quickly as possible—those are the obligations of propriety and love to which apouses bind themselves, by the sweet sanctity of the vows which they have taken before God.

There is a still more rigorous duty for newly-married and well-married persons: they must abstain in public from every overly conspicuous mark of affection and every exclusive attention. Spouses who in society place themselves continually near one another, who converse and dance together, and especially who kiss, do not escape the ridicule to which their feelings blind them. In society, you ought above all to avoid being personal. A husband or a wife is another self; and you must forget that self.

Mothers, in particular, lavish caresses on your children, occupy yourselves entirely with them—unless perhaps you fear to render them proud, demanding, and insupportable! If you fatigue people with their constant presence, if you indulgently encourage or relate their prattle and their sports; or if on the other hand, you treat them severely before strangers, if you scold or punish them, be assured every one will consider you annoying as well as ridiculous.

Domestic propriety, which is at once a duty of justice, religion, and humanity, is also a source of peace and pleasure. Servants treated with proper consideration are attentive, zealous, and grateful, and consequently every thing is done with order and affection. Who does not know the charm and value of this?

Duties of this class require that you never command your servants haughtily or harshly. Every time they render you a service, it claims an expression, a gesture, or at least a look of thanks. It requires you to be still kinder towards the servants of your acquaintances, and especially towards those of your friends, whom you ought always to treat graciously. As to your own servants, carefully beware of addressing to them any confidential or even unnecessary conversation, for fear of rendering them insolent or familiar; but propriety requires you to listen to them kindly, and give them salutary advice when it is for their interest. It commands you also to show them indulgence frequently, so that you may, when there is cause, reprove them firmly, without being obliged to resort to the false energy of anger.

The *ton* of servants ordinarily bespeaks that of their masters. Never suffer them to remain seated while answering distinguished persons who ask for you. Take care that they always do it in a civil and polite manner. Let the servant lose no time, if there is occasion, in relieving a visitor of his over-shoes, umbrella, cloak, &c.; let the servant go before, to save your visitor the trouble of opening and shutting the door. When a visitor is to be announced, the servant should respectfully ask his name, and pronounce it while holding the door of your apartment open for him. If you are not there, the servant should offer a seat, requesting the visitor to wait a moment while he goes to call the master or mistress; it is good practice not to use your name.

When a visitor takes leave, the servant should hasten to open the outer door. He should hold the door by the handle, if you converse a few moments with the person whom you re-conduct. The servant should present him respectfully with whatever garments he may have thrown off, and aid him in again putting them on. The servant should, if occasion requires, light the visitor to the door, going slowly behind him.

Accustom your servants never to appear before you too poorly, or too much dressed; never to sit in your presence, especially while waiting upon the table; not to mingle in the conversation; never to answer by signs, or in coarse terms; and finally to speak to you in the third person.

It is only amongst the ill-bred people of small towns that they say, "the girl," "the boy," "the domestic," or "the servant." Only proud, ill-bred fashionables who ape grandeur say, "the lackey," "the valet," and "my people." Well-bred persons simply say, "the nurse," "the cook," "the chambermaid," &c.; and what is still better they designate their servants by their christian names.

If you have ever met with those merciless housekeepers who give you a whole tariff of the food-stuffs which they have been to market to purchase, attended by their "girl"; who entertain you endlessly with the insults and unfaithfulness of their servants; who fly into a passion before you on account of a glass broken, of which they require the value, and make you witness and judge of pert disputes occasioned by servants' mistakes;

if you have had the misfortune to dine with such persons, and have seen them reluctantly hand their sullen maid-servant one key after another, to arrange the dessert brought out with a good supply of ill-humour; if you have seen them go to the cellar themselves, and when you have scarcely left the table, to anxiously arrange the wine, sugar, and delicacies—tell me, poor guest, if, turning your head away with confusion and disgust, you have not an hundred times said to yourself, "O! what disgusting living models of upstarts *or* provincials!"

——*The Gentleman and Lady's Book of Politeness,*
Manuel complet de la bonne compagnie.

Diversion 1.

Evenings at Home without Company. Mrs. L.—The manner in which I have seen some families pass their evenings at home, when they are not engaged with company, has often appeared to me to be dull, un-interesting, and frivolous. I have beheld the father, mother, and children scarcely keeping up a languid conversation; one lounging in an easy-chair; another listlessly turning over the leaves of a magazine; and all yawning responsively, until the wished-for hour of bed arrived.

If these people were to be seen only at such times, they would be ranked in a very low scale of existence, appearing rather to vegetate than to live. But see them again the next evening in company, and you can hardly credit your senses, which show you the reverse of the family picture you had before contemplated. The father is now all intelligence and anima-tion; the mother brilliant; and the daughters all smiles and good-humour. Is there not something wrong in the habits of individuals who require such excitation to rouse into exertion their talents, their social qualities, and apparently their powers of enjoyment?

Mrs. B.—In such a family party as you describe, the taste for rational pursuits has not been cultivated, to act as a counterbalance to the love of pleasure and variety, which is natural to youth.

The duties of each individual of which a family is composed, being during the earlier part of the day duly performed, the evening should be open for rest or amusement. Where there are young people growing up, who form a part of the evening circle, it is on their account very desirable to render it cheerful and agreeable; varying the amusements, and pro-moting conversation chiefly of an animated and cheering nature; perhaps mingling with it also subjects and reflections of an improving kind, when-ever they can be introduced in any easy and unrepelling manner.

Mrs. L. Should not conversation form the chief amusement of the family evening party?

Mrs. B.—Certainly it should; and therefore to converse *well* is an art of much value to women. It is the most certain means by which they may give a charm to social life; and by which they may banish dulness, the moment in which it attempts to intrude itself. No other talent or amusement has an equal power at all times. Music may often fail to withdraw our thoughts from unpleasant remembrances; and the theatre, ball-room, and card-table are not always in unison with the state of our feelings, which at times renders them irksome or indifferent to us. But it is not thus with conversation. It is scarcely ever so powerless as not to beguile the thoughts from even the most painful recollections, or to release them from that lethargic state in which they are sometimes confined. No one can prize too highly the privilege we possess, in this power of communicating and interchanging our ideas with those of our fellow-creatures. Conversation is at once the medium of affection, consolation, amusement, and instruction.

Mrs. L.—The rules for agreeable conversation will, I think, apply as well to family parties, as to more general society.

Mrs. B.—There are sometimes in family parties other defects than those which I have already mentioned, and which often render the intercourse less agreeable than it might be. These arise from the freedom enjoyed at home, which, though constituting one of the greatest charms of the domestic circle, yet may be also the bane of its comfort, if not properly directed and regulated. I have seen this freedom degenerate into rudeness, petulance, and a total disregard for the feelings of others.

To satirize, without mercy, the failings and weaknesses which may prevail in a family circle, is also not unfrequently the chief amusement of some of its members. Ridicule is a weapon which in domestic life is seldom harmless, either to the person who wields it, or to the individual against which it is aimed. In the former it causes too keen a perception of the failings of our relations; and in the latter it either occasions too great a dread of its power, or too great a callousness to it, according to the disposition of the attacked party. In all such cases, parental authority should check this abuse of a freedom, which if it is not suffered to run riot, is one of the most attractive privileges of home.

Needle-work, the reading aloud of some amusing publication, or occasionally playing at chess and backgammon, may serve to give a pleasant variety to the evening's occupation of the different members of the family circle. Nothing delights the female part of a family so much as the reading aloud of some volume of interest by one of the party, while the others are employed in light and elegant needle-work. In this manner a knowledge of polite literature may be acquired, without any sacrifice of more important duties. Even books of a deeper and more permanent character, which few have the taste or inclination to peruse when alone, are often listened to with great pleasure and much profit, when read aloud in such a circle.

Besides the information and gratification which listening to works thus read aloud afford to a family circle, this custom contributes materially to a never-failing flow of conversation, and sharpens our wit by the opportunities it offers of displaying our critical acuteness, both in pointing out the beauties and in detecting the defects of the work under perusal. It is a species of winter evening employment which I strongly recommend you to encourage.

——*Domestic Duties.*

Chapter XXV.
Propriety in the Street
and in Travelling.

❧❧❧❧❧

Some readers will perhaps be surprised to see me begin a chapter with the duty owed to persons passing in the street; but if they reflect upon it, they will see that there are, even on this subject, enough useful things to say. Though travelling is but remotely connected with the social relations, I have added it to this chapter, as I did not wish to intentionally omit any thing.

Deportment in the Street.

When you are walking along the street, and see coming towards you a person of your acquaintance, or only a lady, a gentleman of exalted rank, or an aged person, you should prepare to give them the wall, that is to say, the side next the houses.

If a carriage happens to stop in such a manner as to leave only a narrow passage between it and the houses, beware of elbowing and rudely crowding the passers-by, with a view to getting through more expeditiously. Wait your turn, and if any one of the persons before mentioned comes up, edge up to the wall, to give them the place. As they pass, they ought to bow politely to you.

If stormy weather has made it necessary to lay a plank across a gutter, which has become suddenly full of water, it is not proper to crowd before another in order to pass over the frail bridge. Further, a well-bred young man should promptly offer his hand to ladies, even if they are not acquaintances, when they cross it.

Pay attention to your manner of walking, for fear of throwing mud around you, and spattering yourself as well as those who accompany you, or who walk behind you. Any person, particularly a lady, who walks in this improper manner, however well-bred in other respects, will always appear awkward and clumsy. (See also Chapters XIII and XXIII.) Every one knows that Parisian ladies are celebrated for their skill in walking. They are seen in white stockings and thin shoes, passing through long, dirty, blocked-up streets, gliding by careless persons, and by vehicles crossing each other in every direction, and yet return home after a walk of several hours without having soiled their clothes in the least.

To achieve this astonishing result, which arouses the wonder and chagrin of provincial visitors on their first coming to Paris, you must be careful to put your foot on the middle of the paving-stones, and never on the edges, for you would inevitably slip into the interstices between the stones. You must begin by supporting your toe before your heel; and even when the mud is quite deep, you must put down your heel but seldom. When the street becomes less muddy, you may compensate yourself for the fatigue this occasions, of which, however, you are hardly sensible in the end.

This manner of walking is strictly necessary when you give your arm to any one. When tripping over the pavement (as they say), you should gracefully raise your gown a little above your ancle. You should hold together the folds of your gown with your right hand and draw them towards your right side. To raise your gown on both sides, and with both hands, is bad *ton*. This ungraceful practice may be tolerated only for a moment, when the mud is very deep.

It is an important thing in the streets of a large city to edge yourself along; that is, to avoid jostling and being jostled by those who are passing. Neglecting this attention will not only make you appear awkward and ridiculous, but you will receive or give dangerous blows. You may edge along by turning sideways, contracting your arms, and watching with your eye the direction which it is best to take in order not to come in contact with the person coming towards you. A little practice and care will soon make this duty familiar.

To make your way along becomes more difficult when you have a parcel or an umbrella to carry, especially if the latter is open. It is then necessary to lower or raise it, or to turn it on one side. If you neglect these precautions, you run the risk of striking it against those who are coming and going, or of seeing it twirled round, and of being thrown against a carriage, or against some one who will complain bitterly of your incivility and awkwardness.

If you have no umbrella, and are surprised by a sudden shower, and any person provided with one is walking in the same direction, you may request him to shelter you. He should receive your request very politely, inform himself of the place where you wish to stop, and offer to conduct you there, unless it is too much out of the way, or he is pressed for business. In that case, he should express his regret at not being able to accompany you so far as you wish.

What I am now about to say, proves that a truly polite person will not wait for you to make this request, but will use every exertion to anticipate it. You must observe, however, whether age, sex, or dress present no objection; for sometimes you would be treated with ill-humour and contempt. If you are a lady, unless you have reached a certain age, it would be extremely improper to accost a person, who on his part ought never to offer this favour nor any other to ladies, and whose air and immodest manners bespeak his vulgarity. It would be equally out of place to address such a request to those of a very low class; but if such a one asks the favour of you, it is proper to receive it politely.

Another not uncommon point of propriety consists of requesting and giving directions. If you have need of this service, salute the person politely, and frankly ask, "Madam *or* Sir, where is such-and-such street, if you please?" Be careful to give this title to persons whom you address, even if they are porters or hucksters. It is particularly to them that you should have recourse, for in addressing passers-by, you are liable to meet those who like yourself are strangers to the neighbourhood, or to hinder those who are busy. It is, moreover, impolite to trouble shop-keepers in their places of business. The direction being given, you thank them, at the same time bowing. Parisians are justly celebrated for the politeness and complaisance with which they show the way to passers-by, and you ought to imitate them every time that occasion offers. If you are a gentleman, and a lady or distinguished person asks this favour of you, take off your hat while answering them.

There are some ill-mannered and malicious persons who take pleasure in misleading strangers by wrong directions. It will be enough to mention such impertinence in order to despise it as we ought.

As to those young men who entertain a false idea that Parisian ladies are coquettes or forward in their manners, and besides that every thing is allowable in a large city, let them be assured that a man who dares (as often happens) to address improper compliments to ladies, follow them, listen to their conversation, or finish a sentence which they have begun, is a model of rudeness, and an object of aversion to ladies and of contempt to true gentlemen. A young man of good *ton* ought not to look at a lady too narrowly, or he will pass for an impertinent fellow who (as they say) stares people full in the face.

It is especially when many persons are assembled in one place that boors play their rude tricks, which they call "hoaxes"; first because they are unperceived, and second because the least bad amongst them think that the crowd are outside the jurisdiction of propriety. This opinion, which is shared by some persons, is an error. Politeness becomes still more indispensable in proportion to the assemblage. Why are crowds usually so disagreeable, and even dangerous? It is because they are composed of ill-bred people, who roughly push against their neighbours with their fists and elbows, who neglect to follow the movement of going and coming, who at the slightest collision, raise lively quarrels, and by their lamentations, cries, and continual trepidation, render insupportable a situation which would be troublesome enough without all this.

When you meet a person of your acquaintance in the street, salute him by bowing and taking off your hat. (However, at Paris a young man ought to avoid approaching, and even saluting a young lady of his acquaintance, out of regard for the natural timidity of her sex.) Sometimes a mere bow is not enough. If you see the person frequently, you must go to him and ask how he is. While you are speaking, if it is a lady, or an aged and respectable gentleman, remain uncovered. It is for the latter, who see how troublesome this politeness is in winter, to insist that you put on your hat.

It also belongs to the person who is the more important of the two to take leave first. In a meeting of this kind, a gentleman never leaves a lady until she bids him good-bye; nor is a young lady allowed to leave first a married or older lady. During this interview, which should be very short, the speaker of least importance should stand on the street side, in order to keep his interlocutor from the neighbourhood of the carriages. It would be supremely ridiculous to enter into a long conversation, and thus detain the person accosted against his will. If you have any thing urgent to say, ask if you may have the honour of accompanying him.

If there is a stranger with your acquaintance, be content with saluting the latter without stopping; otherwise you put his companion in a disagreeable position. This civility becomes a rigorous duty if the companion is a lady. Traditional gallantry required that in this last case, you not only should not stop, but that you should not even salute an acquaintance or friend in passing. This is in order not to force the lady to salute an unknown person (for you should bow every time that the person whom you are with bows) but this custom may be modified. If your acquaintance is a friend or a young man, you may merely make a motion. If it is an aged man, a distinguished person, or a lady, it is necessary to salute him or her, saying to the companion, "I take the liberty to salute Mr. *or* Mrs. Such-a-one." The companion should respond, "And you, Sir."

If a person of your acquaintance is at a window, and you are supposed to perceive him, you ought to address a salutation to him. But it is necessary to avoid speaking to him from the street, or making signs, for that is a custom of bad *ton*.

To enter into a long conversation with common and low people, who make their door-step their drawing-room, shows you to be almost as ill-bred as they are.

Travelling.

If in travelling the duties of propriety are less numerous than in society, they are not therefore less obligatory.

Persons about to travel should make visits of taking leave amongst their acquaintances, whom they should ask if they have any commissions. Unless there is perfect intimacy, it would be inconsiderate to accept this offer, or to ask them to take charge of such-and-such a thing, especially if it is a parcel. If you are very intimate with the person, you may ask for news on his arrival.

Before their departure, the names of passengers are entered in the order of their numbers at the public coach-offices. After this, each one takes the place assigned him. Gallantry, however, requires a gentleman to offer his seat to a lady who is less well accommodated; for it would be improper for him to sit upon the back seat, while she sits upon the front one. Some persons cannot bear the motion of a coach when they ride backwards; and this manner of riding incommodes them extremely. Polite gentlemen will take pleasure in relieving them from this unpleasantness.

Ladies, on their part, ought not to require too much, nor put the complaisance of a gentleman to too severe a test. The latter, however, should at every stopping-place attentively help a lady alight, by offering his hand and directing her feet on the step of the coach. The same thing is necessary in assisting her to get in again.

It would appear ill to take advantage of your superiority of rank, in order to consult your own convenience alone. It is necessary, on the contrary, to take great care not to incommode any one, and to show every civility to fellow-travellers.

Propriety in travelling is not so rigorous as in society. It only requires that you do not incommode your companions; that you are agreeable to them; and that you respond politely when they speak to you. But it leaves you free to read, sleep, look about, or observe silence, &c.

You would be uncivil if you opened or shut the windows of the coach without consulting the people who are with you. Or if you took any light and delicate food, such as fruits, cakes, or confectionary, without offering it to them; but ordinarily they should not accept it. You would appear disobliging if, knowing the route, you did not point out the beautiful sites, and answer any questions concerning them. Finally, you would deserve to be called a fool and a prattler, if you conversed with your fellow-travellers as with intimate acquaintances.

On your return, you should carry or send the commissions which you have received. Slight acquaintances, whose commissions you have offered to take only by writing, should not expect a visit on your return. This right

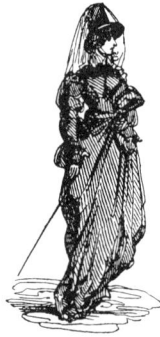

A

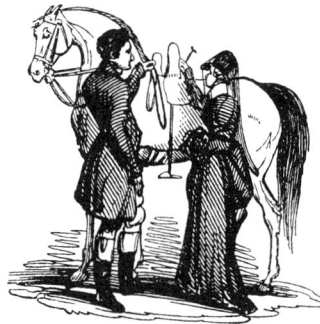

B

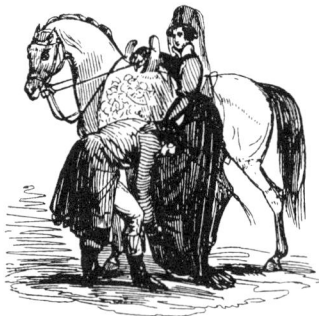

C

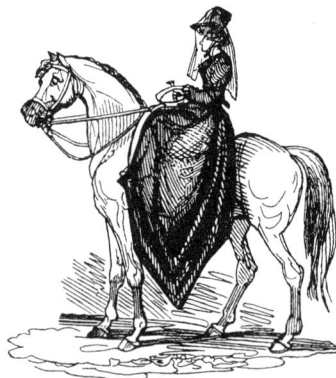

D

Figure 1. How a lady should mount a horse.

belongs only to relations, friends, and intimate acquaintances. Finally, all those for whom you have executed any commissions must pay you a visit of thanks as soon as possible.

If you travel on horseback with a distinguished person, give him the right, and keep a little behind, regulating yourself by his progress. (See Fig. 1, above.) There is one exception to this rule; it is when his horse is skittish, and it is absolutely necessary for yours to pass on first, so that the other will follow.

If you happen to be on the windward side, so that you throw dust upon your companion, change your position. When you pass by trees whose branches are about the height of your shoulders, the person who goes first should take care that the branches, in springing back to place, do not strike violently against the person who follows.

If you are fording a large stream, a small river, or a pool, it is polite to go first. But if you have not taken this precaution, and fall in the rear, keep at a distance, so that your horse's feet may not spatter water or mud upon the gentleman before you. If your companion gallops his horse, you should never pass him, nor make your horse caper, unless he signifies that it is agreeable to him.

——*The Gentleman and Lady's Book of Politeness,*
Manuel complet de la bonne compagnie.

Chapter XXVI.
Propriety in Religious Duties.

❦❦❦

Propriety ought to preside over the highest instructions of morality, just as it regulates the liveliest impulses of pleasure. Therefore, let us consider its connexion with religion.

Respectful Deportment in Churches.

Religious sentiment is an immense difference, perhaps the only one, which is found between man and animals. However it may absorb you by its intensity, exalt you with delight, or withdraw from you in misfortune, this mysterious and sublime sentiment should always command your respect. Therefore, I shall not refer to particular differences of worship, in advising you never to visit a church without submitting to the conventions of religion. Observe silence, or at least speak seldom and in a low voice; take off your hat; walk with a slow and grave step; stop, at the same time making an inclination of your body, if any ceremony engages a pious assembly. Whether the church is Jewish, Catholic, or Protestant, recollect that in this place men honour the Creator of the Universe; that here they seek consolation in their troubles, and pardon for their sins.

If you visit a church or any similar edifice merely to view it, endeavour to do it outside the time of service. (See Fig. 1.) Contemplate silently the pictures, monuments, &c.; beware of imitating those foolish vandals, who in a few moments, deface with their obscure and ephemeral names monuments which are destined to endure for ages. Do not like them forget that the only thing which you can expect is a smile of contempt from all enlightened friends of the arts. Do not wait until the keepers remind you of the gratuity due to their kindness in conducting you; offer it to them with your thanks on taking leave. Pay the price asked for seats without discussion; avoid changing gold and silver; and in order to do so, go always provided with small change. The respect due to the place requires you to abstain from every thing which resembles the cares of business.

I have thus far spoken only the language of tolerance, and of religious worship in general, but I am now going to use that of faith and devotion.

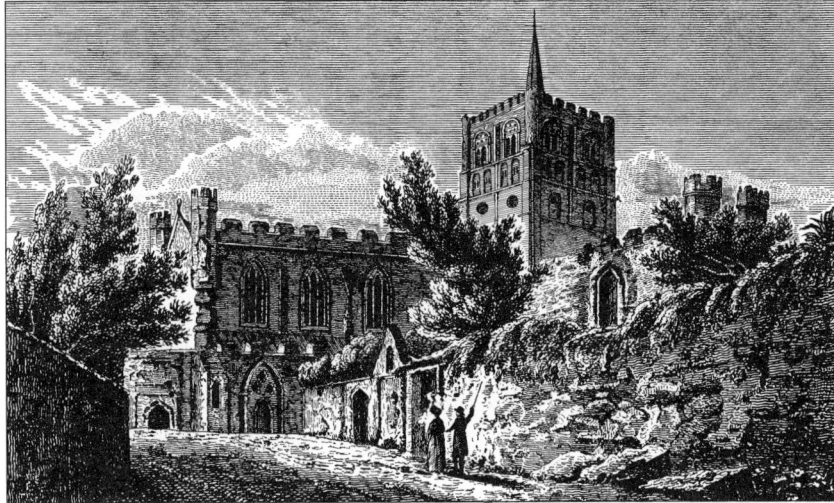

Figure 1. St. Alban's Abbey.

Let the neatness and modesty of your apparel, and your discreet and respectful deportment, show that you perceive what is due to the house of God. Incline your body on entering; take the holy water; then advance by the shortest way, and without precipitation, to the place which you are to occupy. If possible, do not change it; neither put yourself in the passage, nor carry the chairs to a distance. Take two together, to avoid turning your seat as circumstances may require in the course of the ceremony. (See Div. 1.) If on a crowded occasion you have two chairs, it is well to offer one of them to some one who has none; a gentleman should even give his own to a lady who is standing. If the service has commenced before you enter, place yourself in the rear, in order not to disturb those present by your coming. The same motive ought to prevent your going away before the close of the service, except from urgent necessity. During the sermon, it is necessary to endeavour to make no noise, and to bow with profound respect every time the clergyman pronounces the sacred name of Jesus Christ.

If you are accompanied by a lady to whom you owe deference, go before and present the holy water to her; prepare two chairs for her, and place yourself near. In leaving church, clear the passage for her; carry her prayer-book, present her again with the holy water, and hold the door open to let her pass. Indeed, these last two marks of politeness should be shown indiscriminately by well-bred people to any who happen to be near them in entering or leaving the church. Benevolent consideration for your neighbours is a worthy accompaniment of devotion. Whether you give or withhold an offering to the mendicants of either sex, they should be answered by a salutation.

Every one knows that it is contrary to the sanctity of the place to walk in a church as upon a public promenade; to converse there as in a private house; to cast looks of curiosity to one side and the other; to have a mien which displays uneasiness or boredom; to balance yourself upon your seat, or shake in an annoying manner that of the person before you; to carry with you dogs, parcels, &c.

It is entirely contrary to religious propriety to hurry or press forward when going to make an offering, to take the ashes, or when approaching the confessional. Especially in the last case, wait your turn in silence, without trying to supplant those before you. However, should you have any urgent motives, you may make them known softly and politely. The disputes which too frequently arise with regard to this are at the same time an absurdity and impiety. When you take a place at the holy table, lay aside your gloves, book, sword, bag, &c. It is well for ladies to cover themselves with a veil half drawn; this bespeaks piety and modesty.

Religious Propriety in Social Intercourse.

If it is a fundamental principle of propriety not to wound any one in his self-esteem, tastes, or interests, it is even more necessary to respect his religious beliefs. To make sport of faith, that powerful, deep, and involuntary sentiment, before which the law yields; to raise the torment of doubt in hearts just become pious and tranquil; to awaken a spirit of fanaticism and religious excess; to cause yourself to be considered by some as a foolish, by others an unworthy person, and by all as an enemy to politeness and tolerance—these are the sad results of raillery against faith; raillery, too, almost always dictated by a desire to shine as a wit. These results take place without any exception; impious sarcasms constantly do injury to serious people. But they become still more revolting in the mouths of women, who like angels, ought ever to show themselves loving, pure, and free from passion; whom Bernardin de Saint-Pierre designates with much feeling and justice the "pious sex."

However, I do not proscribe entirely delicate and happy allusions, or comparisons drawn from the sacred books, and made in a proper spirit. Thus you may ask some one if he much repents his negligence in visiting or writing to you. If asked how long you have had some habit, you may respond, "For all eternity," &c. It is needless, I think, to provide more examples. Suffice it to add, that rigorism alone can reprove them, and that the occasion sometimes renders them very piquant.

Debates on religion demand the most reserve and care, since without your knowledge conscience frequently becomes in them auxiliary to pride. Therefore, if you are unable to command yourself; if you do not feel enough of logical power, grace, or at least clarity of elocution to contend successfully, avoid controversies. Avoid them through fear of compromising, in the eyes of those of weak faith, that religion which you defend, and of exposing yourself to lasting ridicule. But whatever the skill which you exhibit in evading the arguments of your adversary, whatever your triumph, and though your disposition should urge you, never turn a serious discussion into jest. From that moment you will lose all your advantages; and though overthrown, your antagonist will recover himself with this just reflection, that "nothing is proved by a jest."

Finally, though you manifest on every occasion a sincere and profound respect for religion, beware above all things of making a proclamation of your piety. Avoid talking with those in your parish about your confessor and your religious observances. If you do not distinguish yourself from the crowd, they will take you for a hypocrite, or a person of small mind. If on the contrary you recommend yourself by superior merit, they will think that you take an arrogant pleasure in showing the contrast which exists between your exalted talents and your humble faith. Between ourselves, would they be in the wrong?

———*The Gentleman and Lady's Book of Politeness,*
Manuel complet de la bonne compagnie.

Diversion 1.

Differences between Catholic and Protestant Churches. These directions are more particularly applicable to Catholic churches in foreign countries, where it is not the general custom, as in the United States, to have pews. The whole floor is an open area, and supplied with chairs; during the service each person takes two, one of which he sits on, and places the other before him to kneel upon. This custom of using chairs, however, is not universal even in Europe. The author observes in a note, that it would be desirable for all parts of France to adopt the custom observed at Havre, Dieppe, and other cities of Normandy; where instead of having chairs, the churches are furnished throughout with fixed seats or benches, by which means the service is conducted with much more order and decorum.

———*The Gentleman and Lady's Book of Politeness.*

Chapter XXVII.
Politeness in a Business
or Profession.

Besides general politeness, that ready money which is current with all, there is a characteristic politeness suited to every profession. Interest, custom, and the desire for particular esteem, the necessity of moderating the enthusiasm which almost constantly animates us: these are the motives which determine the different kinds of politeness which I shall consider as regards shop-keepers, people in office, lawyers, physicians, artists, military men, and clergymen. As all this politeness is mutual, I shall necessarily speak of the obligations imposed upon people who have intercourse with these different persons.

Politeness of Shop-keepers and Purchasers.

Politeness in shop-keepers is a road to fortune, which the greater part of them are careful not to neglect, especially at Paris, where we find particularly the model of a well-bred shop-keeper. It is this model which I wish to hold up even to some Parisians, and to the retail dealers of the provinces; as well as to those who are unacquainted with trade, but are destined to that profession.

When a purchaser calls, the shop-keeper should salute him politely, without inquiring after his health, unless they are intimately acquainted. He then waits until the purchaser has made his wishes known, advances towards him, or brings forward a seat; then shows him, with the greatest civility, the articles for which he has inquired. If the purchaser is difficult to suit, capricious, ridiculous, or even disdainful, the shop-keeper ought not to appear to perceive it. In such cases he may, however, show a little coldness of manner.

It must be allowed that the *rôle* of shop-keeper is frequently painful. There are some people who treat them like servants. Some capricious ladies of fashion go into a shop only to pass the time, and to see the new fashions. With this object they make the shop-keeper open an hundred bundles, show heaps of goods, and finish by going out, saying in a disdainful tone that nothing suits them. There are some merciless purchasers who contend for a few cents with all the tenacity of avarice, obstinacy, and pride. Under all these vexations, the shop-keeper must show constant urbanity. He waits upon such imperious purchasers readily, but nearly in silence, for he must be well convinced that the more complying he is to people of this sort, the more haughty and difficult they show themselves.

With a capricious fashionable, his patience should never forsake him. Though he knows perfectly what will be the result of her fatiguing call, he nonetheless should show her his goods, as if he thought she really intended to buy; for indeed this sometimes tempts a lady to purchase. Even though his politeness should be all for nothing, he should still express his regret at not having been able to suit her, and hope to be more fortunate another time. He should then conduct her politely to the door, which he should hold open until her carriage leaves it.

A shop-keeper who wishes to spare himself time, speeches, and vexation, who even feels the dignity of his profession, ought to sell at a fixed price. If he does not announce that he sells in that mode, he ought at least to adopt it, and not to have what is called an "asking price." However, if he has to do with gossips who think themselves cheated unless something is abated, or who design to impose sacrifices on shop-keepers, it is necessary to carry on this ridiculous skirmishing politely, and to yield by degrees, without showing any distaste for these endless debates. But the dealer of good *ton* abstains from lofty assurances, laughable adjurations, and declarations of loss and of preference, such as, "I am making no profit," "This is just for you," and other foolish things, which make a lackey's office of a truly respectable trade.

The clerk should carry the articles purchased to the desk, whither he should politely conduct the purchaser. He then makes up the parcel, which is not handed over until the bill is settled, and the purchaser is ready to depart. If the latter is not on foot, the parcel should not be delivered until he is seated in a carriage, and the door is ready to be shut. If on the contrary, the purchaser is not in a carriage, he must be asked whether he wishes to have the parcel carried home. This politeness is indispensable if the parcel is large, and especially if the purchaser is a lady.

It is further necessary that the person at the counter should offer small change for the balance of the purchase, and apologize if he is obliged to give copper or heavy money. He should present a bill for the articles, and not show any ill-humour if the purchaser thinks proper to look over it.

There is one circumstance which tries the politeness of the most civil shop-keepers; it is when an assortment is wanted. It is indeed irksome enough to show a great quantity of goods, and give patterns of them, with the certainty almost that all this will avail nothing. But it ought not to be forgotten, that like all other qualities, politeness has its trials, and that perhaps the person who has thus chanced to call at the shop, will be induced by this amenity of behaviour to become a regular customer.

I trust that the shop-keepers' clerks, in the advice which I am now about to give them, will not see any pathetic attempt to address them with epigrams. By enjoining upon them to avoid the following—volubility; a disrespectful familiarity towards ladies; extravagant praises of the goods; an affected zeal in serving rich persons; an impolite tardiness, and disdainful inattention to ill-attired ones; the ridiculous habit of wishing to make conversation; urging people to buy whether they wish to or not; and stunning them with the names of all the goods in the shop—I intend less to unite in, then to preserve them from the reproaches of fault-finders.

Every civility ought to be reciprocal, or nearly so. If the officious politeness of the shop-keeper does not require an equal return, he has at least a claim to civil treatment. Besides, if his politeness proceeds from interest, is this a reason why purchasers should add to the unpleasantness of his profession, and disregard the laws of propriety? Many very respectable people permit themselves so many infractions in this particular, that I think it my duty to dwell upon it.

When you enter a shop and find no one there, you must immediately give notice of your presence, either by knocking gently on the inner door, or by calling out, "The shop, if you please." When waited on never say, "I want such a thing," but, "Have the goodness to show me," or "Show me, if you please, that article," or use some other polite form. If they do not show you at first the articles you desire, and you are obliged to examine a great number, apologize to the shop-keeper for the trouble you are giving. If after all you cannot suit yourself, renew your apologies when you go away.

If you make small purchases say, "I ask your pardon," or "I am sorry for having troubled you for so trifling a thing." If you spend a considerable time in the selection of articles, apologize to the shop-keeper who waits for you to decide.

If the price seems to you too high, and the shop has not fixed prices, ask for a reduction in brief and civil terms, and without ever appearing to suspect the good faith of the shop-keeper. If he does not yield, do not enter into a contest, but go away, after saying politely that you think you can obtain the article cheaper elsewhere, but if not, that you will give him the preference.

If the clerk inquires whether you wish for any other article, always answer in a manner to give him hope that you will call again. Never neglect to be agreeable, and always thank him when you go out.

Politeness between Persons in Office and the Public.

This kind of politeness is not much famed; nor can it be, since the desire of pleasing and the expectation of gain have here no influence. Besides, as you remain but a moment with these gentlemen, and as they have business with a great many people, the observances and forms of politeness would be misplaced. The following are points to be observed by them, and are by no means rigid; the greater therefore the reason for conforming to them. (See also Chapter XVIII.)

A man in office is not obliged to rise and salute people, nor to offer them a seat. It is enough for him to receive them by an inclination of his head, and make a sign with his hand, to intimate to them to be seated. The meeting finished, he salutes them on leaving, as before, but never conducts them back to the door. It would be ridiculous to be offended with these bureaucratic forms, and still more so, to wish to enter into conversation, to make inquiries concerning the health, &c. Because of their professional habits, those in office ought, in society, to watch themselves with care.

Politeness of Lawyers and their Clients.

Politeness is a very difficult thing for this respectable class, who constantly see people animated by a sentiment which renders them most unamiable, viz., self-interest. Besides, being in the habit of refuting their adversaries, and being obliged to do it promptly, they acquire in general a kind of bluntness, a decisive tone, and a spirit of contradiction, against which they ought to be on their guard in company, as also in their places of business. The usual inquiries after the health are not customary between lawyers and their clients, unless they are otherwise acquainted. Lawyers are, however, bound to observe attentions which are not practiced by persons in office. They rise to salute their clients, offer them a seat, and conduct them to the door when they take leave; they observe what is due to sex, rank, and age.

As to clients, they ought to conform to the ordinary rules of civility; they ought, moreover, not to exhibit any signs of impatience while waiting until they can be received. They should take care to be clear and precise in the narration of their business, and not to importune, by vain repetitions or passionate declamations, the counsellor who is listening to them. They should also consider that his moments are precious, and retire as soon as they have sufficiently instructed him in their business.

Politeness of Physicians and their Patients.

The conventions adopted in the offices of physicians are the same as those for lawyers; but sympathy should give a more affectionate character to the manner of the former. Well-bred patients beware of abusing it, and keep to themselves all complaints which are useless towards a knowledge of their malady. They answer the physician's questions in a clear, brief, and polite manner. When these questions do not embrace the observations which they may themselves have made on their disorder, they say so, at the same time offering some such excuse as, "I ask your pardon, this observation is perhaps pointless; but being myself ignorant, and wishing to omit nothing, I submit it to your good judgement."

Give frequent and heartfelt thanks to the physician who affords you his advice or attentions. Even if he is unsuccessful, you are not exempt from these testimonies of gratitude. It renders them perhaps more obligatory, for delicacy requires that you should not appear tacitly to reproach him.

Being obliged to speak of different wants and of different parts of the body for which propriety has no appropriate language, a physician ought to avoid being obscure or coarse, particularly when addressing ladies. A forgetfulness of these forms often renders a meritorious and learned man insupportable.

When there is any danger, every one knows with what delicate preparations a physician ought to speak before the patient and his family, of the nature of the illness and the probable consequences; and in what guarded terms he should at last disclose to them a fatal termination, if unhappily it has become inevitable. Every one also knows that however poignant the grief of relations, they ought never to let it appear in their conversations with the physician that they regard him as the cause of their affliction.

Politeness of Artists and Authors, and the Deference due to them.

You may perhaps ask, do artists come under the common rule? I in my turn shall ask: do they live like others? these men, always absorbed in one powerful and single conception, with which they, like the Creator, wish to animate matter? who seek every where the secret of the beautiful which goads, infatuates, and evades them? passionate, absorbed in thought, ingenuous, almost always strangers to calculation, to pleasure, and to the occupations of society? No, they have a separate existence, one which society does not comprehend, and which they ought to conceal from it.

If, as we shall see hereafter, you should avoid speaking of your profession and your personal affairs, for a still stronger reason an artist should be silent about his own labours, successes, and hopes. People will accuse him of arrogance, of vanity, and perhaps even of madness. Enthusiasm is neither included in nor admitted into society, because there the ridiculous is feared above every thing, and "from the sublime to the ridiculous there is but one step." Let him then reserve only for his friends, and for true friends of the arts, his noble and striking bursts of inspiration.

People are also generally prone to suspect artists of jealousy. To escape this accusation, and at the same time preserve the right of expressing their thoughts, they ought to commend warmly what appears to them good, and criticize with much moderation and without any raillery what seems defective.

These observations are addressed equally to authors, but with an important addition. Besides the charge of arrogance, people are much disposed to accuse them of pedantry. Let them therefore be careful, and check constantly the desire of entering into conversation upon the interesting subjects with which they are continually occupied. Let them always be in fear of obtaining the name of a *bel esprit*, which calls up so many recollections of pedantry and affectation.

A graceful simplicity, a happy mixture of elevation and naïveté, should characterize authors and artists, but particularly female ones. Ladies who handle the pen, the lyre, or the pencil, ought to be well persuaded that a vestige of prejudice raises against them, especially in provincial places, a multitude of unfavourable observations. And besides, so many half-instructed women have had so much the air and manners of upstarts, that this opinion is almost excusable. This prejudice lays it down as a rule that every female author or artist may be instantly recognized by her oddities, her want of modesty, and her pedantic prudery. Do away with this unjust prejudice, ladies: it will be both easy and pleasant. You have only to follow the influence of an elevated soul and pure taste; you have but to recall that simplicity is the coquetry of genius.

But if authors and artists ought to apply themselves without reluctance or ill-humour to all the requirements of society; if they ought to strip themselves of all pretension, and forget themselves, others should not forget them. Propriety requires that you converse with an author concerning his works; that you congratulate him on his successes, and bestow upon him suitable and delicate praises. If any of his works is unknown to you, earnestly ask him the loan of it; read it promptly, and prove to him by your quotations that you have a thorough acquaintance with it. If he makes you a present of any of his productions, you owe him a visit, or at least a billet of thanks. Handsome compliments, and lively testimonials of acknowledgment, ought to fill up this visit or billet.

Remember also, that to please an artist it is necessary to flatter at once his taste, his self-esteem, and his worship of the fine arts. Speak to him therefore like a connoisseur, or at least an admirer of painting or music. Ask the favour of seeing his pictures, or of hearing his symphonies. Contemplate the former a long time; listen to the latter with great attention. Address to him enthusiastic compliments mingled with thanks; then by an adroit transition, put to him questions which prove your desire to be initiated into a knowledge of the arts.

When an artist or a writer obtains any honourable distinction, such as a prize, a medal, dramatic success, or an academical title, his friends and acquaintances should lose no time in offering him their congratulations. Those at a distance may perform this duty of propriety by writing.

Not only professional authors, but literary persons who publish a speech, a little work, or a pamphlet should send, in an envelope, a copy to their family, friends, professional brethren, authors who have sent them similar presents, intimate acquaintances, superiors, and persons to whom they owe respect; and according to the nature of the work, people with whom they have relations of pleasure or business. (See Fig. 1.) It is affectionate and very good *ton* for the author to write with his own hand at the top of the first leaf, or of the cover, some kind or respectful words, according to the recipient. These words, which are designed to make of the gift a remembrance or homage, are always written under the name of the recipient, and signed by the author.

I shall speak here of a dedication only to observe that you may not dedicate a work to any one without having previously obtained his consent, either verbally or by writing. When it is to the king, queen, or princes, it is necessary to write to their secretary, to know their wish in this respect. As for any other person of dignity, you may write to him without any intermediary. If the members of the royal family have accepted the dedication, the author is generally allowed the honour of presenting his work to them.

Figure 1. An author presenting his book.

Politeness of Military Men.

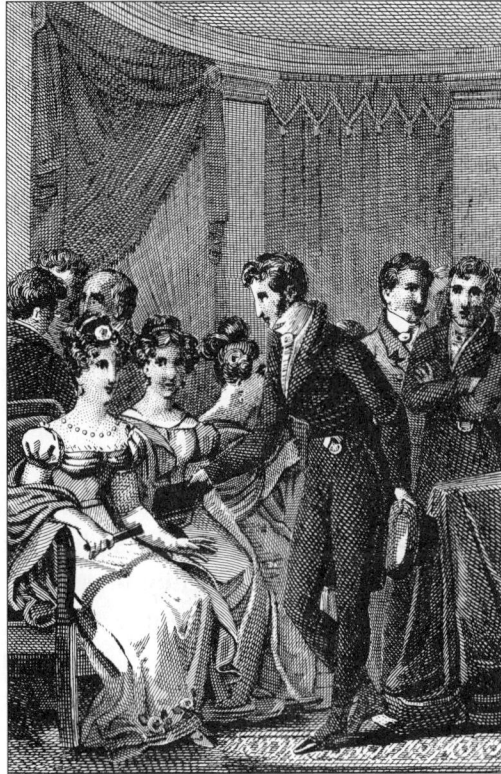

Military politeness has, as is well known, some peculiar characteristics. Officers and soldiers do not uncover themselves on entering a church, if they are under arms; only during the elevation of the host, they raise their right hand to the front part of their helmet, cap, or shako. This motion is their ordinary salute. When soldiers converse with their superiors, they constantly hold the edge of their hand to their forehead.

On entering a drawing-room, an officer lays down his sabre or sword. It is not in good *ton* for a gentleman to present himself before ladies in the uniform of the national guard, unless some circumstance excuses or authorizes this liberty. In a citizen's dress, officers may wear a black cravat.

If you are acquainted with military men, in addressing them call them only "general" or "captain." It would be uncivil to give them the title of an inferior rank; thus you should not say "lieutenant."

Propriety of Clergymen and Nuns, and the Deference due to them.

A clergyman should be considered in two points of view: when he is exercising his holy office, and when he is taking part in the relations of society. In the first situation, he is an object of special respect. Even the title given him, the words addressed to him, and the attitude taken in speaking to him are regulated by the liturgy. But though the clergyman is not now in society an object of religious veneration, he has, as the representative of God, and as a minister of the altar, a claim to much respect and deference. Too light conversation, dancing, and love-songs, would be out of place in his presence.

Clergymen have two shoals to avoid. Their custom of preaching a severe and sacred morality, and of catechizing and censuring the penitent with authority, gives them sometimes a dogmatical and rigid tone, a pedantry of morality altogether contrary to social affability. Sometimes also, to guard against this result, which they feel to be nearly inevitable, clergymen, especially the more aged, indulge themselves in unsuitable pleasantries which they would not dare to allow in men of the world. A mild gravity, a moderate gaiety, a noble and affectionate urbanity—these are the characteristics which ought to distinguish the clergyman in society. (See Div. 1.)

——*The Gentleman and Lady's Book of Politeness,*
Manuel complet de la bonne compagnie.

Diversion 1.

Titles given to Members of Religious Orders. The following material was left out of the original American translation.

——Frances Grimble.

Priests are not ordinarily called "Monsieur," though this title is sometimes added to their particular function. Monks of any order are called "Brother." Nuns receive the appellation of "Sister." Letters sent to a nun are addressed to "My Sister Such-a-one," or "My Dear Sister Such-a-one." If you are not at all familiar with her, so that it would prove embarrassing to call her "My Sister," you may call her "Madame," but never "Mademoiselle"; that would be disrespectful.

——*Manuel complet de la bonne compagnie.*

Chapter XXVIII.
Of Visits.

Visits are a very important part of social relations. They are much more than the simple means of communication established by necessity, since they have at once for their object duty and pleasure, and they enter into almost all the acts of life. (See Div. 1.)

There are many kinds of visits, but I shall confine myself to the principal ones. The first are the visits on new year's day; next, those of friendship and of ceremony. As for those which only occur under peculiar circumstances, visits of business are described in Chapter XXVII, and visits related to weddings, illness, and mourning are described in Chapter XXX.

Different Kinds of Visits.

At the return of each new year, custom and duty require you to present yourself to your relations first; afterwards to your patrons, friends, and those who have done you favours. It would appear ridiculous to wish people a "happy new year" in ceremonious visits.

Other visits are divided into several classes. Those of the evening or afternoon are the most polite; those of the morning are the most friendly and respectful. Then there are visits by cards and presenting yourself, and by cards without presenting yourself. Weekly visits are confined to acquaintances with whom you have not very close relations. Monthly visits are less ceremonious, but partake of coldness: it is especially at Paris that these visits are permitted. Such visits demand much attention to the toilet. They should be as short as possible; a quarter of an hour is long enough, and you should be careful to retire when other persons chance to come in.

I shall not mention friendly visits, except to remind my readers that almost all ceremony should be dispensed with. They are made at all hours, without preparation or dressing. A too brilliant attire would be out of place, and if the engagements of the day carry you in such a costume to the house of a friend, you ought obligingly to give an explanation. Should you not find him at home, do not leave a card; such useless ceremony would astonish your friends. Merely remind the servants to mention your calling, and leave your card only when they are absent; then the card should be rolled up, and put in the key-hole. It is well to call again soon.

With a friend, or relation whom you treat as such, do not keep an account of your visits. The one who has most leisure, calls upon him who has the least. However, this privilege ought not to be abused. Friendly visits should be returned now and then.

On the contrary, a visit of ceremony should never be made without keeping an account of it, and you should even examine the intervals at which they are returned; for it is essential to let a similar interval elapse. People in this way give you notice whether they wish to see you often or seldom. There are some persons whom you go to see once a fortnight, others once a month, and others even less frequently. In order to neither neglect returning visits, nor to accidentally repeat them, persons who have an extensive acquaintance will do well to keep a little memorandum for this purpose.

You cannot make ceremonious visits in a becoming manner, if you have any slight indisposition which temporarily affects your appearance or voice, or which embarrasses your thoughts, and renders your company fatiguing. For instance, a swelled face, a cold, or a slight head-ache; in that case it would appear impolite and familiar. On the contrary, if you make visits of friendship under such circumstances, you will only appear more amiable and zealous.

To choose a suitable time, is as indispensable in visiting, as in any thing else. You may manage this by considering the habits of the person you are going to see; by making your arrangements so as not to visit at meal-times, in moments of occupation, and when your friends are walking. The correct time necessarily varies; but it is customary not to make ceremonious visits either before mid-day or after five o'clock. To present yourself earlier would render you annoying, and to present yourself later might interfere with arrangements which have been made for the evening.

After making their toilet with care, visitors should furnish themselves with cards; that is, with small pieces of card or pasteboard upon which their name is printed or clearly written. Gentlemen simply put their cards in their pocket, but ladies carry them in an elegant little receptacle called a card-case. They hold it in their hand, and it contributes (together with an elegant handkerchief of embroidered batiste, which is carried on this occasion) to an air of good taste. (See Div. 2.)

I shall here make a digression in regard to cards. Formerly it was not considered impolite to take the cards of a cast-off pack, cut them crossways into three parts, and write your name upon them. However, this is now a subject of ridicule, and is only seen in the provinces, where they sometimes also replace these improvised cards with small pieces of thick paper. Next to these come cards made of thin pasteboard, plain, gilt-edged, or embossed, and intended to have the name in writing. These are suitable for young gentleman and young ladies, and they answer for half-ceremonious visits. After these come lithographic cards, then printed ones, and lastly those which are engraved. Some cards are richly embossed, and available in every shade. Every one will choose cards according to his taste; but it is well to observe that cards ornamented with borders, and those of rose-colour and celestial blue, are not proper for gentlemen, nor for ladies of mature years, because they seem too *recherché* and showy.

The title should be placed under the name. In large cities the address is placed at the bottom of the card, in smaller letters. Mourning cards are surrounded by a black margin; half-mourning ones are of a clear grey.

It is bad *ton* to preserve the cards you have received round the frame of a looking-glass; such a display shows that you wish to parade the names of distinguished visitors. At the beginning of a new year, or when some occasion (such as a funeral or a wedding) multiplies visitors at your house, and you are obliged to return these numerous visits, it is not amiss to keep the cards in an obvious place, and save yourself the trouble of writing a list. If all year round your glass is seen bristling with yellowed cards, it will doubtless be attributed to an ill-regulated self-esteem. But let us return to our visitors.

If the visit is made in a carriage, the servant will ask if the person you wish to see is at home. Persons of high *ton* are accompanied as far as the ante-room by one or two footmen, who meet up with them again when they leave. If you call in a hired carriage, or on foot, go yourself to ask the servants. Servants are considered as soldiers on duty. If they reply that the person has gone out, by no means urge the point, even if you are certain it is not the case. If by chance you see the person, you must pretend that you did not; leave your card and retire. When the servant informs you that the lady or gentleman is unwell, engaged in business, or dining, you must act in the same manner. Leave as many cards as there are persons you wish to see in the house; for example, one for the husband, another for the wife, another for the aunt, &c.

When admitted, lay aside your over-shoes, umbrella, cloak, &c. in the ante-room; even ladies should lay aside their cloaks at very grand houses. In the provinces they commonly keep them on. You are then announced by a servant, if it is the custom of the house, or at least you wait until (without announcing you) he opens the door of the room.

If the servants are absent, do not enter immediately, but tap gently with your finger, and wait until some one opens the door or bids you to enter. If no one does either, open the door slowly and softly. Should you find no one, do not go about and open other doors, or pass into an inner room, but retrace your steps immediately, return to the ante-room, and remain until some one comes to show you in. If you are obliged to wait very long, you may leave your card on a piece of furniture or with the porter. This situation very rarely occurs, but it is well to be prepared for it, in order not to be taken unawares.

When admitted, a gentleman presents himself with his hat in his hand, and advancing towards the lady, salutes her gracefully and respectfully. As soon as he observes that the lady is looking for a seat to offer him, he must lose no time in providing one for himself (commonly a chair). He places it towards the door by which he entered, and at some distance from the lady, to whom he thus leaves the most honourable place in the room. He ought by no means to sit, unless she is seated; and holding his hat upon his knee, must not balance himself on the edge of his chair or sink down into it, but preserve an easy, polite, and becoming attitude.

It would be familiar and bad *ton* to put down your hat or walking-stick before the gentleman, and particularly the lady of the house, has invited you to do so. Even then it is well to refuse, and not to do it until asked two or three times. Do not put your hat down carelessly, nor place it on a sopha, for this is impolite. (See Div. 3.) The sopha, which in ancient times was regarded as a sanctuary, must be neither touched nor approached by a man. It is best to put your hat on a console-table, centre-table, &c. The lady of the house does not attempt to take the hats of gentlemen, unless she wishes to treat them with familiarity, which is seldom done in visits of pure ceremony.

These remarks apply also to ladies. For the past fifteen years it has been their custom to take off their hats and shawls. This supposes an intimacy which authorizes their abstaining from it at the houses of distant acquaintances. If you are invited to lay them aside, you should refuse. The short time devoted to a ceremonious visit, and the necessity of consulting a glass in replacing your head-dress, and of being assisted in putting on your shawl, prevent ladies from accepting such an invitation. If you are slightly familiar with the person you are visiting, and wish to be more at ease, ask permission, which should be granted, your hostess rising to assist you in taking them off. An arm-chair or a piece of furniture in a distant part of the room should receive these articles; they should not be placed upon the sopha, unless the lady of the house puts them there. At the house of a person you visit habitually, you may lay them aside without saying a word. You may even adjust your hair and *fichu* before the glass, provided you take only a few moments to do so.

If the person you call upon is preparing to go out, or to sit down at table, you ought, though she asks you to remain, to retire as soon as possible. The person visited so unseasonably should be careful to conceal that she wishes your visit would end soon. Always appear delighted to receive a visitor, and if under these circumstances he leaves quickly, express your regret.

A ceremonious visit should be short; if the conversation ceases without being again continued by the person you have come to see, and she gets up from her seat under any pretext whatsoever, custom requires you to make your salutation and withdraw. If before this tacit invitation to retire, other visitors are announced, you should slip out without saying any thing. If the gentleman of the house, in waiting upon you to the door, asks you to remain longer, briefly reply to him that a pressing engagement calls you, and earnestly entreat him not to detain you. You should terminate your visit by briskly shutting the door.

If on entering the room, you find strangers engaged in conversation, content yourself with the few words which the gentleman or lady of the house addresses to you; stop only a few moments, make a general salutation, and conduct yourself as described earlier. When you have happened to meet the strangers elsewhere, they may unite sometimes with the person you are visiting, to prevent your taking leave. Say every thing which is polite and flattering, but still persist in retiring. If while you are present, a letter is brought to the person you are visiting, and she lays it down without opening it, you must entreat her to read it. She will not do so, and this incident will bind you to shorten your visit.

When you make a half-ceremonious visit, and the person you are visiting warmly insists upon your stopping, it is proper to yield, but after a few minutes you should rise to go. If you are urged still further, and are taken by the hands and made to sit down as it were by force, to leave immediately would be impolite. Nonetheless you must, after a short interval, get up a third time, and then certainly retire. If during your visit a member of the family enters the room, you need not on this account take leave, but content yourself with rising and saluting the person. If the person is a lady, you must not seat yourself until she is seated; if a gentleman, you may accept the invitation made you to take your seat, while the other remains standing.

If you make a visit with others, there are some points to be observed concerning your companions. It is improper for more than three or four to visit together. In mounting the stairs, it is rigorously the custom to give precedence to those to whom you owe respect, and to yield to them the most convenient part of the stairs, which is that next the wall. Above all do not forget this last precaution if you accompany a lady; and a well-bred man, at such a time, should offer his arm. When there are several persons, he should bestow this mark of respect on the oldest. If you meet any one on the stairs, place yourself on the side opposite to the one he occupies.

It would be vexatious and out of place to make an everlasting ceremony as to who should be announced first; the preference must be given to ladies; next to them, to age and rank. The time of taking leave should also be determined by ladies, or by aged or important persons, and those who are of consequence. It would be impolite to wish to retire before they give the signal.

To carry children or dogs with you on a visit of ceremony is altogether vulgar and provincial. Even in half-ceremonious visits, leave your dog in the ante-room, as well as the nurse who holds the infant, for this circumstance alone excuses such a train. As to animals, it is a thousand times better not to have them at all.

Provincials are justly reproached for lavishing salutations and time-worn formulas on people when meeting and in taking leave of them. This custom, which may make people confused or overly familiar, is extremely ridiculous. Is it not difficult to keep your countenance when you see a visitor salute every article of furniture, turn about twenty times as you conduct him, and pour forth at every pause a volley of greetings or fare-wells? My readers will beware of this singular politeness; they will salute the first time at the moment they take leave, and again when the person who conducts them back has stopped at the door.

I said before that when you do not find a person at home, or when you are afraid of disturbing him, to leave a card. But that is not what is particularly called visits by card. In the latter, it is not your object to see the person, since you do not ask for him, and confine yourself to giving your card to the porter or a servant. This custom, which has been introduced necessarily amongst persons of very general acquaintance, and especially at times when every one ought to be visited, as on new year's day, is not considered ridiculous; but it becomes so by the great extension which has been given to it for some time. This consists of making a visit without leaving your drawing-room; that is to say, merely by sending your card by a servant, or even by means of an agency established for this purpose. That practice of visits by cards seems to well-bred persons the most insolent and offensive thing imaginable. Do not therefore permit it, except when it is a matter of returning visits made in this way; and do not use such retaliations, except to prevent these ill-advised visitors from thinking that you put yourself out to oblige them.

You should not merely call upon ministers, heads of the public administration, and very distinguished persons; you must write to them beforehand to request a meeting, and specify the object of your visit. (See also Chapter XXVII.) You must call upon them at the appointed hour; you must refrain from inquiring after their health, and strictly observe the obligations of propriety. These visits, which are the acme of ceremony, ought necessarily to be very short. In Chapter XXXII, you will see what titles are given to these important personages. It is well to be furnished with a letter of admission, so that if necessary you may show it to the guard.

In works devoted to instruction in the rules of politeness, authors think only of fortune and affluence. (See Div. 4.) They entirely forget people of a more modest condition, and when they find themselves in connexion with them, they cry out against their impoliteness. It is an injustice, and in my opinion poor judgement. An injustice, because true politeness pertains less to rank, then to sound morals and a good heart; a poor judgement, for to refuse to initiate people into what renders social relations easy and agreeable is to prepare affronts and annoyances for yourself, and retard the practice of the forms of civilization as much as you can.

Therefore, despising this foolish disdain, I applaud the forethought of persons not in affluence, who having neither porter nor servant, place by their door a slate furnished with a pencil, that in their absence visitors may write their names; for these visitors are seldom such as carry cards. I applaud the benevolent care of persons whose staircase is not lighted, or whose apartment is in the upper stories, and who leave with the porter a candle which every one who arrives takes in order to ascend, and returns it again on descending. If any of my wealthy readers should be tempted to smile at my description of these precautions of the more humble citizens, I would remind them that they are entirely strangers to that spirit of politeness, of which these precautions are a striking example.

The Manner of receiving Visitors.

It is no less important to receive people well than to present yourself well to them. To receive visitors with ease and elegance, and so that every thing in you and about you breathes propriety and pleasure; to endeavour that people may always be satisfied when they leave you, and be desirous to come again: such are the obligations of the gentleman, and especially the lady of a house.

Every thing in the room ought, as far as possible, to offer English comfort and French grace. Perfect order, exquisite neatness, and an elegance which dispenses with splendour, ought to mark the entrance to the house, the furniture, and the attire of the lady.

If your family is in easy circumstances, it is indispensable to have a drawing-room, for it is troublesome and in bad *ton* to always receive visits in a bed-chamber. (See Div. 5.) That may indeed do for a mere call; but it becomes almost ridiculous when, after dinner, it is necessary to pass into this room to drink coffee, when you are receiving a small company, &c. This custom is no longer followed, except in the provinces, and amongst persons who do not pride themselves on their good *ton*.

To receive company in a dining-room is not allowed except amongst persons who cannot bear the expense of furnishing a room or drawing-room. Simplicity, admitted into a room of this kind, suited to the smallness of their means, I cannot but approve, while nonetheless regretting the inconveniences to which such a residence subjects them. But I have, in this respect, an express warning for people who resign themselves to it unnecessarily. It is altogether opposed to the received customs of good society to receive company in a place which you cannot adorn, where you cannot place arm-chairs, a chimney-piece, a looking-glass, a clock, and all things useful to persons who come to see you; where you are exposed to receiving twenty visits during dinner; of being disturbed as many times while the table is being set, since it is impossible to spread the cloth while strangers remain; finally, of having them witness your domestic cares while removing the remains of a repast, the table-cloth, dishes, &c.

Young mothers of families who wish to have their children with them (dangerous guests in a drawing-room, as every one knows) think that they may remain in the dining-room and have strangers conducted into an adjacent room. That this may not be improper, it is necessary to observe three things. First, strangers should be admitted into this room before seeing the lady of the house, because they would not fail to create difficulties, by saying that they did not wish to disturb her. Second, the room should be constantly warmed in winter. Third, in summer it should be furnished precisely like an occupied room, for nothing is more vulgar than to conduct people into a room which seems to be for let.

Unless from absolute inability, you ought to light your staircase. If the practices of good domestic economy, regulated by the needs of civilization, were more wide-spread, an unlighted staircase would not often be found.

When you see any one enter, whether announced or not, rise immediately, advance towards him, and request him to sit down; but avoid the old form of, "Take the trouble to be seated." If it is a young man, offer him an arm-chair, or a stuffed one; if an aged man, insist upon his accepting the arm-chair; if a lady, beg her to be seated upon the settee. If the gentleman of the house receives the visitors, he provides a chair and seats himself at a little distance from it. If on the contrary it is the lady of the house, and if she is intimate with the lady who visits her, she places herself near her. If several ladies come at a time, give this last place to the one most distinguished by rank. In winter, the most honourable places are those at the corner of the fire-place; the closer the seat is to the front of the fire, the more it is considered inferior. When the visitor is a respectable married lady, and one whom you wish to honour, take her by the hand and conduct her to the corner of the fire-place. If this place is occupied by a young lady, she ought to rise and offer her seat to an aged lady who arrives, taking for herself a chair in the middle of the circle.

A lady of a house ought to be solicitous that visitors experience no discomfort. Consequently, take care to present screens to the ladies seated in front of the fire; move tabourets under their feet, or what is better, cushions; but never foot-stoves. If you are alone with an intimate acquaintance, invite her to share yours; but never extend this politeness to a gentleman. If a door or window happens to be open in the room in summer-time, you should ask visitors if it incommodes them.

If you receive a half-ceremonious visit while doing needle-work, leave off immediately, and do not resume it except at the request of the visitor. If you are on quite intimate terms, you may yourself request permission to continue. If a person visits in an entirely ceremonious way, it would be very impolite to work even an instant. Even with friends, you should hardly be occupied with your work, but should seem to forget it on their account.

People no longer practice that frank and kindly hospitality of the provinces, by virtue of which, in the middle of winter, they urged visitors to refresh themselves with some solid eatables. Nowadays such a proposal would excite a smile. Do not make any such offer, except in the following three situations. First, during very hot weather, invite your guest to take a glass of syrup or ice-water. Second, if any one is reading, have him brought sugar-water on a little piece of furniture designed for the purpose. Third, offer orange-flower water to a lady who happens to be suddenly indisposed. Otherwise, if any one wishes to refresh himself, he requests the lady of the house to allow him to ring the bell. After assent is given, he asks whatever he desires of the servant who comes.

As a new visitor enters, the gentleman or lady of the house rises, and any visitors who are already there are obliged to do the same. Some of them may then withdraw. In that case, if the gentleman and the lady of the house have with them any members of their family, after having conducted those who are going as far as the door, they request one of their relations to take their place. Otherwise, it is necessary to choose between the visitors who remain and those who retire. If the latter are superior in rank, age, or consequence, you must give them the preference, and *vice versa*. But however respectable the person who departs, you may dispense with conducting him farther than the door of the room.

The manner in which you should usually re-conduct visitors is regulated in an invariable mode. If it is a lady who is to be accompanied, the gentleman of the house takes her hand, passes it under his arm, and thus leads her as far as the bottom of the staircase, unless the steps are so narrow that two cannot go abreast. It is no longer the custom to give your hand to ladies, but to offer them your arm. This new custom does not at all change the ancient rule of propriety which requires that in descending a staircase, you should give the side next the wall to the lady whom you accompany. You commonly present your right arm to her, provided that necessity does not oblige you, in order to avoid placing her next the banister, to offer your left. If she is to return in a carriage, you should politely hand her into it.

In the provinces, they conduct all or almost all visitors as far as the street-door, unless they are gentlemen and have visited a lady. She ought then to accompany them, as is commonly done at Paris, as far as the door of the room, or the head of the stairs. Parisians add an agreeable civility to this custom; they hold the door open, and standing upon the threshold or edge of the staircase, follow the visitor with their eyes until he turns round to say the last good-bye, or to request the host to return.

——*The Gentleman and Lady's Book of Politeness,*
Manuel complet de la bonne compagnie.

Diversion 1.

New Acquaintance. Mrs. L.—How is a lady who settles at a distance from her own family connexions to select her acquaintance?

Mrs. B.—There are not many women who have the power to select their acquaintance after marriage. Most women must enter, without much discrimination, into the circle in which marriage places them. This is particularly the case with the wives of professional men, whose interest it is not to be forgotten by those from whom they expect employment, nor to remain unknown to the public.

——*Domestic Duties.*

Diversion 2.

Morning Visits. Mrs. L.—I wish to know the forms to be observed in morning visiting; in what manner and at what time, I am to return the attentions of those whose cards are spread upon my table. Some of them, I perceive, have been left by persons whom I very highly esteem; others by individuals with whom I am unacquainted; and some even by those with whom I have no desire to be intimate.

Mrs. B.—A newly-married woman, on arriving at her future home, will have to send her cards in return for those which are left at her house, after her marriage. She may afterwards expect the visits of her acquaintance; for which it is not absolutely necessary to remain at home, though politeness requires that they be returned as soon as possible. But having performed this, any further intercourse may be avoided (where it is deemed necessary) by a polite refusal of invitations. Where cards are to be left, the number must be determined according to the various members of which the family called upon is composed. For instance, where there are the mother, aunt, and daughters (the latter having been introduced to society), three cards should be left.

Morning visits should not be long. In this species of intercourse, the manners should be easy and cheerful, and the subjects of conversation such as may be easily terminated. The time proper for such visits is too short to admit of serious discussions and arguments. The conduct of others often, at these times, becomes the subject of remark; but it is dangerous and improper to express opinions of persons and characters upon a recent acquaintance. A young married woman would do wisely, to sound the opinions and to examine for herself the characters of a new circle of acquaintance, before exposing her own sentiments.

I do not mean that she should be afraid of broaching them, but rather that she may avoid the possibility of unknowingly giving pain and offence. When she is better acquainted with the circle of which she has become a member, she will see more clearly around her; and then, as she thinks fit, she may diminish her caution. Friendships are acquired and secured by qualities of intrinsic value; but amongst mere acquaintance, it is by pleasing manners chiefly that we must expect to obtain a favourable reception. The deportment of a bride, in particular, is so far important to herself, that it may decide in a degree her future estimation in society.

Mrs. L.—I have often thought that morning visits are very annoying, both to receive and to pay. They fritter away so much time, without affording any adequate return; unless indeed, any thing is gained by hearing the little nothings of the day enlarged upon, and perhaps of acquiring myself the art of discussing them as if they were matters of deep importance.

Mrs. B.—And yet, when it is desirable to keep together a large circle of acquaintance, morning visits cannot very well be dispensed with. You must be aware that as time and circumstances seldom permit the frequent interchange of other visits, our acquaintance would become estranged from us, if our intercourse with them were not occasionally renewed by receiving and paying morning visits. A good economist of time will of course keep morning visits strictly for this purpose; and not considering them as intended merely for amusement, will not make them more frequently than is necessary. By the occasional appropriation of a few hours, many debts of this kind may be paid off at once, and thus a season for other pursuits will be provided. The economy of time, so essential to the head of a family, will also prompt certain limitations as to the times of receiving morning visits. To have every morning liable to such interruptions, must be a great impediment in the way of more important avocations, and must occasion the useless dissipation of many an hour. Experience has found this out, or the custom of denial would not have become so prevalent.

Mrs. L.—What is your opinion of denials?

Mrs. B.—This custom cannot be better enforced than towards the idlers of both sexes. If they choose to fritter away their time, they have no right to condemn others to do so too, who may have better notions of the value of existence, and of such pursuits as leave them no time to kill. The gay and fashionable idlers of the other sex, in particular, should without mercy be doomed to the restrictions of formal visiting alone. This is the more desirable when the husband of a young lady is generally absent from home in a morning, because it has lately become fashionable to pay more attention, and to show more undisguised admiration, to young married women (provided they are agreeable) than to the single. The greater intercourse for the last few years with foreigners, and the imitation of their manners, which allow of gallantry to married women alone, may be one cause of this change in English manners. Or it may partly arise from the forwardness of young ladies to be married, and the too evident desire of many mothers to establish their daughters early in life; which by disgusting those they desire to charm and allure, destroy their hopes and defeat their purpose. But to be the object of such gallantry can seldom be either agreeable or flattering to a woman of sense: the superiority of such, indeed, must at once secure her from any attentions inconsistent with the esteem which that superiority claims.

——*Domestic Duties.*

Diversion 3.

Lit in the original French. If unmodified, as in the original text, *lit* means "bed," but that contradicts the advice given later against receiving visits in a bed-chamber.

——Frances Grimble.

Diversion 4.

Visiting amongst Servants. Mrs. L.—Some indulgences should be, I suppose, occasionally allowed to servants.

Mrs. B.—Visiting their relations and friends now and then, but not too frequently, and only when it suits the convenience of the family, can scarcely be denied them. But I think it unfortunate that Sunday should be the most convenient day on which this indulgence is generally granted them. It makes *that* a day of dissipation, which ought at least to be one of rest.

Mrs. L.—What inconveniences are likely to arise from permitting servants to receive the visits of their friends?

Mrs. B.—There are many; and these quite sufficient to induce the lady of a family only to allow it in a very limited degree. To forbid it altogether is to tempt your servants to deceive you. Therefore, I advise you to prohibit any visit beyond a call from their friends, unless they request your permission, upon the occasion of near relations coming to see them from a distance, to entertain them for a longer period.

——*Domestic Duties.*

Diversion 5.

Arrangement of the Drawing-room. Mrs. L.—I think I have perceived some care shown in the arrangement of the drawing-room, when visitors were expected. Is this necessary?

Mrs. B.—Morning visitors are generally received in the drawing-room. To preserve this room neat, and to exhibit good taste in its decorations and the arrangements of its furniture, are of some importance to the young mistress of a house. From these, strangers are apt to form an opinion of the character of its proprietor. The drawing-room is that part of a private house in which decorations and embellishments are most in place.

Every thing, therefore, in the drawing-room should be light and elegant. Mirrors are here in character, and bouquets and flowering plants. On the tables may be displayed some of the labours of the fine arts, such as small specimens of sculpture and engravings. Oil-paintings of a large and more important character are seldom seen upon the walls of a drawing-room, though those of a more light and airy description may there find a place. But in general, the appearance of these in a drawing-room, of which the decorations are of a nature to throw a great variety of reflected lights upon a painting, argues a defect of knowledge of the art in the proprietor. It is agreeable to see the drawing-room tables exhibit a small and choice collection of engravings, or of water-colours; but it is better, I think, to be without them, unless they are specimens of the first character.

It is here that the works of the poet, the dramatist, the novelist, and the traveller may find an occasional resting-place; and while they display, in a degree, the taste and pursuits of the lady of the house, they may tend to give an interest, and afford topics for the transitory conversation of a morning visit. Memoirs, biography, reviews, and journals may be added to the list of books which are not unappropriate in the drawing-room. Nor do I mean to exclude those of a serious and moral nature, though their more suitable place is either in the library or the dressing-room; where in seasons of privacy and abstraction, they are at hand to supply subjects for reflection and mental improvement.

I am convinced it is needless to caution you, my young friend, not to permit any volumes to remain on your table which are at variance with the natural modesty and correctness of our sex, and that delicacy of mind, which I believe has hitherto been considered the great charm of English-women. The works of Beaumont and Fletcher, Rousseau's *Confessions*, Fielding's novels, and some others, however they may be admired by the few, are becoming obsolete, and are therefore not very likely now to make their appearance on the tables of the young and fashionable. But there are many productions from modern pens, the perusal of which I think will afford you little gratification, and the possession of which would do little credit to your taste. Of this kind is *Don Juan,* and some of the other poems of Lord Byron.

In the arrangement of the drawing-room for receiving morning visitors, the chairs should be placed so as to facilitate the colloquial intercourse of the strangers, without the necessity of a servant entering the room to place them; and this arrangement, while it is devoid of formality, should be done with some attention to good order. Ease, not carelessness, should predominate.

Plants and flowers are pleasing ornaments in a drawing-room, and give an exercise for taste in their choice and arrangement. They should harmonize in colour with one another, and with the furniture of the room. If it is white, pale yellow, pink, and white flowers, with abundance of green leaves, should be preferred. If yellow, the most accordant colours will be purple, violet, and crimson; and if blue, white, blue, pink, orange, and red. And let me also observe, that though it may not be necessary for a lady to be a botanist or a naturalist, yet it is awkward if she is ignorant of the names and characters of the flowers which adorn her drawing-room. To learn their names, something of their natural history, and (if they are exotics) of their native soil, is soon done. Such slight knowledge often promotes conversation between those who, from slight acquaintance, have with each other few subjects in common, and between whom conversation consequently flags, and becomes heavy.

It is almost unnecessary to add, that the occupations of drawing, music, and reading should be suspended on the entrance of morning visitors. But if a lady is engaged with light needle-work—and none other is appropriate in the drawing-room—it promotes ease, and it is not inconsistent with good-breeding to continue it during conversation; particularly if the visit is protracted or the visitors are gentlemen.

It was formerly the custom to see visitors to the door on taking leave; but this is now discontinued. The lady of the house merely rises from her seat, shakes hands or courtesies, according as her intimacy is with the parties, and then ringing the bell to summon a servant to attend them, leaves them to find their way out of the house.

———*Domestic Duties.*

Chapter XXIX.
Promenades, Parties,
and Amusements.

Propriety ought, as you have seen, to direct and embellish all the circumstances of life. But it is, if possible, still more necessary in relation to pleasures, which would have no attraction without it.

Promenades.

A young man who walks with an aged person, undoubtedly knows that his companion has not the same strength and agility as himself; he ought therefore to regulate his pace by that of the aged person. The same precaution should be used when you accompany a distinguished person to whom you owe respect.

Propriety demands that a gentleman offer his arm to a lady who walks with him; and gallantry requires him to ask permission to carry any thing which she may have in her hand, such as a bag, a book, or a parasol (if the sun does not shine); and if she refuses, he should insist upon it. If there are more ladies than gentlemen, you should offer your arm to the oldest, and to a married lady rather than an unmarried one. If you are accompanied by two ladies, you cannot dispense with offering an arm to each of them. Place those whom you accompany upon that side which seems to them most convenient, and beware of opposing their tastes or desires.

When occasion presents itself, offer seats to your companions to rest themselves, and do not urge them to rise until they manifest a desire to continue their walk. If they accept your invitation to sit down, and it happens that there are not enough seats, then the ladies should sit, and the gentlemen remain standing. In a large public garden, chairs are seldom wanting. But if it is necessary to go for some to the place where they are kept, that is the business of the gentlemen, who should take care not to place them before persons already seated, for this would be an incivility. When payment for the seats is called for, one gentleman of the company pays for the whole. It would be foolish to offer to reimburse him.

There is also a rule of propriety to be observed with regard to those whom you meet in walking. You ought to offend neither their eyes nor their ears. Take care not to attract their attention by immoderate laughter, nor allow yourself liberties which you cannot take in a private garden. To sing and skip about in walking, would expose you to the jeers of the crowd, and other unpleasant things for which you could blame only your own folly. If you are in a public promenade, converse upon unimportant subjects which can offend no one, in order that your remarks may not be misinterpreted by persons who chance to hear them. Beware on the other hand, of listening to the conversations of those who are not of your party.

If you give your arm to a lady in the street, she ought to be next the wall; and if by chance you are obliged to cross over, you should then change the arm. This attention is likewise due to all who are entitled to your respect. Two gentlemen do not take one another's arms in the street, unless they are young persons and intimate friends.

Never go in advance of the lady whom you accompany. If she stops, do so likewise, and remain with her in looking at whatever attracts her attention. If a mendicant comes to ask for alms, immediately draw out your purse to satisfy his wants, so that the lady with whom you are walking will not be importuned by him.

If you walk in a private garden, and the company is numerous, you may separate, and form distinct groups. If the gentleman of the house or any important person invites you to walk up and down the alleys, take care to give him the right, it being the most honourable side. At the end of each alley, when you must retrace your steps, turn inwards towards the other person, and not outwards, in order to prevent turning your back to him. If you happen to be with two persons who are your superiors, do not place yourself in the middle, for that is the place of honour; the right is the second, and the left the third place.

Be careful also of the choice of places if you take an airing in a coach; yield the first seats to ladies and distinguished persons. The one of most consequence gets in first, and places himself at the right of the back seat; the left of the same seat is occupied next; then the third person seats himself on the front seat, facing the one in the first place; and the fourth person takes the remaining seat, facing the one in the second place. If there is no servant, it is proper for the gentlemen to open the door, arrange the parcels, &c.

In a cabriolet, the right side is reserved for the one who drives, when there are only two persons. If there are three, the driver sits in the middle, even though he may be very inferior to his companions. I should add, it is not customary for a lady to go alone in a hired cabriolet, since she would then be in company with the driver only.

Dinner-parties.

Without intending to adopt the epigrammatic style, I shall say that dining is a great occasion, because the lady of the house and her guests must observe so many points of decorum. (See Div. 1.) When you mean to give a dinner, begin by selecting such guests as may enjoy themselves together, or at least tolerate one another. If it is to be composed of gentlemen, there should be no lady present, except the lady of the house. Give out verbal or written invitations two or three days beforehand. During the Carnival, it is necessary to do it at least five days in advance, on account of the numerous engagements.

When you receive a written invitation, you must answer immediately whether you accept or not, though silence may be considered equivalent to an acceptance. If you decline, give a plausible reason, and do it very politely. When the invitation is verbal you must avoid being urged, for nothing is more foolish and disobliging. Either accept or refuse in a frank and friendly manner, offering some reasonable motive for declining, to which you should not again refer. It is not allowable to be urged, except when you are requested to dine with some one whom you have seen only at the home of a third person, or when you are invited on a visit or other similar occasion. In the former case, if you accept, first leave your card to open the acquaintance. Having once accepted, you cannot break an engagement except for a most urgent reason.

An invitation ought to specify exactly the hour of meeting, and you should arrive precisely at that hour. The table should be ready, and the lady of the house in the drawing-room to receive the guests. When they are all assembled, a servant announces that the dinner is served. Do not rise eagerly, but wait until the gentleman of the house requests you to pass into the dining-room, whither he conducts you by going before. It is quite common for the lady of the house to act as guide, while he offers his hand to the lady of most distinction. The guests also give their arms to ladies, whom they conduct as far as the table, and to the places which they are to occupy. If you are not the principal guest, take care not to offer your hand to the handsomest or most distinguished lady; it is a great impoliteness. Having arrived at the table, each guest respectfully salutes the lady whom he conducts, and who in her turn bows also. Bend forwards a little to see the place-cards on the napkins, but expect that the housekeeper has indicated the place you must occupy according to the shades of rank, political opinion, education, and amiability.

It is one of the most important and difficult duties to arrange the guests properly, and to place them in such a manner that the conversation may always be general during the entertainment. You should as much as possible avoid putting two persons of the same profession next one another, as it would necessarily result in a private conversation, which would injure the general conversation, and consequently the gaiety of the occasion. The two most distinguished gentlemen are placed next the lady of the house; the two most distinguished ladies next the gentleman of the house; the right hand is especially the place of honour. If the number of gentlemen is nearly equal to that of the ladies, take care to intermingle them. Separate husbands from wives, and remove near relations as far from one another as possible, because being always together, they ought not to converse amongst themselves in a general party. The youngest guests, or those of inferior rank, are placed at the lower end of the table.

In order to be able to watch the course of the dinner, and to see that their guests want nothing, the gentleman and lady of the house usually sit at the centre of the table, opposite to each other. As soon as the guests are seated, the lady of the house serves in plates, from a pile at her left hand, the soup which she sends round, beginning with her neighbours to the right and left, and continuing in the order of their distinction. These first plates usually circulate twice, for every one endeavours to make his neighbour accept whatever is sent him.

The gentleman of the house carves the large pieces, or has them carved by some expert guest, in order afterwards to do the other honours himself. If you have no skill in carving meats, do not attempt it; nor should you ever discharge this duty except when your good offices are solicited by him. Neither may you refuse any thing sent to you from his hand.

A gentleman of a house ought never to pride himself upon what appears on his table, nor confuse himself with apologies for the bad cheer which he offers you. It is much better for him to observe silence in this respect, and leave it to his guests to praise the dinner. Neither is it good *ton* to urge guests to eat, nor to load their plate against their inclination.

I shall now give a few words of advice to guests; it may be puerile, but it is well to listen to and observe. It is ridiculous to make a display of your napkin; to attach it with pins upon your bosom, or to pass it through your button-hole; to eat soup with a fork; to ask for "meat" instead of "beef"; to ask for "poultry" instead of "chicken" or "turkey"; to turn up your cuffs before carving; to crush fresh eggs at the pointed end and leave the shell on your napkin, instead of cracking them with the edge of a knife; to take bread, even when it is within your reach, instead of calling upon the servant; to cut your bread with a knife, for it should be broken by hand; and to pour your coffee into the saucer to cool.

At a great house, each guest is accompanied by his own servant, who takes his place behind his chair. The guest should not address the servant during dinner, still less reprimand him. Before sitting down at the table, the guest should direct his servant to serve the other guests also, and to retire as soon as the table is served, because the servants of the house ought to eat apart in the kitchen.

During the first course, every one helps himself to whatever he prefers to drink. But in the second course, when the gentleman of the house passes round choice wine, it would be uncivil to refuse it. You are not obliged, however, to accept a second glass.

If a gentleman is seated by the side of a lady or an aged person, propriety requires him to save her all trouble of pouring out drink, of procuring any thing to eat, and of obtaining whatever she is in want of at the table. He should be eager to offer her what he thinks to be most to her taste.

When at the end of the second course the table-cloth is removed, the guests may assist in turning off that part of it which is before them, and contribute to the arrangement of the dessert-plates which happen to be near, but without attempting to alter the disposition of them. From the time that dessert appears on the table, the duties of the gentleman of the house diminish, as do also his rights.

It would be impolite to monopolize a conversation which ought to be general. If the company is large, you should converse with your neighbours, raising your voice only enough to make yourself heard.

The question whether it is proper or not to sing at table, depends now upon the *ton* of the gentleman of the house. People do not sing at the houses of people of fashion and the high classes of society, but they still sing at the tables of the middling classes. Here I shall repeat what has been said and proved a thousand times, how ridiculous it is to be urged when you know how to sing, or to insist upon hearing a person sing who has an invincible timidity.

At the end of the meal, custom allows ladies to dip their fingers into a glass of plain water, and to wipe them with their napkins. It allows them also to rinse their mouth, using their plate for this purpose; but in my opinion, custom sanctions it in error.

It is for the lady of the house to give the signal to leave the table. All the guests then rise, and giving their arms to the ladies, return to the drawing-room, where coffee and liqueurs are prepared. Coffee is never taken at the table, except at unceremonious dinners. In leaving the table, the gentleman of the house should go last. Do not leave the table before the end of the meal, unless from urgent necessity. If something disagreeable happens to a married lady, she requests some one to accompany her; if a young lady, she departs with her mother.

Propriety requires you to remain at least an hour in the drawing-room after dinner. If you can dispose of an entire evening, it is well to devote it to the person who has so courteously entertained you. After dinner you converse, have music, or what is more common, prepare the tables for cards. In the course of the evening, the lady of the house sends sugar-water or refreshing syrups round upon a waiter.

During the week which follows the dinner, each guest owes a visit to the host. You usually converse at this time of the dinner, the pleasure you have enjoyed, and the persons whom you met there. This visit has received the cant name of *visite de digestion*.

Other Parties and Amusements.

I shall have but few things to say upon the manner of conducting yourself at a party, as I would only repeat the advice already given on propriety in the carriage of the person (see Div. 2), in visits, and in conversation.

When a gentleman enters a drawing-room where there are more than ten persons, he should salute all generally by a very respectful inclination of his head, and present his respects first to the lady of the house, but converse at first only with her husband. The seated ladies answer the salutation by a similar one. Ladies do not rise, except in saluting one of their own sex. The gentlemen usually stand in groups.

However distinguished a person may be, conversation is not suffered to be disturbed by his coming. A new-comer listens for a few moments while observing the persons present, then mingles in the conversation without pretending at all to monopolize it. When conversation is not general, nor the subject sufficiently interesting to occupy the whole company, the circle is divided into several different groups. Every one converses with one or two neighbours on his right and left. If you wish to speak to any one, avoid leaning across the person who happens to be between. A gentleman ought not to lean upon the arm of a lady's chair; but he may, if standing, support himself with the back of it, in order to converse with the lady partly turned towards him.

It is extremely impolite to converse in a loud voice with any one upon private subjects, or to make use of allegories and particular allusions which are understood only by your interlocutor and yourself. It is equally out of place to converse in a foreign language, with any one who is able to speak it.

It is not proper to withdraw abruptly in the midst of a conversation, but to wait until the subject in which you are engaged is exhausted. Then salute only your interlocutor, and depart without taking leave of any one, not even the gentleman and lady of the house.

Card-parties.

The mind has need of recreation; it cannot be always occupied. Hence the custom of passing a few moments in those family and social parties, where you amuse yourself with games which have been invented to relax and divert the mind.

It is needless to observe that I do not mean to speak of those scandalous establishments in which the resources of families are frequently swallowed up, and where a man, led by an unhappy passion, may consume in one evening enough to furnish an annual support for fifty orphans. I design to speak only of those innocent games, in which people are interested in a moderate stake, and sometimes only ambitious of the glory of a triumph. (See Divs. 3 and 4.) To propose to play high would be to expose yourself to contempt. Those who compose the assembly would imagine that you had no other object in view but to enrich yourself at the expense of others, and that you are accustomed to frequenting those abominable houses of which I have just spoken.

When the lady of the house has prepared the tables for playing, she takes as many cards as each game requires players, and presents them to persons in the company, beginning with the one whom she wishes especially to honour. To accept a card is considered an engagement to play. The distribution of the players requires all her attention, as there are some persons not to be desired for partners. Besides bad players, there are persons who being little accustomed to playing, stop a long time to think; bite their lips; strike their feet together under the table; drum upon it with their fingers; pretend that a certain person being near them brings them bad luck; and request out of their turn to shuffle the cards, in order to change their luck, &c.

The lady of the house experiences, besides the embarrassment of arranging these poor players, sufficient trouble in keeping from the same table, those who have any antipathy to one another. Remember not to unite members of the same family, who necessarily find no pleasure in winning money from each other. You may, without impropriety, ask any one if he plays a certain game, even if he plays well; and you may ask those invited to play, whom they desire as partners. The most honourable set, namely that in which the lady of the house plays, may never be refused, except by one unacquainted with the game.

When you commence playing, salute by an inclination of your head, the persons with whom you play, while dealing the first card to them. The gentlemen should collect the cards at the end of each hand, shuffle, and present them to the lady who is to deal.

People have a bad opinion of a player who shows excessive joy when he wins, or betrays the least chagrin when he loses. You ought to remember that it is only for amusement that you play. If you are winning, do not quit the game when you perceive that your adversary wishes to finish it. If on the contrary you are losing, withdraw if it seems well to you, good-humouredly paying the amount agreed upon without being asked. The debts of play are inviolable, which is why they are called debts of honour. Conduct yourself without letting the least word of dissatisfaction escape, and be good-humoured even if you are unlucky. When you leave off playing, converse with your adversary, and do not seem to avoid him. But be careful never to speak to him of his good luck in playing, unless it is with a frank gaiety; otherwise you would seem to be inspired by anger.

Play fairly, and do not endeavour to see the hands of your adversaries in order to profit by it. Pay attention to your game, and do not converse with others; this inattention would necessarily render you insupportable to those who play with you. If any play is contested, do not discuss it warmly, but refer to disinterested persons, explaining the point in dispute to them calmly and politely. In playing, you must always preserve an even temper. Neither should you devote too much time to play, for the amusement would then become irksome, and be soon changed to a fatiguing occupation.

You should generally resist the desire to bet for one player and against another. The one whom you back and whose cause you espouse, and who perhaps does not risk much for himself, will be intimidated if he knows that you hazard a considerable sum on your faith in his luck. The player against whom you bet may, on his side, be humiliated by this species of challenge.

In houses where it is customary to pay for the cards, each player, on finishing the game, silently places his compensation under the candlestick.

Parlour Games with Forfeits.

Those games, called innocent, generally please young persons of both sexes, because they are lively, and require exercise of the memory and the mind. However, it is necessary in this, as in every thing else, to manifest attention, delicacy, and propriety. You ought not to endeavour to be noticed for your too great vivacity or freedom. Be satisfied with showing your talent at playing in your turn, and taking part in the common gaiety, without pretension or excessive zeal. Above all, avoid throwing out any vindictive remarks, bestowing misplaced compliments, and imposing mortifying forfeits, or ones which may wound the feelings of any person in the company.

The selection of different games belongs to the ladies. The person who receives the company should be careful to vary them; and when she perceives that any game loses its interest, she should propose another. There are almost always persons in a company who wish to take the lead, and give the *ton;* this is a caprice or a fault in politeness which should be avoided. You may modestly propose any game, and ask the opinion of others in regard to it; but never pretend to dictate, nor even urge having your own proposal accepted. If it does not please generally, be silent, and resign yourself with a good grace to the decision of the majority.

In these games, the forfeits which are imposed too often consist of embracing the ladies of the company. (See Div. 5.) As they cannot refuse, since you follow the rule of the game, take care to do it with such propriety, that modesty may not be offended. If you are ordered to impart confidences to a married or young lady in a low voice, make them very short, so as to arouse no suspicion that they are any thing but compliments.

A young man should never take a young lady by the waist, nor seize her riband or bouquet. He must not attach himself exclusively to any one person, but be amiable and cheerful with all.

Balls, Concerts, and Public Performances.

These amusements require a fortune and good *ton,* therefore the customs of society. Consequently, a forgetfulness of the precepts of propriety in respect to them, would be truly preposterous.

Balls. I was going to say, let us begin with private balls; but I recollect that this term is no longer fashionable. You do not say, "a ball at Mrs. Such-a-one's," but "an evening party" (soirée). When you wish to give a dance, send out invitations a week beforehand, that the ladies may have time to prepare articles for their toilet. (See Chapter XI and Div. 6.) The toilet of all the assembly should be made with great care. A gentleman who appeared in a riding-coat and boots would pass for a person of bad *ton*.

If it is to be a simple evening party, in which you may wear a summer promenade costume, the lady of the house gives verbal invitations and does not omit to apprise her friends of this circumstance, or they might appear in unsuitable gowns. If on the contrary, the soirée is to be in reality a ball, the invitations are written, or what is better printed, and expressed in the third person. At the bottom of the billet you put this sufficiently ridiculous announcement, "There will be a violinist."

You might as well add, "There will be a card-table," because this is an essential piece of furniture in the drawing-room near the ball-room. A cloak-room furnished with *porte-manteaux* to hang up the shawls and other garments of the ladies, is also almost indispensable. The servants who have been stationed there, aid the ladies in taking off their out-door garments.

You are not obliged to go exactly at the appointed hour; it is even fashionable to go an hour later. Married ladies are accompanied by their husbands, unmarried ones by their mother or a chaperon. These last ladies place themselves behind the dancers. The gentleman of the house then goes before one and another, procures seats for them, and mingles again amongst the gentlemen who are standing, and who form groups or walk about the middle of the room.

When you are sure of a place in the dance, go up to a lady, and ask her if she will "do you the honour" to dance with you. This formula is *de rigueur*. If she answers that she is engaged, invite her for the next dance. Take care not to address yourself afterwards to any ladies near her, for these not being able to refuse you, would feel hurt at being invited after another. Never wait until the orchestra gives the signal to seek a partner, for nothing is more impolite than to invite a lady hastily, and when the dancers are already in their places; it can be tolerated only when the set is incomplete.

A lady cannot refuse the invitation of a gentleman to dance, unless she has already accepted that of another, for she would be guilty of an incivility which might occasion trouble. She would, moreover, seem to show contempt for the gentleman she refused, and would expose herself to receive a slighting remark from him.

The gentleman of the house should see that all the ladies dance. He should take notice particularly of those who seem to be what are called wall-flowers, and see that they are invited to dance. But he must do this wholly unperceived, in order not to wound the self-esteem of the unfortunate ladies. The gentlemen pressed into service should be ready to accede to his wish, and even appear delighted to dance with a person thus recommended to their notice.

In a private ball or party, it is proper to show still more reserve, and not manifest more preference for one lady than another. Dance with all indiscriminately; you may, however, invite the same lady more than once.

Ladies who dance much, should be very careful not to boast before those who do not, of the great number of dances for which they are engaged in advance. They should also, without being perceived, recommend gentlemen of their acquaintance to these less fortunate ladies.

Persons who have no ear for music, that is to say a false one, ought to refrain from dancing. When not dancing, it would be uncivil to take the seat of some one who is. Never hazard taking part in a quadrille unless you know how to dance tolerably; for if you are a novice or but little skilled, you would bring disorder into the midst of pleasure. Once engaged to take part, if the figures are unfamiliar, be careful not to advance first. You may in this way govern your steps by those who go before you. Beware also of taking your place in a set of dancers far more skilful than yourself.

Dance with grace and modesty; do not affect to make a parade of your knowledge; refrain from great leaps and ridiculous capers which would attract the attention of all. When an unpractised dancer makes a mistake, you may apprise him of his error; but it would be very impolite to have the air of giving him a lesson. In giving your hand for the ladies' chain or any other figure, smile politely, inclining your head in the manner of a salutation.

The waltz being a rather voluptuous dance, unmarried ladies should refrain from it altogether, at both public and private balls. However, very young married ladies may waltz at private balls, if it is very seldom, and with persons of their acquaintance. It is indispensable for them to acquit themselves with much dignity and modesty.

Avoid talking too much; it would occasion remarks and have a bad appearance to whisper continually into the ear of your partner. In these assemblies, you should conduct yourself with dignity and propriety towards all present, even those unknown to you.

At the end of the dance, the gentleman reconducts the lady to her place, bows, and thanks her for the honour which she has conferred. She also courtesies in silence, smiling with a gracious air.

Married or young ladies cannot leave a ball-room or any other party alone. The former should be accompanied by one or two other married ladies, and the latter by their mother, or by a lady to represent her.

At public balls, a gentleman offers his partner refreshments, which she very seldom accepts, unless she is much acquainted with him. But at private parties, the hosts send round cordials and cakes, to which every one helps himself as he pleases. In the middle of the evening, there is a punch. Later there is a supper, at which the gentlemen nearly always stand behind the ladies, who are seated. In a soirée without great preparation, the punch and even the supper may be dispensed with, but refreshments are essential; not to offer them would be the greatest impoliteness.

In speaking of public balls, as opposed to private ones, I might have said society balls by subscription. In regard to the public balls of Paris and other large cities, I have nothing to advise my readers but to shun them. Masked balls are an amusement altogether to be condemned, except those of the Opera. Neither should you appear there except in a domino.

You should retire incognito, in order not to disturb the gentleman and lady of the house. Pay them a visit of thanks during the week, at which you speak much of the pleasure of the ball, and the good selection of the company.

Concerts. The received conventions for concerts differ little from those for any other assembly or for public shows; for concerts partake of the one or the other, according to whether they are public or private. In private concerts, the ladies occupy the front seats, and the gentlemen are generally in groups behind, or at the side of them. You should observe the most profound silence, and refrain from beating time, humming the airs, applauding, or making ridiculous great gestures of admiration. It often happens that a dancing soirée succeeds a concert; and billets of invitation distributed two or three days beforehand, should give notice of it to the persons invited.

When a lady is going to perform, it is good *ton* for a gentleman to stand behind her chair and turn over the leaves attentively, if he knows how to read music. (See the frontispiece to Part III.)

After an invitation to a concert, you should pay a visit of thanks.

The Theatre, Opera, Ballet, &c. It would be a mistake to imagine that there exist no rules of propriety to be observed in public places, where persons assemble together, and at theatrical performances. (See Fig. 1 and Div. 6.) There are some general attentions which you should show to persons whom you meet there. It would be impolite to jostle continually, and in an annoying manner, those near whom you are

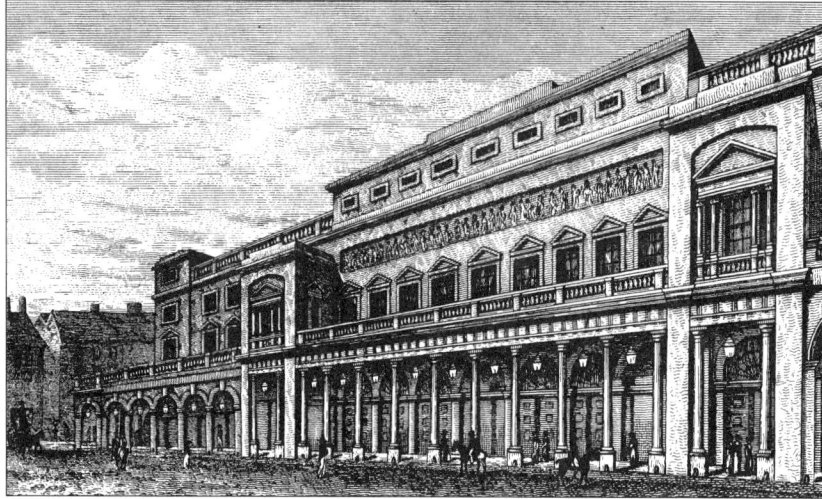

Figure 1. The Opera House, Haymarket.

placed, to step upon a lady's gown, or run against those who are walking at a moderate pace.

If you go with a party to the theatre, one of the gentlemen should carry the tickets to the door-keeper, to spare the ladies any trouble on entering. Gentlemen should address themselves to the attendants at the boxes, give them a gratuity, and place under their care their hats, and the ladies' cloaks and other articles of dress; you must not hang these over the boxes, whether it is a pocket-handkerchief, a tippet, a shawl, &c. (In certain theatres at Paris, however, this is allowed.)

When the box is open, the gentlemen should place the ladies in the front row, according to age, or the consideration they deserve. When ladies enter a box where a gentleman is seated in front of them, propriety requires that he offer his seat, even if they are strangers to him; he should insist upon their taking it, even after they have once refused. Young persons should occupy the seats behind, and avoid leaning over too much, and disturbing those who are seated in front of them. If the heat incommodes you, do not open the door of the box, without the consent of those who occupy it. Do not turn your back to the stage; for in that case you expose yourself to the derision of the pit, and to hear disagreeable remarks. Then the eyes of all would be fixed upon you; and your imprudence would excite a disturbance, which would be troublesome to the audience.

Be very reserved at the theatre, in order not to trouble those who are near you. Maintain a profound silence when the actors are on the stage, that you may not interrupt the attention of persons who take an interest in the performance. When a spectator of tender feelings is affected at seeing the misfortunes which the heroes of the play suffer, or has his sympathy touched by the virtues which are displayed, nothing can be more annoying to him than to have a morose critic constantly at his side, who mercilessly finds fault with the finest parts of the performance, sees nothing to his taste, and changes a resort consecrated to amusement and pleasure into a place of fatigue and ennui. It is, moreover, almost as ridiculous to place no bounds to your applause. It is improper to pass too positive and severe a judgement on the performance or the playing of the actors, whether to praise them, or to find fault with them. You may meet persons of a contrary opinion, and engage yourself in a controversy which it is prudent to avoid.

Between the acts, the gentlemen should ask the ladies if it is agreeable to them to walk in the corridors, or the foyer, or to take refreshments. They should also ask them if they wish for a journal of the theatres or an opera-glass; and if bouquets are sold at the door of the theatre, it is amiable and gallant to present them with one.

On leaving, when you arrive at the outer door of the theatre, if you have a carriage, you must take care to have all your party ready at the very moment it drives up. It is necessary to do the same thing, if you send a porter to get a hired coach.

The Duties of Hospitality.

Those of my readers who, from habit or instinct, fear the least appearance of constraint, and perhaps even in this work think they have found overly strict lessons on propriety, and say that civilization has augmented these beyond measure, will doubtless apply the same remark to this article. But what indeed are the slight duties of modern hospitality, compared to the rigorous ones of former times?

When a letter of announcement has informed you, as is customary, that a previous invitation on your part will bring guests to your house, you must commence by having a bed-chamber carefully arranged for them. They should have a good bed, armoires, a fire in the winter, and every thing which may contribute to their comfort: a washbasin, water, glass tumblers, a flask of Cologne water, a sugar bowl filled, or better a glass of sugar-water prepared, and several towels. In short, every thing which will contribute to neatness or elegance ought to be placed in the room.

These preparations finished, a little before the appointed hour of their arrival you must go and wait upon your guests; a servant should go with you to bring their baggage to the house. Embrace your friends, express your pleasure in receiving them, inquire kindly about the incidents of their journey, conduct them attentively, and show them in, begging them to make your house their home. This finishes the second class of the duties of hospitality.

The third class of duties, is assiduity to your guests; otherwise it would seem to them that their presence was troublesome. To you belongs the care of kindly offering to their view every thing in your house, in the city, or in the country, which is interesting; and of making parties in their honour, such as dinner-parties of their acquaintances, or persons you presume will please them. (See Div. 8.) These are duties of hospitality which you cannot omit.

To do the honours of your own house, it is necessary to have tact, address, knowledge of the world, great evenness of temper, and much affability. It is necessary to forget yourself, in order to be occupied with others, but without bustle or affectation; to encourage timid persons, and put them at their ease; and to enter into conversation, directing it with address rather than sustaining it yourself. The lady of a house ought to be obliging, even-tempered, and attentive in accommodating herself to the personal habits of every one. She should especially appear delighted that they are with her, and make themselves perfectly at home.

When visitors show any intention of leaving you, affectionately endeavour to retain them. Nonetheless, if their resolution seems immovable, send to engage their seats at the coach-office; offer them delicate refreshments, and accompany them thither. When taking leave of them, embrace them. Renew your invitations for another visit, and your regret at not having been able to succeed better at retaining them.

Guests, on their part, should show themselves contented and grateful for the reception which is given them. They should, on departing, give generous vails to the servants. (See Div. 9.) Immediately on arriving at home, they should write a letter of cordial thanks to their hosts.

The duties of hospitality are demanding, fatiguing, and expensive; but they are an indispensable obligation. To omit them is to be willing to pass for a person of no breeding or delicacy, because it places people in a most embarrassing and painful position.

——*The Gentleman and Lady's Book of Politeness,*
Manuel complet de la bonne compagnie.

Diversion 1.

Dinner-parties. Mrs. L.—How are dinner-parties to be managed?

Mrs. B.—Cards for a dinner-party should be issued a fortnight, three weeks, or even a month beforehand; and as dulness is less tolerable at one's own table than at any other, care should be taken in the selection of the party, which cannot be otherwise than heavy and dull, if incongruously assembled. A very large party is not likely to be so lively and sociable, as one of moderate size. A remark has somewhere been made, that a dinner-party should never be less in number than the Graces, nor more than the Muses; but certainly more than ten or twelve in number is not desirable. When a table is very long, the conversation, witticisms, and pleasantries at one end must be lost at the other. When from prudential motives, it is an object to have a restricted number of dinner-parties, they cannot of course be of so limited a size: it being settled by all strict economists, that the expense of dinner-parties is in proportion to the number given, and not to the size of them.

The extent of a party being determined, the next point to be considered is the selection of the guests. It is fatal to good-humour and enjoyment, to invite those to meet who are known to be disagreeable to each other. The lively and reserved should be mixed together, so as to form an agreeable whole, the one amusing, and the other being amused. An equal number of ladies and gentlemen, neither all old, nor yet all young, should be so mingled, that the conversation may be as varied as the party, uniting the sense and experience of age with the vivacity and originality of youth.

The conversation must, however, be regulated in a great degree by the host and hostess; who should be always prepared to rouse it when it becomes heavy, or to change it skilfully, when it is likely to turn upon subjects known to be unpleasant to any of their visitors. This kind of tact is the effect of habit and of associating with good company; though I see no reason why it may not soon be acquired by those who have been brought up in retirement, unless indeed an unfortunate degree of timidity exists, which must prove an obstacle in acquiring easy and fashionable manners, though it generally attends a pleasing and amiable mind.

Mrs. L.—When the party is formed, how is the table to be regulated?

Mrs. B.—The regulation of the table is a concern of some nicety; and in this every lady must first exercise her judgement as to its expense, and then show her taste in its arrangement, whatever her establishment may be. Whether she has to fix upon her bill of fare with a housekeeper, or with a cook of fewer qualifications, her superintendence will still be necessary.

She is the best judge of what dishes may be too expensive, too heavy, or too unsubstantial. To provide the wines is the province of the gentleman of the house. In general, preserves form a part of the dessert, whether West Indian or English; and when the latter are made at home, they are usually better in quality, and one-half cheaper than those purchased at the confectioner's.

Mrs. L.—Will you give me some idea of the best method of setting out and arranging a dinner-table for a party of sixteen, or twenty?

Mrs. B.—Fashion, the great arbiter of every thing connected with social life, varies the nature of the courses, and the quantity of viands which must be placed at one time upon the table; so that the dinner which might be considered as elegant at one time, would have the air of vulgarity at another. Particular directions, therefore, on this part of your inquiry can scarcely be given. By describing a dinner of three courses for the present time, some idea may be given, which may be modified to any future change of fashion.

In the middle of the table is generally an epergne, filled with either real or artificial flowers, or it may contain a salad ornamented. A dish of fish is placed at each end of the table, one boiled and the other fried or stewed; the requisite sauces being placed between these dishes and the epergne. Two tureens of soup, one white and the other brown, may be placed on a line with the fish, or on each side of the epergne. This is the usual plan of the first course.

The second may consist of roasted and stewed meat, at the top and bottom of the table—the choice of these must depend upon what happens to be in season. On each side of the epergne, where the soup was placed in the first course, may now be boiled chickens and a tongue, or a small ham, varnished and decorated. Between the top dishes and the epergne two small made dishes, or tureens with sauce, may fill up that space. The four corners must have covered dishes, which may contain either curry, patties, palates, fricassée of mutton-chops, stewed rump-steaks, stewed mushrooms, stewed cucumbers, or any similar viands. Other vegetables are on a side-table, to be handed round by the servants. On removing this course, the epergne may be taken away; and at some fashionable parties, a small table-cloth or napkin, which covers part of the table only, is also withdrawn.

A third course generally consists either of two dishes of game, or of some kind of poultry, at each end of the table; or there may be but one dish of game at the bottom of the table, and at the top a large dish of asparagus, sea-kale, or peas; in the centre may be a trifle, or some kind of confectionary. The intermediate spaces, in the length of the table, may be occupied by a dish of prawns at one end, neatly set up, and at the other by lobster-salad or a prepared crab. On one side of the centre dish may be a light pudding, on the other a tart or macaroni. At the corners put jellies, blanc-mange, tartlets, creams, or any other fancy confectionary.

The wines are placed upon the table at first, in six decanters, one of each being placed at each corner of the table, and one on each side of the epergne; while two bottles of some light French or Rhenish wine, undecanted and corked, fill up a space between the epergne and each end of the table. Small decanters of water, covered with an inverted tumbler, should be placed by every second guest; but malt liquors, cider, soda-water, ginger-beer, or similar beverages are handed by the attendants when called for. In the interval of each course, champagne, hock, burgundy, or barsac are handed round to each guest. Cheese, with a fresh salad, follows the third course, and a glass of port wine is generally offered by the servants to each of the gentlemen.

When according to the Continental fashion, the cloth is allowed to remain on the table, or according to the more general custom of this country, before it is removed, a silver, china, or glass dish containing rose-water is passed round the table, into which each guest dips the corner of his table napkin, for the purpose of refreshing his mouth and fingers, prior to the appearance of the dessert.

The dessert necessarily varies with the season. When that will admit of ripe fruits, the most important, such as grapes, pine-apples, peaches, or apricots, must of course occupy the ends of the table; while the inferior fruits, such as strawberries and raspberries, with preserves and dried fruits, fill the corners and sides of the table. A Savoy cake, on an elevated dish, is very proper for the centre; wafers, and any other cakes, may fill up the spaces in the length of the table. In the summer a china pail of ice is generally placed at each end of the table, and served out on glass plates before the wine is circulated. Sometimes Noyau, curaçoa, Danzig, Constantia, or some other liquor, is handed to the guests in small glasses, immediately after the ice has been served; the pails and glass plates are removed before the servants leave the room.

The decanted wines placed on the table during dinner are white wines; either Madeira, sherry, or Bucellas; those circulated after dinner are port, Madeira, and claret. Claret is generally contained in a decanter with a handle, and of a peculiar form.

Mrs. L.—But when dinner is announced, what form then takes place?

Mrs. B.—When dinner is announced, the gentleman of the house selects the lady most distinguished by rank, or respectable by age, or the one who is the greatest stranger in the party, to lead to the dining-room, where he places her by himself. If her husband is of the party, he takes the lady of the house to her place at table, and seats himself beside her. The rest of the party follow in couples, and the hostess arranges them according to their rank, or according to what she imagines may be their expectations; always, however, placing the greatest strangers amongst the gentlemen near herself. This arrangement should be effected in an easy, gentle manner, and with as little form as possible.

The trouble of carving generally devolves on the gentlemen next the lady. The gentlemen around the table are supposed to pay every attention to the ladies next them; and it is the duty of the servants to hand round the fish and soup, which are presumed to be generally eaten. It is not now the fashion for the hostess to pay those very particular attentions to her guests, which formerly was a formidable task. In this point, however, some discrimination must be shown; too much attention has the appearance of effort, and annoys; too little may offend. The lady of the house should never be so much engaged with these attentions as to render her unable to listen to conversation, or to keep it alive. Her aim should be to give it an easy transition from one topic to another, and to guard it from dwelling long on one which is not likely to excite general interest.

In fact, a gentlewoman is known in her own house. She may pass unnoticed elsewhere, because there may be nothing striking in her appearance; but at home, and at her own table, she is instantly discovered. It is with her manners as with her gown; she does not follow fashion blindly and immoderately, but rather moulds it into the superior form of good-breeding.

It is customary in some houses which are regarded as fashionable, for the host and hostess to sit together at the head of the table, leaving the lower end in charge of a son, or some male relation or friend. But this custom has never been sanctioned by general use, and is so objectionable, as regards the attention and comfort which every guest has a right to expect from his host, that it is not likely ever to prevail. It is true that bad health, advanced age, or accidental circumstances may place a gentleman as a guest at his own table; but when these do not exist, his appropriate situation is certainly at the lower end of the table.

The same objections do not apply to a lady resigning her situation to the gentleman who would otherwise be placed at her right hand; because if he is to carve, he can do so with more ease when situated at the head of the table, and the lady is left more free to distribute her attention and conversation to those who surround her. To a young woman in particular this is allowable; the graceful deportment of a lady at her own table, which is generally so pleasing to her husband, would be much diminished if she were obliged either to carve, or her attention were directed too much to supplying the plates of her visitors. However, ladies who have been married some years generally prefer to carve for themselves; and as habit has made them expert, they manage it without being too much engrossed by it.

Mrs. L.—Can a lady refuse to take wine with a gentleman when requested?

Mrs. B.—It is not the custom to refuse the request, nor is it considered polite; though I think it may be done, provided the manner in which it is done is so tempered by politeness as to avoid the unpleasantness of offending.

Mrs. L.—What is your opinion with regard to the discontinuance of the old custom of drinking healths?

Mrs. B.—I think the total omission of the old custom not altogether defensible; for though the routine of drinking healths by every individual is a formality which may well be dispensed with, yet I should prefer the ancient fashion to be preserved, as far as regards the friends at whose social board we are guests, and whose attentions seem to claim some acknowledgment and tribute of respect on our parts. There is to my mind an apparent heartlessness in the present fashion; and a little of that honest warmth which characterised the rude hospitality of our forefathers would not detract from the refinement of the present age, but would increase the pleasures of the social table.

Toasts, on the contrary, are properly exploded; for they restrained the liberty of the guest, and forced him to take more wine than he might desire; and though few were ever given in the presence of the ladies, yet those which passed after they had retired, kept the gentlemen from the drawing-room in the evening, which you may think a sufficient reason why the female part of society should discountenance the drinking of toasts.

Mrs. L.—Will you permit me to say that I think the ladies retire, in general, too soon from the dining-room. I have frequently perceived the lady of the house restless and uneasy until she could find an opportunity of carrying off the female part of her visitors; and as every gentleman to whom I have spoken on this subject has condemned this fashion, I wish to hear your opinion as to the time at which the withdrawing should take place.

Mrs. B.—The custom for the ladies to retire soon after dinner is the relic of a barbarous age, when the bottle circulated so freely, and toast upon toast succeeded each other so rapidly, that the gentlemen of a company soon became unfit to conduct themselves with the politeness essential in the presence of the female sex. But in the present age, when temperance is a striking feature in the character of a gentleman; and when delicacy of conduct towards the female sex has increased with the esteem in which they are now held, on account of their superior education and attainments, the early withdrawing of the ladies from the dining-room is to be deprecated. It prevents much conversation which might afford gratification and amusement, both to the ladies and the gentlemen. The truth of this remark is now almost universally acknowledged in polite circles; and it is not now customary for the ladies to retire very soon after dinner. A lapse in the conversation will occasionally indicate a seasonable time for the change to take place.

I may take this opportunity of remarking, that servants should be instructed to attend to the drawing-room fire, and to prepare the lights after dinner. Prints, periodical works, or other publications of a light kind ought to be dispersed about the room, and are sometimes useful to engage the attention when any thing like ennui is observable. Coffee should be brought up soon, and the gentlemen summoned.

——*Domestic Duties*.

Diversion 2.

The chapter on the carriage of the body in the *Manuel des dames* is very similar to the short chapter on the subject in the *Manuel complet de la bonne compagnie,* except that the former adds details peculiar to ladies. Therefore, I have included all the most pertinent information on the carriage in Chapter XIII.

——Frances Grimble.

Diversion 3.

The original American translation systematically omitted remarks indicating that its readers might be playing cards for money.

——Frances Grimble.

Diversion 4.

Card-parties and Conversaziones. Mrs. L.—How are card-parties conducted?

Mrs. B.—The invitations to these are similar to those issued for routs and balls, with the change of the word "quadrilles" to "cards." (See Fig. 2, below.) As many should be invited as will fill up a certain number of whist-tables, with the addition of a loo or round table. Tea and coffee are handed to the guests on their arrival, and wine, cakes, and ices are handed round to the players at intervals during the evening. Each whist-table should be furnished with at least two new packs of cards, differently coloured on the backs, besides counters for markers. The lady of the house generally fixes the value of the points which determine the game; and she should also be prepared to change the players at table as soon as the rubber is declared to be over. As all the company is not always engaged in play, the lady of the house, as well as her husband, should remain disengaged, to lead into conversation those who are strangers to one another, and to promote the general amusement of the guests.

Mrs. L.—Are conversaziones conducted in the same manner as routs?

Mrs. B.—Not exactly. Conversaziones are more select meetings in respect to both the number and the characters of the individuals who are invited. To routs the invitations are general and unlimited; to conversaziones they are limited, and the individuals are at least supposed to possess a taste for information, whether obtained from books or from conversation.

However, this description of evening amusement is not general, but is confined either to literary circles, or to those persons of rank and fortune who wish to patronize literature. When you wish to give a conversazione, the party should be selected with some care; and though persons of the same pursuits should be brought together, yet individuals of the most opposite characters and acquirements should also be invited, to give variety and interest to the conversation which is the object of the assembly. The tables should be spread with the newest publications, prints, and drawings. Shells, fossils, and other natural productions should also be introduced, to excite attention and promote remark.

Mrs. L.—According to your account, conversaziones and card-parties may be united?

Mrs. B.—Certainly; and these are perhaps the most rational description of evening entertainments in the metropolis. The introduction of cards takes off the air of pedantry which is supposed to pervade a pure conversazione, while the introduction of conversation at card-parties sets aside the character of gaming, which might be attached to a party met solely for the purposes of play. Many of our ablest men of science and in literature are fond of a hand at whist, and would willingly go to such a mixed party, though they would hesitate to attend a party purely conversational, or convened solely for card-playing.

——*Domestic Duties.*

Diversion 5.

Forfeits. The divers movements of parlour games, their variety, the graceful and playful ideas which they inspire, and the decent caresses which they permit, unite to make them true diversions. These caresses do not know how to alarm either modesty or prudence, because a kiss honestly received and given in front of numerous witnesses is often an act of propriety; however, it is well not to multiply it, and these forfeits are in such abundance that nothing will be easier.

To kiss the Four Corners of the Room. The player for whom this forfeit is commanded, who follows it to the letter, prepares for laughter at his expense: he must beseech four ladies who are willing to stand in the four corners of the room, then he kisses them in turn. Or taking one lady firmly by the hand, he conducts her to the corners of the room and kisses her in each corner.

To kiss the Candlestick. This is not a question of kissing a candlestick. The player begs a lady to hold a lighted candle for a few moments, then he kisses the lady thus metamorphosed into a candlestick.

To kiss the Bottom of the Candlestick. This is the same thing. The player holds a candlestick over the head of a lady, whom he kisses at the same time.

To kiss your Shadow. The player stands between the lamp, to which he turns his back, and the lady he wants to kiss.

To kiss the Earth. A clever player who is given this command takes good care not to prostrate himself on the floor and kiss the planks. He knows that God has drawn man to the earth, and consequently woman; therefore he will give a kiss to a lady.

To kiss the Image of God. The player who must endure this forfeit does not petition Christ, or an image of Our Father. If a gentleman he kisses a lady, if a lady she kisses a gentleman, like the image of the Creator.

To kiss the Person you prefer, without appearing to. This forfeit consists, for a gentleman, of kissing all the ladies in the company, and for a lady, receiving a kiss from all the gentlemen.

The Deceitful Kiss. The lady who has been sentenced to this forfeit approaches a young man, who advances eagerly to kiss her; but he finds himself driven away, and this favour is granted to his neighbour. When this manœuvre is known, the young man who advanced at first cannot be deceived, therefore he is not the only one she seeks to fool, but the neighbour who, believing he is the only one wanted, approaches . . . . The lady, who has a free choice, repulses him and gives a kiss to the player situated near him; sometimes she returns to the first whom she deceived initially, and the game is even more piquant.

To kiss the Back of the Door. The young man on whom this forfeit is imposed, does not kiss the back of the door any more than his precursors kissed the floor or the candlestick. He begs a lady to accompany him near to a door, and there he gives her a kiss.

To kiss the Top of the House. For a gentleman, this is the sweet obligation to kiss a lady on the forehead. For a lady, it is likewise to kiss a gentleman on the forehead.

To kiss the Hare. The gentleman for whom this forfeit is prescribed thinks himself very fortunate. He must take a length of thread long enough to sew with between his teeth, and he begs a lady to likewise take the other end. Both of them must chew their end of the thread, and their two mouths are going to meet . . . but the lady is well informed, and as soon as the thread comes closer, she breaks it with a penknife or scissors. It is always best to abstain from this forfeit.

——*Manuel complet des jeux de société.*

Diversion 6.

Balls. Mrs. L.—How long before a ball is given should the invitations be issued?

Mrs. B.—A month at least, or even six weeks; and the invitation (printed from a copper-plate on cards) is usually in the form of either *A* or *B* in Fig. 2.

As the company is generally numerous at balls, it is neither necessary, nor is it expected, to be so select as at smaller parties. On these occasions the rooms may be well filled, though too great a crowd should be avoided. The majority ought, of course, to be juvenile; and

Mrs. T—— and Family.

Mrs. S——

At Home.

Tuesday, the 27th June.

QUADRILLES.

A

Mrs. M——

Requests the honour of Mr. and Mrs. N's

Company at a Quadrille Party,

on the 15th of April.

R. S. V. P.

B

Figure 2. Forms of invitations for a ball.

the number of gentlemen should be equal to, or even exceed, that of the ladies.

I need scarcely remind you of the great advantage of being beforehand in all the necessary preparations for parties of every kind. Early in the day, the sophas, chairs, and tables should be removed, as well as every other piece of furniture which is likely either to be in the way or to be injured. Forms should be placed round the walls of the room, as occupying less space than chairs, and accommodating more persons with seats. A ball-room should be brilliantly lighted, and this is done in the best style by a chandelier suspended from the centre of the ceiling, which besides adds much to the elegant appearance of the room. Lustres placed on the mantel-piece, and branches on tripods in the corners of the room, are also extremely ornamental.

Mrs. L.—I hope you also recommend chalking the floor, which is not only very ornamental but very useful, as I know by experience, in preventing those awkward and disagreeable accidents which a slippery floor inevitably occasions amongst the votaries of Terpsichore.

Mrs. B.—A chalked floor is useful too in disguising, for the time, an old or ill-coloured floor, which would otherwise form a miserable contrast to the elegant chandeliers, and the well-dressed belles and beaux. When the season will allow it, do not forget to fill the fire-place with flowers and plants; which indeed form an appropriate and pleasing ornament on the landing-places, and in other parts of the house through which the guests may have to pass.

In consulting the beauty of the fair visitants, those flowers should be selected which reflect colours in harmony with the human complexion; as for example the rose, the early white azalea, the white and pink hyacinth, and other flowers of similar tints. There should not be an over-proportion of green; for as this colour reflects the blue and yellow rays, it is by no means favourable to the female complexion. Sill worse are yellow and orange-coloured groups, whether of natural or artificial flowers. In some degree, however, the flowers should be chosen to harmonize also with the colour of the paper, or the walls of the ball-room.

The music should always be good, as much of the pleasure of dancing depends upon it. Violins, with harp and flute accompaniments, form the most agreeable band for dancing.

The lady of the house, who is expected to appear in rather conspicuous full dress, should be in readiness to receive her guests in good time; allowing herself a few minutes' leisure to survey her rooms, to ascertain that every thing is in proper order, and nothing defective in any of her arrangements. The arrival of her guests will be between the hours of nine and twelve.

A retiring-room should be in readiness for ladies who may wish to disburden themselves of shawls and cloaks; and here a woman should be in attendance to receive them, and to perform any little office of neatness which a lady's gown may accidentally require. Tea and coffee may also be presented in this room, if any are deemed necessary; but of late the custom of introducing these refreshments at balls has been nearly abolished.

At least three male servants are necessary, and as many more as the sphere of life of the individual who gives the ball sanctions. One servant should attend at the door of the house. Receiving the names of the company as they arrive, he should transmit them to another, who should conduct the party into the ante-room. He in turn communicates their arrival to a third at the drawing-room door, who should announce them to the lady of the house. Her station should be as near the entrance of the room as possible, that her friends may not have to search for her to whom, of course, they wish first to pay their respects, and from whom they expect their welcome.

As soon as a sufficient number of dancers are arrived, the young people should be introduced to partners, that they may not, by any unreasonable delay of their expected amusement, lose their self-complacency, and cast the reflection of dulness on the party. When the lady of the house is a dancer, she generally commences the dance; but when this is not the case, her husband should lead out the greatest stranger, or person of highest rank present. While one dance is proceeding, the *maîtresse du bal,* if a French term is allowable, should be preparing another set of dancers to take the place of those upon the floor, as soon as they have finished. Nothing displays more want of management and method, than a dead pause after a dance; while the lady, all confusion at so disagreeable a circumstance, is begging those to take their places who perhaps have never been introduced to partners. There should be no monopoly of this delightful recreation, but all the dancers in the party should enjoy it in regular succession.

Refreshments, such as ices, lemonade, negus, and small rout-cakes, should be handed round between every two or three dances, unless a room is appropriated for such refreshments. Supper should be announced at half-past twelve or one o'clock, never later. Each gentleman should then be requested to take charge of a lady to the supper-room. Both with regard to the pleasure of her company, and her own comfort, the *maîtresse* would do well to discountenance the habit, which is sometimes sanctioned, of gentlemen remaining long in the supper-room after the ladies have retired.

Mrs. L.—Indeed, I entirely agree with you in this opinion. When the gentlemen remain in the supper-room, it frequently causes a formal party of silent and listless fair ones, who seem to consider this temporary suspension of their amusement as an evil of sufficient magnitude to rob their countenances of the smiles of cheerfulness and good-humour, which they had worn during the preceding part of the evening. As our gentle islanders lose half their charms when they lose their good-humour, it is charitable to them to prevent, if possible, this half-hour of discomfiture.

Of what, my dear madam, should a supper for such a party consist? Is it an expensive addition to the entertainment?

Mrs. B.—The variety of little delicacies of which suppers generally consist, makes them rather expensive. The table is usually crowded with dishes, which contain nothing of a more solid nature than chickens, tongue, collared eels, prawns, lobsters, trifles, jellies, blanc-mange, whips, fruit, ornamental confectionary, &c. French wines are frequently presented at suppers. As it would be scarcely possible to seat a very large party at once at a supper-table, it is advisable to keep one part of the company dancing in the ball-room, while another is at supper. Even in this case, the gentlemen need not be seated, nor sup until after the ladies have retired.

Very little apparent exertion is necessary in the lady of the house. Yet she should contrive to speak to most of her guests some time during the evening, and to the greatest strangers she should pay more marked attention.

Mrs. L.—What ceremonies are to be observed at routs?

Mrs. B.—The preparations for a rout, with the exception of lifting the carpet, chalking the floor, and providing music and a supper, are similar to those for a ball. The same announcements are requisite; the lady of the house is required to receive her guests in the same manner; and refreshments are provided in the waiting-room. But further, the assembled groups are left to amuse themselves, if amusement can be found in a crowd resembling that which fills the lobbies of a theatre on the first night of a new performance. To a person unacquainted with fashionable life, nothing can appear more extraordinary than the influence of fashion in these gregarious assemblies.

The secret is this: few expect any gratification from the rout itself. The whole pleasure consists of the anticipation of the following days' gossip, which the faintings, tearings of gowns, and elbowings which have occurred are likely to afford. To meet a fashionable friend next day in the Park, without having been at Lady A—'s, would be sufficient to exclude the absentee from any claim to *ton*, while to have been squeezed into a corner with the Marchioness of B—, or the Duchess of C—, is a most enviable event, and capable of affording conversation for at least ten days.

——*Domestic Duties.*

Diversion 7.

Amusements for Servants. I cannot do better than present you with the sensible remarks of Mrs. Taylor on the subject of amusements. "There are fairs, and other places of amusement, which require a word of caution. If a fair were only a few gay stalls, offering to your notice a little fruit and gingerbread, ribands, and gloves, with perhaps a show of wild beasts, and some music; and if the company were all decent people, who once a year assembled together to shake hands, and treat each other to a slice of plum-cake, or to purchase some useful article which could not be had in their own village or neighbourhood, it might all be very well.

But if ever you have been to a fair, you must have perceived that this is not all. What crowds of drunken men are there, who will hardly suffer a modest girl to pass unmolested! What profaneness and wicked conversation, and lewd songs are to be heard! But especially, if you have been tempted to see one of their plays, as they are called, if you have any sense of propriety, you will be deterred from going again. Indeed, you may judge of what is going forward within, by that which is seen without. What uncouth figures and shocking grimaces there are, twirling their tambou-rines, and winding their hurdy-gurdys! What bold and impudent women, who ought not even to be looked at but with a sigh of pity or a frown of disapprobation! And what figures of children, brought up to the same trade, tossed to and fro, and trundling over and over."

Do they look like reasonable beings, or can you suppose them to be wise and good, and sober people? They may produce great fun; but fun is a thing that does not always lead to the best consequences; and it is possible to be very happy and cheerful without it. I advise you therefore, if after all you are disposed to visit a fair, that you at least avoid such places as these, where there is much to corrupt, but nothing to instruct you; that you go with decent company; that you do not stay until a late hour, when drunk-enness and revelling are at their height; and that you are not too lavish in spending your money, by purchasing unnecessary things because they may seem cheap, or articles which you do not want, for they are bargains only to those who really want them. She who indulges in all the excesses of such a place, is not one whom we would expect to behave well when at home.

What has been said relates entirely to *country* fairs, for a discreet ser-vant would hardly wish to be seen at those which are in or near London.

——*The Duties of a Lady's Maid.*

Diversion 8.

Evenings at Home with Company. Mrs. L.—When there is com-pany at home, reading and working must give place to amusements of more general interest. Here, I suppose, you will tell me musical skill in the lady of the house may be agreeably employed in giving entertainment to her guests, or in inducing others to join their powers to hers. Music and dancing for the younger, and cards for the older visitors, are the only amusements which seem to unite in one common interest a whole party.

Mrs. B.—Certainly; and however much these amusements may be censured by the *few* as excluding conversation, they are undoubtedly suitable to the *many*, who without them would, in the midst of a party, be as it were shut up in themselves; some from notions of etiquette, and others from pride or timidity. But by throwing open the dancing-room, and preparing the card-tables, these symptoms of coldness and formality vanish. All are at once free, easy, and sociable, mingling one with another in the quadrille, or cheerfully associating themselves at the card-table. No lady who wishes to see her guests smiling and pleased, will discard these amusements from her evening parties.

——*Domestic Duties.*

Diversion 9.

Gifts to Servants from Visitors. Mrs. L.—Would you permit your servants to receive presents from friends visiting at your house?

Mrs. B.—It is not a pleasant idea that our friends should pay for the few attentions and services they may receive under our roof. I am happy to find it is a custom growing into disuse, and is actually prohibited in many houses, where the servants would instantly lose their places, if they were known to receive vails (as such gratuities are called). It never does any good to the servants themselves; indeed it has a tendency, by giving them the power, to increase their extravagant inclinations.

Vails are objectionable also, inasmuch as they regulate the comfort and convenience of the friends who visit you, by the extent of their purses, and their inclination to reward your servants. An individual who is not rich, or who refrains from bribing servants to do their duty, may be rendered so uncomfortable in his visits to you, as to decline future invitations. Thus the cupidity of your servants, and the existence of a bad custom, will deprive you of the society of a friend whom you highly esteem. It may be extremely difficult to check the practice at once; but the reform might be accomplished by a small addition to wages, given on the express condition that no vails will be taken.

——*Domestic Duties.*

Chapter XXX.
Propriety in the Happiest and Unhappiest Circumstances of Life.

The subjects of marriage and christening have peculiar claim to the precepts of propriety; for the first is the closet of the social relations, and both furnish occasions for the most brilliant entertainments. Nor can propriety remain a stranger to misfortune. That which takes possession of all our feelings, cannot forget to pity. It is in this light that it is moving, almost religious, since it even contributes to bind closer this most important and powerful tie of human nature.

Weddings.

A profound secret is usually made of the preliminaries of marriage, because if it were broken off, there might be unfortunate interpretations. (See Div. 1.) But as soon as the first promises are exchanged, it is necessary to make it known in confidence to intimate friends, and those to whom you are under these obligations. Later, give intelligence of it by letter to your connexions.

A young man who solicits a lady in marriage, should be extremely devoted and respectful. He should appear a stranger to all the details of business which the two families discuss. He converses with his intended particularly of their future establishment, her tastes, the selection of a residence, furniture, wedding-presents, &c. Avoiding all misplaced familiarity, he calls her "Miss" until returning from church on the wedding-day. He accompanies her in all assemblies, and shows himself a devoted suitor.

At Paris, when the banns have been published, it is customary for a flower-seller of the neighbourhood to come and congratulate the bride by presenting her with a bouquet. This attention requires a gratuity.

The marriage is announced into two ways. Three or four days beforehand, you invite your acquaintances to the religious ceremony, and specify precisely the time and church where it will be performed. Only witnesses and near relations are present at the civil ceremony.

Propriety requires that a person invited to the ceremony should come, or send an excuse if it is impossible to be present. If a person is invited to the repast or entertainment which follows the ceremony, you make express mention of it at the bottom of the letters of invitation. (These letters are usually duplicated, as the invitation should appear to be given by the parents of both the engaged parties.)

Communicate simply the fact of the marriage to those who have been invited neither to the ceremony, nor to the entertainment. These letters of announcement are sent a few days afterwards. Such a letter requires only a visit or two in return; the first of which is made by card.

Presents are usually given before the wedding. Those which the groom makes to the bride are called wedding-presents and consist of different articles of the toilet, a parure of diamonds, &c., which are sent in a basket. Some persons content themselves with sending a purse containing a sum of money in gold, for the purchase of these things; the bride then spends it as she thinks proper. The groom also makes a present to each of the brothers and sisters of his intended.

The bride, on her part, gives some present to her bridesmaid. She often presents her with a gown or some ornament, and receives in her turn a belt, gloves, and a bouquet of orange-flowers. Since I have spoken of wedding-presents, I shall add that at Paris the bride receives a gift from her sisters and female cousins; but in the provinces, on the contrary, she must offer them some token.

Let us now pass on to the ceremony. After the civil ceremony, which may be some days previous, the bride and groom, followed by their relations, commonly go to the church in the carriages which conducted them to the civil ceremony; for at Paris, whatever their circumstances, wedding parties never go on foot. The bride goes in one carriage with her relations and the bridesmaid; the groom in another carriage with his parents, or his nearest relations.

The acquaintances of the bride and groom repair to the church at the appointed hour. The friends of the groom place themselves on the right, those of the bride on the left, on chairs prepared beforehand, which have been paid for. The wedding procession then advances in the following order. The bride gives her hand to her father, or to one who represents him. Then comes the bridegroom with his mother, or the lady who represents her, and afterwards the members of the two families in couples. As the couple and their relations approach the altar, every one bows to them in silence. The relations place themselves in the same order as the acquaintances, and before the latter, in the front rows, which have been reserved for them.

The couple to be married are placed in the middle. Though it is polite to always present your right hand to the lady whom you conduct, or to give her the right when you are next her, yet the bridegroom takes the right of the bride. In this act, which is at once religious and civil, man ought to preserve the prerogative which both human and divine law have conferred upon him. Besides, as the bridegroom is to place the wedding-ring on the bride's right finger, it is more convenient for him to be on her right side than her left. When the clergyman puts the ritual questions to them, each should consult their relations by a respectful sign of the head, before answering the decisive "yes."

The canopy is held over the couple's heads by two children whose parents they wish to honour. The bridesmaid is usually a sister or very intimate friend of the bride. Her business is to preside at the toilet of the bride, designate the places at the religious ceremony, and take up the collection for the church. Afterwards, at the ball, she supplies the place of the bride, who may take no active part. The groomsman, for there should be one or even several, looks well to the list of those invited to the ceremony, to see what persons are absent, as it is the custom of married persons not to make the wedding visit to any one who has been guilty of this impoliteness.

After the benediction, the married couple salutes the assembly again, and then receives the congratulations of every one. In some families of the middling classes, the bride is then embraced by all at the marriage ceremony. In the upper classes, she embraces only her father, mother, and new relations, and only in the vestry. The groom must give numerous gratuities to the attendants at the church, the poor, &c.

The groom gives his hand to the bride when returning from the church. At dinner he should be placed between his mother and his mother-in-law, while the bride is seated between her father and father-in-law. However, if there is a supper, the married couple sit next each other. The bride opens the ball with the most distinguished person in the assembly. She retires mysteriously, accompanied by her mother, and one or several near relations whom they wish to honour.

The newly-married couple make wedding visits in the course of a fortnight, in a carriage and wearing full dress. They should make these visits alone. They only leave their cards for those with whom they do not wish to be intimate.

Such are the received usages in the capital. In the provinces, many of the old-fashioned and common customs are still preserved, such as an engagement gift of a laced shirt-bosom from the bride to the groom, co-loured ribands or garters for the bride, two colours of ribands with which they decorate some of the young persons at the wedding, &c.

Christenings.

Several months beforehand, the godfather and godmother of the child that is to be christened must be invited. If the ties of blood have given you a right to this onerous duty, you cannot dispense with it. If not, you may seek a specious excuse.

When you have consented to hold the infant at the font, you should do the thing properly, and according to your own condition and that of the child's parents. A present should be given to the mother, which usually consists of confectionary. The godmother receives a pair of white gloves and sugared almonds; and if she is a young person, she also receives a bouquet of white flowers. If the godfather wishes to show her any atten-tion, he may add to the presents an elegant and graceful article, such as a fan; in which case it is good *ton* for the godmother to send in return some rich and tasteful present. She has also the honour of giving the child the christening cap, and frequently the christening robe. To her also belongs the duty of putting the first dress on the child.

The attendant and the nurse have also a right to some present. At the church the clergyman, the verger, and the poor should each receive a gratuity proportionate to their condition. Simply put a piece of money into the hands of the humbler persons; but present the clergyman with a box of sugared almonds in which is enclosed pieces of gold or silver.

Persons of a very high class, in order to free their friends from these expenses, send servants to present their children at the font. This is a most unbecoming custom. It seems to regard this holy consecration as a slav-ish ceremony, and destroys at its source the sentiments of respect and affection that a godson or god-daughter should inspire in those who have adopted them before God.

At the hour appointed for the ceremony, you go to the church in a carriage at the expense of the godfather. He and the godmother pass in first; next comes the infant borne by its nurse or the midwife; and then the father, who accompanies the other persons invited. After returning from the christening, it is the custom in many families to give a grand repast, at which the godfather and godmother receive all the honour.

Above all, they should give their godchild new year's gifts while it is a child, and manifest their affection during the whole of its life.

The mother's confinement is announced by a printed letter. You should respond with a visit, which she returns after her churching.

Duties to the Sick, Infirm, and Unfortunate.

When any one of your acquaintance is ill, you should regularly send a servant to inquire after his health, every day or every other day, according to the virulence and nature of the disease. If there is immediate danger, send even twice a day. Now and then ask the servant to find out whether the sick person can receive any one, because in that case, you must go and testify all your interest in person. Continue to obtain information about the sick person's health until his recovery or death.

Your visits to a sick person should be extremely short, quiet, and diffident. Express your interest in few words and a low voice, and converse softly with the family member who attends him. Ask who is the physician, what is the treatment, and urge every ground for consolation and hope; you ought hardly to reply to the questions the person in attendance asks regarding your own health or affairs. Retire reiterating the proofs of your interest.

If the person is convalescent or only indisposed, address a thousand questions concerning his complaints, sympathize with him, praise his patience, and describe to him the pleasant image of returning health. Take good care not to say that you find his features much changed, that his recovery may be slow, &c. To speak these truths is very malapropos, and with reason; you would pass for having an unfeeling heart, or instead, a limited understanding.

When sufferings and indispositions are prolonged, and resist all the efforts of medical skill, they are infirmities indeed. The most absolute and rigorous silence should be observed respecting them. Not only ought you never to speak to an infirm person of his misfortune, also carefully avoid mentioning any person who is afflicted in the same way, thus reminding him of his own case. This is only allowed when you can make it appear to him that the benefits of which he is deprived are not so permanent but that you have experienced some similar inconveniences. Thus to a lame person, you might say that you yourself are fatigued with walking, that your own legs are not firm, &c.

If the infirmity is not too visible, and the poor subject speaks to you of it, assure him earnestly that you would not have observed it. If he complains, offer him grounds for solace. Take care that you change the subject of conversation before he does, otherwise he might think you are importuning him about his malady. Finally, do every thing in your power to comfort him. If he is afflicted with imperfect sight, place objects near him, but without affectation, and without making him think that he requires your assistance, or permitting him to thank you. If he is troubled with deafness, you must not speak unreasonably loud. Bring his attention back to the subject of your conversation by skilful and delicate transitions. Do not abruptly say, "We are speaking of thus-and-so." Perhaps you will say this is much trouble. Trouble to console people? Why, you take more to please them!

Some persons who are reduced in circumstances, keep up in their misfortune (at least in society) their habits of opulence, and to manage with such persons requires not a little skill. If they invite you to their frugal repasts, or offer you any presents, let not the fear of occasioning them expense induce you to refuse warmly and obstinately; you would wound them deeply. Accept, but seek an opportunity of repaying these proofs of their politeness with interest. Never speak to them first of their sad situation; but if they introduce the subject themselves, receive their confidence with a respectful and affectionate attention. Show how much you are affected with that which grieves them; and without forgetting discretion, endeavour, at least in appearance, to render them confidence for confidence.

Funerals and Mourning.

When you have lost any one of your family, you should give intelligence of it to all persons who have had relations of business or friendship with the deceased. This letter of announcement usually contains an invitation to attend the funeral service and burial.

Unless you are in full mourning for some one else, it is impolite not to accept the invitation. On receiving it, you go to the house of the deceased, and follow the body as far as the church. You should appear in mourning. You are excused from accompanying the body to the graveyard, unless it is a relation, a friend, or a direct superior. If you go as far as the graveyard, cede the first carriages to the relations and most intimate friends of the deceased. Walk with your head uncovered, silently, and with a sad and thoughtful mien. It is not proper for relations to give themselves up too much to their grief.

At a burial or funeral service, the members of the family are entitled to the first places; they are nearest to the coffin, whether in the procession or in the church. The nearest relations wear very deep mourning, with a black mantle which has white borders on the sleeves. At the funeral, as well as the burial, the male relations go first, and then those invited; the female relations go next, and are followed by the other ladies.

It is not customary at Paris for women to follow the procession; and nowhere do they go quite to the graveyard, unless they are of a very low class. A widower or widow, a father or mother, are not present at the burial or funeral of those whom they have lost. The first are assumed to be unable to support the afflicting ceremony; and the second ought not to show this mark of deference.

You owe a visit to persons who have invited you to a funeral, if you were unable to accept their invitation. If you did attend, then they are the ones who owe the visit. Visits paid to the bereaved are called visits of condolence. In making them, observe silence, and never inquire about their health; that would be out of place. A gentleman offers them his hand, but a lady embraces them, even though they are but slightly acquainted. Refrain from conversing on too gay or personal subjects. If you are at a distance, testify by letter all your sympathy for the misfortune which afflicts them. Their grief cannot excuse them from answering you, though it is not immediately necessary.

There are two kinds of mourning, full mourning and half-mourning. (Also see Chapter XI.) Full mourning is worn for a father, mother, grandfather, grandmother, husband, wife, brother, or sister. It is divided into three periods. (Several of the particulars which follow are not observed in the United States.) For the first six weeks, wear only woollen garments. In the six weeks following, you may wear silk, and the last three months mingle white with the black. In full mourning, you should wear neither curls nor perfumes.

Half-mourning is worn for uncles, aunts, first cousins, and second cousins. The first fortnight you wear black silk, and the last week white mixed with black.

Custom requires that a widow wear mourning for a year and six weeks, while that of a widower is only six months. This difference, which may appear singular, is founded upon reasons of convenience and social relations.

In the first three months of mourning, a widow wears only woollen garments. During the first six weeks, her head-dress and *fichu* are black crape or *gaze de laine;* in the following six weeks, they are white crape and a *fichu de lingère*. The next six months, she dresses in black silk; *gros de Naples* in winter and taffety in summer. Her head-dress is white crape. The last three months, she wears black and white, and the last six weeks, white only.

For a widower, mourning is a black cloth coat without buttons, bronzed shoes, black buckles, woollen stockings, and a crape sword-knot, if he carries a sword. At the end of six weeks, he may wear a black cloth coat with buttons, black silk stockings, silver buckles, and a black riband upon the sword. The half-mourning of the last three months is a black suit, white silk stockings, silver buckles, and a black and white sword-knot.

If you marry a person who is in mourning, put on black the day after your wedding; the time preceding is reckoned as if the mourning had been worn. On the contrary, if you yourself remarry at a time when the death of a relation by your former marriage requires this sombre dress, leave it off immediately, since your new union annuls the former alliance. If you assist at a marriage, leave off mourning that day and resume it the next.

It is altogether contrary to propriety to select articles of mourning for yourself at the shops, to have them made in your presence, or to make them yourself. For a fortnight at least, and sometimes even for the first six weeks, you ought not to do needle-work, even while receiving relations and intimate friends, so much are you supposed to be overcome by your affliction.

During the first forty days, do not leave the house, except to go to church. It would be very improper to visit, dine out at a restaurant, or go to any assembly during first mourning. To be present at a funeral, or even to look at one passing, are forbidden. Attending a funeral service, other than that of the person you are mourning, is equally prohibited.

When this time has expired, you may return visits of condolence, and go out a little more; but you cannot yet appear at public promenades, at spectacles, or at balls. Neither may you sing, even at home. It is only at the time of half-mourning that you resume by degrees your former habits of life.

For at least ten days after the death of a very near relation, it would be very reprehensible for people whose profession recalls ideas of pleasure, such as musicians or dancing-masters, to return to their employment.

——*The Gentleman and Lady's Book of Politeness,*
Manuel complet de la bonne compagnie.

Diversion 1.

Love and Courtship. This is an affection of the mind, compounded of desire, esteem, and benevolence, which forms the bond of attachment and union between individuals of the different sexes; and makes them feel in the society of each other, a species of happiness which they experience nowhere else.

It is a maxim laid down amongst ladies, and a very prudent one it is, that love is not to begin on their part, but is entirely to be the consequence of an attachment of the other sex to them. As Nature has not given you that unlimited range in your choice which the men enjoy, she has wisely and benevolently assigned to you a greater flexibility of taste on this subject. Some agreeable qualities recommend a young man to your common good-liking and friendship. In the course of his acquaintance, he contracts an attachment to you. When you perceive it, it excites your gratitude, this gratitude rises into a preference, and this preference perhaps at last advances to some degree of attachment, especially if it meets with crosses and difficulties; for these, and a state of suspense, are very great incitements to attachment, and are the food of love in both sexes.

The effects of love amongst men are diversified by their different tempers. An artful man may counterfeit every one of them, so as easily to impose on a young maid of an open, generous, and feeling heart, if she is not extremely on her guard. The finest parts of such a girl may not always prove sufficient for her security. The dark and crooked paths of cunning are unsearchable and inconceivable to an honourable and elevated mind.

The following are the most genuine effects of an honourable passion amongst men, and the most difficult to counterfeit. A young man of delicacy often betrays his passion by his too great anxiety to conceal it, especially if he has little hope of success. True love renders a man not only respectful, but timid, in his behaviour to the woman he loves. To conceal the awe which he feels, he may sometimes affect pleasantry, but it sits awkwardly on him, and he quickly relapses into seriousness. He magnifies all her real perfections in his imagination, and is either blind to her failings, or converts them into beauties.

His heart and his character will be improved in every respect by his attachment. His manners will become more gentle, and his conversation more agreeable; but diffidence and embarrassment will always make him appear to disadvantage in the company of the object of his affections.

When you observe these marks in a young man's behaviour, you must reflect seriously what you are to do. If his attachment is agreeable to you, if you feel a partiality for him, you will do well not to discover to him the full extent of your love. Your receiving his addresses shows your preference: which is all, at that time, he is entitled to know. If he has delicacy, he will ask for no stronger proof of your affection, for your sake; if he has sense, he will not ask it for his own.

If you see evident proofs of a young man's attachment, and are determined to shut your heart against him; as you ever hope to be used with generosity by the person who will engage your heart, treat him honourably and humanely. Do not suffer him to linger in a state of miserable suspense, but be anxious to let him know your sentiments concerning him.

Beware of acting the part of a coquette. There is one case perhaps, and but one, where a young lady may do it justifiably, to the utmost verge which her conscience will allow. It is where a young man purposely declines to pay his addresses until such time as he thinks himself perfectly sure of her consent. This at bottom is intended to force a woman to give up the undoubted privilege of her sex, the privilege of refusing. It is intended to force her to explain herself, in effect, before he himself designs to do it, and by this means to oblige her to violate the modesty and delicacy of her sex, and to invert the clearest order of Nature.

It is of great importance to distinguish whether a young man who has the appearance of being your lover, delays to speak explicitly from the motive above mentioned, or from a diffidence inseparable from true attachment. In the one case you can hardly use him too ill, in the other you ought to treat him with great kindness: and the greatest kindness you can show him, if you are determined not to listen to his addresses, is to let him know it as soon as possible.

It appears necessary to be more particular on the subject of courtship, because it may and does commonly take place at an early period of life, when young ladies have but little experience or knowledge of the world; when their passions are warm, and their judgement not arrived at such full maturity as to be able to correct them. It is very desirable that every lady should possess such principles of honour and generosity as will render her incapable of deceiving, and at the same time to possess that acute discernment which may secure her against being deceived.

It is a generally received opinion, founded in fact, that women may attain a superior degree of happiness in a married state to what they can possibly find in the other. What a forlorn and unprotected situation is that of old maids! What chagrin and peevishness are apt to infect their tempers! And how great is the difficulty of making a transition, with dignity and cheerfulness, from the period of youth and beauty, admiration and respect, into the calm, silent, unnoticed retreat of declining years! A married state, if entered into from proper motives of esteem and affection, is certainly the happiest. It will make you most respectable in the world, and the most useful member of society.

Advice previous to Matrimony. If a young man makes his addresses to you, or gives you any reason to believe he will do so, before you allow your affections to be engaged, endeavour, in the most prudent and secret manner, to procure from your friends every necessary piece of information concerning him; such as his character, as to sense, morality, religion, temper, and family; whether it is distinguished for parts and worth, or for folly and knavery. When your friends inform you of these, they have fulfilled their duty; and it behooves you to hearken to their counsel, and to attend to their advice.

Avoid a companion who may entail any hereditary disease on your posterity, particularly that most dreadful of all human calamities, madness. It is the height of imprudence to run into such a danger; and further it is highly criminal.

Do not marry a fool: he is the most untractable of all animals; he is led by his passions and caprices, and is incapable of hearing the voice of reason. It may probably hurt your vanity, to have a husband for whom you have reason to blush and tremble every time he opens his lips in company.

A rake is ever to be avoided by a prudent woman; he always makes a suspicious husband, because he has only known the most worthless of your sex. He likewise entails the worst diseases on his wife and children, if he has the misfortune to have any.

If you have a sense of religion yourself, do not think of a husband who has none. If you marry an infidel, or an irreligious character, what hope can you entertain of happiness? If you have children, you will suffer the most bitter distress, in seeing all your endeavours to form their minds to virtue and piety, all your endeavours to secure their present and eternal happiness, frustrated and turned into ridicule.

As the choice of a husband is of the greatest consequence to your happiness, be sure you make it with the utmost circumspection. Do not give way to a sudden sally of passion, and then dignify it with the name of love. Genuine love is not founded in caprice; it is founded in nature, on honourable views, on virtue, on similarity of tastes, and sympathy of souls.

If you have these sentiments, you will never marry any one when you are not in that situation which prudence suggests to be necessary to the happiness of either of you. What that competency may be, can only be determined by your own tastes: if you have as much between you as to satisfy all your demands, it is sufficient.

Marriage may dispel the enchantment raised by external beauty; but the virtues and graces which first warmed the heart, may, and ought ever to remain. The tumult of passion will necessarily subside; but it will be succeeded by an endearment which affects the heart in a more equal, a more sensible and tender manner.

Considerations before Marriage. If a union about to take place or recently contracted between two young persons, is mentioned in conversation, the first question asked concerning it is, whether it is a "good match." The very countenance and voice of the inquirer, and of the answerer, the terms of the answer returned, and the observations, whether expressive of satisfaction or of regret, which fall from the lips of the company present in the circle, all concur to show what, in common estimation, is meant by being well married. If a young woman is described as thus married, the terms imply that she is united to a man whose station and fortune are such, when compared with her own or those of her parents, that in point of precedence, in point of command of finery and of money, she is more or less a gainer by the bargain. In high life they imply that she will now possess the enviable advantages of taking place of other ladies in the neighbourhood; of decking herself out with jewels and lace; of inhabiting splendid apartments; rolling in handsome carriages; gazing on numerous servants in gaudy liveries; and of repairing to London, and other fashionable scenes of resort, all in a degree somewhat higher than that in which a calculating broker, after poring on her pedigree, summing up her property in hand, and computing, at the market price, every item which is contingent or in reversion, would have pronounced her entitled to. A few slight and obvious alterations would adapt the picture to the middling classes of society.

In the same manner a diminution of power as to the supposed advantages already enumerated, is supposed to be a bad match, and is universally lamented in polite meetings with real or affected concern. The good or bad fortune of a young man in the choice of a wife is estimated according to the same rules.

——*The Female Instructor.*

Chapter XXXI.
The Art of Conversation.

Conversation is the principal, though not the only, means of pleasing and succeeding in society. How does it happen then, that so many persons converse without being troubled by the ridicule thrown upon themselves, and the ennui they occasion their auditors? Without inquiring into whether they have not some physical qualities which present greater or lesser obstacles to the art of conversing well, or without seeking the means of correcting them?

Physical Concerns.

I shall first point out some faults and the means of remedying them.

Divers Faults. It is essential in speaking to be well on your guard not to protrude your tongue too near the edge of your lips. This bad habit has many great inconveniences. It occasions a kind of disagreeable hissing, produced by the immediate contact of this organ as it passes the teeth; it hinders pronunciation; and it exposes you to throw out saliva. (When this accident happens to some one else, you must appear not to perceive it.) When an unfortunate habit, or too great a development of the tongue, produces these accidents, take care to keep this unlucky organ out of the way on one side of your gums or the other.

As to the opposite fault, that is stammering, owing to an overly small tongue, practice speaking distinctly when you are alone. To declaim, and to exert yourself upon the words which present the greatest difficulties, is a useful exercise. There are some persons in whom the saliva is so abundant, that it makes their pronunciation thick; they should accustom themselves to swallow it before beginning to speak.

Propriety in accordance with hygiene, requires that your teeth be perfectly clean. A yellow and foul set of teeth, which emit an odour, will not suffer any one to be sensible to the grace or eloquence of your language. (See Chapter II for the means of remedying this.) A judgement of disgust is without appeal. Some persons who have fine teeth, have the lamentable fault of displaying them in speaking. This ridiculous vanity excites laughter, and besides, injures the physiognomy. It is unnecessary to conceal your teeth to the utmost, but always show them without affectation. To use a toothpick while speaking, to carry your fingers to your gums, and to hold a flower between your teeth are habits of bad *ton*.

To open your mouth widely when you speak, especially when making an exclamation of wonder or surprise; to draw your mouth to one side to give yourself an original air; to purse your lips; to roar with laughter in a foolish and boisterous manner; to impart trembling and convulsive motions to your lips when any one relates or reads something sad or terrible; to force your breath into the face of your interlocutor—all these are shocking faults, and insupportable grimaces.

Gestures. To act a pantomime with every word cannot be tolerated. Large or numerous gestures, which do not accord with the conversation; mysterious signs accompanying the announcement of the simplest thing; abrupt gestures in friendly conversation; mincing gestures in serious conversation; rapid movements of the person, sitting or standing, which make you seem to perform a kind of dance—all these are equally great faults against sense and taste.

You should not entirely forego gestures, which according to the Abbé Delille, give physiognomy to conversation. Moderate gestures corresponding to your words, and by turns a little comic, lively, and graceful, are allowable and even indispensable. (See also Chapter XIII.) Your left hand must not move, but an intelligent and well-ordered co-operation of your right should never be wanting in conversation. Often you may add much art and grace to listening by gesturing gently. For example, by counting upon your fingers, or by making a motion of surprise, assent, or admiration. This is a tacit manner of saying, "Ah, I recollect, you are right," and charms the narrator without interrupting him.

I must censure dialogists who put their hands into their pockets or work-bags, or who constantly rest them joined or crossed, without making any movement. Such persons give themselves the air of automatons, but excessive gesticulators have the appearance of lunatics. Persons who in conversing, violently seize hold of the arms of their chair; play with little objects which come under their hands; amuse themselves by scratching or defacing furniture; revolve their hat in both directions; or twist and untwist the strings of their bag, or the corners of their handkerchief, are doubtless ignorant how opposed to propriety are these displays of familiarity, childishness, and awkwardness. I shall briefly add, that those who witness all these ridiculous actions should never point them out by laughing or speaking, unless they wish to be still more ridiculous.

Pronunciation.

Pronunciation is even more indispensable in conversation than in elocution. Before selecting your expressions, you must make them understood, and you can do this but imperfectly if you pronounce badly. From this fault arise forced repetitions, the loss of relevant points, fatigue, disgust, the impatience of both persons speaking, and in short, all the sad results of deafness. Should you not make every effort to rid yourself of it?

Volubility. This is the greatest impediment to pronouncing well. By speaking too fast you mutter, producing inarticulate and unintelligible sounds, which without dispute is quite unbearable. You know very well that to speak too slowly, and (as they say) to listen to your own words, is a caprice which seems to denote pride or listlessness, and that in certain cases it is necessary to speak quickly. But you ought never to speak precipitately, even on subjects which require you to be brief. Besides the physical inconvenience, indistinctness has moral inconveniences; it implies heedlessness, loquacity, or foolishness.

Hesitancy. This is scarcely less troublesome, for it fills the conversation with ridiculous and painful efforts. This defect, though sometimes owing to too much forethought, results still more frequently from neglecting to think before you speak, from timidity, from some lively emotion which obliges you to stammer, or from a pretentious concern for employing choice phrases. This last motive is nearly an eccentricity. With the object of pleasing people, you bore them with repetitions or far-fetched mincing words, and in order to appear clever, you render yourself excessively annoying.

Bad Habits. Habits acquired in childhood and in small towns are frequently obstacles to good pronunciation; here are some examples. It is not uncommon to hear, even amongst well-educated people, such misuse of words as the following: "Me," for "I," "Miss" for "Mrs.," "set" for "sit," "sat out" for "set out," "expect" (of a past event), "lay" for "lie," "shew" for "show," "would" for "should," "hadn't ought" for "ought not," &c.

According to Rousseau, over-nicety of pronunciation, or purism, should also be condemned. He (and many others like him) could not tolerate people who are particular in sounding every letter of a word. For example, some persons are scrupulous in the distinct pronunciation of every letter in such words as "extra-ordinary," "Wed-nes-day," &c.

Accents and Tones. As to accent, each province has its own. To recognize it, shun it, and modify it by an opposite effort, are the means of avoiding these shoals. But however ridiculous you may appear in running upon them continually, you are an hundred times less so than people who, like real schoolmasters, stop you in the midst of an affecting recital, to repeat with a sardonic smile a vulgar phrase, a badly-pronounced word, or a wrong accent which happens to escape you.

Besides a general accent, there is also a distinctive tone which gives a shade to the words when you express a sentiment. I feel all its delicacy and charm; but I feel also that it ought to be in perfect harmony with the language, that it should be free from all affectation and exaggeration. To utter hard things in a mild tone; to display proud pretensions in a humble voice; to broach a political discussion in a caressing tone; to recount an affair of pleasantry with a melancholy accent, are ridiculous in the highest degree. It is no less so to force your tone, and pervert it into irony; or introduce into the discourse a kind of declamation or chant.

People cannot judge the accent of a person who speaks too loud or too soft. But they decide in the first case that he is vulgar, and in the second that he is disdainful.

Correct Grammar and Language.

As Nicolas Boileau-Despréaux says, "Above all, language in your discourse." In addressing this advice to readers, I shall beware of believing them strangers to the rules of grammar. It is so disgraceful at the present day to be ignorant of your own language, that it would be no less so to suspect others of not knowing it. But though you may not be deprived of this indispensable knowledge, it is still necessary to carefully beware of contracting bad habits in language; of using incorrect phrases, and even of using terms which you do not understand. (See Div. 1.) A little study and attention will afford a certain remedy to the awkwardness which you may experience. Young people cannot be too much on guard against these faults, which bespeak an education which has been little attended to. They will succeed at this by studying the speech of a good grammarian, and by paying attention to the sense of their words.

If in the silence of the study, you have much trouble with correctly rendering a long sentence, how must it be in society, when the fervour of conversation prevents you from reflecting? To make long phrases is to be willing to make mistakes in language. If you take time to present interminable sentences in a correct form, you only appear more clumsy, or more affected. Conversation ought never to seem laboured, and your expression and thoughts should be of the same nature.

Avoid over-using the pronouns "who" and "which," particularly when they are interrogatives. Though grammar does not absolutely condemn their frequency, yet as it is useless and disagreeable to the ear, you should endeavour to avoid it. Thus instead of, "Who is it who did such a thing?" or, "What is this thing which is here?" say, "Who did such a thing?" or, "What is this thing?"

Persons who are careful of their conversation, avoid, like faults of language, expressions which injure clarity, elegance, and harmony. Thus they abstain from uniting words which, having conflicting meaning and pronunciation, create ambiguity except when written. They carefully beware of amassing a profusion of synonyms and epithets, or at least of forgetting the laws of gradation with regard to the latter. They avoid multiplying adverbs, which burden and weaken discourse. They pay great attention to the requirements of euphony. In order to do so, they avoid bringing similar sounding words close together, and repeating similar words even of the same meaning, such as, "At present we offer a present," and, "It does a good deal of good."

These scrupulous and excellent conversationalists are particularly careful of the connecting particles, for they know how much their omission injures euphony; how it causes persons who are little charitable, to believe that it is a veil under which doubt or ignorance is adroitly concealed. This opinion is not always a prejudice.

Skilful conversationalists endeavour not to furnish opportunities for puns by fortuitous coincidences of words. In the mode of their conversation, they avoid rhymes which are unfortunate and even ridiculous in prose. They dread repetitions of phrases and axioms, like the repetitions of words. By short and judicious pauses, they mark punctuation in spoken as in written language. Finally, they endeavour to render their conversation clear, correct, and elegant.

But these conversational models are in less danger of defeating their object, if they have not in the slightest the mannered air of the schoolmaster. Far from it; if a grammatical error escapes them, they quickly correct it, but with ease and gaiety. If they hear a gross grammatical error, they do not permit themselves even a smile or a look which might show up or embarrass the culprit. If some one else attempts to play the schoolmaster, giving a lesson in syntax, the judicious conversationalist hastens to say that he also sometimes happens to make mistakes.

Customary Formalities in Conversation.

Goodness, moderation, and decorum—these are the motto and the spirit of moral propriety in conversation. A solicitude to be always agreeable and obliging; of observing a proper medium in every thing; of respecting the rights of others, even in the most trifling things; susceptibility for every thing which is connected with delicacy, piety, and modesty—all the qualities which belong to propriety are included in those expressive words.

Inquiries concerning the Health. It is proper to vary the phraseology of these commonplace questions as much as possible. You must abstain from them entirely towards a superior, or a person with whom you are but little acquainted, as such inquiries presuppose some degree of intimacy. In the last case, there is a method of manifesting your interest without violating etiquette. It consists of making these inquiries of the servants, or other persons of the house, and of saying afterwards when presenting yourself, "I am delighted, Sir, to hear that you are in good health."

Custom forbids a lady to inquire after the health of a gentlemen, unless he is ill or very aged. To compensate for this, a lady who addresses a gentlemen should be earnest in her inquiries after the health of his family, however little intimacy she may have with them. A great many persons ask this question mechanically, without waiting for the answer, or else hasten to reply before they have received it. This is bad *ton*. Inquiries about the health, it is true, are frequently of little consequence, but they should appear to be dictated by attention and kindness. However, you must not be deceived, but be careful not to mention a slight indisposition to persons who are strangers to you, because their interest can only be formal.

After you are informed of the health of the people you are visiting, it is proper to inquire after the health of their family; but it would be wearisome if you made a long enumeration of its members. You may put a general question, designating, however, the most important individuals. If near relations are absent, ask the people you are visiting if they have heard from them lately, and if the news is favourable. They, on their part, ask the same of you.

When you are not on a visit of great ceremony, when you take leave you are commonly charged with the compliments and regards of the persons you are visiting, to those with whom you live. You should reply briefly, but give them assurances of your regard, and thank them.

Forms of Address. Propriety infuses into visits of some little ceremony, a colouring of modesty, grace, and deference, which should be preserved with the greatest care. In speaking, it is always proper to use the title of "Mr.," "Mrs.," or "Miss," and if the sentence is tolerably long, the title should be repeated. If the question requires an affirmative or negative answer, never curtly say, "Yes" or "No." (See Div. 2.) It is, however, impolite to join the person's name to the title of "Mr." or "Mrs." You may do this only when the person you are addressing is distracted or turned the other way, and it is necessary to get his attention. If the person has a title of nobility or that of a distinguished profession, it is even more proper to call him by it. If several persons present follow the same profession, you may then add the name. Every one knows that it is very coarse to refer to a third person by saying, "he" or "she"; you must say, "Mr." or "Mrs." You may also refer to him by his title or name.

A lady does not say, "My husband," except amongst intimates. In all other circumstances, she should address him by his name, calling him "Mr." It is equally good *ton* that except on occasions of ceremony, and while she is quite young, to designate him by his christian name. The same rules apply to a husband, with one exception: in society it would be ridiculous to say, "Mrs. Such-a-one, my wife." You should simply say, "My wife." When you speak to a gentlemen of his wife, do not say, "Your wife," unless you are intimately acquainted. "Mrs. Such-a-one" is the most proper. The rules of propriety are the same when referring to a husband. (See Div. 3.)

It is positively half-witted to form a sentence which may be taken in the wrong way, by using some disagreeable word near "Mr." or "Mrs."

When you speak of yourself and another person, whether he is present or absent, propriety requires you to mention yourself last. Thus you should say, "he and I" or "you and I." (See Div. 4.) When you relate a personal experience, the circumstances of which are creditable to yourself, and a very distinguished person has also a share in the credit, you should only mention him. Instead of the plural form, "we resolved," or, "we did such a thing," you should forget yourself, saying, "Mr. Such-a-one resolved or did thus and so." Delicacy will dictate this degree of modesty to you, and your superior in his turn will proclaim your merit on the occasion at his own expense.

Greetings, Apologies, &c. Some persons invidiously say that forms avail much in society. I agree with them, but in a favourable sense.

It is only to inferiors that you say, "I wish you good morning," or especially, "Good morning." If you are a gentleman say, "I have the honour to greet you" to an aged lady, a married one, or a young lady. You should never ask a thing of any one without saying, "Will you have the goodness," "Will you do me the favour," "Will you be so good," &c. To a question which you do not fully comprehend, never answer, "Ha?" or "What?" but, "Be so good as," &c., or, "Pardon me, I did not understand." If you strike against any one in the least, ask pardon for it immediately. The other should reply, "It is nothing, nothing at all," &c., even if the blow was violent.

In a circle, do not pass before a lady; neither should you present any thing by extending your arm over her, but pass round behind, and present it. In case you cannot do it, say, "I ask your pardon," &c. Never disdainfully refuse a pinch of snuff, and rather than disoblige people, accept one, even if you throw it away after having pretended to take it. When you hear a sneeze, do not flinch away, or do so imperceptibly and silently. Beware of presenting a box of bon-bons to ladies in balls or assemblies, under penalty of having the air of a caricature.

It is customary to employ the few moments of a visit of mere politeness in looking at the portraits which adorn the fire-place, and even taking them down, if you are invited to do so. It would be the extreme of impoliteness, to say that they were flattering, or to pretend to recognize in the portrait of a young lady, the likeness of an aged lady, or one less favoured by Nature. It is also improper to make long compliments; indirect and ingenious praise is all that is proper.

Dialogues.

This article comprises both the choice of elegant language, and the rules of propriety for praises, complaints, questions, and disputes.

Suppositions and Comparisons. The two shoals to be avoided in this form of language are directly opposed to each other. The one is triviality, the other bombast. The object of supposition, which is already antiquated, and sometimes too simple, is to increase the force of reasoning, and to carry conviction to the mind of the auditor. Comparison tends to make an image, or to place the object described before the eyes. When supposition and comparison are regulated by reason, custom, and taste, it is all very well; but how seldom is this the case!

They are not properly used if, in the course of a discussion, you suppose a respectable person to supply the place of a lunatic, an ignorant person, or a robber. Or if you suppose him to be in a disgraceful or even ridiculous situation. For example, "If you had been this scoundrel," or "Suppose that you had committed this base act," or, "Suppose that you were laughed at," &c.

Comparisons are also misplaced, whenever, being satisfied with avoiding shocking ones, you endeavour to single out some one as contemptible, by comparing his appearance with that of some other person in society. For example, "This wretch is of your size, sir; he has your features, your general appearance," &c.

They are again misplaced, if used in the presence of people of a profession upon which the injurious comparisons fall, for instance, "quackish as a doctor," "greedy as a money-lender," "loquacious as a lawyer," &c.

Finally, propriety and taste cannot at all exist in comparisons if they are trite and trivial, such as, "pretty as a picture," "black as a chimney," "high as one's hand," &c. Or if they are in a turgid and pretending style, such as, "accomplished as the Muses," "fresh as the dawn," &c.

Frequently Recurring Expressions. Madame Necker ingeniously observes that those favourite and frequently-repeated terms with which conversation is filled, serve ordinarily as a mark of people's character. "Thus," says she, "those who exceed the truth are in the habit of saying, 'You may rely upon it, it is the truth'; the long-winded say, 'In a word, to be brief'; and the proud say, 'Without boasting.'" This striking observation is well founded, and consequently you ought to take good care not to expose the secrets of your peculiarities. But independently of this motive, it is necessary to carefully avoid frequently recurring words, as in time habit multiplies them to an inconceivable degree. They embarrass and overwhelm your conversation, avert the attention of your auditors, and render you ridiculous and unwelcome without your being able to perceive it.

If habitual words, which on no other account are reprehensible, may become so troublesome, what results may old-fashioned turns of phrase, trite phrases, trivial expressions, and vulgar transitions produce, when they become frequent! For example, "To put yourself in his place," "To begin at the beginning," "If things come to the worst," &c.

Quotations and Proverbs. The insupportable pedantry of a horde of quoters without taste or wit has justly thrown quotations into disrepute for a long time. But if quotations are well chosen, few, and short; if they are apropos, "What puts time to flight, what pleases like the graces," if they are altogether new, and used by a person possessed of modesty, elegance, and taste, and having perfect breeding, quotations have much success and charm. But without these qualifications there is little safety; and in this matter there can be no mediocrity. You will either be a good model, or an insupportable pedant. Consider whether you will rashly take this risk, especially on making your debut in society, when young men ought so carefully to avoid parading a vain college erudition, and seeking the reputation of a man of learning by employing words borrowed from foreign languages, or scientific terms unknown to people in society.

Popular sayings and proverbs, as well as other quotations, require some care; and except in familiar conversation, are altogether misplaced. If they are frequent, conversation becomes merely tedious chatter. If introduced without a brief preparation, one of two things will take place. They will either prevent the speaker from being understood, or give him the air of Sancho Panza. The necessary notice need be but short, for example, "As the proverb says," or, "As the wisdom of nations has it." A proverb well applied, and placed at the end of a sentence, frequently makes a very happy conclusion.

Pleasantries. If society is not a school for exercising pedantry, neither is it an arena for the use of those perversely clever people, who think themselves licensed to insult with grace. Whatever may be the keenness of their sarcasms, the piquancy of their observations, or the smile which they elicit from me, I nonetheless refuse to call these caustic spirits and mocking wits polite persons, or ones of good *ton;* for in politeness there must be good-will. Those who incessantly study to trouble and wound people without taking any precaution except to deprive them of the right or means of complaining; who are ready to catch at the slightest error, exaggerate it, envenom it, and present it in the most ridiculous light; who meanly attack those who cannot answer them, or expose themselves every day for a sarcasm to sport with their own life and that of another in a duel—such people, what are they? In truth, I dare not say. (See Div. 5.)

Such a picture, which certainly is not highly coloured, would render pleasantries always odious. But to indulge in pleasantry is not to resemble such mischievous persons. Thank God! it is far otherwise; for mild, amiable, and light-hearted pleasantry should be taken in good part even by those who are the subjects of it. It is a friendly and sportive contest, in which sarcasm, distrust, and resentment should never appear. Whenever you perceive the least trace of them, the pleasantry is at an end; desist, then, the moment they appear.

As to hoaxing, that sarcasm of fools, and that silly merriment excited by the ingenuousness or politeness of people whom you deceptively cause to believe the most foolish things, because they do not let you know that they see through this pleasure of stupid fellows, I have nothing to say—except that I have too good an opinion of my readers to suppose that they do not despise hoaxes as I do.

I speak only to censure; I therefore entreat my readers not to manufacture puns, and to despise this foolish wit, this childish method of eliciting a passing smile. Not that you cannot repeat in good company one of those rare political *bon mots* which are happy in both form and meaning. Nor that you ought to deprecate puns before people who are fond of them, still less to tell them what they hear every day, "That is poor." To have taste does not authorize you to be impolite.

I must be much more severe on another kind of équivoques; viz., those which offend modesty. Propriety allows and furthermore requires you not to listen to, and even to interrupt an ill-bred person who troubles you with those indecent witticisms which a man of good society ought always to avoid. These are the ones which cover certain jests with a veil so transparent that they are the more obvious. What pleasure can be found in causing ladies to blush, and people to believe that you keep bad company?

There are those who think that they may permit themselves every kind of pleasantry before certain females; but a man of good *ton* ought to preserve it wherever he is. I could cite more than one example of persons who have lost politeness of manners and language by adopting the habits and conversation of all kinds of society into which chance may have carried them. It requires but a moment to lose those delicate shades of character which constitute a man of the world, and which cost so many pains to acquire.

It is a great error to suppose that you must always shine in conversation, and that it is better to be admired for a lively and ready repartee, then to content yourself sometimes with silence, or with an answer less brilliant than judicious. Do not imagine that all traits of wit are in the class of politeness. A vain and triumphant air spoils a *bon mot;* moreover, when you repeat a thing of this kind of which you are yourself the author, beware of saying so to your auditors.

That a repartee may be truly pleasing, it is necessary that he who makes it has a right to do so, and that it may be quoted without doing him any wrong. Otherwise people would laugh at the repartee, and despise its author. There are repartees which are pleasing in the mouth of a military man, but which would be ridiculous in that of a magistrate. A young lady may make lively and brilliant repartees, which would be insupportable in a woman in the decline of life; as the latter might make such as would be unsuitable in a young lady.

Eulogiums and Complaints. One of the most improper things, is to praise excessively and unseasonably. Extravagant and misplaced eulogiums honour neither the person who bestows them, nor the one who receives them.

An infallible method of giving a person of merit the air of a fool, is to address him to his face and without disguise, in exaggerated eulogiums; it is indeed not a little embarrassing to reply. If you remain silent, you appear to be inhaling the incense with complacency; and if you repel it, you seem the more to encourage it. Thus are seen, even amongst very clever persons, those who reply by silly exclamations and by rude assertions. "You are laughing at me," they say; but this cannot be tolerated, for it is to be supposed that the person who praises you is incapable of such an act. I think it better to say, "If I did not know you were so kind (or so good) I would really think you were jesting with me." Or else say, "Your partiality blinds you."

Men who are unacquainted with society, commonly think that they cannot address a lady without first assailing her with compliments. This is a mistake, gentlemen, and I can reveal to you what my sex prefers to these banal eulogiums. It is bad *ton* to overwhelm with insipid flattery, every lady that you meet, without distinction of age, rank, or merit. It may indeed please unthinking women, but will disgust sensible ones. Carry on with them a lively, piquant, and varied conversation; and recollect that they have a too active imagination, and a too great versatility of disposition, to support conversation for a long time upon the same subject.

But is it then necessary to proscribe eulogiums entirely? Not at all— society has not yet arrived at that degree of philosophy. Eulogiums are and will for a long time be a means of success. But they should be true, or at least probable, in order not to have the appearance of outrageous insult. They should be indirect and delicate, that the person praised may listen to them without being obliged to interrupt. And they should be tempered with a kind of judgement, the skilful use of which is itself praise.

As I have often said, let there be moderation in every thing. Should you not regard as vulgar and ridiculous, that exaggeration which is frequently used in praise as well as in censure? It seems that true propriety in language consists principally in a certain moderation of expression. It is much better to cause people to think more than you say, than to exaggerate, and run the risk of exceeding what you ought to say.

Whatever your connexion with your auditor, complaining has always a bad grace. Banish bitterness and animosity from your complaints. Let your anger be only an expression of the wrong you have suffered, and not of that which you would cause. This is the surest means of winning to your side persons who might perhaps be doubtful whether to favour your adversary or yourself. Propriety is no less opposed to making excessive complaints to the first person you meet who sympathizes with you, then to the frequent and extravagant praises which you bestow improperly upon those from whom you expect a favour in return.

Tactlessness and Prejudices. Though there are divers kinds of tactlessness, I speak here of a want of due regard to, and forgetfulness of, the delicate attentions which seem to identify you with the situation of others. Here are some examples. To accost sad people with a smiling face and sprightly manners, which prove to them the little interest which you take in their situation; to trouble by a whimsical and cross ill-humour, and misanthropic declamations, the pleasure of contented persons; to extol the advantages of beauty before ladies who are aged or naturally unfortunate; to speak of the power which wealth bestows in the presence of people scarcely arrived at mediocrity of fortune; to boast of your strength and health before a valetudinarian, &c.

When speaking of "prejudices," I do not mean to discuss those erroneous judgements, acknowledged as such, which though undermined and shaken, are still credited by the society which they plague. I wish only to warn my readers against those anti-social prejudices of nation against nation, city against city, and neighbourhood against neighbourhood; that spiteful disposition which fills the mouth of a Frenchman with malicious observations on the English; with which a Parisian makes the name "provincial" synonymous with awkwardness and bad *ton;* and which, in the drawing-rooms of the Chaussée-d'Antin, allows no favour to persons lodging in the Marais—especially since the people of the Marais, provincials, and Englishmen consider it no fault to return prejudice for prejudice, and contempt for contempt.

Questions. It is an axiom of propriety that you should never speak of yourself (except to intimate friends) and that you should converse with strangers about themselves, and every thing which may interest them. Questions are therefore necessary, but they demand infinite delicacy and tact, in order neither to fatigue, nor to wound the feelings. If instead of expressing a gentle and heart-felt interest, you ask a dry question dictated by a cold curiosity; if you seem to pay no attention to the answers which you call forth; if you maladroitly take a patronizing tone; if you prolong without bounds this kind of conversation; or if you embarrass some one who instead of keeping silence, vainly endeavours to save himself by an evasive answer, be assured that both your questions and yourself will be considered a torment.

Discussions and Disputes. Whatsoever the subject of conversation, propose your opinion with modesty; defend it with composure, and in a mild tone if you are opposed. Yield with a good grace if you are wrong; and even if you are in the right, if the subject of discussion is of little importance, and especially if the one who opposes you is a lady or an aged person. If love of truth, or the desire to improve your mind, compels you to enter into a dispute, do it with address and politeness. If you cannot win over your opponent, you will at least gain his esteem. (See Div. 6.) But if you have to do with one of those people who, possessed with a mania for dispute, commence by contradicting before they listen, and who are always ready to sustain the contrary opinion, yield to him; you will have nothing to gain with him. Be assured that the spirit of contradiction may be conquered only by silence.

Narrations. There are some conditions indispensable to the success of a narration. These conditions are, first, novelty; the best anecdotes weary when they are repeated too often, because every one wishes to be an actor in his turn upon the stage of society. When you have any thing excellent to relate, consult less your own desire to tell it, than the wishes of others to hear you. There are but too many people who discover the secret of wearying while telling very good things, on account of their over-eagerness to tell them.

The next thing is to choose a suitable opportunity. Let your narrative spring naturally from the conversation. Let it explain a fact, or come in support of an opinion; let it never appear to be introduced by the foolish pleasure of talking, or by a no less foolish desire to display your wit. Recollect that the most mediocre narratives, when they are apropos, frequently please more than the best things in the world, when they are said out of time. Even endeavouring to monopolize the conversation is bad *ton*, particularly for young gentlemen and ladies, especially if it is but a few moments since they occupied the attention of the company.

It is all-important that your language correspond to the different forms which the narration requires; that under pretext of adorning your story, you do not wander into far-fetched comparisons, dull details, or interminable dialogues; and that if you relate any thing amusing or striking, you keep the greatest composure. Finally, before commencing a recital of this kind, keep in mind these lines of La Fontaine (see Div. 7):

"Beware of saying, 'Lend an ear,'
    To something marvellous or witty,
To disappoint your friends who hear,
    Is possible, and were a pity."

For want of observing these rules and many others, some narrators fail of the expected effect, and believing they can tell the story over again, remark on the comic part, and labour to repeat it thus, "Do you not think this excellent *or* wonderful?" Alas! they only add to their own defeat, and to the ennui of their poor auditors.

When your narrations have had success, keep a modest countenance; leave others to point out the striking parts which have pleased them. The surest means of not gaining the approbation of others, in your actions as well as your discourse, is to solicit it, whether by looks or words.

As every auditor is obliged to listen and attend without objecting, it follows that you should feel your ground before speaking, and ask if such-and-such a thing is known to the company. When a story has been published in the newspapers, so that it is not altogether new, or seems borrowed from a compilation of *anas,* if you attribute it to some person of your acquaintance (of course one who is absent) an ineffaceable ridicule will very properly stigmatize you.

It is an agreeable and modest attention to request some one to relate an anecdote of the day, of which you have made mention, and the circumstances of which you desire to know. This is well suited to persons of distinguished talents. The person called upon bows and apologizes in a few words before acceding to your request.

Literary Critiques. I now come to what seems to me the most difficult part of conversation. If you are not certain that you can arrange your ideas in order, and express them with great clarity and an easy elegance, do not have the temerity to wish to analyze a book or a play. You would be laying up for yourself a rude mortification, which would have an unfavourable influence on your *entrée* into society. You would be wrong, however, to conclude that I condemn you to perpetual silence. I wish only to inspire you with a salutary diffidence, in order to preserve you from such a complete failure, and to put it in your power some future day to answer, in this particular, the wishes of a distinguished and brilliant assembly.

Begin by jotting down a rough outline of a short piece, as for instance a vaudeville, or a little comedy. Do this until, being sure of the manner in which you would encompass the whole, and arrange the details, you can produce your analysis of it without embarrassment. When you arrive at this point, abstain from such analyses, which though indeed more correct, seem laboured. They have besides less freedom, appropriateness, and grace. Know this, and remember it well, that every other preparation than thinking about what you will say, will make you acquire two intolerable faults: affectation and stiffness.

I give this advice only to persons who, by a quick and penetrating perception, by a love of the fine arts, and a peculiar readiness, find themselves able to speak knowledgably of literary productions. Those who are less engaged in these things should content themselves with simply and briefly explaining a subject, and of mentioning the emotion they felt; with speaking of some brilliant passage, and adding that they do not pretend to pronounce judgement.

Digressions. The first degree of digression is the aside. Provided it is short, natural, and seldom repeated, and that you always take care to announce it, and moreover not to abuse it, you may make skilful use of it. The second degree of digression becomes more nice. It includes those accessory reflections, those common but agreeable or established expressions, and those general or particular allusions, which are only to be used with a peculiar emphasis, which is to language what italic type is to printing. This manner of speaking in italics may be striking and artless, but it often becomes obscure and trite. The habit is dangerous, and you should use this difficult digression only before intimate friends.

I now come to the third degree, to what is properly called digression; it is usually involuntary. Often in a lively and animated dialogue, the impetus of conversation carries you, as well as your interlocutor, far from the point where you started. If it is a question of pleasure or interest, return to your point by employing a polite expression such as, "Pray let us not lose sight of our business." But if it is an affair of nothings succeeding nothings, let it flow on.

Voluntary digression, when it is not mere loquacity, may be employed in serious discourse, such as political, philosophical, or moral discussions. But it is important to treat it with infinite reserve and care. Never introduce a personal justification or a domestic incident, which is altogether out of place, as those persons do who, in narrating any event relative to an individual, recount his life, their connexion with him and his whole family, and make an hour seem like an eternity. Lawyers, literary men, military men, travellers, invalids, and aged ladies ought to have a prudent and continual distrust of the abuse of digressions.

The Art of Listening.

To converse is not to talk continually, as prattlers suppose. (See Div. 8.) It is to listen and speak in your turn; you must not acquit yourself less well in the one than in the other. To do this, attend half the time to the person who is addressing you (on this account it is impolite to work while talking); if he hesitates or is embarrassed, appear not to notice it. If you are tolerably intimate with him, after a few moments you should, very modestly, supply the expression which seems to have escaped him.

Repetition. If some one relates an anecdote which you already know, permit him to finish it, and do not in any way draw off the attention of those who are listening. If your opinion is asked, give it frankly, and without wishing to appear better informed than the narrator himself. Moreover, if you happen to be in a *tête-à-tête* with the same narrator, observe silence and listen with an air of interest. If he happens to impart to you what he related the previous day, or what he had from you yourself, likewise appear to listen as if for the first time. Frequently, in the midst of a recital, the narrator, through forgetfulness, hesitates and thinks that he can recall it. Look at him attentively. If he is in doubt, declare that you are altogether ignorant of the matter. If his memory returns, request him to continue, saying, "I always listen to you with new pleasure." This delicate politeness is particularly to be observed towards aged persons.

Interruptions. If your interlocutor is interrupted by any incident, when the cause of the interruption has ceased, do not wait until he resumes the conversation, but with a benevolent smile and an engaging gesture, invite him thus to proceed, "Please to continue; you were just saying . . . " If you are obliged to palliate any interruption, much more ought you never to allow yourself to cause one. This is so rigorous a rule, that if in the warmth of conversation two persons commence speaking at once, both ought to stop the moment they perceive it, and each, while excusing himself, to decline proceeding. It is proper for the one worthy of the most respect to resume the conversation.

Novices in the customs of society think they may simply interrupt a conversation which is begun, by asking for an explanation of some incident which they have not understood, or for a name to be repeated. This may be done only under certain circumstances, and then with much tact. If the narrator pronounces badly; if you see that other auditors are in the same situation as yourself; if you foresee that for want of having followed him in his narration, you will not be able to reply politely, you may interrupt. Here is the proper form: "I ask your pardon, I fear I have lost some part of your interesting conversation, will you be kind enough to repeat it?" &c. It is necessary also to choose a favourable moment, as for instance when the narrator pauses, hesitates over a word, or stops to take his handkerchief.

It may sometimes happen that you foresee some incident in an interesting story; and the pleasure which you take in this, the desire of showing that you have guessed correctly, and the intention of proving your interest, induce you to interrupt suddenly in this manner, "I follow you, it is like this." Such an interruption, though well meant and natural, will offend aged persons, who like to tell a story at full length, and will confound formal narrators, who will be in despair at being deprived of a showy phrase. These interruptions are only allowable amongst intimate friends, or inferiors. Otherwise you will receive an ill-humoured response, or a triumphant one such as, "No, you are quite mistaken," &c., which is exceedingly awkward.

The very worst kind of interruption is that dictated by arrogance. A clever person seizing hold of a story which another is telling, with the intention of making it more lively, becomes, despite his eloquence, a model of impertinence and vulgarity. It is doubtless hard to see a fool spoil a good anecdote, of which he might have made something interesting; but if propriety does not restrain you from expressing your feelings, interest should. Now auditors of delicacy will remain silent to the conclusion of the recital, and will address themselves with good-will to the poor narrator who is injured in his rights.

Interruption is pardonable if it is made to prove or clear up a fact in favour of a person who is absent. When they accuse you, you may if need be interrupt by an exclamation, but it is better to do it by a gesture. In a lively, animated, and friendly dialogue, people may interrupt each other by turns, in order to finish a sentence which is begun, or to improve an epithet. This contributes to vivacity in discourse; but it ought not to be too often repeated.

If a person relates any thing to you, who without having any pleasantry, makes attempts at it; or without being affecting, endeavours to move you, however bored you may be, appear pleased and assume an air of interest. If the narrator wanders into long digressions, have patience to let him extricate himself from the labyrinth of his story. If the history is interminable, be resigned, and do not appear less attentive. This forbearance is especially to be observed if you are listening to an aged person, or another deserving of respect. If the merciless story-teller is your equal or friend, you may say to him, in order to induce him to finish his narration, "And finally . . ."

Falsehoods. When a person relates to you an obvious falsehood, the art of listening becomes embarrassing. If you seem to believe it, you will pass for a fool, and if you appear to doubt it, you will pass for a boor. (See Div. 9.) A cold air, a slight attention, an expression such as, "That is astonishing," will extricate you honourably from the situation. When an event is narrated which is only extraordinary or doubtful, your manner should be otherwise. Your countenance should express astonishment, and you should reply with an expression such as, "If I did not know your strict regard for the truth" or, "If any person but you had told me this, I should scarcely have believed it." In any event you should not stop him.

When you are obliged to deny the assertion of any one, employ apologetical forms. The most proper ones are, "I may be mistaken," "I am undoubtedly mistaken, but," "Be so good as to excuse my mistake, but it seems to me," "I ask pardon, but I thought," &c. Those persons are but ill-bred, who think to soften down a denial merely by expressions of doubt. They say, "If what you advance is true," "If what Madam says is positive," &c. With these forms, they think they comply with the rules of propriety. It is incivility with affectation.

Additional Remarks. There are many shoals to be avoided in listening, which always betray inexperience in society. To say from time to time to the narrator, "Yes, yes" either by nodding your head, or by motioning with your hand, a habit of aged persons, which is a good representation of a pendulum; to keep your eyes fixed and your mouth gaping open; to have an absent-minded or pensive air; to point your finger at persons designated by the narrator; to yawn without concealing it with your hand or handkerchief, which is by no means flattering to the speaker; to cast your eye frequently towards the clock: all these habits are offences against good *ton*.

——*The Gentleman and Lady's Book of Politeness,
Manuel complet de la bonne compagnie.*

Diversion 1.

Swearing. There is one offence committed in conversation, of much too serious a nature to be overlooked, or to be animadverted on without sorrow and indignation; I mean, the habitual and thoughtless profaneness of those who are repeatedly invoking their Maker's name on the most trivial occasions. There is perhaps hardly any sin so frequently committed, so slightly censured, so seldom repented of, and so little guarded against. On the score of *impropriety*, too, it is additionally offensive, as being utterly repugnant to female delicacy, which often does not see the turpitude of this sin, while it affects to be shocked at swearing in a man.

——*The Female Instructor.*

Diversion 2.

The material from here to the end of the paragraph was omitted in the original American translation.

——Frances Grimble.

Diversion 3.

Of addressing Relations in French. The following material was omitted from the original American translation.

—————Frances Grimble.

When you do not say to parents, "Mademoiselle your daughter," it is customary to say "your young lady" *[demoiselle]*. The expression "your daughter" *[fille]* is no longer employed, because it is usual to give this title to courtesans, who have nearly been banished from society. In speaking of family members, avoid saying, "your father" or "your mother"; add the title "Monsieur" or "Madame." It would be affected to say "Messieurs your parents," in speaking in a general manner, but you may very well say, "Messieurs your brothers" or "Madames your sisters." If you are not well acquainted with these relations, this attention is less necessary, and you may say, "your cousins" without being impolite.

It would appear ridiculous in the highest degree to call your parents "Monsieur my father" and "Madame my mother." However, when speaking of your relations, it is good *ton* to call them by their names, adding the customary title. Thus you may say, "Monsieur Such-a-one" or "Mademoiselle Such-a-one." You may say of your in-laws, "my daughter-in-law," "my sister-in-law," &c. Only workmen have the habit (even within the household) of designating their relations by their family name, without being joined with the title of "Madame" or "Mademoi-selle," or even indicating the degree of relationship. Therefore they should say, "my aunt N" or "my cousin N," and never "the N," which is completely unacceptable.

—————*Manuel complet de la bonne compagnie.*

Diversion 4.

The Use of the Third Person in French. The following material was omitted from the original American translation.

—————Frances Grimble.

. . . or even better, "Monsieur and I," because do not forget that to speak in the third person is more polite and respectful. Sometimes it is necessary to be circumspect in employing this mode, because under some circumstances it has an air of servility. Between gentlemen it is seldom used. Besides, however estimable the person, it should not be used con-tinually. The only situation in which it is always perfectly proper, is when it is a question addressed to a lady. You may very well say, "Does Madame wish to join us?" or, "Does she wish to take the air?" &c.

——*Manuel complet de la bonne compagnie.*

Diversion 5.

Raillery. Some women indulge themselves in sharp raillery, unfeeling wit, and cutting sarcasms, from the consciousness, it is to be feared, that they are secured from the danger of being called to account; this license of speech being encouraged by the very circumstance which ought to suppress it. To be severe, because they can be so with impunity, is a most ungenerous reason. It is taking a base and dishonourable advantage of their sex; the weakness of which, instead of tempting them to commit offences because they may commit them with safety, ought rather to make them more scrupulously careful to avoid indiscretions, for which no reparation can be demanded. What can be said for those who carelessly involve the injured party in consequences from which they know themselves to be exempted, and whose very sense of their own security leads them to be indifferent to the security of others?

——*The Female Instructor.*

Diversion 6.

Arguments. If difficulties arise in your mind, and constrain your dissent to the things spoken, represent what objections some persons would be ready to make against the sentiments of the speaker, without telling him you oppose. This manner of address carries something more modest and obliging in it, than to appear to raise objections of your own by way of contradiction to the speaker.

When you are forced to differ from some one who delivers his sense on any point, yet agree as far as you can, and represent how far you agree; and if there is any room for it, explain the words of the speaker in a sense to which you can in general assent, and so agree with him. Or at least, by a small addition or alteration of his sentiments, show your own sense of things. It is the practice and delight of a candid auditor, to make it appear how unwilling he is to differ from the speaker. Let the speaker know that nothing but truth constrains you to oppose him; and let that difference be always expressed in few, and civil, and chosen words, such as give the least offence.

——*The Female Instructor.*

Diversion 7.

This verse was left in French in the original American translation. The version here is from Elizur Wright's 1841 translation of La Fontaine's *Fables*.

——Frances Grimble.

Diversion 8.

Listening. A certain Roman orator observed, that silence was so important a part of conversation, that there was not only an art, but an eloquence in it: how peculiarly does this apply to the modesty of young ladies! But the silence of listless and vapid ignorance, and the animated silence of sparkling intelligence, are two things almost as obviously distinct as the wisdom and the folly of the tongue. An inviolable and marked attention may show that a woman is pleased with a subject, and an illuminated countenance may prove that she understands it, almost as unequivocally as language itself could do. This, with a modest question, which indicates at once rational curiosity and becoming diffidence, is in many cases as large a share of the conversation as it is decorous for female delicacy to take. This would prove also a flattering encouragement for men of sense to pursue useful topics in the presence of women, did you yourself discover that desire of improvement which liberal-minded men are pleased with communicating.

——*The Female Instructor.*

Diversion 9.

Exaggeration. Out of a restless desire to please, grows the vain desire to astonish; for from vanity, as much as credulity, arises that strong love of the marvellous, with which the conversation of the ill-educated abounds. Hence that fondness for dealing in narratives hardly within the compass of possibility. Here vanity has many shades of gratification: those shades will be stronger or weaker, whether the relater chances to have been an eye-witness of the wonder she recounts, or whether she claims only the second-hand renown of its having happened to her friend, or the still remoter celebrity of its having been witnessed only by her friend's friend. To correct this propensity to "elevate and surprise," it is well in mixed society to abstain altogether from hazarding stories, which though they may not be absolutely false, yet lying without the verge of probability, are apt to impeach the credit of the narrator.

——*The Female Instructor.*

Chapter XXXII.
Epistolary Composition.

Next to social communications by means of visits and conversation, are those by means of letters and billets. It is not only absence, but a multiplicity of business and a great number of relations, which give a very great extension to this part of social relations. (See Div. 1.)

My readers have too much judgement to think that I wish to give them lessons in style, or teach them how they should write letters of friendship, congratulation, condolence, encouragement, apology, recommendation, invitation, complaint, or censure. This enumeration alone shows the impossibility of it. Some general reflections on epistolary conventions, and scrupulous details of the forms and ceremonial parts of letters, will compose this important chapter.

General Observations.

Letters, as I have said, supply the place of visits in bestowing presents, or on occasions of weddings, funerals, and other ceremonies; and to neglect to write in such a case, is gross impoliteness.

Letters for new year's day and other holidays, are usually written beforehand, in order to arrive on the previous or very same day. This is particularly required towards relations. For friends and intimate acquaintances, the following week will do, and for other persons, any time within the month.

It is as indispensable to respond when you are written to, as when you are spoken to, and the indolence which so many correspondents allow themselves in this respect is an incivility. And if after all they decide to answer, they begin with apologies so constantly renewed, that these become commonplace. You must use much care so that such excuses may not appear ridiculous. Conciseness, and some new terms of expression, are in this case indispensable. The same observation applies to reproaches for not writing.

The rules of propriety ought to decide as to the expense of postage. (See Div. 2.) They require you to defray the expense of the letter if it is written to a distinguished person, or to one of whom you ask any favour. But it would be an incivility, and sometimes a want of delicacy, to do it when you write to a friend, an acquaintance, or a person of little fortune, whose feelings you should fear to wound. Therefore, in order to both save him the expense and avoid dissatisfaction, endeavour to make some excuse of business.

The Appearance of Letters.

The choice of materials for writing, without being the most important thing, is yet necessary. To write on very coarse paper is allowable only for the most indigent; to use gilt-edged and perfumed paper for letters of business would be ridiculous. The selection of paper ought always to be in keeping with the person, age, sex, and circumstances of the correspondents. Ornamented paper, of which I have just spoken; paper bordered with coloured vignettes and embossed with ornaments in relief upon the edges, or slightly coloured with delicate shades, is designed for young ladies, and those whose condition, taste, and dignity presuppose habits of luxury and elegance. Many distinguished people, however, sensibly prefer simplicity in this thing, and make use of very beautiful, yet unornamented paper.

People of business, heads of companies or establishments, and persons of distinction with many titles, use paper printed at the top, that is, having the name of their residence, the first three figures of the date of the year, their address, and the words, "Mr. A— (here follow the titles) to Mr.—."

Letters of petition or request should be in folio, that is to say, upon a sheet of paper in its full size. The margin should be half the breadth of the page. The spaces and blanks which should be left between the upper edge of the paper and the salutation, and between the salutation and the first line, differ greatly according to the degree of inferiority or superiority. The greater the spaces, the more respect they indicate. The first line ought always to begin below the middle of the page, when you write to a person to whom you owe much respect; the second page should begin one line below the salutation. A blank space should always be left between the last words of the signature, and the lower edge of the paper. If there is not sufficient room, it is better to carry one or two lines over to the next page, than to fail in this respect.

For a familiar letter, it has become fashionable to leave no margin at all. However, it is only in these letters that margins may be used, namely, to receive a vertical line when all the paper is filled.

It is extremely impolite to write upon a single leaf of paper, even if it is a billet; it should be always double, even though you write only two or three lines. It is still more vulgar to use for an envelope, paper on which there are one or two words foreign to the letter itself, whether they are written or printed. Billets, letters folded lengthways, and half-envelopes are little used. A letter folded in quarters, especially if written upon vellum paper, should be pressed at the folds by means of a paper-knife.

Two persons should not write in the same letter, by one writing upon the first, and another upon the second leaf, unless you are intimate with the correspondent. The same is applicable to postscripts.

When you use no envelope, and the third page of the letter is all written upon, you should leave a small blank space where the seal is to be put; as without this precaution, some very important words may well be covered.

Every letter to a superior ought to be folded in quarters at the most. It should always have an envelope. It shows a want of respect to seal with a wafer; you must use sealing-wax. Gentlemen ordinarily select red; but young ladies use gilt, rose, and other colours. Both use black wax when they are in mourning. Except in this last case, the colour of the seal is immaterial, but not the size, for very large ones are in bad taste. The smaller and glossier, the better *ton* they are. Though sealing-wax is preferable, still you should avoid using it at times when you are afraid that the seal may be opened.

You should not seal a letter of respect with an antique device. It is more polite to use your coat of arms or initials. Persons of taste who have no coat of arms, adopt a seal bearing some ingenious device, in keeping with their profession, sentiments, &c.

When the letter is closed with or without an envelope, put only a single seal upon it; but if the letter is large, use two. If it contains important papers, it should have three seals or more, according to the kind and size of the envelope, and be sent insured. If a person takes charge of a letter as a favour, it would be very impolite to put more than one seal upon it. If the letter is folded so as to be open on one side, so that part of its contents may be read, it is equally impolite to put a little wax upon the edges. You may use this precaution only when the letter is sent by the post or by a servant. (See Div. 3.) It is only conscripts and peasants who fold a letter like an apothecary's packet, and omit to seal it with sealing-wax, or secure it all over with pins.

A letter which is to be shown, such as a letter of introduction or recommendation, should not be sealed, since the bearer ought necessarily to know the contents. To seal it without having first allowed the bearer to read it would be impolite. You should prove to the person recommended that you have spared no pains to render him a service.

Never seal petitions which are to be presented to the King, and to the members of the royal family.

The Style of Letters.

When you write upon any subject, consider it fully before putting it upon paper, and treat of each topic in order, that you may not be obliged to recur to any one again, after having spoken of another thing. If you have many subjects to treat of in the same letter, commence with the most important. If the person to whom you write is interrupted while reading it, he will be the more impatient to read the remainder, however little interesting he may find it. It is useful and convenient to begin a new paragraph at every change of the subject.

If in conversation you ought to attend to propriety of language, its choice and graceful euphony, it is even more necessary to endeavour to make your style in writing clear, precise, elegant, and appropriate to all subjects. The vivacity of discourse frequently forces the sacrifice of happy though tardy expressions, to the necessity of avoiding hesitancy. But this obstacle in speaking does not interfere with the use of the pen. Therefore, avoid repetitions, erasures, insertions, omissions, confusion of ideas, and laboured construction. If you write a familiar letter to an equal or a friend, these blemishes may remain; otherwise you must commence your letter again. The most exact observance of the rules of language is strictly necessary. A fault of orthography, or an incorrect expression, are not allowable even in the least careful letter or the most unimportant billet. Even correction is not admissible; for besides being a blemish on the letter, it betrays the ignorance or inattention of the writer.

For these reasons, it is well to make a rough draft, if you are little accustomed to epistolary style, and if being very young you cannot perfectly remember the rules of syntax and the dictionary. Some persons, it is true, censure this precaution, which they say marks the style with affectation and stiffness. This censure does not seem to me well founded. The loss of time which this method entails, is a more real inconvenience; and for this reason, and because of the difficulty which you may find in it, it is well to accustom yourself to writing a letter extempore neatly, elegantly, and correctly.

You may use a lofty style towards persons to whom you owe respect; an easy, trifling, or even jesting style towards a friend; and a courteous style towards ladies generally. You should not write in a trifling style to persons of higher rank. It sometimes happens that a great man honours with his friendship a man of lower rank, and is pleased that the latter writes to him without ceremony. In this case you may use the privilege which is given you; but take care not to abuse it, and to make known from time to time that you are ready to confine yourself within respectful bounds.

Take care, when writing to a person worthy of respect, not to send compliments to any one. Instead, write to this third person whatever you wish him to know.

Figures are used only for sums and dates. Numbers of men, days, weeks, &c., are to be written at length.

The Forms for Formal and Informal Letters.

In addressing the Pope, say at the top of the letter, "Holy Father" or "Most Holy Father"; and instead of "You" say, "Your Holiness." To a prime cardinal say, "My Lord" and "Your Most Eminent Highness." To a cardinal say, "My Lord" and "Your Eminence." To an archbishop or bishop say, "My Lord" and "Your Grace." To an emperor or empress say, "Sire" or "Madam," and instead of "You," say, "Your Imperial Majesty." To a king say, "Sire" and "Your Majesty." To a queen say, "Madam" and "Your Majesty." To the brother of a king say, "Your Royal Highness." To an Elector of the Holy Roman Empire say, "Your Electoral Highness." To a sovereign prince say, "Your Most Serene Highness." To a prince say, "Your Highness." To an ambassador or minister say, "Your Excellency." To the Chancellor of France say, "My Lord" and "Your Lordship." The title "Excellency" is not given to ladies. The daughters of the King of France are called "Madame" from the cradle. To a lieutenant-general or brigadier say, "General."

Titles of respect, such as "Lordship," "Majesty," "Highness," "Excellency," "Honour," "Madam," &c., ought never to be abbreviated, either in writing to the persons themselves, or to any one acquainted with them.

Persons who have an exact knowledge of the language and customs of the court, know the most proper manner of expressing themselves. Here are some examples in which the different degrees of respect may be readily perceived. "I have received the letter with which you have been pleased to honour me," "which you have done me the favour to write to me," "which you have done me the honour to write to me," "which you have taken the trouble to write to me," or, "I have received your letter of the 12th of this month."

The Forms for Letters.

Some persons commence their letters with the words, "I have received yours of the 12th." This is a fault; you should say, "your letter." The first is the style of merchants, who being pressed with business, are obliged to make abbreviations. You must, in the common customs of life, beware of imitating them in this respect. I may say the same in regard to persons who express their pleasure in writing to you, or who put at the top of their letters, "I have received your honoured letter of such a date," or "In answer to your honoured letter," or "I write you these few words." All these forms are objectionable.

Never repeat in the first sentence of a letter, the names "My Lord," "Sir," or "Madam," with which you began. But if you write to a prince, or even to a minister, after the first line use the words, "Your Majesty," "Your Highness," or "Your Excellency," and repeat them from time to time in the course of the letter, if it is of some length.

After having written "Sir" or "Madam" at the top of the letter, do not commence with one of these phrases, "Sir, Mrs.—, your sister, has written to me that . . . " You should say, "I understand by a letter which Mrs.—, your sister, has written to me . . . "

As to the conclusion of a letter, do not say simply, "I am," without adding some such phrase as, "With the most profound respect," "with profound respect," "with the highest regard," &c. To persons who have the title of "Majesty," "Highness," "Eminence," &c., say, "I am your Majesty's" or "your Highness's," &c. "very humble," &c.

The words "esteem" and "affection" are used alone, only in letters to friends or acquaintances, because they are too familiar; but when accompanied by words which relieve them, they do not offend. As for example, "I am with profound respect, and the highest esteem," &c. The following forms may be used with elegance: "Accept, Sir, the assurances of high consideration," "Be pleased to accept the assurances," &c.

It is not allowable, except to familiar friends, to use expressions borrowed from foreign languages, for instance the Italian phrase, "I kiss your hands," &c. The language of gentlemen who write to ladies ought always to have a polish of respect, with which the latter may dispense in answering. Except for the most ceremonious letters, a lady ought not to address to a gentleman such phrases as, "I have the honour to be," &c., while the latter should use the most respectful formulas, such as, "Deign, madam, to allow me," "Allow me the honour of presenting you my respects," &c.

I have not the folly to regulate the sentiments of the heart by any ceremonial. But there is in reality nothing more cold and ridiculous, than accumulations of such epithets as, "Your tender, sincere, and constant friend," "A thousand kisses," &c.

The date of a letter may be put at the beginning when you write to an equal. But in writing to a superior, it should be at the end, in order that the title at the head of the letter may be entirely alone. In letters of business, on the contrary, it is necessary to put the date at the top and on the first line, that persons may conveniently know the chronological order of their communications. The date is often necessary to the understanding of many passages of your letter, or to explain the sense of one which your correspondent may have received at the same time from another person.

A letter is generally addressed to one person only. If it is written to all the members of a family, the address may be given, with the addition of all their names.

It is well to add the recipient's name, title, or profession, in order to prevent any mistake. However, if circumstances have obliged any one of your acquaintance to act in an inferior situation, it would be a want of delicacy to join his name to that of his business.

Some distinguished persons are flattered by your omitting to precisely designate their address when writing to them. This is an error; you should clearly indicate the town, province, state, &c. if there is more than one town of the same name. In a large city, it is well to write the name of the street and number, as well as the district where the street is. People of business abbreviate this by putting "N" and the number, or the number alone; but this practice is more expeditious than polite.

When you write to the King, put simply in the address, "To the King." To foreign kings you say, "To his Catholic Majesty," "To his Britannic Majesty," &c. To persons who have the title of "Highness," say, "To his Highness," and then their position. To ministers and ambassadors, say, "To his Excellency, the Minister" or "Ambassador." If a person has several titles, select the highest, and omit the others.

Billets.

Do not write a billet to ladies or to superiors, as this custom was introduced only to avoid ceremony.

Put the date of the day, "Monday," &c. at the top of the paper. It is well sometimes to add the hour. Begin the letter about two inches below. The word "Sir" is put in the first line. Conclude with one of these phrases, "I am, Sir, yours"; "I am truly yours," &c.

The most unceremonious billets, contrary to common sense, are written in the third person. They contain very little, and begin thus, "Mr. *or* Mrs. Such-a-one presents his respects, or compliments, to Mr. Such-a-one, and requests," &c. After having made the request, end with, "and will oblige his humble servant." If the recipient is of the same profession, say "colleague," because you should seize every opportunity for politeness. In this kind of billet, it is best not to use the pronoun "he" or "she," for independently of the incivility, it might result in confusion. Sometimes it would be difficult to know whether the pronoun referred to the recipient, or to the writer.

——*The Gentleman and Lady's Book of Politeness,*
Manuel complet de la bonne compagnie.

Diversion 1.

Time devoted to Correspondence. Mrs. L.—If a newly-married lady happens to be at a great distance from her family connexions, how far is it proper, or essential in reference to her new character, to maintain with them an extensive epistolary correspondence? Would it not very much interfere with her domestic duties?

Mrs. B.—After marriage, various may be the impediments in the way of personal intercourse, and but for the communication which writing affords, we should lose a source of happiness arising from keeping up mutual interest in the welfare of relations. Still, an extensive correspondence cannot be continued after marriage, consistently with the increased duties in which domestic concerns and good neighbourhood involve many married women. The constant locomotion these require tends to destroy also the relish for such tacit conversation, and for the still life which, in idea, an absent spot presents, and which are opposed to the active scenes and employments in which the married woman finds herself called upon to take her share. It may therefore seem needless to guard her against the attempt to carry on an extensive correspondence; a few months may perhaps see it gradually diminished, and her letters become, "like angel visits, few and far between," until they cease altogether. As it is not, however, pleasant to incur the charges of "changeableness" and "forgetfulness," to which this natural death of her correspondence would render her liable, the young married woman should select a chosen few from amongst those friends whom sterling qualities render valuable, and whose friendship she may hope not only to retain herself to the end of her life, but to bequeath to her children.

——*Domestic Duties.*

Diversion 2.

Expense of Correspondence. Mrs. L.—Do any other disadvantages attend an extensive correspondence?

Mrs. B.—In a pecuniary point of view, an extensive correspondence may prove a serious evil in the marriage state. It is one of those enjoyments which, however agreeable, is not essential; and a wife is not less responsible for squandering money, under certain circumstances, on the trifling gossiping of an extensive epistolary correspondence, than in the purchase of superfluous ornaments. No postage may be regarded as extravagant, when it is the means of conveying intelligence of the welfare of our relations and friends; but to a gentleman of limited income the expense of daily packets addressed to his wife, which contain nothing but commonplace remarks, or every-day news, is both an oppressive and injurious tax.

——Domestic Duties.

Diversion 3.

Discretion in Correspondence. Mrs. L.—Is it necessary for a married woman to permit her letters to be opened by her husband?

Mrs. B.—A sensible man, who has confidence in the prudence of his wife, will have no desire to assume that privilege, which his situation as a husband confers upon him; nor to infringe on the sacredness of her correspondence. The slightest tincture of suspicion is incompatible with the mutual happiness of a husband and wife. A married woman therefore, though her husband may not desire it, should voluntarily place her letters in his hands, feeling that in so doing she is merely sharing with him the pleasure they may bestow, or alleviating the poignancy of grief their intelligence may impart. It is always preferable, however, for both parties to hold the correspondence of the other sacred, and not even to desire to become a party in it.

Mrs. L.—But is it not impossible for a married woman to have any correspondence which should be concealed, under any circumstances, from her husband?

Mrs. B.—It is certainly more advisable to have none which he cannot inspect; but circumstances may arise, in the progress of life, to involve the married woman in a correspondence of which it might not be proper to make her husband a party. A letter may convey to her communications relative to an early friend or acquaintance, which are confidentially imparted to her. Under these circumstances, though she might not be willing to betray the confidence of her friend, she ought to satisfy the mind of her husband, with sufficient reasons for not being more explicit towards him. If she can convince him that the correspondence has no reference to herself, but relates to the private concerns of her friend, it will scarcely be sufficient to excite any interest in his mind, or to create the slightest suspicion unfavourable towards his wife.

——*Domestic Duties.*

Chapter XXXIII.
Additional Rules
for the Social Relations.

Here I include proper conduct for friendly attentions, such as services, loans, presents, and advice; and also for discretion, regarding conversations, letters, secrets, confidences, &c.

Advice.

Advice is a very good thing, it is true; but in society it is one of the least pleasing things. A giver of advice who is incessantly repeating, "If I were in your place, I would do thus-and-so," repels every one by his arrogance and indiscretion. Such an impertinent person should know that he ought not to give advice unless he is asked, and that the number of those who ask for it is very limited.

However, I am not speaking here of gratifying vanity, but of advice whose kindness and affection gives it a claim to attention. It is important to use much reserve and care. Otherwise, you would seem to have a tone of superiority which would array your friend's self-esteem against your wisest counsels. Of the forms of modesty, not one is superfluous here. You may say, "It is possible that I am mistaken," "I should be far from having the courage to ask of you," &c. If a person makes any objections, do not say, "You do not understand me" but "I have expressed myself badly."

Discretion.

The duties of discretion are so sensibly felt by well-bred persons, that they do not violate them except through forgetfulness. It will, therefore, be enough to enumerate them, without pointing out their necessity.

Discretion requires in the first place, respect with regard to conversation. If when you enter the house of any one, you hear people talking animatedly, step more heavily, in order to give them notice. If in an assembly, two persons retire by themselves to speak of business, be careful not to approach them, nor to speak to them until they have separated.

Discretion.

People who have lived a little in the world, know how essential it is not to inquisitively interfere in the business or habits of persons whom they visit; nor are they ignorant of how to behave in case they surprise some one by an unexpected visit. But young persons may not know, and I beg them to give their attention to it.

When you see a person occupied, you retire, or at least make signs of it. If he detains you, step aside, and appear to be contemplating a picture, or looking out of the window, to prove that you take no notice of what engages him. But the desire to find for yourself some such occupation, should not lead you to leaf through books placed upon the chimney-piece or elsewhere; to run over a pamphlet; or to handle visiting-cards or letters, if only to read the superscription. If the person you are visiting is opening an armoire or drawers, it would be rude curiosity to approach in order to see what was contained there. If amongst a number of valuable things, he takes out one to show you, be satisfied with looking at that alone, without appearing to think of the others.

If before the person you are visiting comes in, you encounter another visitor, who to pass the time takes a journal or a book from his pocket, it would be extremely impolite to read over his shoulder, and likewise to read what a person is writing.

It is not allowable to take down the books from a library. But you may, and even ought to read the titles, in order to praise the good taste which has been shown in the choice of the works.

If it happens that any one exhibits to a circle some rare and valuable object, be not in haste to ask for it, or reach out your hand for it. Wait modestly until it comes to you. Do not examine it too long when you have it, and if by chance any ill-bred person requests it before you have seen it, do not detain it; for it is better to suffer this small privation than to appear ill-bred yourself. However insignificant the boasted object may be, do not criticize it. If your opinion is asked, respond with a few words of praise; if the thing is really curious, abstain from exaggerated compliments.

To violate the secrecy of letters, under any pretext whatever, is so base and odious, that I hardly dare to say a word about it. I think, however, I ought to say, that it is also very reprehensible to endeavour to read any part of a letter folded so that the ends are open. (See Chapter XXXII.) When a certain passage in a letter concerning yourself is handed you to read, put your finger below it in order not to read any thing more. If you are allowed to add any thing to a letter, have the discretion not to cast your eyes over the rest, and be expeditious so as to avoid any suspicion that you take advantage of the opportunity.

Propriety is also opposed, in certain cases, to excessive haste to know any thing concerning yourself. For example, if a person brings you a letter, do not hasten to open it, but consider whether the letter concerns the bearer at all, or only yourself. In the first case, you should open it, and read it while he is present; in the second, lay it aside.

Propriety does not, however, impose such restraints upon curiosity in small matters, and leave you free in important ones. Therefore, I shall not say that you ought religiously to keep a secret, or that confidence received is a sacred trust. But I shall say to persons who have the curiosity to know any private circumstance, that they ought to be filled with shame if they do not desist from all importunity as soon as they hear the phrase, "It is a secret."

Favours.

Polite persons are necessarily obliging. A smile is always on their lips, an attentiveness in their countenance, when you ask a favour of them. They know that to render a service with bad grace, is in reality not to render it at all. If they are forced to refuse, they do it mildly and delicately; they express such feeling regret, that they still inspire you with gratitude. In short, their conduct appears so perfectly natural, that it really seems that the opportunity which is offered them of obliging you is obliging themselves; and they refuse all your thanks without affectation or effort.

This amiable character, a necessary attendant of perfect civility, is not always found with all its charms. There are besides some obliging persons who force you to extort their services, who feel of great consequence, and like to be supplicated and thanked to excess. Do not imitate them: they render you ungrateful in spite of yourself, and make gratitude a torment and a burden. When some one asks any favour of you, reply kindly, "I am at your service, and shall be very happy to render you any assistance in my power;" or else, with a sad manner, lament that there is such-and-such obstacle, &c. Then consider the means of overcoming the obstacle, even if you are assured beforehand that there are none.

Other persons, pretending to be polite, make declarations of their services and zeal, without taking the trouble to abide by their offers when an occasion is afforded them. So great is their trifling in this respect, that they may be justly compared to those false heroes who are always talking of fighting, but who would be put to flight at the sight of a drawn sword. These professions of zeal are suspicious when they are employed every moment and without any reason; a knowledge of the world teaches you to discern them, and to give them the degree of confidence which they merit.

Sometimes you may congratulate people, wish them well, and appear to take an interest in the recital which they are making of their affairs, without really feeling the slightest interest in them. You cannot always command your indifference in this respect; but you are obliged to spare them that constraint and ennui, which would infallibly arise if you displayed to them the coldness which they inspire. It belongs to persons who know the world, not to confound this forbearance with the pretended zeal of the Don Quixote of the drawing-room, of whom I spoke earlier.

For a service to be rendered perfectly, it is imperative for it to be rendered quickly, nothing being more disobliging than tardiness, and offering the person the choice between addressing new solicitations to you, or suffering by your delay. Your slow assistance may perhaps be detrimental, for some would suffer a long time before resolving to importune you anew. If any circumstance prevents you from acting, inform the person, apologize, and promise to make reparation for your neglect. On his part, the person who will be under the obligation to you, should be careful not to use a single term of reproach, or accost you with an air of dissatisfaction.

Loans.

When any one who is visiting you has need of a shawl, a handkerchief, or a hat, offer it with a complaisant zeal, resist the refusal which may be made (and which propriety does not require), select the best you have, and finish by urging the person not to be in haste to return the articles. If it is very bad weather, and there is occasion, offer your umbrella or even your carriage. The articles thus lent are returned the next day by a servant, who is charged to thank you for them. But if they are linen, they should not be returned without having been washed.

When a lady has borrowed jewels of another, the latter should always offer to lend her many more than are asked for. She ought also to keep a profound silence about the articles which she has lent, and even abstain from wearing them for some time afterwards, to prevent their being recognized. If any one, perceiving they were borrowed, spoke to the parties of it, he would pass for an ill-bred character. If the borrower speaks to you of it, it is well to reply that no one recognized them. All this advice is minute, but what kind will you have? It concerns female self-esteem.

One species of borrowing which occurs daily, very often to the loss of the owners, is the borrowing of books. People are so wanting in delicacy in this regard, that book-fanciers who are very obliging in other respects, are forced to refuse these troublesome loans. And yet the thing is difficult. You cannot say, "I am not willing to lend you this work." But if the borrower is a suspicious person, you may say that you have need of it, to your very great regret, but that you will lend it to him in a few days. However, you do not lend it at all.

Well-bred persons do not make a bald request for a book. They wait until it is offered, and then accept the offer hesitantly; they find out the length of time they may keep it, and return it punctually on the appointed day. In order to prevent every accident, they cover it with cloth or paper, since the favour should render them more careful than the value of the book. They also take care not to turn down the leaves, or make marks, marginal notes, &c.

If any accident happens to a borrowed article, without saying any thing, you must repair the loss immediately. I shall not speak of more important loans, which are outside the jurisdiction of propriety.

Presents.

In the eyes of persons of delicacy, presents have no value, except from the manner in which they are bestowed. Therefore, in my advice I shall strive to give them this value.

Presents are offered first to relations and then to friends. This is done under divers circumstances: on your arrival at a place from which you have been absent for a long time; when your intimate friends leave the town in which you reside; on your return from a journey, particularly to the capital, or to remarkable and remote countries; and on birthdays, name-days, and new year's day.

But such a day is not only the occasion of exchanging presents in a family. It is a day for acknowledging services and civilities; of paying your respects to ladies, and to superiors whom you wish to honour. It also offers you a tactful means of succouring the unfortunate. At harvest time, if you own land; and in the hunting season, if a hunter, it is good *ton* to send your intimate friends fine fruits, rare flowers, or some choice cuts of game.

Next to fitness of time for presents, comes fitness in the selection of them; generally, luxury and elegance ought to reign in the latter. But this rule has numerous exceptions. Though it would be out of place to offer purely useful things (which in some circumstances would have the appearance of charity), still you would be in error to suppose that a present is suitable, which is brilliant alone. It must by all means be adapted to the taste, age, and profession of the person, and his connexion with you. Thus to superiors, you present fruit, game, &c.; to a studious man, books; to a friend of the arts, music or engravings; to young married ladies, delicate and graceful articles of the toilet, &c. (It is not polite to offer books after you have cut the leaves.)

The most delicate presents are the productions of your own industry; a drawing, a piece of needle-work, ornamental hair-work, &c. But such offerings, though invaluable amongst friends, are not used on occasions of ceremony.

Presents should excite surprise and pleasure; therefore you ought to involve them in a little mystery, and present them with an air of joyful kindness. When you have made your offering, and thanks have been returned, do not bring back the conversation to the subject: particularly avoid making your present of consequence. On the contrary, when its merit has been extolled, and the person who has received the present has evinced a lively satisfaction, say that the present receives all its value from his opinion of it.

However slight the charm a present may have, or even if it is preposterous, you would be ill-bred not to manifest much pleasure in receiving it. It is also necessary, when an opportunity offers, to speak of it, and not fail to tell the donor how useful or agreeable his present is to you. The more time has passed, the more amiable this attention is; it proves that you have preserved the object with care. And this reminds me to say that you should never give away a present which you have received from another person—or at least you should so arrange it, that it may never be known.

It is well to mingle some reproaches on the high value of the present with your expressions of gratitude, but not to dwell a long time on the subject, or to exclaim earnestly about it. Under some circumstances, these declamations may seem dictated by avarice and indelicacy; and they are in bad taste at all times.

A present is often made to some one through his children or wife, especially on new year's day, when it is the custom to present at least confectionery to young families of your acquaintance. At Paris, such presents are made to married ladies; in the provinces, they are not.

Above all, when some one has received a present of some value, he calls upon the donor, or if the distance is great, sends him a letter of thanks. Every one knows that custom requires you to give the servant who carries the present a gratuity of proportionate value.

With this subject, I shall conclude my treatise on propriety, hoping that, having arrived at this point, my readers will say, "Evidently this work is comprehensive and methodical." I shall not dare to flatter myself with more; but that is enough, for it is assurance that my labour has been useful.

I trust therefore, that I have rendered an essential service to young people in making them acquainted with these rules, which have become so necessary. In truth the propriety on which we pride ourselves at the present day is a virtue which you ought never to renounce, since it gives to the intercourse of life that sweetness, pleasure, elegance, and charm which may be truly felt only by those who possess it. The learned Madame Lambert put it very well: "Politeness is the desire of pleasing those with whom you are obliged to live, and in a manner causing all around you to be satisfied with you; superiors with your respect; equals with your esteem; and inferiors with your kindness." (See Div. 1.)

——*The Gentleman and Lady's Book of Politeness,*
Manuel complet de la bonne compagnie.

Diversion 1.

The Manners of the French. The following material was left out of the original American translation.

——Frances Grimble.

Young people, I appeal to you in the name of your homeland; it is in your own interest. Strive, by your politeness, consideration, and propriety, to nourish in the minds of other nations, that high ideal of manners which we have formed. Foreigners will be able to report their feelings of esteem for the peoples amongst whom they have lived. But they will always remain enchanted by the manners full of affability and grace which they encountered only in the French.

——*Manuel complet de la bonne compagnie.*

Finis.

Glossary, Bibliography, and Index.

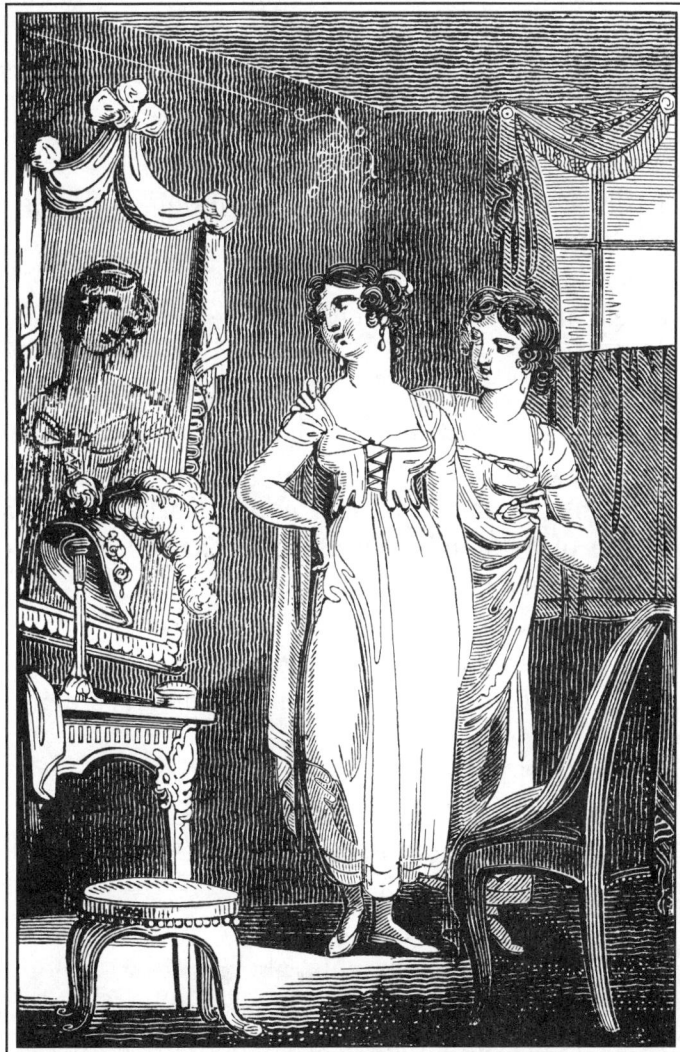

Glossary.

Most definitions below are rewritten or translated from sources which are contemporary, or as near to it as possible. In addition to the books listed in the first part of the bibliography, the principal sources are: the sixth edition of the *Dictionnaire de l'Académie Française*, 1832–1835, the first edition of Samuel Johnson's *Dictionary of the English Language*, 1755, and John Walker's *Critical Pronouncing Dictionary*, 1835. Most terms defined in the main body of the text are not included here.

À baguette. Shaped like a stick.

À cheval. Literally "astride." Refers to the positioning of a tape or riband when binding an edge.

À crochet. Shaped like a hook.

À dentelle. Dentelle means "lace." To mend *à dentelle* is to mend with lace stitches.

À étoile. Star-shaped.

Affiquet. A narrow hollow stick used by knitters to support the needle on which they make the first stitch, when they wish to make a new one.

Aigrette. An upright bunch of feathers used to ornament a head-dress. Or, a bunch of diamonds, pearls, &c. disposed in the shape of an aigrette and used similarly.

À la Madonna. A simple coiffure with a centre part.

À la paresseuse. Literally *paresseuse* means "lazy woman." A species of stays which is not laced, but is fastened with straps tightened by the wearer.

Alembic. A vessel used in distilling.

Alkanet. This plant is a species of bugloss, with a red root, from the Levant and the southern parts of France.

Alum. A kind of mineral salt, of an acid taste.

Amaranth. A dark reddish-purple.

Ambergris. A fragrant drug, which melts almost like wax, commonly of a greyish or ash-colour, used as both a perfume and a cordial.

Ambrette. This seed emits simultaneously an odour of amber and of musk, which is very agreeable, peculiar, and diffusive.

Angel-water. Take a pint each of orange-flower water and rose-water, and half a pint of myrtle water. To these put a quarter of a drachm of distilled spirit of musk, and a drachm of spirit of ambergris. Shake the whole well together, and preserve for use.

Antique oil *à la jonquille.* Jonquil-scented hair-oil.

Antique oil *à la tubéreuse.* Tuberose-scented hair-oil.

Antique oil *au cédrat.* Citron-scented hair-oil.

Antique oil *au citron.* Lemon-scented hair-oil.

Antique oil *au girofle.* Clove-scented hair-oil.

Apollo knot. A loop of plaited hair, of which one or several may compose a coiffure.

Aquafortis. The nitric acid of commerce.

Archil. Any of divers lichens which yield a coloured dye, and the colouring matter prepared from them.

Artificial flowers. These are sometimes made of very fine coloured paper, sometimes of the inside linings upon which the silkworm spins its silk, but principally of cambric.

À tuyaux. Fluted.

Bag. A kind of pocket made of leather, toile, or material, which is sewed at the bottom and sides, leaving only the top open to put in what you will. Formerly called a reticule or ridicule.

Balm of Mecca. This is a liquid resin, of a whitish colour, approaching to yellow, with a strong smell resembling that of a lemon, and a pungent and aromatic taste. It is one of the most highly-esteemed cosmetics, though very dear, and in its genuine form extremely difficult to procure. That sold in Paris and London is made by the perfumers of those cities, and is a mixture of the finest turpentine with the aromatic oils, whose aroma approaches nearest to that of the genuine balm.

Bandeau. A band which is used to encircle the forehead and the head.

Barège. A material of light, untwilled woollen used to make shawls, *fichus,* gowns, &c.

Barwood. A red wood imported from Africa, used chiefly for dyeing.

Batiste. A species of very fine, tightly-woven linen.

Baumé. A kind of hydrometer, of which the scale is uniformly graduated, or the aforesaid scale.

Beetle. A heavy mallet, or wooden hammer.

Belt. The French *ceinture* can mean either belt, sash, or waist-band; or sometimes fancy braces, or a pair of short stays. Unless something else is clearly meant, it is always translated here as "belt."

Benzoin. A medicinal kind of resin, imported from the East Indes.

Bergamot. This most useful perfume is procured from the *Citrus bergamia* or bergamot orange, by expression from the peel of the fruit. It has a soft sweet odour.

Bergère. A species of arm-chair wider and deeper than ordinary arm-chairs, and furnished with a cushion on which to sit.

Bias. Sloping; contrary to the straight-way of the material. To obtain a perfect bias, fold the material slantways so that the bottom of the material, all along the width, is laid on one selvage. Also, a piece of material cut out on the bias; such are frequently used for trimmings.

Bismuth. A hard, white, brittle, mineral substance, of a metalline nature, found at Misnia. White rouge is made of this metal.

Bite. *Mordre* in the French. The action of taking stitches more or less deeply into the material.

Black points. Blackheads.

Blond. A silk bobbin-lace, which may be either cream-colour or black.

Body *à la Marie Stuart*. A tight body with a pointed waist in front, and a bone down the middle of the front.

Body *à la Sévigné*. With plaited folds across the top of the front, divided in the middle.

Body *en gerbe*. The front, and sometimes also the back, is plaited or gathered so as to fan out from the waist to the shoulders.

Bombasine. A light silken material whose manufacture has been brought from Milan to France. Used for mourning.

Book-muslin. A plain clear description of muslin.

Borax. An artificial salt, prepared from sal ammoniac, nitre, calcined tartar, sea-salt, and alum, dissolved in wine.

Bouillons. Large round plaits made in certain materials for attire or ornament. Puffs.

Bourré. Raw silk.

Bouteille. Literally "bottle," and generally considered equivalent to either an American pint or quart.

Braid. The French *ganse* can refer to either a cord or a braid, depending upon how the word is modified. In this work it is usually translated as either "round braid," or "flat braid."

Brandenburgh. An ornamental loop or frog, usually of braid. Used for both fastening and decoration.

Breadth. An indefinitely long piece of material across the full width, between the two selvages. Also, the straight pieces of a skirt.

Broché. Embossed linen or figured materials.

Bucellas. A kind of Portuguese white wine.

Buckram. A kind of strong linen cloth, stiffened with gum, used by tailors and stay-makers.

Bullion. Gold embroidery thread.

Burat. A light, plain-woven material for gowns; used for mourning.

Buttons. There are several kinds; some are made of gold or silver lace, others of mohair, silk, horse-hair, thread, metal, glass, &c.

Cache-peigne. A loop of hair which serves to conceal the comb or riband which holds a woman's coiffure. Or, flowers, ribands, or pearls placed behind the head as if to conceal the comb.

Cajeput oil. The fragrant oil of the cajeput tree.

Calcareous. Containing lime or lime-stone.

Calcine. To burn in the fire to a calx, or friable substance.

Calendering. A finishing process, which produces a smooth and glossy surface by passing the material between heated steel rollers.

Calico. An Indian material made of cotton; sometimes stained with gay and beautiful colours.

Cambric. A kind of fine linen.

Cambric muslin. An imitation of cambric, made of cotton instead of flax.

Camion. A very small pin.

Camwood. A hard red wood imported from West Africa, and used for dyeing.

Canezou. A woman's garment, like the body of a gown without sleeves.

Caoutchouc. India-rubber.

Carbonic acid. A solution of carbon dioxide in water; a weak acid.

Carmine. A bright red or crimson colour, bordering on purple.

Carpenter's stool. A saw-horse.

Cassas. A soft fine India muslin.

Castile soap. A fine hard soap.

Catarrh. A defluxion of a sharp serum from the glands about the head and throat.

Centime. The hundredth part of a franc.

Cerate. A medicine made with wax, which with oil, or some softer substance, makes a consistence softer than a plaster.

Chamberlye. Urine.

Chatelaine. A massive gold chain attached to the belt by an ornament of the same metal, and falling considerably below the waist. A gold key ornamented with jewels is attached to the chain, as are also some other trinkets of an antique form; but the key is *de rigueur*.

Chauffe-pied à lampe. A foot-warmer which uses an oil-lamp and a heat reservoir placed over it, rather than a fire.

Chaufferette. A kind of box lined with sheet tin, with holes pierced in the top, into which a fire is put to keep the feet warm.

Chemisette. A garment which is worn over the chemise, and which ordinarily extends from the shoulders to the hips.

Cherry-tree gum. An exudation yielded by the cherry, plum, apricot, and almond trees. Similar to gum-arabic.

Chilblains. Sores made by frost.

Chip. Wood, or a woody fibre, split into thin filaments to make hats and bonnets.

Chrysolite. A precious stone of a dusky green, with a cast of yellow.

Cinnabar. Cinnabar is native or factitious; the factitious cinnabar is called vermilion.

Citrate of potash. Citric acid combined with potash to produce a salt.

Citronella. Under this name there is an oil in the market, chiefly derived from Ceylon and the East Indes. Its true origin is unclear; in odour it somewhat resembles citron fruit, but is very inferior. Probably it is procured from one of the grasses of the *Andropogan* genus.

Civet. The civet is a little animal, not unlike our cat. The perfume is formed like a kind of grease, or a thick scum, in an aperture or bag under its tail. It must be used in very small quantities, for unless the odour is greatly diluted it is offensive; but mixed in minute proportions with other perfumes, it strengthens their energies.

Cloth. A general term for any material, but especially woollens.

Cochineal. An insect, gathered and dried, from which a beautiful red colour is extracted.

Coiffe. The lining of the crown of a hat or bonnet.

Collerette. A kind of linen collar, covering the throat and shoulders.

Cologne water. Though this was originally introduced to the public as a kind of "cure-all," a regular "elixir of life," it now takes its place, not as a pharmaceutical product, but amongst perfumes.

Comb *à papillottes.* Literally "curl-paper comb."

Comb *du cou.* Literally "comb for the neck."

Combs. The commoner sorts are generally made of bullocks' horns, or of elephants' and sea-horses' teeth. Some of are made of tortoise-shell, and others of box, holly, and other hard woods.

Constantia. A sweet dessert wine.

Consumption. Tuberculosis.

Copperas. A name given to several sorts of vitriol, the blue being sulphate of copper, the green a native iron sulphate, the white copiapite, and the yellow sulphate of zinc.

Cord. The French *ganse* can refer to either a cord or a braid, depending upon how the word is modified. In this work it is usually translated as either "round braid," or "flat braid." Only occasionally are cords referred to by *cordon*.

Cordon. A French term for cord, made of divers materials; used for trimming.

Cordonnet. A raised rim, like that of a needle-lace.

Cornette. A kind of head-dress which women wear in dishabille.

Côte-pali. A light material, of silk and goat hair.

Coulis. Strong broth, gravy, jelly.

Court plaster. Take half an ounce of isinglass, and a drachm of Turlington's or friar's balsam. Melt the isinglass in an ounce of water, and boil the solution until a great part of the water is consumed. Then gradually add the balsam to it, stirring them well together. After the mixture has continued a short time on the fire, take the vessel off. While the mixture is yet fluid with heat, spread it onto the extended silk with a brush.

Coutil. A species of toile made of hemp or linen thread, very tight and smooth.

Crape. A very light transparent material, in some respects like gauze. However, it is made of raw silk, gummed and twisted on the mill, and woven without crossing. It is used for mourning, and is now a very fashionable article in court gowns.

Cravat. A close neck-cloth.

Crêpe aerophane. A finely-crimped crape.

Crêpe de chine. A crape made of raw silk.

Crêpe gaufré. Crimped crape.

Crêpe lisse. A kind of crape which is not crimped, commonly used for women's head-dresses.

Cross-way. Though "on the cross" is a British term for "bias," in this work "cross-way" means straight across the material or the garment; that is, along the weft threads.

Cudbear. A purple or violet powder used for dyeing, prepared from divers kinds of lichens.

Curaçoa. An orange liqueur.

Cyprus crape. A thin transparent black material.

Danzig. A kind of brandy.

Deal. Firwood; the wood of pines.

Delft. A kind of glazed earthenware.

Demi-saison. Autumn.

Demi-tasse. Literally half a cup. Unhappily no definition of the exact quantity, at this time and place and for this use, has been found.

Dentelle en carreaux. Lace with square openings.

Diachylon. A kind of ointment composed of vegetable juices.

Diatomaceous earth. Formed of the fossil remains of diatoms, that is, algae which lived in salt or fresh water; it is a chalky substance.

Dimity. A ribbed material whose warp is of linen and the weft of cotton.

Dishabille. Partially or carelessly dressed.

Dorea. A kind of striped muslin from India.

Douillette. A garment made of wadded silk, which is worn on top of the others, in winter.

Drachm. The French *drachme* is here translated as "drachm." The *drachme* is about 3.19 grams. The English drachm is about 3.89 grams. The avoirdupois drachm is about a sixteenth of an ounce, or 1.77 grams.

Drap. Any woollen (or occasionally silk) material; used to distinguish properties of such materials when little precision is wanted. Also, a middling-weight, much-fulled worsted.

Dresden-work. A kind of white-work embroidery.

Drop. A unit of volume in the apothecary system, equal to about 0.0592 millilitres in England.

Dropsy. A collection of water in the body.

Dyer's-weed. Any of several plants which yield a dye, including weld, dyer's green-weed, and dyer's woad.

Ear-pick. An instrument for clearing the ear of wax.

Écarlate. A woollen material dyed red.

Écru. An unbleached silk or toile, or the natural colour of same. For sewing, a raw silk thread.

Elecampane. A plant also called horse-heal; it has very large yellow flowers and bitter aromatic leaves and root.

Ell. *Aune* is translated here as "ell." In the Systéme Usuelle used in the 1820s, the *aune* is 1.2 meters, or about forty-seven and a quarter inches. The English ell is forty-five inches.

Embonpoint. Plumpness.

En casque. Shaped like a helmet.

En cheveux. Literally "in hair." A coiffure which may be ornamented with flowers, &c., but is not covered by a hat or cap.

En girandole. An earring usually with a central stone or part, and three ornaments depending from it.

Engrêlure. The straight edge of lace which is sewed to the material; also known as the footing.

En sautoir. In the shape of an X—the cross of St. Andrew.

Entre-deux. Literally "between two"; an insertion of lace or a trimming made of material.

Esparto. Also called Spanish grass; a plant fibre imported from the Mediterranean countries and made into, amongst other things, hats.

Esprit. An aigrette of feathers sometimes put on head-dresses.

Essence. Any essential oil.

European *courtrai.* A superior Belgian flax.

Excipient. That ingredient in a compound medicine, the business of which is to receive all the rest.

False colour. A fugitive dye.

Fancy-shops. Haberdashers and others in the fancy line.

Faveur. A kind of very narrow silk riband.

Felon. A small abscess or boil, an inflamed sore, or a whitlow (a tumour formed between the bone and its investing membrane, very painful).

Fichu. A little piece of material of a triangular shape, with which woman cover their bosom and shoulders.

Fichu-pelerine. A garment like a pelerine, but with long ends descending as far as halfway to the knee.

Finger. A measure referring to the width of a finger (three-quarters of an inch).

Fish-glue. A strong glue obtained by heating fish parts (especially the skin, fins, and bones) with water.

Fixed alkaline salt. Solid potassium carbonate.

Flesh-brush. Used to rub the body, to excite the circulation.

Flora indigo. One of several plants called indigo and yielding a blue dye.

Florence. A slight taffety which was formerly brought from Florence.

Fluting. Frill ornaments, with plaits shaped like a flute.

Fold. As a trimming, this can be either a tuck or a folded band of material applied to the garment.

Foot. *Pied* is here translated as "foot." In the Système Usuelle used in the 1820s, the *pied* is 33.3 centimeters, or approximately thirteen and a sixteenth inches.

Footing. For lace, the straight edge which is sewed to the material; also known as the *engrêlure*. For stockings, it is a term employed when the feet, having been worn out, are replaced with others knitted onto the original legs.

Form. A seat for several persons, without a back.

Franc. A monetary unit of the metric system, divided into ten parts called décimes, and an hundred parts called centimes.

Frankincense. A dry resinous substance in pieces or drops, of a pale yellowish-white colour; a strong smell, but not disagreeable; and a bitter, acrid, and resinous taste.

Freeze. From the French *glacer*. To freeze a lining to the material, is to sew them so that they are completely joined together, and appear as smooth as ice.

French cambric. A very superior make of cambric, fine in quality, and very silky in appearance.

Full. To finish woollens by cleansing, shrinking, and thickening them.

Fuller's earth. A marl of a close texture, extremely soft and unctuous to the touch. When dry it is of a greyish-brown colour, in all degrees, from very pale to almost black, and generally has something of a greenish cast in it. Used to full cloth.

Fuller's teasel. A teasel having hooked prickles between the flowers. Used to tease cloth, that is, to raise the nap.

Galbanum. It is soft like wax, and ductile between the fingers; of a yellowish or reddish colour; its smell is strong and disagreeable; its taste acrid and bitterish. It is of a middle nature between a gum and a resin.

Gall. Bile; an animal juice remarkable for its supposed bitterness.

Gallery. The horizontal part of an ornamental high comb.

Gallipot. A pot painted and glazed, commonly used for medicines.

Gauze. A very thin, transparent material, woven sometimes of silk, and sometimes only of thread.

Gaze brillantine. A very light silk material with a high lustre.

Gaze de laine. Though the literal translation is "woollen gauze," Mme. Celnart clearly describes this material as being of silk.

Gaze d'Italie. A gauze made of natural silk thread.

Gigot sleeve. A leg-of-mutton sleeve.

Gingham. A thin linen or cotton material, chequered, striped, or plaid.

Glacé, or glazed. For material or leather, having a smooth surface with a high polish or lustre.

Gland à œuf. An egg-shaped tassel.

Glossary.

Glass. *Verre* is here translated as "glass." The *verre* of the 1820s is equal to about three-eighths of an American cup. However, the *verre* of the Ancien Régime is equal to about three-quarters of an American cup.

Goffer. To crimp, plait, or flute with a heated goffering-iron.

Gonflé. Inflated.

Gore. A wedge-shaped or three-cornered piece of material let into a skirt, or any part of a garment, to widen it.

Grafting. The insertion of a sound piece of stocking-web into a space from which an unsound piece has been cut out.

Grain. In the Système Usuelle used in the 1820s, the French grain is about 54.253 milligrams. The traditional English grain is about 64.798 milligrams.

Granite. A kind of weave producing a small irregular surface similar to that of crape.

Grenadine. An open silk, or silk and woollen material, plain or with stripes, chequers, or other patterns.

Gros. In the Système Usuelle used in the 1820s, the *gros* is equal to an eighth of an *once* and to seventy-two grains. In modern measures it is about 3.9 grams, or about an eighth of an ounce.

Gros de Chine. A mixture of silk and stuff, warm and appropriate to the winter.

Gros de Naples. A stout silk material with cross-ribs.

Gum-arabic. A kind of gum obtained from several kinds of acacias, used to make glue and finish textiles.

Gum-dragon. A kind of plant sap which is dried, then when water is added to it, becomes a gel which may be stirred into a paste. It is tasteless and odourless.

Gum guaiac. A resin used to reduce the severity of disease, move the bowels, and promote discharges by sweat and urine.

Gum-senegal. A kind of gum-arabic.

Gusset. A small gore, for the under arms of shifts and the like, which may be square or three-cornered.

Haberdasher. *Mercière* is here translated as "haberdasher." The *mercière* sells a little of everything, but principally all the little articles required for the toilet and the habitual work of lades: needles; pins; all kinds of ribands; thread, cotton, and silk for sewing and embroidery; and an infinity of other things too numerous to mention.

Hand. Translated from *main*. The hand is a traditional English unit of measurement equal to four inches; the *main* may be the same.

Handle. By handling over is meant passing the goods through your hand end to end, to make the dye communicate equally through the piece.

Heading. The edge of the lace which is left free when the lace is sewed to the garment (as opposed to the footing). Also, an edge of a flounce left free above the gathers.

Hollow. To cut inwards to form the shape of a crescent, or a portion of a circle.

Inch. *Pouce* is here translated as "inch." In the Système Usuelle used in the 1820s, the pouce is 27.75 millimeters, or about an inch and a sixteenth.

India paper. A very thin, but strong, printing paper of a cream or buff-colour.

Isinglass. Sheet mica. It is found in broad masses, composed of a multitude of extremely thin plates or flakes. The masses are of a brownish or reddish colour, but when the plates are separated, they are perfectly colourless, and more bright and pellucid than the finest glass.

Ispahan. A deep shade of red typically used in Ispahan carpets.

Ivy-gum. The resinous juice exuded by ivy.

Jaconet. A thin, yet close cotton material, of a quality between muslin and cambric, being thicker than the former and slighter than the latter.

Jaspé. A material with irregular colouring produced by yarn with coloured slubs, or printed warp threads.

Jujube. A fruit which appears something like the date, and tastes something like the crab-apple.

Lace-woman. *Passementière* is here translated as "lace-woman." The *passementière* makes and sells passements, or braids to ornament clothing and furniture. Celnart indicates that the domains of the *passementière* and the *mercière* overlap.

Lamé. A material enriched with strips of gold or silver.

Lamp-black. This is the soot of oil, collected as it is formed from burning lamps. For the purpose, a quantity of oil is burned, in various large lamps in a confined place, where no part of the fume may escape. The soot formed by these fumes being deposited against the top and sides of the room, may be swept together and collected.

Lapis. A rich azure blue.

Lavallière. A shade of brown, more or less that of a dead leaf.

Lawn. A very clear, thin kind of linen.

Leghorn straw. Hats of Leghorn straw are much sought after, because of the elegance of the workmanship. They are made of a particular variety of wheat, of which the stubble is very sturdy and fine. This variety is cultivated in the arid soil of Tuscany.

Letting-in lace. Lace insertion.

Leucoma. A white scar in the horny coat of the eye.

Levantine. Levantine is a stout, close-made, and twilled silk.

Lime-water. Put some quicklime in a well-glazed pan; cover it with clear water; let it remain so for one day. Then strain off the water, and keep it for use. By means of this water, sap-green may be changed into blue. Lime-water in dyeing browns or black, especially browns, is found to be a good corrective.

Line. The French *ligne* is here translated as "line." In the Système Usuelle used in the 1820s, it is a twelfth of a *pouce*. In the English system, it is a twelfth of an inch.

Lingère. The *lingère* makes and sells every kind of article in toile, to serve for clothing, the bed-chamber, and the table.

Litharge. Properly lead vitrified, either alone or with a mixture of copper. This recrement is of two kinds, litharge of gold and litharge of silver. It is collected from the furnaces where silver is separated from lead, or from those where gold and silver are purified by means of that metal. The litharge sold in the shops is produced in the copper works, where lead has been used to purify that metal, or to separate silver from it.

Liver of sulphur. Produced by heating potash with sulphur.

Logwood. The heart-wood of a Central American and West Indian tree, or an extract of it, used for dyeing. Also, a blackish-purple to purplish-black colour.

Love-riband. A narrow gauze riband with satin stripes. It may be had in both black and white.

Madapolam. A kind of strong calico.

Madras. A material with a silk warp and a cotton weft.

Mancheron, or sleeve top. An ornament or trimming at the top of the sleeves of a woman's gown.

Manganese. An iron-ore of a poorer sort; the most perfect sort is of a dark iron-grey, very heavy but brittle.

Mantua-maker. There are four kinds of *couturière,* whom Mme. Celnart does not distinguish by title. The *couturière en habits de femme,* here translated as "mantua-maker," occupies herself with gowns and all the other principal parts of a woman's attire. She uses paper patterns to cut out the body, but hardly ever for sleeves, skirts, or trimmings, as their styles change continuously. She is expected to have much taste and experience, intelligence, and a knowledge of the fashions; but not always to make the seams very sturdy, as that is less important. The *couturière en corps d'enfant et en corsets*, here translated as "stay-maker," cuts out (using paper patterns), fits, and makes up stays for both adults and children. The *couturière en linge* sews every kind of body and household linen, and marks it. The *couturière en habits* makes up waistcoats, pantaloons, &c. previously cut out by a tailor.

Marceline. A silk material, a kind of florence, but wider and stouter.

Marchande de modes. These artists occupy themselves principally with every thing which concerns the superficial ornaments of ladies' attire. They work only with the lightest materials: lace, blond, tulle, gauze, fine batiste, taffety, satin, ribands of all kinds, all sorts of embroidery, artificial flowers, feathers, &c. Often they only trim gowns made by other artists. Their great talent consists in inventing new modes.

Margin. The material allowed for the seams of a garment.

Marli. A kind of gauze net, used for attire and embellishments.

Mastic. A kind of gum gathered from trees of the same name.

Measures. About twenty years ago, tailors took the measures with the aid of a doubled strip of paper, which each workman marked in his own manner by cutting with scissors. To recognize it, he inscribed the name of the customer at the end of the measure. The workshop was cluttered with a host of these measures, any one of which was troublesome to locate. Some one then thought to substitute one measure only, divided evenly into inches or centimetres. Clever tailors adopted it, and the idea was gradually welcomed.

Mechlin lace. A delicate bobbin-lace.

Megrim. A head-ache.

Melilot. A plant much used for plasters, poultices, &c.

Merino. A thin woollen twilled material.

Merveilleuse. A female fop.

Mille-fleur. A mixed floral scent.

Milliner. *Modiste* has here been translated as "milliner," as that is the sense in which Mme. Celnart uses the word. However, at this time the *modiste* is also defined as being the same as the *marchande de modes*.

Minim. A measure for a very small quantity of liquid; a drop. The English minim is equal to about 59.194 microlitres.

Minium. Either vermilion or red lead.

Miniver. The fur of a kind of squirrel, grey on the back, and white underneath and on the neck.

Moiré. A mode of dressing some materials of silk, woollen, cotton, or linen. The grain is crushed by calendering to impart variations in lustre, and a waved appearance.

Mordant. A substance used for fixing dyes in material.

Mucilage. A slimy or viscous body; a body with moisture sufficient to hold it together.

Muriate. Chloride.

Muriatic acid. Hydrochloric acid.

Musk. An animal secretion, contained in excretory follicles about the navel of the male musk-deer. It is strongly and agreeably odorous.

Muslin. A very clear, ordinarily very fine, cotton material. It may be plain, embroidered, figured, or striped.

Nankeen. A firm-textured, durable cotton material. It is commonly a buff-colour, either the natural colour of a certain Chinese cotton, or an imitation woven elsewhere and afterwards dyed. To produce the pale-reddish buff dye so much in use for nankeen, boil equal parts of arnatto (an orange-red dye) and common potash in water until the whole are dissolved.

Negus. A drink consisting of wine, port, or sherry, hot water, sugar, and flavourings.

Neroli. An oil distilled from the flowers of the bitter orange, which is pale yellow in colour.

Nervous consumption. A wasting or decay of the whole body, without any considerable degree of fever, cough, or difficulty of breathing. It is attended with indigestion, weakness, want of appetite, &c.

Nœud. A bow or knot.

Nouveautés. The newest and most fashionable things.

Noyeau. A brandy flavoured with almonds, or the kernels of peaches, plums, or cherries, and tasting like bitter almonds.

Ochre. The earths distinguished by the name of "ochre" are of various colours, such as red, yellow, blue, green, and black. The yellow sort are called ochres of iron, and the blue sort of copper.

Oil of behen, or ben. This oil is extracted by expression from the nuts known by the same name. It possesses the property of never becoming rancid; it has neither taste nor smell. In consequence of this latter quality, perfumers make use of it with advantage to take the scent of flowers, and to make very agreeable essences.

Oil of origanum. Oil of wild marjoram.

Oil of tartar. Take a pound and a half of white-wine tartar, two ounces of saltpetre, and an ounce of rock alum. Pound them all together, put them into an earthen plate, and expose them to a reverberating fire until they are calcined quite white. Then put an ounce of this substance into a pint of brandy.

Oil of vitriol. Sulphuric acid.

Open-work. A term employed in knitting, embroidery, and fancy-work of all kinds. It simply means that the work is made with interstices between several portions of close work, or of cut or open material.

Orange-flower water. Take two pounds of orange-flowers, and twenty-four quarts of water, and draw over three pints. Or, take twelve pounds of orange-flowers, and sixteen quarts of water, and draw over fifteen quarts.

Organdy. A kind of muslin of strong clear cotton.

Orpiment. Arsenic trisulphide. It is of a fine and pure texture, remarkably heavy, and its colour is a bright and beautiful yellow, like that of gold.

Orris. The powered root of the Florentine iris. It has a very pleasant odour which, for want of a better comparison, is said to resemble that of violets. Take best dried and scraped orris-roots, free from mould. Bruise or grind them; the latter is best, as being very tough, they require great labour to pound. Sift the powder through a fine hair-sieve, and put the remainder in a baker's oven, to dry the moisture. A violent heat will turn the roots yellow. When dry, grind again, and sift; and repeat the same until the whole has passed through the sieve.

Ounce. The French *once* is here translated as "ounce." In the Système Usuelle used in the 1820s, the *once* is 31.25 grams, or about an ounce and an eighth. Both French and English original sources use the ounce as a unit of measure for liquids as well as for solids.

Oxygenated muriatic acid. Chlorine.

Paris white. A fine kind of whiting; powdered calcium carbonate.

Parma violet colour. A deep or medium purple.

Parure. Attire, dress, finery, ornament, or a set of jewels. Or, costume for full dress.

Passé. Outmoded.

Patte. A tab, strap, or flap.

Pearl ash. Purified or partially-purified potash.

Pelerine. A lady's garment made in the form of a great turned-down collar, which covers the shoulders and bosom.

Pelisse. An out-door coat or cloak.

Pelisse-robe. A gown fastened down the front.

Percale. A fine, closely-woven cotton material, originally made in the Indes, but now imitated throughout Europe.

Percaline. A slight lustrous cotton material, used principally for linings.

Perry. Perry is made in the same manner as cider, only from pears, which must be quite dry. The best pears for this purpose are such as are least fit for eating, and the redder they are the better.

Petite-maîtresse. A woman who is fashionable to the point of being ridiculous.

Petticoat. An under skirt concealed by the gown; an under skirt discovered by clear fabric or openings in the upper skirt; or a skirt worn independently of a gown body.

Picots. Little loops or bobs which ornament needle-made laces of all kinds, and which are often introduced into embroidery.

Pinking. A mode of decorating trimmings by means of a sharp stamping instrument. This is used to evenly cut out pieces of the material at the edge in scollops, points, or other designs.

Pins. Pins are now chiefly made of brass wire. For persons in mourning, they are sometimes made of iron wire, rendered black by a varnish of linseed-oil with lamp-black. There are also pins with double heads used by ladies to fix their curls for the night, without the danger of pricking. The sizes of pins are distinguished by numbers.

Pint. *Chopine* is translated here as "pint." The *chopine* is equal to 1.006 American pints; only negligibly larger.

Pipe-clay. A fine white clay used to cleanse leather.

Plait. The French *pli* can refer to a plait of any kind soever, or to a tuck, or to a separate fold placed on the material for decoration, or to a wrinkle. Sometimes it is used to refer to gathers. The best possible effort has been made to determine what is what.

Points, or notches. A decorative edge with points, scollops, crenellations, &c., either cut into the edge or woven into the piece (as for lace). Large points or notches are called Vandykes.

Pomatum. Pomade for the hair, or ointment for the skin.

Ponceau. A very vivid and full red, a poppy-red.

Poplin. A material with a silk warp and a worsted weft, with fine crossways ribs.

Porte-montre. A flat, embroidered little cushion, against which you suspend a watch. Or, a little piece of wooden or metal furniture in the shape of a pendulum, in which you may place a watch in such a manner that only the dial appears.

Portugal water. Some say this is the same as angel-water.

Potash. An impure fixed alkaline salt, made by burning from vegetables.

Pot-pourri. A mixture of divers kinds of dried flower petals and spices, used for its scent.

Pound. *Livre* is translated here as "pound." In the Système Usuelle used in the 1820s, the *livre* is equal to 500 grams, or approximately a pound and an ounce and a half. Both French and English original sources use the pound as a unit of measure for liquids, as well as for solids.

Precipitation. The separation of a solid substance from a liquid, in the form of a powder or crystals.

Prie-dieu. A kind of desk with a step at the bottom, on which you kneel to pray.

Provence rose. Cabbage rose.

Prunella. A twilled worsted material, frequently dyed a plum-colour, and used for shoes.

Purse. A little bag of leather, material, or any other tissue, in which you put the money you wish to carry.

Quart. *Pinte* is translated here as "quart." The *pinte* is equal to 1.006 modern American quarts; only negligibly larger.

Quarter. Unless a quarter of something else is specified (for instance the distance round a skirt), this means a quarter of an ell.

Quicklime. After burning the stone, when lime is in its perfect and unaltered state, it is called quicklime.

Quicksilver. Mercury; a naturally fluid material, and the heaviest of all known bodies next to gold.

Quilling. Small round plaits made in lace, tulle, or riband, lightly sewed down, with an occasional back-stitch, the edge of the trimming remaining in open flute-like folds. The name was probably given to this description of plaiting because it is just sufficiently large to admit of a goose or turkey quill.

Quina. A name for cinchona bark, which yields quinine.

Reagent. A substance employed in chemical reactions.

Realgar. A red-orange arsenic sulphide.

Recherché. Sought-after; extremely stylish.

Recoquillée. Turned up.

Redingote. A garment longer and wider than a gown, used chiefly as an outer garment to shield against cold or rain.

Red lead. A red oxide of lead obtained from litharge.

Reseda. A kind of plant known as dyer's rocket. Also, a greyish-green colour.

Retort. A chemical glass vessel with a bent neck to which the receiver is fitted.

Revers. Lappels; the two parts of a garment which join over the chest, and which are, or seem to be, folded over to discover a portion of the under side or the lining.

Rheum. A thin watery matter oozing through the glands, chiefly about the mouth.

Riband. The French *ruban* can mean either riband or tape, where no fibre is specified. In such cases the best possible effort has been made to identify which is which.

River-water. Snow-water contains a little muriate of lime, and some slight traces of nitrate of lime; rain-water has the same salts in a larger quantity, and also carbonic acid; spring-water most frequently contains carbonate of lime, muriate of lime, muriate of soda, or carbonate of soda. River-water has the same substances, but in less abundance. Well-water contains sulphate of lime or nitrate of potash, besides the above-named salts. This information is of the most essential benefit to the art of dyeing, as from this, a judgement may be pretty accurately formed of the causes of the frequent failures in producing fine colours with certain waters; and the difference of colours, which frequently arises even from the same ingredients, water excepted.

Robe aux deux fins. A gown made to serve two purposes.

Robings. A trimming in the form of bands or stripes.

Rosette. A collection of bows of riband, arranged to form a circle.

Sadden. To make dark coloured.

Safflower. An herb with large red or orange flowers, used to prepare rouge and red dye for materials.

St. Lucia wood. This wood comes from Switzerland. It is reddish-violet, and of an agreeable odour, increasing with its age.

Salep. A nutritive starchy product named salep is prepared from the roots of certain orchids, and its infusion or decoction was taken generally in this country as a beverage before the introduction of tea and coffee. Sassafras chips were sometimes added to give the drink a flavour. It may be purchased as a powder, but not readily miscible with water, so that many persons fail in making the decoction. The powder should be first stirred with a little spirit of wine. Then the water should be added suddenly, and the mixture boiled. A drachm by weight of the salep powder in a fluid drachm and a half of the spirit, to half a pint of water, are the proper proportions. Sometimes amber, cloves, cinnamon, and ginger are added.

Salt of lemon. Potassium hydrogen oxalate.

Salt of sorrel. The salt of sorrel of commerce is oxalic acid.

Salt of tartar. Potassium carbonate.

Salt of vinegar. Impure potassium sulphate.

Saltpetre. This salt (potassium nitrate) is used in the preparation of fragrant pastilles. The nitre has a cooling saline and piquant taste, and promotes the secretion of saliva.

Sandal-wood. A precious kind of Indian wood, of which there are three sorts, red, yellow, and green.

Sanguine. Consisting of or containing blood.

Sarcenet. A fine thin silk material, which may be had plain or twilled.

Scabiosa. A kind of herb.

Scarlet composition. Take a pound of aquafortis duplex and a pound of water, and put them in a glass vessel. Add an ounce of salt of ammonia, and gradually, having pounded it fine, add half an ounce of salt of nitre, in the same manner. Shake them together until the salts are dissolved. Then add to the compound three ounces of granulated tin; introduce it gradually, until it is all in. It is well to set, or mix it in the morning; then it will be ready for use the next morning. So soon as the tin is principally dissolved, make the vessel close, with a glass or beeswax stopper. This is then called the composition for scarlet.

Scruple. The French *scrupule* is translated here as "scruple." The *scrupule* is equal to 1.0623 grams. The English scruple is equal to 1.2960 grams.

Seam fold. *Pli-rentré* is translated as "seam fold" throughout this work. It is the seam margin folded under by a few lines at the raw edges to prevent fraying, often before rather than after sewing the seam.

Serge. A twilled woollen material.

Serous fluid. A thin watery fluid resembling serum.

Serre-tête. A riband or cap which fits tight on the head.

Silk tulle. A fine silk net.

Sleek. To render soft, smooth, or glossy by rubbing.

Sleeve *à la Mameluke.* A sleeve which is very full from the shoulder to the upper part of the wrist.

Sleeve *à la Marie.* A sleeve which is full from the shoulder to the wrist, but divided into a varying number of compartments by means of bands round the sleeve.

Sleeve *à l'imbecile.* Even fuller than the Mameluke, to the middle of the wrist, with a short cuff.

Slip. An under gown for wearing under clear material.

Soapwort. An herb from which—most especially the root—a soap may be obtained, by plunging into hot water.

Soda of Alicante. A Spanish mineral soda made by burning the dried barilla plant.

Sou. The twentieth part of the former livre, being worth twelve deniers. Also, a copper coin of this value. Also commonly, the copper coin worth five centimes.

Southernwood. This plant agrees in most parts with the wormwood, from which it is not easy to separate it.

Spangles. Small, thin, round leaves of metal, pierced in the middle, which are sewed on as ornaments to clothes.

Spanish brown. A kind of reddish-brown earth used as a pigment.

Spanish white. A finely-powdered chalk used for cleansing or as a pigment.

Spencer. A garment shaped like a gentleman's coat, but cut between the waist and the tails. It is worn over the gown.

Spermaceti. A particular kind of whale affords the oil whence this is made; and which is very improperly called sperma, because it may only be made of the oil which comes from the head. It is changed from what it is naturally, the oil itself being very brown and rank. After treatment it becomes perfectly pure, inodorous, flaky, smooth, white, and in some measure transparent.

Spirit. The chemists apply the name to so many differing things, that they seem to have no settled notion of the thing. In general, they give the name of "spirit" to any distilled volatile liquor.

Spirit of hartshorn. Ammonia, or its aqueous solution.

Spirit of nitre. Nitric acid.

Spirit of wine. Alcohol.

Spring. A belled or flaring effect.

Stomacher. An ornamental piece worn at the centre of a gown body.

Stone, the. Kidney-stones.

Storax. A resinous and odiferous gum.

Straight-way. The direction of the grain parallel to the selvages and along the warp threads of the material.

Straw. As a support, a thin strip of wood.

Stuff. Textures of woollen slighter and thinner than cloth. Also, material of any kind.

Sulphur alkali. Potassium sulphide.

Sulphuric acid. The union of oxygen and sulphur.

Sulphuric ether. The liquid resulting from the action of sulphuric acid upon alcohol.

Sumach. The flowers of this tree are used for dyeing, and the branches for tanning.

Swiss. A fine clear crisp cotton material.

Tabinet. A poplin of rich character, the warp being of silk, the weft of wool, with a watered surface.

Tablier. A part of a gown, or a trimming on it, resembling an apron.

Taffety. A thin silk of a plain weave.

Talc. The kinds of talc suitable for the perfumer's use are called Venetian talc and French talc. These talcs in powder are used as the basis or body of rouges or paints.

Tape. The French *ruban* can mean either riband or tape, where no fibre is specified. In such cases the best possible effort has been made to identify which is which.

Ternaux cachemire. Cachemire manufactured by the firm founded by Ternaux, in imitation of India cachemire.

Thread. As well as denoting the finest description of manufactured fibre, this term is also distinctively applied to flax, or linen.

Tippet. A fur which women wear on their necks in winter.

Toile. Any linen, hemp, or cotton material; used to distinguish properties of such materials when little precision is wanted. Sometimes, linen in particular.

Toile d'Orange. A fine strong calico.

Ton. The fashion, and people of fashion.

Toque. A kind of hat with a narrow brim, covered with velvet, satin, &c., flat on top, and plaited all round.

Torsade. An ornament resembling a twisted rope; also used of hair.

Tour. A term for divers things used for attire which are put on in a circle.

Tuberose. The scent extracted from the tuberose flower is as it were a nosegay in itself, reminiscent of that delightful perfume observed in a well-stocked flower-garden at evening close.

Tucker. An edging of lace or fine material worn round the neck of a gown.

Tulle. A kind of netted tissue, very fine and light, which is given some firmness by means of a dressing, and which is principally employed in ladies' attire. It may be made of silk, cotton, or linen.

Tuyaux d'orgue. Organ plaits.

Valenciennes. A delicate flat bobbin-lace, with figures on a fine mesh ground.

Vandykes. Large notches cut into collars, trimmings, &c. as a decorative border.

Vapour-bath. A chemist's bath, or heat, wherein the body is placed so as to receive the fumes of boiling water.

Velvet. A kind of stuff, or silk; the nap of which is formed of parts of threads of the warp, which the workman puts on a channelled ruler, and then cuts, by drawing a sharp steel tool along the channel of the ruler, to the end of the warp.

Venetian talc. A hydrous silicate of magnesia.

Verbena. The plant vervain, or a perfume obtained from its leaves.

Vermilion. The red pigment obtained from cinnabar.

Volatile alkali. Most commonly, some solution of ammonia.

Vulnerary. Useful in the cure of wounds.

Wadding. A kind of cotton finer and silkier than ordinary cotton; there is also silk wadding. Wadding is placed between the outer material and the lining of a garment. If not quilted, it is necessary to attach it to the lining, or it is apt to form lumps.

Watch-key. A key with a square hole used to wind watches.

Watch-seal. A seal or decorative ornament at the end of a watch-chain, used to pull the watch out of the pocket.

Water-bath. A vessel full of hot, but not boiling water, into which you put the vessel containing the substances which you wish to cook, heat, or distill.

Whip. A dessert made with whipped ingredients—cream, eggs, and the like.

White copper. An alloy of copper, arsenic, and zinc.

White iron. Sheet tin.

White lead. Any of several white pigments which contain lead.

Whiting. White chalk, or a clay finely powdered, cleansed, and made up into balls.

Young fustic. The wood of the Venetian sumach, used to dye yellow.

Bibliography.

⁂

Many of the early 19th-century books used as sources for *The Lady's Stratagem* were read longer and more widely than modern readers may initially assume. This bibliography, therefore, provides a range of publication dates and places, for different printings and editions. However, this represents the information readily available, which is not necessarily the full publication history. Little attempt is made here to distinguish between what is now called a reprint, and what is now called a new edition—a substantially altered work. Contemporary publishers commonly called reprints "editions." When a work was revised, the publisher trumpeted the fact with a title featuring the word "new," and trailing off into a list of information corrected, plates added, &c. On the other hand, entirely unchanged works were re-titled to appear to more advantage, though the word "new" was less commonly used.

References.

Adams, Samuel and Sarah. *The Complete Servant; Being a Practical Guide to the Peculiar Duties and Business of All Descriptions of Servants, from the Housekeeper to the Servant of All-Work, and from the Land Steward to the Foot-Boy; with Useful Receipts and Tables.* London: Knight and Lacey, 1825.

Reprinted by Fairleigh Dickinson University Press in 2000.

Anonymous. *The Art of Beauty; or, the Best Methods of Improving and Preserving the Shape, Carriage, and Complexion.* London: Knight and Lacey, 1825.

No other editions found.

——. *The Art of Preserving the Hair, on Philosophical Principles.* London: Septimus Prowett, 1825.

The author is probably James Rennie, whose *The Art of Preserving the Hair, on Popular Principles; Including an Account of the Diseases to Which It Is Liable* was published by Prowett in 1826.

——. *The Book of English Trades, and Library of the Useful Arts.* London: Shackell and Arrowsmith, 1825.

Also titled *The Book of Trades*, and sometimes has the sub-title *A Circle of the Useful Arts*. Numerous editions were published in England and the United States between 1804 and 1861.

——. *The Duties of a Lady's Maid; with Directions for Conduct, and Numerous Receipts for the Toilette.* London: James Bullock, 1825.

Also published in 1829.

——. *Instructions on Needle-work and Knitting; as Derived from the Practice of the Central School, Baldwin's Gardens, Gray's Inn Lane.* London: Roake and Varty, F. Rivington, and Hatchard and Son, 1829.

There are also 1832 and 1838 editions, by the National Society for Promoting the Education of the Poor in the Principles of the Established Church.

——. *The Toilette of Health, Beauty, and Fashion; Embracing the Economy of the Beard, Breath, Complexion, Ears, Eyes, Eye-Brows, Eye-Lashes, Feet, Forehead, Gums, Hair, Head, Hands, Lips, Mouth, Mustachios, Nails of the Toes, Nails of the Fingers, Nose, Skin, Teeth, Tongue, &c. &c.* Boston, Allen and Ticknor, 1834.

Several editions were published in England and the United States between 1832 and 1837.

——. *The Young Lady's Book; A Manual of Elegant Recreations, Exercises, and Pursuits.* London: Vizetelly, Branston, and Co., 1829.

A number of editions were published in England and the United States between 1829 and 1876. The 1829 edition was reprinted by Adamant Media Corporation in 2001.

——. *The Young Woman's Companion, or, Female Instructor; Being a Sure and Complete Guide to Every Acquirement Essential in Forming a Pleasing Companion, a Respectable Mother, or a Useful Member of Society.* London: G. Virtue, 1828.

Numerous editions were published in England and the United States between circa 1811 and 1856, some with the title *The Female Instructor; or, Young Woman's Friend & Companion.*

Burtel, Mme. *Art de faire les corsets, les guêtres et les gants.* Paris: Audot, 1828.

No other editions or English translations found.

——. *Art de la couturière en robes.* Paris: Audot, 1828.

No other editions or English translations found.

Byfield, Robert. *Sectum: Being the Universal Directory in the Art of Cutting; Containing Unerring Principles upon which Every Garment May Be Made to Fit the Human Shape with Ease and Elegance.* London: H. S. Mason, 1825.

No other editions found.

Celnart, Mme. [Elisabeth-Félice Bayle-Mouillard]. *The Gentleman and Lady's Book of Politeness and Propriety of Deportment, Dedicated to the Youth of Both Sexes.* Boston: Allen and Ticknor, 1833.

This is the first American translation of the *Manuel complet de la bonne compagnie* (the sixth edition, published in 1832). It was reprinted up to 1863. The French version went through a number of editions between 1818 and 1863. Mme. Celnart revised the French manual in 1832, but was not its initial author.

———. *Manuel complet d'économie domestique, contenant toutes les recettes les plus simples and les plus efficaces sur l'économie rurale et domestique, à l'usage de la ville et de la campagne.* Paris: Roret, 1829.

At least three editions were published, in 1827, 1829, and 1837.

———. *Manuel complet de la bonne compagnie; ou, guide de la politesse et de la bienséance.* Paris: Roret, 1832.

Several editions were published between 1827 and 1852.

———. *Manuel complet des jeux de société, renfermant tous les jeux qui conviennent aux jeunes des deux sexes.* Paris: Roret, 1836.

Several editions were published between 1827 and 1846.

———. *Manuel des dames; ou, l'art de la toilette, suivi de l'art du modiste, et du mercier-passementier.* Brussels: Aug. Wahlen, 1829.

Several editions were published in France and Belgium between 1827 and 1833.

———. *Manuel des demoiselles; ou, arts et métiers qui leur conviennent, et dont elles peuvent s'occuper avec agrement.* Paris, 1827.

Several editions were published between 1826 and 1837.

Cluz, M. and Jean-Sébastien Eugène Julia de Fontenelle. *Manuel complet des fabricans de chapeaux en tous genres.* Paris: Roret, 1830.

No other editions found.

Francoeur, Louis-Benjamin et al. *Dictionnaire technologique; ou, nouveau dictionnaire universel des arts et métiers, et de l'économie industrielle et commerciale par une société de savans et d'artistes.* Paris: Thomine et Fortic, 1822–1825, and Paris: Thomine, 1826–1835.

The term *nouveau* in French encyclopædia titles often does not indicate that this is a new edition of the work, but seems added to distinguish the encyclopædia in question from others on the market.

Golding, J. *Golding's Guide; or, New Edition of The Tailor's Assistant, and Improved Instructor; Containing a Synthesis of the Art of Cutting to Fit the Human Form with Ease and Elegance.* London: E. Wilson, 1820.

At least three editions of *The Tailor's Assistant* were published between 1815 and 1823.

Hewlett, Esther [Esther Copley]. *Cottage Comforts, with Hints for Promoting Them.* London: Simpkin and Marshall, 1830.

Several editions were published between 1825 and 1844.

Huish, Robert. *The Alphabetical Receipt Book and Domestic Advisor.* London: John Williams, 1827.

Huish's 1826 *Female's Friend and General Domestic Advisor* seems by description to be much the same thing. Both books went through later editions between 1830 and 1839.

Joseph Robins. *The Ladies' Pocket Magazine of Literature and Fashion.* London: Joseph Robins, 1824, 1827, and 1829.

This magazine was published from 1824 to 1840. The descriptions seem to discuss the fashions of a month or so previously, and at least some are from French sources.

Pariset, Mme. *Manuel de la maîtresse de maison; ou, lettres sur l'économie domestique.* Paris: Audot, 1822.

There is also an edition of 1825.

Parkes, Mrs. William [Frances Byerley Parkes]. *Domestic Duties; or, Instructions to Young Married Ladies on the Management of Their Households and the Regulation of Their Conduct in the Various Relations and Duties of Married Life.* London: Longman, Hurst, Rees, Orme, Brown, and Green, 1825.

A number of editions were published in England and the United States between 1825 and 1838.

Rudolf Ackermann. *R. Ackermann's Repository of Fashions.* London: R. Ackermann, 1829.

This magazine was published from 1809 to 1829.

Tucker, Willam. *The Family Dyer and Scourer; Being a Complete Treatise on the Arts of Dyeing and Cleaning Every Article of Dress, Bed and Window-Furniture, Silks, Bonnets, Feathers, &c., Whether Made of Flax, Silk, Cotton, Wool, or Hair; also Carpets, Counterpanes, and Hearth-Rugs.* Philadelphia: E. L. Carey and A. Hart, 1831.

Several editions were published in England and the United States between 1817 and 1841.

Villaret, P. *Art de se coiffer soi-même, enseigné aux dames; suivi du manuel de coiffeur.* Paris: Roret, 1828.

Reprinted by Leonce Laget in 1981.

Further Reading.

Arnold, Janet. *Patterns of Fashion 1: Englishwomen's Dresses and Their Construction 1660–1860.* New York: Drama Book Publishers, 1972.

Contains patterns taken from seven original 1820s garments: a pelisse, a pelisse-robe, two evening gowns, a wedding gown, and two chemisettes.

Ashelford, Jane. *The Art of Dress: Clothes and Society 1500–1914.*

A history of costume which includes some descriptions and pictures of 1820s styles.

Bissonnette, Anne. *Fashion on the Ohio Frontier 1790–1840.* Kent: Kent State University Museum, 2003.

A scholarly study which includes colour photographs of seven surviving women's garments from the 1820s, and some men's.

Blum, Stella, ed. *Ackermann's Costume Plates: Women's Fashions in England, 1818–1828.* New York: Dover Publications, 1978.

Contains fashion plates for most kinds of women's garments (excepting undergarments), a few in colour.

Bradfield, Nancy. *Costume in Detail: Women's Dress 1730–1930.* Boston: Plays Inc., 1983.

Drawings of original garments and accessories with rough measures, with a chapter on the 1800–1835 period.

Burnham, Dorothy K. *Cut My Cote.* Toronto: Royal Ontario Museum, 1973.

Includes a pattern diagram of an 1831 shift, and another of an early 19th-century man's shirt.

Further Reading.

Corson, Richard. *Fashions in Hair: The First Five Thousand Years*. London; Peter Owen Ltd., 1991.

A large book encompassing women's and men's coiffures, which of course includes the early 19th century. For each period there are drawings of the styles, modern descriptions, and where available long quotations from period sources.

——. *Fashions in Makeup from Ancient to Modern*. London; Peter Owen Ltd., 1972.

A large and detailed discussion of cosmetics from "ancient civilizations" to 1970. Contains information on ingredients, application, social attitudes, and advertising. Includes substantial information for the early 19th century.

Cunnington, C. Willett. *English Women's Clothing in the Nineteenth Century*. New York: Dover Publications, 1990.

A detailed, decade-by-decade survey covering 1800 to 1899, with many quotes from period sources.

de Dillmont, Thérèse. *The Complete Encyclopedia of Needlework*. Reprint: Running Press, 1972.

An early 20th-century translation of the late 19th-century *Encyclopédie des ouvrages des dames*. Includes illustrated instructions for hand-sewing, mending, embroidery, knitting, &c.

Dreher, Denise. *From the Neck Up: An Illustrated Guide to Hatmaking*. Minneapolis: Madhatter Press, 1981.

Practical, step-by step instructions for various kinds of historic millinery.

Fukai, Akiko, Tamami Suoh, Miki Iwagami, Reiko Koga, and Rii Nie. *The Collection of the Kyoto Costume Institute: Fashion: A History from the 18th to the 20th Century*. Köln: Taschen, 2002.

Not a genuine history, but a large anthology of colour pictures of surviving women's garments. These include several styles of 1820s stays, gowns, and some accessories.

Hunnisett, Jean. *Period Costume for Stage & Screen: Patterns for Outer Garments, Book I: Cloaks, Capes, Stoles and Wadded Mantles*. Studio City: Players Press, 2000.

Contains pattern diagrams based on surviving garments. For the 1820s, includes six women's cloaks and mantles.

Bibliography.

——. *Period Costume for Stage & Screen: Patterns for Women's Dress 1800–1909*. Studio City: Players Press, 1991.

For 1820–1830, the patterns include a pair of stays, a petticoat, high and low bodies, divers sleeves, and three skirts.

Johnston, Lucy. *Nineteenth-Century Fashion in Detail*. London: V & A Publications, 2005.

Consists of colour photographs, sketches, and descriptions of women's and men's garments. Only a small proportion are from the 1820s, but the book is notable for its close depiction of trimmings, embroidery, &c.

McMurray, Elsie Frost. *American Dresses 1780–1900: Identification and Significance of 148 Extant Dresses*. New York: Cornell University, 2001. CD-ROM.

A study of styles decade by decade, based on surviving garments. For each garment, it provides colour photographs, drawings with rough measures, and a technical description. One chapter focuses on the 1820s.

Pointer, Sally. *The Artifice of Beauty: A History and Practical Guide to Perfumes and Cosmetics*. Phoenix Mill: Sutton Publishing, 2005.

Though this book contains little information about early 19th-century cosmetics specifically, it is useful for its detailed descriptions of old ingredients and implements.

Tarrant, Naomi. *The Rise and Fall of the Sleeve 1825–1840*. Edinburgh: Royal Scottish Museum, 1983.

An overview which includes a number of photographs of original 1820s garments.

Waugh, Norah. *Corsets and Crinolines*. New York: Theatre Arts Books, 1970.

Contains a pattern taken from an original late 1820s pair of stays.

——. *The Cut of Women's Clothes 1600–1930*. New York: Theatre Arts Books, 1968.

The patterns taken from original garments include an 1820s pelisse and an evening gown.

Index.

A

accents, 669

acquaintances, 577–579, 619–620

advice, 698

affiquets, 436

age

    and chaperons, 573–574,
        576–577

    and deference, 591, 614, 618,
        624, 628, 636, 682–683

    and dress, 106–109, 236,
        543–545, 571–572

agrafes, 334, 419–420, 539,
    546–547

aigrettes, 549, 557

alterations, 415–423, 534,
    536–537

anecdotes, 679–680

apologies, 672–673, 688

aprons

    knitted, 459

    making, 416–417, 426

    styles, 186, 213–214, 570

    turning, 416–417

arguments, 599, 678–679, 686

arms, 193, 254–255, 354

artists, 604–606

authors, 605–607

B

back-stitch, 306, 311

bags

    crocheting, 465

    laying out, 116

    lining, 450, 465

    styles, 188, 193, 212

baldness, 15

ball-rooms, 648–649

balls. *See also* dancing

    dress for, 190–193, 226–232,
        470, 633, 649, 673

    private, 632–635, 647–650

    public, 634–635

bandeaux

    jewellery, 106, 232–233

    night, 94, 117, 184, 569

baptism, 657–658

bargaining, 601–603

basting stitch, 345

bathing-gowns, 41

baths

    and dieting, 71

    and health, 23, 41–44, 83

    and modesty, 41, 583

    perfuming, 78–79

batistes, 147, 156–157, 200

battlement indents, 207

bed-chambers, 613, 634

bedgowns, 251–252

belts

    à chou, 485–486

    à la duchesse, 491

    with corded piping, 489

    elastic, 489

fastened in back, 484–485
with fringed ribands, 361,
    363–364, 484–485
lined, 486
with metal buckles, 487
putting on, 100
with sewed loops, 486
with shoulder-straps, 364,
    487–489, 508–509
storing, 123
styles, 221, 242
berets
    for full dress, 189, 193, 225,
        570
    for home, 187
    knitted, 444–445
    millinery, 534
biases
    on *fichus*, 501
    on gowns, 230–231, 329–330
    in hair, 99, 189
    on millinery, 545
billets, 694–695
binders, 91
blackheads, 59–60
bleaching, 147–148, 155–158, 180
blond. *See* lace
blouse gowns, 189, 198, 226, 232,
    350
blouse pelisses, 207
blueing, 144–145
bodies
    à la Circassienne, 210, 215, 217
    à la Diane, 230
    à la Marie Stuart, 192
    à la Raphaël, 351
    à la Sévigné, 224, 226–228,
        231, 350
    à la Vierge, 223
    à l'Edith, 230

à l'enfant, 192, 201
Anglo-Greek, 220
boning, 347, 349, 352
Castilian, 220
cutting out, 345–347
décolletage, 192, 221, 223,
    226, 239, 347
with draperies, 354–355
en chevrons, 198
en fourreau, 347–351, 360, 364
en gerbe, 198, 200, 215, 217,
    221, 228–229, 351
fitting, 347, 349
Gallo-Greek, 227
laced, 221
length, 239
making up, 318–319, 347–349,
    385–386
padding, 348
patterns, 345–347, 383–385
for pelisses, 379–383
piping, 350
plain tight, 345–347
for riding habits, 373–379
separate, 241
bones
    for bodies, 347, 349, 352
    for bonnets, 528, 530
    for *fichu* collars, 495–496
    and health, 89–90
    preparing, 294–295
    re-curving, 85
    for stays, 262, 267–272,
        294–295
bonnets. *See also* hats; strings
    à bouillons gonflé, 528
    à tuyaux d'orgue, 528–530
    with curtains, 531–532
    making, 527–530
    with puffed crowns, 527

for servants, 249
styles, 187, 426–427, 555–556
boots, 103. *See also* gaiters
bosom, 40–41, 74, 85, 101, 272
bouillons
 à gueule-de-loup, 357–358
 on *fichu* collars, 499
 on gowns, 219–220, 227
 making, 327–328, 353, 357
bouquets, 637, 654, 657
bows
 fringed, 484–485, 543–544
 large, 482–483
 materials, 484
 for millinery, 487, 502–504,
  538–542, 552–553
 with one loop, 483
 with several loops, 482
 supporting, 483, 541, 543
 with two loops, 481–483
box-plaits, 334–335, 357, 496–498
bracelets, 84, 467–468
braids, 204, 330, 476–478
Brandenburghs, 198
breasts. *See* bosom
bridesmaids, 656
bullock's gall, 148–149, 158–160,
 179, 429
bureaucrats, 603, 615
busk pockets, 118, 261–262,
 268–269, 277, 288, 295
busks, 84–85, 271, 288, 295
button-holes, 183, 312–314, 487,
 494
buttons, 211, 501, 552

C

calicoes, 146–147, 195–196,
 421–422

calling cards, 609–612, 614–615,
 619
calls. *See* visits
cambrics, 199
canezou-pelerines, 224, 418
canezous, 210, 213, 350, 418–419,
 502
canezou-spencers, 198, 200,
 209–210, 426–427
caps. *See also* strings
 cornettes, 197, 208–209,
  503–505, 553
 for *demi-négligé*, 189
 and health, 66
 lace, 200, 249, 570
 making, 418, 503–507,
  512–521
 materials, 534–535, 569–570
 mourning, 235, 515, 517,
  519–520
 night, 117, 123, 183–184, 519,
  521
 stiffening, 512, 515
 storing, 122–123
 trimming, 325, 483, 503–507
 washing, 125, 152–153
card games, 629–631, 633,
 645–646, 653
carriage of the body, 254–259
carriages, 572, 592, 601, 611, 637.
 See also coaches
carving, 624, 639–640
casings. *See* bones; straw-cases;
 string-cases
casting on, 431
Catholicism, 568, 599, 608
ceintures. *See* belts
cerceaux, 529, 543
chain-stitch, 312, 314
chaperons, 573–577, 633

chaps, 60

charity, 249–251, 442, 625, 656

charlatans, 12, 24, 29, 46

chatelaines, 213

cheating at cards, 631

chemises. *See* shifts

chemisettes, 100, 115

chilblains, 41

children, 584, 614, 616–617, 703

chintzes, 200

choux, 485–486

christenings, 657–658

churches, 596–598, 607, 655–657,
    659–660

clergymen, 608, 657

cloaks, 204, 207, 211–213, 611.
    See also mantles

clogs, 83–84

closets, 130

cloth. *See* materials

clothes-lines, 170

clothing. *See also* specific garments
    choosing, 236–239, 242–247,
        252–253, 340–341,
        571–572
    and economy, 238, 241,
        248–251, 261, 282,
        337–338, 371, 408–430, 571
    and health, 86–87
    for the lower orders, 127,
        249–251, 585
    and propriety, 247–249, 597
    putting on, 115–118
    second-hand, 238, 251
    storing, 120–127, 129–130, 407
    taking off, 116–117

cloth-work, 396, 398, 400–401

coaches, 593

coat-hangers, 121, 160

cockades, 543

coiffures
    à cache-peigne, 95
    à Chinoise, 95
    à chou, 95–96
    à la chevalière, 109
    à la Grecque, 108
    à la Madonna, 108–109
    à l'Anglaise, 98
    à la Ninon, 16, 96
    à l'enfant, 106
    à l'Inca, 106
    Apollo knots, 94, 96–98, 108,
        226
    choosing, 106–109, 236–237
    en cheveux, 10, 16, 106, 187,
        189–190, 236, 572
    en chignon, 95
    en couronne, 95
    Lesbian, 508–509
    Vandyke, 107

collars for *fichus*
    à la Medicis, 364–367
    with biases, 501
    with blond net, 364–366, 499
    falling double, 500, 502
    hemming, 499, 501
    with puffs, 499
    with ruches, 496–498,
        501–502
    patterns, 500
    setting on, 496, 499
    standing double, 495
    standing single, 494–496
    standing square, 495–496
    stiffening, 495–496, 498
    Vandyked, 501–502

collars for gowns
    à la chevalière, 208
    en paladin, 217
    with *entre-deux,* 333

mourning, 509–510
patterns, 509–510
for pelisses, 381, 383
collars for men, 368, 509, 511–512
collerettes, 115, 122–123, 186, 197. *See also* collars for *fichus*
Cologne water, 76–77
colours, 237, 242–246. *See also* dyeing
combing mantles, 115, 186
combs, 8, 25, 98, 106–107, 109, 113–114
commissions, 251, 593–595
comparisons, 673–674
complaints, 677
complexion, 38–40, 57–61, 237, 242–244, 246. *See also* face; skin lotions
compliments, 575, 591, 606, 627, 677
concerts, 635
confessionals, 598
confinements, 658
conversation
with artists, 605–606
at assemblies, 628–631, 634, 639
for the clergy, 608
dialogues, 673–681
and discretion, 698
family, 583–584, 586–588
about health, 600, 603–604, 671
listening, 681–684, 687
about religion, 598–599
and servants, 584–586
in the street, 591–593
when travelling, 593–594
with the unfortunate, 658–659, 660

during visits, 613, 619–620, 671–673
during walks, 625
conversaziones, 645–646
cordonnets, 475
cords, 477–478
cornettes, 197, 208–209, 503–505, 553
corns, 68–69, 102, 110
corsets. *See* stays
cosmetics, 45–56. *See also* paints
courtesans, 676, 685
courtesying, 257–259
courtship, 654, 661–665
crapes
for evening, 217, 223, 230–232
for mourning, 234, 501, 660–661
shawls, 207, 210, 215
cravats, 607
critiques, 605, 637, 680–681
crocheting, 465, 539
cuffs, 84, 238, 314, 352, 382, 417
curling-irons, 10, 17
curl-papers, 10, 17, 92–94, 114, 569
cuticles, 68
cutting-tables, 338

D

dancing, 256, 258, 584, 633–634, 650, 653. *See also* balls
dandruff, 8, 62
darning, 408–409, 455–456
darts, 348, 350, 379, 383
death, 604, 658–661
debts of honour, 631
décolletage, 192, 221, 223, 226, 239, 347

dedications, 606
deformities, 281, 301–302
demi-jarretières, 356
demi-négligé, 187–189. *See also*
    the descriptions of costumes
denials, 611, 620–621
dentifrices, 27–33, 35
dents de harpie, 331–332
dents de loup, 208, 233, 331–332
depilatories, 12–13, 23
dessert, 628, 641
dieting. *See* weight
digressions, 681
dining-rooms, 616
dinners, 189–190, 217, 626–629,
    639–644, 656
dinner-tables, 639–641
dipping. *See* dyeing
discretion, 573, 584, 696–670
disputes, 599, 678–679, 686
douillettes, 187, 240, 324, 572
draperies, 241, 333–334,
    350–351, 354–355
drawers, 73
drawing-rooms, 616, 622–623
Dresden-work, 392–393
dress. *See* clothing
dresses. *See* gowns
dressing-gowns, 185, 569
dressing-rooms, 104, 113
dressing-tables, 104, 113, 115
dress-making. *See* mantua-making
dress shields, 82–83
drives, 203–217, 625–626
drunkenness, 643–644
duels, 575, 675, 686
dyeing
    hair, 16–17, 24–26
    hats, 554–555
    feathers, 562–564

gloves, 474–475
gowns, 420–421, 429
repairing colours, 166–167
tools, 172–173

E

ears, 65–66, 81
economy
    in cosmetics, 21–22, 24,
        27–28, 46, 76–77
    in dress, 238, 241, 248–251,
        261, 282, 337–338, 371,
        408–430, 571
    in entertaining, 639
    in foot-wear, 102–103
    in millinery, 522
    of time, 620
    in washing, 140, 168–170
elastics
    in belts, 489
    in bracelets, 467–469
    in garters, 467–469
    in gloves, 473
    in stays, 89–90, 262, 280–281,
        299–301
embroidery. *See also* cloth-work;
    Dresden-work; tambour-work
    on caps, 512, 514
    cleansing, 154–155, 179
    on collars, 387–388, 509–512
    on flounces, 227–228,
        325–326, 399–401, 407
    on gloves, 314, 472–473, 475
    with gold thread, 395–396
    on muslin, 387–394
    on net, 394–395
    patterns, 386–387, 395–407
    on purses, 450
    re-using, 419

on shirts, 314
styles, 224, 230, 232
engagements, 654
entre-deux
dents de harpie, 331–332
dents de loup, 208, 233,
331–332
height for, 241
making, 330–333
on pelisses, 208, 233
on sleeves, 353
trou-trou-popoye, 332–333
envelopes, 690
esprits, 193, 549
exaggeration, 687
expectorants, 81
eyebrows, 62, 72–73
eyelashes, 64–65, 72
eyelet-holes
in embroidery, 389–391
for gowns, 347–348
for stays, 269–270, 277–279,
288, 292–293, 297–298
eyelids, 63
eyesight, 63–64

F

face, 236–237, 667. *See also* complexion; skin lotions
fainting fits, 188
fairs, 651–652
falbalas, 323
falsehoods, 683–684, 687
fans, 124, 232–233, 193
farewells, 591, 614, 618, 623, 635, 638
favours, 700–701
feathers
cleansing, 562
curling, 119–120, 562
drying, 119–120, 562
dyeing, 562–564
in hair, 99
for millinery, 545, 548–550
feet, 83–84, 253. *See also* corns; shoes
fichu-canzeous, 213, 418, 492, 502–503
fichu-pelerines, 190, 200–202, 209, 236, 503
fichu robings, 228–229, 232
fichus. See also collars for *fichus*
à la duchesse, 191, 491
à la neige, 205
in hair, 99
as hat trimming, 548
and health, 66–67
kinds, 490–492
making, 366, 489–494
and modesty, 192, 220, 239
mourning, 194, 498, 501, 660
night, 117, 183–184
putting on, 100–101, 117
of riband, 489–490
storing, 122–124
three-cornered, 116, 502
trimming, 325, 332, 507
for walking, 207
washing, 125, 152–153
fillings, 34, 37
finger-nails, 41, 67–68, 70, 82
finger-stalls, 67, 303
finishes, 151, 153–155, 561
fish-glue, 153–154
flasks, 188, 203
flat-irons, 174
flat seam, 308–310
flattery, 579, 606, 621, 676–677

fleas, 38, 86

flesh-brushes, 43, 74

flounces

   à la fille d'honneur, 325–326

   altering, 419

   embroidered, 227–228,
      325–326, 399–401, 407

   en if, 324

   with headings, 325–326, 358

   hemming, 323–325

   lace, 218–219, 224–225, 230,
      233, 241

   pinked, 220, 480

   setting on, 324–326, 358

   Vandyked, 323

flowers

   colours, 245–246, 649

   in hair, 98, 107–109, 237

   for millinery, 545, 550–552

   repairing, 119

   storing, 123–124

folds, 241, 328–329, 419–420

foot-warmers, 84, 617

forfeits, 632, 646–647

freckles, 49, 61

fringes

   on gowns, 223, 330

   on pelerines, 213

   on purses, 449–450

   on ribands, 363–364,
      484–485, 543–544

frocks, 430

funerals, 659–660

furs

   glazing, 130

   lining, 423

   mending, 422–423

   preserving, 126–127

   re-styling, 423

   styles, 207, 211, 213

G

gaiters, 103, 110–112

galoches, 570

gaming, 630–631, 646

garlands, 99, 109, 124, 552–553

garments. *See* clothing

garters

   elastic, 467–468

   knitted, 432

   with slip-knots, 103, 479

   on stays, 85–86, 290–291

   taking off, 116

   wedding, 657

garter-stitch, 431–432

gathering, 320, 325, 358

gauzes, 147, 153, 155, 228, 308,
   325, 345

gestures, 255–256, 667, 684

gifts. *See* presents

gloves. *See also* mitts

   for balls, 193

   and christenings, 657

   cleansing, 120, 470, 474

   colours, 246, 470

   dyeing, 474–475

   elastic, 473

   embroidering, 472–473, 475

   knitting, 438–439

   lengths, 473–474

   for morning, 185

   perfuming, 79–80

   putting on, 116

   re-using leather, 118–119

   sewing, 472–475

   silk, 41

godparents, 657

gold-thread embroidery, 395–396

good matches, 665

gooses, 371–372

gossip, 574–579, 651

gowns. *See also* bodies; mantua-making; skirts; trimmings
   à la Robin des Bois, 238
   altering, 415, 417–422
   cutting out, 314–315, 341–347, 351, 354, 360, 369, 371
   dual-purpose, 208, 240–241, 350
   dyeing, 420–422, 428–429
   fastenings, 240, 361
   folding, 116
   lining, 320–322, 360–361
   mending, 408, 410–415
   patterns, 337, 372, 383–385
   poplin, 200
   putting on, 100–101
   storing, 121–122, 124–126, 407
   turning, 417
   wadding, 322, 361

grammar, 669–670, 691

gratuities, 596, 653, 656–657

grease-spots, 160–163

greetings. *See* salutations

groomsmen, 656

gros de Naples, 197–211, 213–216, 220–222, 228

guimpes, 66, 100, 491–502

gums, 27, 29, 32, 34

H

hair. *See also* coiffures
   cleanliness, 8–9, 11–12, 22–23, 185
   curling, 10, 16–17, 21–22, 92–94
   cutting, 9, 15–16, 93
   dressing, 8–10, 92–99, 104–105, 115

   false, 10, 93–94, 97, 106
   growth, 14–17
   ornaments, 98–99
   pomatums, 9–11, 15, 17–19
   removing, 12–13, 23–24

hair-brushes, 113–114

hair-dyes, 16–17, 24–26

hair-oils, 10–11, 15–17, 19–21

hair-pins, 9, 118

hair-styles. *See* coiffures

half-veils, 527, 547–548

handkerchiefs
   carrying, 188, 193
   embroidering, 393–394
   folding, 116, 121
   knitted, 459
   perfuming, 79
   as *tournures,* 100–101

hands, 40–41, 60, 83, 303

hang-nails, 67–68

hat-boxes, 122–124

hat forms, 116, 152, 522, 525, 527, 531, 547

hats. *See also* caps; berets; bonnets; strings; toques; turbans
   assembling, 531–532
   beaver, 543–544
   bodies, 523–525
   brims, 525–528, 536–537
   chip, 535–536
   choosing, 193, 236–237
   crocheting, 539–540, 561
   crowns, 528–530
   dressing, 554, 561
   dyeing, 554–555
   esparto, 538
   gauze woven with straw, 538
   kinds, 522, 555–557
   Leghorn, 187–188, 193, 201, 215, 536–538, 552

lining, 530–531
marli, 539
materials, 522–523
mending, 119–120
patterns, 524–525
putting on, 101, 116
straw, 531, 535–538,
    540, 548
taking off, 612–613
trimmings, 541–554
washing, 554
hat-stands, 116, 522
healths, 643
hems
    for flounces, 323–325
    renewing, 417
    for skirts, 318, 330–331
    working, 306, 310–311, 345
herbs, 551
herring-boning, 312–313
hesitancy, 668
hoaxes, 591–592
home dress, 186–187, 197–201
hoods, 362–363
house guests, 637–638
Hungary water, 80

I

illness
    and hair, 14–15
    and mouth, 34
    and perfumes, 79
    and physicians, 604
    and visits, 39, 655, 668
imperial water, 80
infirmities, 658–659
ink-spots, 163–164
insoles, 83–84
interruptions, 682–683

invitations
    to balls, 632–633, 647–648
    to card-parties, 645, 648
    to dance, 633–634
    to dinners, 626, 639
    to funerals, 659–660
    to weddings, 654–655
ironing, 145–146, 174, 177, 303,
    326–327, 336

J

jardinières, 550
jarretières, 355–356
jewellery
    borrowing, 701
    cleansing, 118–119
    choosing, 194, 237, 243–244
    for demi-négligé, 188
    for full dress, 190–193, 217,
        219–221, 226, 228–230,
        232
jokes, 608, 675–676
jumps, 442

K

kisses, 581, 629, 643–644
knife-plaits, 357
knitting. See also specific garments;
    stitches, knitting; stockings
    binding off, 438, 440, 462
    casting on, 431
    commercial, 458–459
    decreasing, 433–434
    increasing, 433–434
    joining on yarn, 435
    mending, 452–458
    patterns, 432–452, 460–465
    tension, 435–438, 442

knitting moulds, 451–452
knitting needles, 431, 439–440, 451, 458–459, 462

L

lace
    choosing, 193, 236, 241
    cleansing, 152–154, 178–179
    sewing, 308–309
laced stitches, 411–413
lace seam, 308–309
lace-work, 394–395
lacing cords, 99, 289, 478–479
lady's maids, 92, 113, 118, 127–129, 252–253, 289–290, 369, 371, 407
lasts, 123
laundresses, 120, 168–169
laundry
    bleaching, 180
    blueing, 144–145
    equipment, 135–136, 169–170, 172–173
    experiments, 139–142
    fine, 131, 137
    ironing, 145–146, 174, 303, 326–327, 336
    rinsing, 125–126, 132, 135
    soaping, 143
    sorting, 131–132, 172
    starching, 142, 146, 175
    stays, 302–303
    storing, 125
    wringing, 143, 172–173
laundry-maids, 168–170
lavender-water, 80
lawyers, 603–604
letters
    addressing, 694

appearance of, 689–691
billets, 694–695
closings, 693–694
of congratulation, 606
and discretion, 696–697, 699–700
frequency, 695
kinds, 688
to parents, 582
postage, 688–689, 696
reading, 613, 690–691, 695
responding to, 688
salutations, 692
style, 691–692
of thanks, 638
liens, 356–357
linens. *See also* laundry; toiles
    buying, 195
    marking, 170–171, 369
    mending, 408–413
    perfuming, 75, 77–78
    storing, 125
    undergarments, 248–249
listening, 681–684, 687
loans, 701–702
Lord Byron, 623
lorgnettes, 188
love-ribands, 234–235, 515
luce water, 80

M

Macassar oil, 21
make-up. *See* paints
mancherons, 205, 224, 232, 353
mantilla-canezous, 210
mantles
    à la Witzchoura, 213
    cachemire, 205, 208
    for full dress, 190

linings, 203–204
making, 361–363
mourning, 234, 659
for walking, 203–204, 208
mantua-maker's seam, 310
mantua-making
    at home, 248, 337–338, 366
    by lady's maids, 252–253,
        369, 371
    methods, 305–363, 383–386,
        415–416
    by the poor, 249–251
    by professionals, 335–336
    tools, 305, 338–339
marital status, 193–194, 535, 571,
    573–575, 672
marking stitch, 369
marmottes, 504
marriage, 654–657, 661–665.
    See also weddings
materials
    cutting out, 251–252, 264,
        314–315, 371
    re-glazing, 151
    washing unbleached, 147
    water-proofing, 87–88
measures
    for gowns, 338–339
    for riding habits, 372–374
    for skirts, 342–343, 346
    for stays, 283–284, 303–304
    for trimmings, 325
measuring-glasses, 35–36
mending
    à dentelle, 413
    darning, 408–409, 455–456
    elastics, 468–469
    furs, 422–423
    invisible, 413–415
    kinds, 408

with laced stitches, 411–413
    patching, 408–411
    shoes, 423–426
    stockings, 452–458
    when to do, 117–118, 128–129
merinos, 151–152, 200–201, 205,
    420–421
metal ornaments, 551–552
millinery. See berets; bonnets; caps;
    hats; strings; toques; turbans
mitts, 443–444, 459
modesty
    in conversation, 672, 676, 687
    in deportment, 256–257,
        580–581
    in dress, 192, 239, 297, 597
    and marriage, 583–584
    when being measured, 283
Moravian work, 389
morning clothes. See also slippers
    for men, 569
    preparing, 118
    in public, 569–570
    stays, 185, 279–280, 299–300,
        569
    styles, 185–186, 196–197,
        569–570
mosquito-bites, 62
moths, 126–127
mourning
    caps, 235, 515, 517, 519–520
    cards, 611
    collars, 509–510
    dress, 194, 232–235,
        660–661
    fichus, 498, 501
    jewellery, 194–195
mouth-washes, 30–31, 34
muslins
    altering, 418–419

embroidering, 387–394, 404–406

for evening, 222–224, 230–231

for home, 199–200

sewing, 323, 325, 413–415

washing, 175–177

N

nankeen, 147

narrations, 679–680

neatness, 7–8, 10–11, 183, 247–249, 185, 297, 337

neck, 66–67, 236, 255

neck-lines, 192, 221, 223, 226, 239, 347

needle-books, 338

needles

    beading, 448

    embroidery, 386

    knitting, 431, 439–440, 451, 458–459, 462

    for mending, 414, 425, 455

    sewing, 293, 338, 344, 447

needle-work. *See also* embroidery; knitting; mantua-making

    and cleanliness, 83, 303, 407

    and health, 63, 67, 73, 281, 301–302, 305

    and industry, 247, 452, 458

    for lady's maids, 128–129, 252–253, 369, 371, 407

    during mourning, 661

    presents of, 703

    as recreation, 587–588

    tools, 338, 372, 450–451, 467, 522

    during visits, 617, 623

négligé, 98, 187, 196, 538, 570

new year's day, 582, 609, 657, 688, 702–703

night-caps, 117, 123, 183–184, 519, 521

night-clothes, 117, 120–121, 183–184, 301

night jackets

    folding, 117, 120–121

    knitting, 441–442, 461–464

    for morning, 185, 569

    sewing, 184, 310, 325, 368–369, 419, 422

night-shirts, 366–368

nose, 81

notes, 694–695

nuns, 608

O

old maids, 193, 573, 663

open-work, 442–443

opera-glasses, 226, 637

organdies, 156, 230

over-casting, 306–308, 475

over-shoes, 570, 585, 611

P

paints, 45–47, 51–55

panes, 336, 547

pantaloons, 222, 464

parasols, 61, 124

parcels, 590, 593, 598, 601

parents, 582

parlour games, 632, 646–647

pastilles, 78–79

patches, 58

patching, 408–411

patterns

    for bedgowns, 251–252

for caps, 511–521

for collars, 381, 383, 500, 509–512

for embroidery, 386–389, 395–407

for *fichus*, 492–493, 500

for gowns, 337, 371, 383–385

for hats, 524, 532–533, 536–537

for knitting, 432–452, 460–464

for pelisses, 379–383

for riding habits, 372–379

for shifts, 369–370

for stays, 262–264, 284–285, 303–304

payments, 598, 601–603, 624

pearls, 191, 194, 551

pelerines

on gowns, 196, 200, 213, 215–216, 221, 231–232

making, 334–335, 362–363, 379–380

on out-door garments, 203, 205, 207–208, 210–212, 215–216

separate, 209, 215–216, 213–232, 234

pelerine-tippets, 213

pelisse-robes, 196, 198–200, 203, 210, 213. *See also* pelisses; redingotes

pelisses

à la maîtresse, 216

à l'Autrichienne, 360–361

cachemire, 216

making, 219, 361–363, 379–382

merino, 212

muslin, 205, 210, 215–216

Prussian, 203

silk, 210–213, 216

tunic, 216

Witzchoura, 211

perfumes, 11, 17–21, 55–56, 75–80

perspiration, 10, 38, 82–83, 303, 348

petticoats. *See also* skirts

folding, 115, 121

knitted, 152, 439–441

making, 251, 417, 421–422

for morning, 185

under pelisse-robes, 199, 203, 216

post-partum, 91

putting on, 99, 101, 117

worn with spencers, 200, 209, 215–217, 426–427

physicians, 604

piety, 599

pimples, 17, 40, 48, 57–60

pince-nez, 188

pincushions, 114–115, 339

pinking, 480, 546

piping, 323–324, 355

pleasantries, 598, 608, 675–676

pockets, 223, 416, 426

pock-marks, 47, 72

poignées, 467

pomatums, 9–11, 15, 17–19, 39, 47–48, 129

pompons, 544

poplins, 200, 223

porte-manteaux, 121, 123–124, 633

postage, 686–689, 696

pregnancy, 90–91, 250–251, 279, 298–299

prejudices, 678

presents, 582, 606, 653–655, 657, 659, 702–703

prick-stitch, 311–312
priests, 608
promenades. *See under* walking
pronunciation, 666, 668–669
proverbs, 675
puffs. *See bouillons*
punches, 335, 480, 546
puns, 670, 675–676
purl-stitch, 432
purses, 188, 445–452

Q

questions, 671, 678, 700
quilting, 463
quotations, 674–675

R

rags, 133
raillery, 598, 686
rakes, 664
reading aloud, 128–129, 587–588, 618
redingotes, 185, 240, 317–318, 324, 360–361. *See also* pelisse-robes; pelisses
refreshments, 591, 618, 626, 632, 634, 650
relations, 570, 579–580, 583–585, 606, 656–661, 699
repartees, 676
repetition, 674, 682
reputation, 573–581
reticules. *See* bags
retiring-rooms, 649
ribands. *See also* bows; *fichus*
    fringing, 363–364, 484–485, 543–544
    for mourning, 234, 515

plaiting, 478
washing, 155
for weddings, 657
ridicule, 569, 572, 580, 587, 605, 667
riding, 594–595
riding habits, 205, 210, 213, 371–379
root canals, 36
rouge, 46–47, 52–54
rouleaux
    on collars, 499, 301
    on gowns, 226–227
    making, 326–328, 420
    on pelisses, 204–205
    turned, 356–357
    tuyaux-de-pipes, 356
    wadded, 218, 225–226, 328, 357
routs, 651
ruches
    on *fichu* collars, 496–498, 501–502
    on gowns, 221, 241
    making, 334–335, 359–360, 496–498
    making into rouleaux, 420
    on millinery, 546
    pinking, 335, 480, 546
running stitch, 304–305
rusma, 12–13
rust spots, 163–164

S

sachets, 56, 78
saluations
    at assemblies, 629
    of shop-keepers, 600
    in the street, 592–593

for visits, 603–604, 614, 617–618, 637, 672

salutes, 607

salves. *See* pomatums

sautoirs, 209

scarfs
- *à la Dame du Lac,* 238
- cachemire, 193, 206, 215
- choosing, 236–237
- gauze, 190, 215
- lace, 193, 226, 228
- silk, 208, 213, 215
- as turbans, 184, 558–560

scissors, 338, 341, 371

scouring, 131, 148–150, 158–160, 172–173, 180–182

scurvy, 30–31

seals, 690

seams. *See also* specific seams
- *à la reine,* 308
- for biases, 330
- on edges, 306, 308–309, 312
- for *entre-deux,* 330
- for knitting, 440–441
- with laced stitches, 411–413
- on silks, 308
- top-stitched, 310–312

seating
- at dinners, 627–628, 642–643
- in theatre boxes, 636
- in vehicles, 593, 625–626, 655
- of visitors, 617, 623
- during walks, 624
- at weddings, 655–656

secrets, 700

sedan chairs, 572

séducteurs, 490

seductions, 575

self-love, 567

serre-têtes, 117, 152–153, 184, 422

servants. *See also* lady's maids; laundry-maids
- clothing for, 127, 249–250, 585
- duties to visitors, 585, 611–612
- as godparents, 657
- at parties, 628, 644, 649–650
- politeness towards, 584–585, 638
- recreations for, 621, 651–652

shaving, 24

shawls
- cachemire, 123, 190, 193, 203, 205, 208, 211, 213, 216
- crape, 207, 210, 215
- exchanging, 251
- folding, 115
- gauze, 210
- hanging, 123
- for home, 186
- ironing, 120
- lace, 193, 236, 503
- lending, 701
- mending, 413–415
- *négligé,* 187
- night, 184
- putting on, 101
- taking off, 255, 612–613, 636
- three-cornered, 236
- as turbans, 560–561
- for walking, 203, 205, 207–208, 210–211, 213, 215–216
- washing, 151–152

shifts
- folding, 120, 123
- making, 100, 369–370, 419
- for morning, 185
- for night, 86, 183–184

putting on, 99

shoes. *See also* gaiters; slippers
- choosing, 102, 186, 246, 570

Index.

cleansing, 570
dancing, 190–191, 425
and health, 70, 83–84, 102, 110
repairing, 84, 117–118, 423–426
storing, 123
taking off, 116–117
shopping, 195, 261, 600–603, 661
side-stitch, 306, 309–310
silks
bleaching, 148
cleansing, 177–178
dyeing, 148–150, 420–421, 429
finishing, 153–154
sewing, 308, 344
washing, 147–149, 178
singing, 628, 661
sitting, 254–255
skin lotions, 38–41, 49–50
skirts. *See also* petticoats
cutting out, 314–315, 341–344, 360
length, 236, 239, 339–340, 373
lining, 320–322, 334
making up, 315–318, 322, 344–345, 415
openings, 317–318, 344
for pelisses, 379–380
plaited all round, 206–207, 213, 223–224, 232, 415
for pregnancy, 344
for riding habits, 373, 378–379
setting on, 319–320, 385
wadding, 322, 361
width, 317
sleeves. *See also* cuffs; mancherons
à l'Amadis, 202–203, 224
à la Mameluke, 197, 202–203, 221
à la Marie, 200, 211, 213, 215, 221

à l'Espagnole, 226
à l'evêque, 206
à l'imbecile, 200, 202–203, 215–216, 224–225, 232, 426–427
cutting out, 351–354, 383–385
en beret, 221–222
engageantes, 224
extra, 350, 416
gigot, 193, 201, 209, 220–221, 228, 237–238, 353–354, 383–385, 427
and health, 82, 84
knitted, 84
lengths, 220, 350, 354
lining, 321–322
long, 350–354
patterns, 375, 378–379, 380–385
Persian, 207
renewing, 417–418
setting in, 319, 350, 352
short, 193, 350, 354
stiffening, 201–203, 238, 352
trimming, 332, 353–354
washing, 132
wristbands, 238
slippers, 83, 132–133, 185, 436–438, 570. *See also* shoes
slips, 185, 190–192, 228–232
small-pox, 47, 72
smelling-salts, 79, 188
soaps
laundry, 137–139, 168–170, 172
for spot removal, 161, 165–166
toilet, 50, 55–56
social class. *See also* servants
and dress, 208, 242, 249–252, 339–341, 570
and manners, 591–593, 615

soldiers, 607

somnambules, 190–191, 236, 503

Spanish-stitch, 369

spencers, 189, 205, 209–210, 215–217, 379–383

sponges, 31–32, 113

spots, 117–118, 131, 160–167

sprigs, 389–392, 402–403, 405

stairs, 614–615, 617

stammering, 666

starch, 125, 142, 146, 174–175

stationery, 689–690

stays. *See also* bones; busks; eyelet-holes

    à la paresseuse, 278–279, 297–298

    basting, 265

    binding, 261, 270–271, 277, 292

    brassières, 301

    brassières de Venus, 298–299

    cleansing, 294, 302–303

    cutting out, 264–265, 286–288

    elastic, 89–90, 262, 280–281, 300–301

    fitting, 266, 289–291, 303–304

    furnishings, 261–262

    gores, 262–267, 272–276, 291

    half-stays, 185, 277–278, 569

    and health, 84–85, 88–91, 300

    jubilee, 303–304

    kinds, 262, 286

    lacing, 84, 90–91, 94, 99, 115, 278–279, 288–289

    lined, 275–277, 281, 296–297

    making up, 266–271, 291–294

    materials, 261, 275, 282–283, 286, 304

    measuring for, 283–284, 303–304

    mending, 118

    modesty-piece, 274, 295–296

    night, 301

    with one bosom gore, 262–271, 296

    padded, 90–91, 281, 301–302

    parts, 262, 285–288

    patterns, 262–264, 284–285, 303–304

    pieced, 274–275

    for pregnancy, 90–91, 277–281, 298–299

    shoulder-straps, 265, 272–274, 292

    with straps, 277–278, 298

    taking off, 109, 116

    with two bosom gores, 271–272, 284–285

    and weight loss, 73–74

sticks, 551

stitches, knitting

    à baguette, 442

    à crochet, 442

    à jour, 442

    de Valois, 445

    garter, 431–432

    purl, 432

    seam, 432

    turn, 432, 458

    twisted, 443

    varié, 443

stitches, needle-work. *See also* specific stitches

    embroidery, 312–314, 369, 388–396, 475

    knitting, 431–432, 442–443

    mending, 408–415

    sewing, 305–314, 320–321, 338, 344, 411–413

stockings

    attaching pairs, 132–133

bleaching, 148, 155
choosing, 102–103
cleansing, 117, 155, 180, 465
commercially-made, 458–459
darning, 408–409
for *demi-négligé,* 189
dyeing, 465–466
fit of, 70, 103
footing, 456
and garters, 85–86
grafting, 453–454
and health, 83–84, 102
knitting, 432–435, 442–445, 458, 464
missing stitches, 436, 452–453
re-cutting, 456–458
re-enforcing, 454–456
stomachers, 220, 227, 233
straw-cases, 527–529
string-cases, 100, 184, 493–494, 507, 515, 517, 519–520
strings, 490, 505, 537–538, 553–554
stripes, 317–318
suitors, 654, 661–665
sulphuring, 147–148, 155
sun-burn, 49
suppers, 635, 650–651
swearing, 684
sweat. *See* perspiration
swords, 598, 607, 661

T

tabliers, 360
tact, 658–659, 678, 698
tailoring, 371–383
tambour-work, 386–387
tartar, 27–29
tassels, 481

teeth. *See also* tooth-aches; tooth-brushes
cleansing, 27–35, 628
decayed, 28, 33–37
displaying, 666–667
false, 37
uneven, 33
theatres, 635–637
thimbles, 338
thread. *See also* yarn
for basting, 344
for embroidery, 386–387, 394–396
for mending, 414
for millinery, 356–357, 525, 527
for sewing, 293, 356–357
tinsel, 190, 192, 550–551
tippets, 208, 211–212, 221, 423, 636
titles, 607–608, 672, 692–693
toasts, 643
toe-nails, 70
toiles, 155–158, 171
toilet-tables, 104, 113, 115
tongue-scrapers, 32
tooth-aches, 35–36
tooth-brushes, 29, 31–32, 115
toothpicks, 28, 32–33, 114, 667
toques, 190, 193, 532–533, 556–567
torsades, 506–507, 546
tournures, 100–101
travelling
cases, 104, 122
etiquette, 593–595
and presents, 702
stays, 278–279, 297–298
trimmings. *See also* embroidery and specific trimmings
choosing, 240–241, 253

colours, 245–246
  positioning, 325, 327–329
  renewing, 418–420
tuckers, 218–219, 223, 226, 228–231
tucks. *See* folds
turbans, 184, 218–219, 533–534, 547, 556–557
turn-stitch, 432, 458
tuyaux-de-pipes, 356
tweezers, 23–24, 114

U

umbrellas, 88, 124, 585, 590–591, 611

V

Vandykes
  embroidered, 396–397, 404
  on *fichu* collars, 500–503
  on gowns, 198, 217, 220, 323
  on millinery, 546
veils
  bleaching, 148
  for church, 598
  for *demi-négligé,* 189
  half-veils, 527, 547–548
  making, 394–395, 480–481
  for protection, 61, 63
  riding, 205
  washing, 152–154
  wedding, 481
velvets, 151, 193, 200, 220, 344
venereal diseases, 664
visits. *See also* conversation; farewells; salutations
  business, 603–604, 615
  by card, 614–615

ceremonious, 610–614
  after childbirth, 658
  of condolence, 660
  denials, 611, 620–621
  and discretion, 699
  dress for, 201–203, 570–571, 609–610
  after entertainments, 629, 635
  half-ceremonious, 613–614
  informal, 609–610
  kinds, 609
  lengthy, 637–638
  morning, 619–620
  and reputation, 574–575, 578
  and servants, 585, 611–612, 621, 638
  to the sick, 658
  and travelling, 593–595
  wedding, 656
volubility, 668

W

waist-bands, 240–241, 318, 346, 349–350, 386
waistcoats, 213, 459–463, 569–570
walking
  dress, 103, 189, 203–217
  manner of, 103, 257, 570, 573, 589–590
  promenades, 624–625
walking-sticks, 478, 612
waltzing, 634
warts, 68
washing. *See* laundry
washing-machines, 137, 169
wash-liquor, 135–139
wash-tubs, 135, 169
wash-water, 172
watches, 119, 188, 477–478, 570

water-proofing, 87–88

weddings, 654–657

weight, 66, 70–71, 73–74, 236–237, 272

weights, 302, 338

whale-bones. *See* bones

whipping, 358

white paints, 47, 51, 53–55

widowhood, 577, 659–661

wigs, 15–16, 572

wines, 628, 641, 643–644

woollens

    beating, 173

    bleaching, 148

    dyeing, 181–182

    finishing, 153–154

    reviving colours, 148–150

    scouring, 158–160, 180–182

    washing, 142–143, 151–152

work-rooms, 338

work-tables, 338

wrinkles, 47, 49, 62

wristbands, 238

Y

yarn

    for berets, 444

    kinds, 431, 458

    for night jackets, 442

    for open-work, 442

    for petticoats, 439–440, 479

    for purses, 446, 448, 451, 465

    for waistcoats, 460

Books published by Lavolta Press.

The Lady's Stratagem; or, The Manual of Respectable Coquetry; A Systematic Treatise on the Whole Art of Pleasing as Laid Down by a Frenchwoman, in its various branches, Faithfully Translated; with many Interesting and Useful Additions from Rare French, English & American Works; also, Annotations, Introductory Remarks, Garment & Embroidery Patterns, Appropriate Illustrations and explanations of same; altogether a compendium of matters with which each Early 19th-Century Costumer, Re-enactor, Costume Historian & Historical Novelist should be Familiar. $75.

After a Fashion; Wherein Beginners of Both Sexes are Led to the Temple of Historic Costuming and Vintage Clothing; including Descriptions of all kinds of Styles from Middle Ages to Art Deco, with many Approved Methods explained in a Clear, Methodical, and at the same time Familiar Style; Elegantly Illustrated by one of the most Distinguished Artists. $38.

Reconstruction Era Fashions; A Choice Collection of 1867 and 1868 Patterns Needful for Ladies, for Dress-making, Millinery & several branches of Fancy Needle-work; Illustrated by a series of Plates on a Large Scale, by Numerous Engravings on Wood & by Scaled Pattern Diagrams; to which is added, by way of appendix, a Full and Clear Display of the Art of Dress-making. $45.

Fashions of the Gilded Age, Vols. 1 & 2; Being the Largest and Most Perfect Collection Ever Formed of Patterns for 1877 through 1882, for Sewing, Millinery, Needle-work Trimmings & Divers Trifles; containing Scientific Systems for Fitting the Female Form with Ease and Elegance, enabling Every Lady to be Her Own Cutter; together with a Plain, Practical & Familiar Treatise on Dress-making and Millinery; with upwards of 800 Engravings on Wood and Steel. Both Volumes Systematically Arranged for Separate Use; $49 per volume.

The Voice of Fashion; Forming a Complete Cyclopædia of Dress-making Patterns for 1900 through 1906; together with Plain and Practical Directions for Making Up, Plates and Diagrams; and a Short and Easy Mode of Cutting the Patterns in Different Sizes for the Female Form, with Directions affording the means of acquiring a Competent Knowledge Without the aid of a Master. $42.

The Edwardian Modiste; Being a Grand Display of Ladies' Patterns for 1905 through 1909, with an Infallible Self-varying System of Enlarging them to Different Sizes; prepared also as a Handbook and Work of Reference on Dress-making; Especially adapted to Self-instruction; illustrated with numerous Lithographs and Engravings; the whole being a Signpost to the Road of Elegance and Fashion. $42.

Prices do not include Shipping and are subject to change without notice. For further information, please visit www.lavoltapress.com.